Neuro-ophthalmology
Focus 1980

J. Lawton Smith, M.D.

Professor of Ophthalmology
Bascom Palmer Eye Institute
University of Miami School of Medicine
Miami, Florida

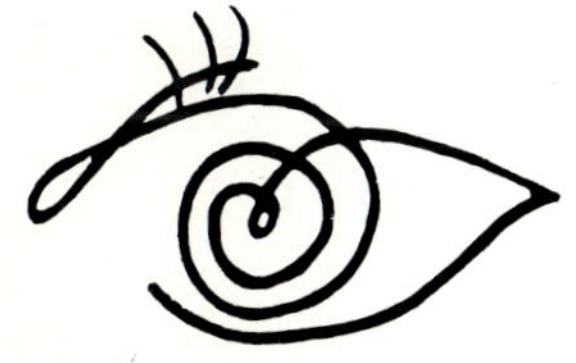

MASSON Publishing USA, Inc.
New York·Paris·Barcelona·Milan·Mexico City·Rio de Janeiro

PREFACE

Neuro-ophthalmology continues to be bombarded with changing technologic knowledge as does the entire field of medicine. This book is an attempt at presenting the state of the art in this field as the 1970s go out and as the 1980s come in. The editor is grateful to the many contributors who have supplied chapters for this book. Initially, I had considered writing one or two more large chapters for the book myself. However, Dr. John Costin impressed me that it might help the practitioner more to give an editorial comment on each chapter. I have tried to do that in order to give a broader and more unified clinical perspective to the points made in the book. This book is really aimed at the practitioner—to that ophthalmologist, neurologist, or neurosurgeon who is busy all day yet who wants to get an update on what is going on in the neurologic sciences. One of the blessings of neuro-ophthalmology is that a neurologist writing for an eye man, does so in a simplified manner. The neurosurgeon writing for another specialty tries to present things a bit more concisely, and I believe that medicine is hard enough, if we try to make it as simple as possible. It is just about impossible, if one tries to make it hard! Therefore, several things have been done in this book that are different from many of the journals today. We have removed the abbreviations whenever possible. I asked each contributor to delete those "DKAs" (doctor killin' abbreviations) because I don't know anything that makes the current journals harder to decipher than that. Also, we have included the commercial names of the medications used. I think it is better to call it the "Thypinone" test rather than the thyrotropin-releasing hormone (TRH) test, because the prescription that you write is for "Thypinone." I see nothing wrong with calling a medication by the name that you write on the prescription. In fact, I see a lot right with that! Furthermore, we have included the zip codes and costs of some of the tests, so that you can even figure out where to mail the blood tests from this book. I realize that inflation will change the cost of some of these tests, but that shouldn't stop us from trying to give you late, practical office information. One thing that will not change, however, is the importance of a good history and complete office neuro-ophthalmologic examination. A good history continues to be over 85% of any diagnosis, and no matter how they hook the patient up to mad scientist machinery, you are still going to need that *good history*. I believe that is a major difference between a *doctor* and a *physician*. Several years ago a famous ophthalmologist was in the hospital himself as a patient and was being seen by quite a few medical doctors. I asked him about the medical care he was receiving. He replied—"I have four doctors but only one physician!" We hope this book will help you to be a better physician.

J. Lawton Smith, MD
Miami, Florida
February 1979

Contents

Contributors

Frank M. Anderson, M.D.
Division of Neurological Surgery
Children's Hospital of Los Angeles
The Division of Surgery (Neurological)
University of Southern California School of
   Medicine
Los Angeles, California

Michael Aptman, M.D.
Wilford Hall Air Force Medical Center
San Antonio, Texas

Frank J. Bajandas, M.D.
Department of Ophthalmology
University of Texas Medical School
San Antonio, Texas

Barbara D. Barnes, M.D.
Assistant Professor of Neurology
University of California
San Francisco Medical Center
San Francisco, California

Charles C. Barr, M.D.
Bascom Palmer Eye Institute
University of Miami School of Medicine
Miami, Florida

Michael E. Barricks, M.D.
Department of Ophthalmology
University of Texas Health Science Center
   at San Antonio
San Antonio, Texas

David Bouda, M.D.
Department of Medicine
University of Texas Health Science Center
   at San Antonio
San Antonio, Texas

James R. Boynton, M.D.
Department of Ophthalmology
Warsaw Medical Group, P.C.
Warsaw, New York
Department of Ophthalmology

University of Rochester School of Medicine
Rochester, New York

J. Raymond Buncic, M.D., F.R.C.S. (C)
Neuro-ophthalmology
555 University Avenue
Toronto, Ontario, Canada

Thomas J. Carlow, M.D.
Associate Professor of Neurology (Neuro-
   ophthalmology)
University of New Mexico School of Medi-
   cine
Chief, Neuro-ophthalmology Section
Veterans Administration Medical Center
Albuquerque, New Mexico

Steven Coker, M.D.
Department of Neurology
Walter Reed Army Medical Center
Washington, D.C.

James J. Corbett, M.D.
Neuro-ophthalmology Unit
Wills Eye Hospital
Departments of Ophthalmology and
   Neurology
University of Pennsylvania
Philadelphia, Pennsylvania

John A. Costin, M.D.
Bascom Palmer Eye Institute
University of Miami School of Medicine
Miami, Florida

Kenneth R. Davis, M.D.
Lahey Clinic
Boston, Massachusetts

Bernard H. Doft, M.D.
Bascom Palmer Eye Institute
University of Miami School of Medicine
Miami, Florida

Carl Ellenberger, Jr., M.D.
Assistant Professor of Medicine

Division of Neurology
The Milton S. Hershey Medical Center of
  The Pennsylvania State University
Hershey, Pennsylvania

Alistair R. Fielder, F.R.C.S.
Derbyshire Royal Infirmary
Derby, England

Edward Fineberg, M.D.
Department of Ophthalmology
Medical College of Georgia
Augusta, Georgia

John Forest, Jr., M.D.
Yale University School of Medicine
New Haven, Connecticut

Lars Frisén, M.D.
Department of Ophthalmology
University of Göteborg
Sahlgren's Hospital
Göteborg, Sweden

Terry W. George, RBP, FBPA
Neuro-ophthalmology Unit
The Wilmer Ophthalmological Institute
The Johns Hopkins Hospital
Baltimore, Maryland

Joel S. Glaser, M.D.
Associate Professor of Ophthalmology
Bascom Palmer Eye Institute
University of Miami School of Medicine
Miami, Florida

Murali Guthikonda, M.D.
Division of Neurological Surgery
University of Vermont College of Medicine
Burlington, Vermont

Mark Hallett, M.D.
Department of Neurology
Harvard Medical School
Section of Neurology, Department of Med-
  icine
Peter Bent Brigham Hospital
Boston, Massachusetts

Maurice Hanson, M.D.
Department of Neurology
Cleveland Clinic Foundation
Cleveland, Ohio

W. Bruce Jackson, M.D.
Department of Ophthalmology
McGill University
The Royal Victoria Hospital
Montreal, Quebec, Canada

Lawrence R. Jenkyn, M.D.
Division of Neurology
Department of Medicine
Dartmouth-Hitchcock Medical Center
Hanover, New Hampshire

Bruce L. Johnson, M.D.
Department of Pathology
University of Pittsburgh School of Medi-
  cine
Pittsburgh, Pennsylvania

Gerald N. Kadis, M.D.
Department of Neurological Surgery
Columbia College of Physicians and Sur-
  geons
The Neurological Institute of New York
Columbia-Presbyterian Hospital
New York, New York

Tulay Kansu, M.D.
Neuro-ophthalmology Unit
Wills Eye Hospital
Departments of Ophthalmology and Neu-
  rology
University of Pennsylvania
Philadelphia, Pennsylvania

Raananah S. Katz, M.D.
Bascom Palmer Eye Institute
University of Miami School of Medicine
Miami, Florida

Robert Katzman, M.D.
The Saul R. Korey Department of Neurol-
  ogy
Albert Einstein College of Medicine
Bronx, New York

Shahram Khoshbin, M.D.
Department of Neurology
Harvard Medical School
Section of Neurology, Department of Med-
  icine
Peter Bent Brigham Hospital
Boston, Massachusetts

Lanning B. Kline, M.D.
Assistant Professor of Ophthalmology
School of Medicine
The University of Alabama at Birmingham
Birmingham, Alabama

Robert A. Laibovitz, M.D.
Neuro-ophthalmology
3301 Northland Drive
Austin, Texas

Edward R. Laws, Jr., M.D.
Associate Professor of Neurologic Surgery
Mayo Medical School
Rochester, Minnesota

Juan-Martin Leborgne, M.D.
Assistant Neuroradiologist, Section of Neu-
    roradiology and Computed Tomography
Chief, Section of Mammography
Department of Radiology
Mount Sinai Medical Center
Assistant Professor of Radiology
University of Miami School of Medicine
Miami, Florida

Daniel B. Levin, M.D.
Department of Ophthalmology
Warsaw Medical Group, P.C.
Warsaw, New York

Lois Lloyd, M.D., F.R.C.S. (C)
Neuro-ophthalmology
170 St. George Street
Toronto, Ontario, Canada

Sheila Margolis, M.D.
Department of Ophthalmology
Institute of Plastic and Reconstructive Sur-
    gery
New York University Medical Center
New York, New York

Barry J. Materson, M.D.
Department of Medicine
University of Miami School of Medicine
Miami, Florida

William A. Meriwether, M.D.
Department of Pathology
University of Texas Health Science Center
    at San Antonio
San Antonio, Texas

Neil R. Miller, M.D.
Neuro-ophthalmology Unit
The Wilmer Ophthalmological Institute
The Johns Hopkins Hospital
Baltimore, Maryland

Lester A. Mount, M.D.
Department of Neurological Surgery
Columbia College of Physicians and Sur-
    geons
The Neurological Institute of New York
Columbia-Presbyterian Medical Center
New York, New York

**Patrick S. O'Connor, M.D., Major,
    USAF, MC**
Ophthalmology Branch
USAF School of Aerospace Medicine
Aerospace Medical Division (AFSC)
Brooks AFB, Texas

Linda S. Orr, M.D.
Neuro-ophthalmology Unit
Wills Eye Hospital
Departments of Neurology and Ophthal-
    mology
The University of Pennsylvania
Philadelphia, Pennsylvania

Robert H. Osher, M.D.
Bascom Palmer Eye Institute
University of Miami School of Medicine
Miami, Florida

Thomas R. Pheasant, M.D.
Division of Ophthalmology
Milton S. Hershey Medical Center
Hershey, Pennsylvania

M. Judith Donovan Post, M.D.
Assistant Professor of Radiology
University of Miami School of Medicine
Miami, Florida

Robert M. Quencer, M.D.
Associate Professor of Radiology and Neu-
    rological Surgery
University of Miami School of Medicine
Miami, Florida

Alexander G. Reeves, M.D.
Professor and Chairman

Division of Neurology, Department of Medicine
Dartmouth-Hitchcock Medical Center
Hanover, New Hampshire

Peter J. Savino, M.D.
Neuro-ophthalmology Unit
Wills Eye Hospital
Department of Ophthalmology
Thomas Jefferson Medical College
Philadelphia, Pennsylvania

Norman J. Schatz, M.D.
Neuro-ophthalmology Unit
Wills Eye Hospital
Department of Ophthalmology
Thomas Jefferson Medical College
Philadelphia, Pennsylvania

Henry Schmidek, M.D.
Professor of Surgery
Chief, Neurosurgical Service
University of Vermonth College of Medicine
Burlington, Vermont

Norman G. Schneeberg, M.D.
Professor of Medicine (Endocrinology and Metabolism)
Hahnemann Medical College and Hospital
Philadelphia, Pennsylvania

James Sharpe, M.D.
Neuro-ophthalmology Unit
Division of Neurology
Toronto Western Hospital
University of Toronto
Toronto, Ontario, Canada

Harold E. Shaw, Jr., M.D.
Neuro-ophthalmology
7-B Cleveland Court
Greenville, South Carolina

Jerome J. Sheldon, M.D.
Chief, Section of Neuroradiology and Computed Tomography
Department of Radiology
Mount Sinai Medical Center
Associate Professor of Radiology

University of Miami School of Medicine
Miami, Florida

Irwin M. Siegel, M.D.
Department of Ophthalmology
Institute of Plastic and Reconstructive Surgery
New York University Medical Center
New York, New York

Harold W. Skalka, M.D.
Associate Professor in Ophthalmology
Combined Program in Ophthalmology
The University of Alabama in Birmingham
Eye Foundation Hospital
Birmingham, Alabama

Robert Smallridge, M.D.
Department of Neurology
Walter Reed Army Medical Center
Washington, D.C.

J. Lawton Smith, M.D.
Professor of Ophthalmology
Bascom Palmer Eye Institute
University of Miami School of Medicine
Miami, Florida

Steve Stevens, M.D.
Wilford Hall Air Force Medical Center
San Antonio, Texas

Barbara W. Streeten, M.D.
State University of New York
Upstate Medical Center
Syracuse, New York

John O. Susac, M.D.
Neuro-ophthalmology
222 East Central Avenue
Winter Haven, Florida

Edward Tarlov, M.D.
Department of Neurosurgery
Lahey Clinic Foundation
Boston, Massachusetts

H. Stanley Thompson, M.D.
Professor of Ophthalmology
University of Iowa Medical School
Iowa City, Iowa

Robert L. Tomsak, M.D.
Bascom Palmer Eye Institute
Department of Ophthalmology
University of Miami School of Medicine
Miami, Florida

Jonathan D. Trobe, M.D.
Assistant Professor of Ophthalmology
University of Florida Medical School
Gainesville, Florida

Joan L. Venes, M.D.
Texas Neurological Institute at Dallas
Dallas, Texas

Maurice Victor, M.D.
Professor of Neurology
Case Western Reserve University
Cleveland Metropolitan General Hospital
Cleveland, Ohio

Thomas J. Walsh, M.D.
Professor
Ophthalmology and Neurology
Yale University School of Medicine
New Haven, Connecticut

Clark Watts, M.D.
Professor and Chief
Division of Neurosurgery
University of Missouri School of Medicine
Columbia, Missouri

Ronald L. Young, M.D.
Assistant Professor
Department of Obstetrics and Gynecology
Baylor College of Medicine
Houston, Texas

Timothy Ziegler, M.D.
Division of Ophthalmology
Milton S. Hershey Medical Center of The
    Pennsylvania State University
Hershey, Pennsylvania

FOREWORD

There are many *gaps* evident in medicine today. There is a gap between the amount of time that many patients need in the doctor's office and what he or she really receives. Another obvious gap is in the realm of continuing and undergraduate medical education. There is a notable disparity between the information that the practitioner really needs to help his patients, and the facts that are put out from the teaching institutions. However, one thing that has impressed me over the years is the fact that the *truth* is not defined by popular opinion. This bears repetition—the truth is not defined by the majority vote! If it is true, it is true—and will stand against the winds of opinion.

An important truth today is that America needs to turn back to the Bible. Consider the words of prophet Zechariah from the Old Testament (14:1-3): "Behold, the day of the Lord cometh, and thy spoil shall be divided in the midst of thee. For I will gather all nations against Jerusalem to battle: and the city shall be taken, and the houses rifled, and the women ravished; and half of the city shall go forth into captivity, and the residue of the people shall not be cut off from the city. Then shall the Lord go forth, and fight against those nations, as when he fought in the day of battle." Now consider the gap that will occur in the next verse! "And His feet shall stand in that day upon the mount of Olives, which is before Jerusalem on the east, and the mount of Olives shall cleave in the midst thereof toward the east and toward the west, and there shall be a very great valley; and half of the mountain shall remove toward the north, and half of it toward the south." Verses 8 and 9 tell us—"And it shall be in that day, that living waters shall go out from Jerusalem: half of them toward the former sea and half of them toward the hinder sea: in summer and in winter shall it be. And the Lord shall be king over all the earth: in that day shall there be one Lord, and His name one." If you really want to know the truth, consider carefully John 14:6—"Jesus saith unto him, I am the way, the truth, and the life: no man cometh unto the Father but by me." Doctor, this is a terribly strong statement—The Lord Jesus Christ says categorically that He is the truth! I have learned from personal experience that what the Holy Bible says is true. I want to commend to you the following verse (Romans 10:9)—"That if thou shalt confess with thy mouth the Lord Jesus, and shalt believe in thine heart that God hath raised him from the dead, thou shalt be saved." May the Lord bless you, your family, and your practice!

J. Lawton Smith, M.D.

1 Fifty Neuro-Ophthalmological Pearls

J. Lawton Smith, M.D.

The purpose of this book is to summarize the state of the art in clinical neuro-ophthalmology as the 70's go out—and the 80's come in. Things are changing so rapidly that this is a large order, but I am indebted to all the many contributors who have really sent in good material for this book. However, in the past I have taken the liberty of simply tabulating some red hot gems and pearls so that if you are tired from a long day in the office or hospital when you pick up this book, you might simply want to read down these short pearls and pick out a nugget or two to help you, and can then defer a more meticulous reading until next weekend (or never, as often happens—unfortunately!). At any rate, not all of the points below are really new, but it seems to me to be appropriate to emphasize them again at this time, and I hope they will help you. They are in no particular order, except as they pop into my mind while writing this. Some of them are from this book, too, and you'll find more detail about them elsewhere in the volume. Certainly there are more gems in this big book than these few—but, let's go!

1. Be sure to get *CORONAL* cuts on your computed tomography scan when you suspect a tuberculum sellae or planum sphenoidale meningioma. You may completely miss such a lesion without them!

2. Don't expect to get good *CORONAL* cuts on a computed tomography scan if the patient has any appreciable number of dental fillings! *Filled teeth* give *horrible artefacts* on *coronal* scans!

3. Do not bypass getting plain skull films and go straight to a computed tomography scan in a patient with visual loss. This is poor economy! You are going to miss many good points—that early hyperostosis from the meningioma—that eroded clinoid that is not as well seen on the computed tomography scan—that early enlargement of the optic canal or superior orbital fissure on one side. Remember—*always* get *plain films before* a *computed tomography* scan!

4. Be sure to order your computed tomographic scans from a physician who will send *YOU* a *copy* of the *PICTURES*! It is not enough to simply send you a nice typed up report. The reason you need a set of the pictures is twofold: (1) You can look at them and see if the study is of good quality or not, and (2) you can learn from your own cases. You'll never learn by reading reports—but you'll sure learn from looking at the actual x-rays themselves! Simply call him up on the phone and nicely ask him to please send you a set of the films—either the polaroids or the actual films. The field is sufficiently competitive now that he'll be glad you asked!

5. Be sure you tell the neuroradiologist what you are looking for. Many patients getting a computed tomography scan ordered by an ophthalmologist will have a study primarily of the *ORBIT*—simply because you are an eye man! That will do no good at all if you suspect the problem is in the *BRAIN*. These are TWO different examinations—it's just like telling the radiologist whether you want a small bowel barium study or an air-contrast barium enema! You really need to know whether you suspect regional ileitis or a descending colon carcinoma!

6. A common error in office neuro-ophthalmology is to see a patient with progressive visual loss in one eye who has had several sets of plain films and several computed tomographic scans but who has not had *optic canal polytomography*. There are many, many optic nerve sheath meningiomas that you simply cannot diagnose any other way than by optic canal tomograms—and generally base view tomography with hypocycloidal tomography is indicated in such cases. If the radiologist calls you up and says—"All the x-rays are absolutely negative in this case!"—then you should ask him—"Well, how about hypocycloidal optic canal polytomes on her?" Most often, you'll get either a stunned silence or some stammering about not having that equipment in town from the other end. You still need them!

7. It is *very* important for any case with progressive unexplained visual loss for you to actually look at the x-rays yourself in the presence of the radiologist or neuroradiologist. Now, you may ask—"Are you crazy? I'm an eye man and I just got through sewing in three intraocular lenses and I don't know ANYTHING about x-rays!" Well, all I can say is that the commonest error I believe I have made in neuro-ophthalmology over the years is to accept that "blue sheet" stamped, nicely typed-up report from the radiologist—without checking those films with him personally. If you can't get a good check-out with your x-ray man, then borrow the films, and mail them to some terrific neuroradiologist and ask for an independent review. It'll pay off time after time! I saw four patients from Texas in one year with progressive visual loss who had bilateral carotid arteriograms read by board men out there as negative—and when those films were put up on the view box at our conference, several men on the front two rows immediately pointed out: "Why, there's the meningioma!" Remember, have the *films reviewed!*

8. A major teaching point is this—"*AL-WAYS GET A CF BEFORE A CT!*" What that says is simply: Always get a confrontation field before a computed tomographic scan. I continue to see cases regularly who have had x-rays and computed tomographic scans time after time that are called negative, while they have bitemporal field defects obvious to gross confrontation that

have been present for 3 to 5 to 8 to 10 years or more before the x-ray changes are obvious!

9. I have come to appreciate more and more what I call a *"HISTORY FIELD."* What this simply means is that I am attempting to extrapolate an Amsler grid test all the way across the examining room by history. Thus, I ask the patient to close her left eye—and look at me (sitting about 6–8 feet away on my office stool) and simply tell me what she sees. If she notes that she can see the top of my head and the bottom of my chin, but nothing in between—why, that is a central scotoma you can drive a Mack truck into! However, if she can see my eyes and my mouth but not my nose, that is a small, distinct central scotoma, such as you might get from a macular hole. Ask her if she can see BOTH of your ears across the room. If she sees only your ear that is in her nasal field, but misses that ear of yours that belongs to her temporal field, LOOK OUT! If she sees the top of you, but nothing from your waist down—you have a lower altitudinal defect, and, in one eye only, you are already thinking of ischemic optic neuropathy, for example. This takes about 30 seconds per eye but really pays off more and more, as I use it.

10. A helpful point is to check the central field with the projectorlite technique all the way across the room in some patients. You can no longer get those small Ednalite pointers, but you CAN get those large Ednalite pointers as used in most hospital lecture rooms. If you send a check for $23.45 to Alpha Photo Products, Inc., 560 20th St., Oakland, Calif. 94612 and ask for a Rowi 530 pointer, they will send you the best one now available on the market. You will want to change the bulb to a GE #14 bulb when you get it, but believe it's worth your trying anyway.

11. If you have the patient fix on a door knob, or light switch, or some specific target across the room, you will enlarge that central field so much that it is a "neat" way to find out if that scotoma is a CENTRAL scotoma or a CENTROCAECAL scotoma. If you throw a spot of light into the "waist" (i.e., equidistant between fixation and the blind spot) and the patient misses this spot, you have a centrocaecal (or caecocentral)

scotoma until proven otherwise in that case!

12. The differential diagnosis of *TUBU- LAR FIELDS* consists, in my experience, of seven things: (1) glaucoma, (2) retinitis pigmentosa, (3) syphilitic chorioretinitis and/or syphilitic optic nerve disease, (4) bilateral homonymous hemianopias with macular sparing, (5) functional, (6) toxins (typically quinine now, and years ago try-parsamide), (7) bilateral central retinal artery occlusions with intact cilioretinal arteries. Now, it is obvious that ALL of these have ABNORMAL FUNDI except the differentiation of *FUNCTIONAL* from *OC-CIPITAL LOBE* DISEASE. I advise a good CT scan with enhancement with emphasis on the occipital lobes in such cases. You can readily detect all the others with a good "OV" (office visit). A good neurological exam may also give some tips in such cases—does he swing his arms asymmetrically on walking? Is the plantar response suspicious on one side? The workup of such cases, therefore, is in addition to a complete eye exam—FTA–ABS test, ERG, neurologic exam, blood pressure check, and CT scan. I don't think photic driving or a visual evoked response helps *UNLESS* the patient has no light perception, and then you can diagnose it at the office visit.

13. A *computed tomographic scan* is a good way to confirm the ophthalmoscopic diagnosis of a *choroidal osteoma* ("bone in the eye"). See the two papers on this topic in this book. Obviously, this is a more common fundus entity than had been appreciated before Dr. Gass put it on the map! Obviously, you should tell the neuroradiologist you are interested in an orbital study primarily here—not an intracranial one!

14. If you have a small infant and find a gross transillumination problem on examining the skull in a dark room, don't write this child off as a case of hydranencephaly! This might be a simple arachnoidal cyst that could be surgically relieved. Be SURE to get a good computed tomography scan in that case, and read Dr. Anderson's chapter in this book to let you know about such cases!

15. Optic nerve drusen and migraine—run together! Dr. Webb and Dr. McCrary found that 38% of a series of patients with hyaline bodies of the optic discs had a history of migraine. That is very important! I also think there is a higher incidence of migraine in patients with Adie's tonic pupils. These points are of obvious clinical significance. Thus, if you saw a patient with a blurred disc who had no headaches, you might not worry so much and could look at it more objectively and could call it pseudopapilledema or buried drusen. BUT, if she were complaining about headaches, you might get nervous! Likewise, if you saw a patient with a large, dilated, and fixed pupil who had no other complaints, you might tune in on this being an Adie's tonic pupil. But *IF* she also were having headaches, again you might get nervous! The moral of the story is that you need to take a good *history* in both of these cases. Finally, the Hruby lens exam will tell you about those optic disc drusen if you really look carefully!

16. A *right* homonymous hemianopia to confrontation in a *right-handed* person with *no other* neurologic *defect* is *occipital*—until proven otherwise. And, after it has been proven otherwise, it is still usually occipital. This is a very valuable rule. The converse from that non-dominant hemisphere does *not* hold, however.

17. Do *NOT* put Fresnel (paste-on) prisms on *BOTH eyes*. These plastic prisms are VERY helpful in office practice, but they do blur the vision a bit in the eye looking through them. I have never seen a patient really comfortable with bilateral paste-on prisms, so just don't order those. If you really need to combine some vertical with some horizontal prism, you can get together with your optician, and, in moderate degrees of correction, he can rotate that prism before one eye and come up with an acceptable correction. However, don't put paste-ons before BOTH eyes—you're asking for trouble!

18. INDERAL is the drug of choice in treating *migraine* in my experience. Take her off the "pill," first (or premarin)—and then start with one 10 mg tablet a night the first night, one at 8 AM and 8 PM the next day, one at 8 AM, 1 PM, and 8 PM the third day, and one at 8 AM, 12 noon, 4 PM, and bedtime a day for the next four days. Many of these patients will respond to only 40 mg/day. Don't give up at that dose, however, if they do not. You might have to go up to 80 mg/day. That dose is quite safe, however, for the cardiologists use much, much larger doses without batting an eye. Remember, you should *NOT* use Inderal if they have a history of *asthma,* and you *SHOULD taper* it off when you stop it if they have a history of angina or any form of heart disease. With those exceptions, it is beautifully tolerated and often helpful in the dosage listed for office eye work.

19. I have found that *TIMOPTIC* (0.5% timolol) is really a terrific medication for glaucoma. We had a patient with ischemic glaucoma on top of a mixed glaucoma (i.e., she had had a peripheral iridectomy before but still had a tension of 36 when I saw her). We put one drop of 0.5% timolol in that eye, and, in one hour, the tension fell from 36 to 18. Dr. Costin suggested using timolol drops in a lady with pathologic lid retraction due to thyroid eye disease. She reported on the phone that it helped her. This might be worth trying in some cases. I'd appreciate hearing from others about their experience with this, as this is too early for me to be sure.

20. There is a higher incidence of *hypertension* in *alcoholics.* I advise that someone in your office check the brachial blood pressure on every one of your new patients. This really pays off in neuro-ophthalmologic office practice! I see patients regularly complaining with headaches or about their eyes, and when my associates take their blood pressure, it may be 210/125 and the patient often tells me that they had never known that! This is a word to the wise for the eye man!

21. *OLD PHOTOGRAPHS*—this continues to be a red hot office pearl! It is amazing how often a patient is referred in for a neuro-ophthalmologic evaluation of ptosis (unilateral or bilateral or asymmetric) which is said to have been present for eight months—yet that ptosis is quite evident on that driver's license picture in their wallet made two years ago! Furthermore, you can even see it to a lesser degree in her wedding album picture made 25 years ago! Ocular muscle dystrophy (Kiloh-Nevin syndrome) (chronic progressive external ophthalmoplegia) is quite common and is so slowly progressive they don't know they

have it. I have found that the neck flexors are much weaker than the neck extensors in most of these cases. That is a quick pearl to check as well as testing for weakness of the orbicularis, in such cases. Lock your examining chair, put their head back in the head holder, and put your hand on their forehead, and ask them to push against your hand as hard as they can. You can overcome this readily and can just push them right back there in ocular muscle dystrophy syndromes.

22. *Bromocriptine* is a new drug that is now being used in the treatment of amenorrhea-galactorrhea. In fact, there have been two recent reports that it cured a case of acromegaly and made a pituitary tumor shrink up and go away within three months that came out this month. The references to these are discussed elsewhere. A quick note, however, is: (1) Spark, R. F. *et al.* Complete remission of acromegaly with medical treatment. *J. Am. Med. Soc.* **241**(6):573, Feb. 9, 1979. (2) McGregor, A. M., *et al.* Reduction in size of a pituitary tumor by bromocriptine therapy. *N. Engl. J. Med.* **300**(6): 291, Feb. 8, 1979.

23. Dr. Simmons Lessell has done it again! He had done a good *prospective* study of optic neuritis and has found out that there is a *28%* chance of definitely developing multiple sclerosis after an attack of optic neuritis. The reference to this work is in *Neurol.* **29**(2): 208–213, Feb. 1979.

24. The *ERG* (electroretinogram) is a *MUST* in the workup of a child with unexplained visual loss. You will often find an essentially normal fundus in Leber's congenital amaurosis early in the course of the illness, but the ERG will be essentially extinguished. Two to three years later, the fundus is obviously abnormal, however. Likewise, in the disseminated unilateral subacute neuroretinitis syndrome of Dr. Gass—formerly called the "unilateral wipeout syndrome"—you will need an ERG to make that diagnosis. You'll find a normal ERG in the good eye, and a significantly depressed ERG in the involved eye in that syndrome. A reference to that is in *Ophthalmol.* **85**(5): 521, May 1978.

25. The *optokinetic nystagmus* responses are, interestingly enough, usually

perfectly *normal*—if properly tested—in a patient with tubular fields, or so-called gun-barrel fields, even with bilateral hemianopias with macular sparing. It has always been interesting to me to see those good crisp optokinetic responses when they are looking down a 1–2 degree tube!

26. Declomycin may be helpful in the treatment of the inappropriate antidiuretic hormone secretion syndrome. Dr. Venes has suggested this point, and if that is true, one might consider the use of declomycin as a prophylactic antibiotic after those craniotomies where inappropriate antidiuretic hormone secretion might be expected. One must remember that declomycin has cause photosensitivity (more important in south Florida than New England!)—and, more significantly, that it can mar the appearance of the teeth when used in youngsters, and the latter can be permanent and distressing to the family. However, this is not a problem in adults and this clinical tip may be helpful in some cases.

27. Don't forget that you can diagnose the syndrome of *superior oblique myokymia* usually by history (often over the phone!)—and certainly at a good office visit. This is usually a middle-aged adult who suddenly notes *monocular oscillopsia*. They will tell you that suddenly things begin to jump up and down with their right eye (or their left eye). It is always in *only one eye*, in my experience, and these patients are always able to tell you which eye it is. They may describe it "as if the vertical adjustment on the television is off!" They have no other complaints for practical purposes, as a rule. The next gem is that their examination is usually completely negative. Furthermore, they may even be having the attack while the physician is seeing them and it can be missed! What you have to do is repeatedly have them look down and in (i.e., in the field of the superior oblique) and if you do, you'll see the finest little rotary nystagmic movements of that eye—which are not present in the other eye. Another way to see it is when you are looking at the disc with direct ophthalmoscopy, particularly while they are in the position of looking down and in. Once you recognize the history and are not concerned

because you don't see the eye moving at your office visit (particularly, if they are not having the complaint while you see them), you should start them on a trial with *TEGRETOL.* Tegretol is terrific in the treatment of this condition. Many patients (and doctors) become alarmed when they read the package insert and read about Tegretol. They shouldn't be because you only need a much, much smaller dose of this medicine than is commonly suggested. I have them start on only one-half tablet a night for two days, then one-half tablet morning and night for three days, and then one-half tablet three times a day for four days. Many, many of these cases will be controlled on extremely small doses of Tegretol. We have had a few cases who had a permanent remission after a short course of Tegretol. Don't jump in and do muscle surgery on these cases right off the bat, or without a really good trial with Tegretol. Muscle surgery is really indicated in only a very, very few of them—in my experience.

28. Always remember to get a *sedimentation rate* in any patient above 60 with neurologic complaints and/or headaches. Remember—particularly episodic complaints that sound vascular, for example—amaurosis fugax attacks after 60, get a sed rate! Mild, infrequent headaches after 60, get a sed rate! There are more and more cases of proven giant cell arteritis being reported in whom the sedimentation rate was found to be normal—and there is no question that this occurs. However, the sedimentation rate is still THE BEST office screening test for the disease that we have, and you do NOT want to miss this. So, get that sedimentation rate drawn in the office—WHILE you are waiting for the drops to work—and this will help you not to miss this important and frequent neuro-ophthalmologic problem. Finally, I believe it is helpful for the ophthalmologist to learn how to do temporal artery biopsies himself. For years, I have had the fellows and residents working with me do temporal artery biopsies on these patients in the office as an out-patient procedure. This allows you to get the test readily when you need it, and saves the patient an awful lot of money. We hope to make a tape on the technique of doing a temporal artery biopsy soon on

Neuro-ophthalmology Tapes. There are some fine points about this that will help you. Remember to get the pathologist to do serial sections across the lumen of your specimen—a longitudinal cut is NO good—and you should submit a good length of the artery.

29. Temporal arteritis can be an unusual case of recurrent *pulmonary edema* in the elderly. This is important to recognize because if a 70-year-old man keeps getting pulmonary edema, you would think you should *NOT* give him steroids because of fluid retention. However, *if* this is due to giant cell arteritis involving the myocardium and/or pulmonary vessels, then he *NEEDS* steroids or you will not be able to control it any other way. We have been informed of three cases of this, and I don't know how you will be able to diagnose it definitely unless you do those temporal artery biopsies, whenever a good clinical suspicion comes up!

30. Downbeat nystagmus is a tightly localizing neuro-ophthalmologic sign for brain stem disease. The lesion is usually low in the stem at the *cervicomedullary junction.* Less often, it is at a midbrain (mesencephalic) level. Remember that the cervicomedullary junction is a "weak" spot for computed tomography! Further experience with downbeat nystagmus has shown us that only about one-third of these cases are due to *surgical* lesions near foramen magnum. Thus, about two-thirds of them are due to *medical* lesions at the stem or near the outlet. You do NOT want to miss those surgical lesions there, however. The pearl is this—the *FIRST* thing you do after your office visit discloses downbeat nystagmus is to *examine the* patient's *relatives* sitting out in the waiting room with a pencil and a flashlight. *Familial* downbeat nystagmus due to spinocerebellar degeneration is now about the *commonest* cause of it that I see. *Most* of the involved relatives do *not* know that they have downbeat nystagmus—or that anything is wrong for that matter! The *second* thing that you do with downbeat nystagmus is order a good set of *ROUTINE SKULL FILMS* and inform the radiologist that you are specifically interested in the cervicomedullary junction. Thus, you want a GOOD, TRUE LAT-ERAL of the skull showing a bit of the upper cervical spine and the foramen magnum region well—as you don't want to miss basilar impression, Arnold Chiari, Klippel-Feil, other anomalies at this junction, etc. Finally, you *MAY* have to go to a pneumoencephalogram with PA and lateral tomography at this area. You should read Dr. Shaw's chapter in this book for more details on these cases!

31. In my experience, *90% or more* of patients with *ocular myasthenia gravis* can be well controlled with one Mestinon timespan a day in the morning and gradually increasing use of oral prednisone according to the Seybold–Drachman regimen. I think EVERY patient with myasthenia gravis deserves at least a six weeks trial with Mestinon and Prednisone BEFORE considering thymectomy (unless, obviously, they have a large thymoma on their chest x-rays—which they almost invariably do NOT have)—or any other therapy, as plasmapheresis. I start these patients on one Mestinon timespan by mouth every morning for a week or 10 days. If not controlled, I then start them on prednisone 25 mg at a dose, given as a single dose every 48 hours, and increase this by 10 mg every third dose (i.e., every six days). Usually by the time they get up to taking a "teen" number of prednisone pills (i.e., using the 5-mg dose tablets)—or at about 65–80 mg every other morning as a single total dose—they very often call in that they just "clicked in" and everything is under control. One can then begin to very, very slowly taper the dose off, and I have quite a few patients who have been perfectly controlled in this medicine for three, five, or eight or more years using this technique. Many physicians hasten to point out that the doctor treating the myasthenia gravis should be capable of taking care of acute crises, respiratory involvement, and the like. I think the problem is that many physicians are not comfortable treating myasthenia at all—whether they be internists, neurologists, or whatever. I believe you should get the patient to someone who is familiar and comfortable with treating myasthenia unless you want to try the above regimen yourself.

32. Don't forget the possibility of a *vitrectomy* for *TERSON'S SYNDROME!*

Terson's syndrome is the occurrence of a vitreous hemorrhage in one or both eyes of a patient who has sustained an acute subarachnoid hemorrhage. A reference to this disorder is: Shaw, H. E. and Landers, M. B. Vitreous hemorrhage after intracranial hemorrhage. *Am. J. Ophthalmol.* **80**(2): 207–13, Aug. 1975. It is rather rare but is so treatable you shouldn't forget it! The way it usually presents itself in my experience is for a patient to be admitted on neurosurgery with an acute subarachnoid hemorrhage in coma. When the patient regains their senses in a few days, they ask the nurse to turn the lights on in the room. The nurse is horrified to hear that—because the lights ARE on in the room! The neurosurgeon is promptly called, finds that the patient has essentially no vision, but then notes that the pupils DO react to light. He immediately suspects that this is CORTI-CAL blindness and calls for the ophthalmologist! You see the patient in bed—find that they have light perception with the indirect ophthalmoscope wide open, and that the pupils really do work with that light—but you cannot see the fundus! When you dilate them, you'll find a "blackball" vitreous hemorrhage on both sides. The thing to do is to reassure the patient, her family, and the neurosurgeon that this will usually clear spontaneously. It nearly always does on its own—usually within six weeks to a few months. HOWEVER, if it doesn't, or if this is the patient's only good eye, and after six months the vitreous is still nearly opaque, they are IDEAL candidates for a surgical vitrectomy. Dr. Clarkson has done two of these for me, and they went from hand movements or finger counting to 20/40 on the first postoperative day! The vitreous surgeon loves these cases because the prognosis is particularly good for him in that this is occurring in the presence of an essentially normal retina. In other words, he doesn't have that horrible retinitis proliferans and the like back there behind the scene that usually plagues him. This is an important one in therapy, folks, so don't miss it!

33. The *THYPINONE TEST* merits emphasis for the diagnosis of "euthyroid thyroid eye disease." The *Werner* triiodothyronine suppression test is a good test, helpful in about half the patients with "euthyroid Graves disease," *BUT* it requires the patient to have *FOUR VISITS* over at least 7–10 days. The *THYPINONE* test may be just about as good. *Thypinone* is Abbott's name for synthetic *TRH* (thyrotrophin-releasing hormone).

What is done in this test is simply this— a serum TSH (thyroid stimulating hormone level) is drawn. The patient is then given an injection of THYPINONE (a 1-ml ampoule of 500 mcg) is given intravenously as a bolus over 15–30 seconds, with the patient in supine position and remaining supine for an additional 15 minutes. A *repeat TSH* (thyroid stimulating hormone) is drawn *30 minutes later*. This has the advantage that the entire test is done at one visit. It is probably just about as good as the Werner test, although the final precinct in thyroid eye disease about that isn't in. The disadvantage of the test is that the patient must pay for two serum TSH levels plus the medication, so that when the smoke clears, the final cost of the test to the patient is about $100. The Werner test will be more than that, however. The only BETTER way to diagnose thyroid eye disease is by a careful "OV" (office visit), for you can usually diagnose them sitting in the waiting room or with a hand-light examination.

34. The *CEA* (carcinoembryonic antigen) *test* is a good blood test to help you tell if a mass lesion is primary or metastatic. Usually, you make that differentiation by your examination. However, if still in doubt, you can have this blood test drawn. Normal values are 0–5. Anything above 10 is very suspicious. Anything above 20 is considered diagnostic of metastatic disease. Details on how to get this test are in the chapter by Dr. Barricks in this volume.

35. The *dynamic carotid scan* or *radionuclide scan* is another name for the old radio-isotopic brain scan that was commonly used *BEFORE computed tomography* came in. One should *NOT* confuse these two tests. Both may be loosely referred to as a *"brain scan."* However, there is about as much difference as between coryza and chloroma (even though both begin with a "c"). In my experience, the *ONLY* indication for a radionuclide brain scan now is when you are trying to evaluate the patient for a *high grade carotid stenosis* (without an invasive procedure) *OR* (even better!) for an *intracavernous aneurysm*. It really is very helpful in confirming the clinical suspicion of an intracavernous aneurysm and may spare that elderly lady an arteriogram in such a case. Otherwise, you *always* want a *computed tomographic* scan. I prefer the *DELTA* scan pictures to the *EMI scan* pictures. Others are pushing the AS&E scanner. However, in our area the difference in quality between the pictures we get back from the delta scan units over the EMI scan units is really impressive. You should send your patient to the facility providing the best quality computed tomographic scan at the most rapid service to you and the patient and at the best price to the patient. That is very important, and one should not get involved in any "politics" in making that decision.

36. Do *NOT* use a *cornea* from a patient dying with *dementia* for *corneal transplantation*! Remember that Jakob-Creutzfeldt disease has been transmitted via corneal transplantation, and although that is very rare, it would be prudent to avoid using the corneas from anyone dying with *dementia* for transplantation.

37. Congenitally *tilted optic discs* can cause *upper bitemporal* visual field defects that are typically seen on tangent screen but spare the extreme peripheral fields. Such discs may be seen in some patients with craniofacial dysostoses or craniosynostosis syndromes. However, if there is a Marcus Gunn pupil in one eye, or the history is abnormal, or the acuity (corrected) is asymmetric, you should still get a good set of *routine skull films* in such a case (see the case reported in this volume by Drs. Osher and Schatz).

38. Do *not* order a *VER* (visual evoked response) to make the diagnosis of *multiple sclerosis until* after that patient has had a good refraction, a good set of visual fields, and a reasonable fundus examination. Remember—any form of organic eye disease can reduce the amplitude or prolong the latency of the occipital response obtained from stimulating that eye as compared to its normal fellow. Therefore, you don't want to make the mistake of getting a "high on the hog" expensive test (just because it's new and available) and missing the fact

that you simply had a young girl with functional visual loss who wasn't looking at the pattern too well. She needed a good eye "OV" (office visit) more!

39. I still think that *subtenon's steroids* are very, very helpful in the office management of *optic neuritis.* I use a 1-cc tuberculin syringe (or a 2–3-cc syringe) with a #25 needle that is ⅝ in. long. A drop or two of Ophthaine is placed in the eye, the lower lid is wiped off with an alcohol syringe, and the patient is instructed to look up and to the opposite side. In other words, you give this just as you would a retrobulbar injection for cataract surgery. The bevel of the needle is up, and you should inject through the lower lid at the junction of outer and middle thirds of the lid. You should go along the floor of the orbit and up and in only a little bit to make sure you do NOT inject this into the globe. That HAS happened, but any ophthalmologist who can give a retrobulbar injection can give a subtenon's injection, in my opinion. When the needle is at the "hub," you should suck back a bit to make sure there is no blood, and then rather slowly give 1 cc (40 mg) of aqueous Kenalog (triamcinolone). I then put a patch over the patient's eye and ask her to massage this gently behind the globe for a minute or two. One can then put a patch on the eye for two hours, if desired, or it can be omitted entirely, whichever is indicated in your patient. You can use aqueous decadron, if you like. However, this injection lasts for one to two weeks (at times up to four to six weeks!), avoids the systemic side effects of large doses of oral steroids, and you have given the medicine around that optic nerve where it is needed, without filling up their liver, intestines, and everything else with the medicine. It is seldom necessary to have to repeat this treatment—occasionally, you will need a second treatment in two weeks—and only very rarely, a third one will be needed. Dr. Bird's study showed that the patient with optic neuritis will regain the same acuity without steroids that he will with steroids— however, the time course is shortened on steroids. I believe that the "treatin' doctor" will want to shorten the time course for his patients. Of course, the "diagnosin' doctor" might prefer to get *HLA* antigen typing and follow them. I must admit that when I hear someone speaking on the *HLA* system come in the front door, I have a strong temptation to go out the back door, however!

40. Permanent homonymous *hemianopias can* follow *migraine* attacks! These are rare but I have seen or have notes on at least five such cases now. The history is particularly helpful in diagnosis. One should get a good computed tomographic scan with emphasis on the occipital lobes in such a case. After a few months, this will show a "pear" or "tear" shaped occipital softening on the involved side. A follow-up scan should be obtained 6–12 months later, and this will be the same. Do *NOT* overcall this diagnosis, however—that is the temptation!

41. Many physicians are still not aware of the *"moment of truth"* maneuver in diagnosing an *ADIE'S TONIC PUPIL.* The usual Adie's pupil is a unilaterally large pupil that makes you think the patient had dilating drops or Cyclogyl in that eye yesterday. It is larger than the good eye, reacts essentially nil to light, and also is essentially nil to near. You question the patient repeatedly about "drops" and they always respond "negative!" The thing to do at that point is to have them look at the muscle light across the room, in a semidarkened room but with enough light for you to see the pupils well, and then you should take the tip of one of their fingers, hold it up close to their nose, tap on that finger a bit, and urge them to look at that finger like crazy! In other words, you want to use exhortation, edification, comfort, reassurance, and everything else you can to get a maximum near response. Keep them at near—wiggle that finger—move it around—exhort them to keep looking at it at near. Do NOT use a light at near, but their finger! After you have elicited that maximum near response for about 20 seconds at least (and you usually will have seen NO pupillary constriction to near that you can be sure of), then—HERE IT COMES!—the "moment of truth"!!! Now, have them promptly look down at the end of the room at that muscle light again. Lo and behold, you will see that the pupil you thought really hadn't constricted to near, obviously had done so to a bit, for now you will see that pupil slowly and tonically re-

dilate back to distance. This phenomenon—"tonic redilatation from near to distance"—is the hall-mark of the office exam of an Adie's pupil, and will usually knock the diagnosis out of the ball park! If you're not sure after that (and after tapping their knee and ankle jerks, usually using your hand-light handle since you may not be able to find a reflex hammer, if you are an ophthalmologist), you can try using ⅛% pilocarpine. Take a 2-cc syringe, pull the plunger out, put seven drops of Dacryose, sterile saline, Contactisol or what have you in there first, and then put 1 drop of 1% pilocarpine in and restore the plunger. Shake this mixture up thoroughly and then put exactly one drop of this in the involved eye. I usually take a picture before and after. Some like to put the ⅛% pilocarpine in BOTH eyes at the same time—I can't argue with that too much but my practice has been to do one eye, and then do the other—with pictures before and after. If the involved eye comes down to ⅛% pilocarpine (using the home-made technique just described) and the normal eye does NOT come down to this strength, that is evidence for cholinergic hypersensitivity and favors the diagnosis of Adie's pupil. Remember, however, that it takes several months for this to develop. If you have a FRESH Adie's—as occurs, say, six weeks after the chickenpox or a viral infection—this test may be negative. Don't let that throw you— just repeat it a year later! To save the time, however, the "moment of truth" maneuver will let you make the diagnosis without having to do the other fancy tests. I haven't seen tonic redilatation from near to distance with any other pupillary abnormality and believe it is THE WAY to diagnose Adie's!

42. Remote history of head trauma, some chronic sinusitis, unilateral proptosis with or without cranial nerve palsy (as diplopia)—makes me think of a mucocele. Be sure to get serial sections of that biopsy specimen of the mucocele—because some of them harbor occult sinus carcinomas that may not be evident hiding behind that mucocele! See *Am. J. Ophthalmol.* **80**:943, Nov. 1975.

43. Dr. Glaser has a good test he emphasizes in optic nerve disease. Cover the involved eye, and shine a bright flashlight in the patient's good eye. Tell them—"This is $1 worth of light!" Now, cover the good eye, shine that same light in the involved eye and ask—"Now, how much is this amount of light worth?" *Some* astute patients will immediately reply—"15 cents!" However, many patients do not comprehend this too well, so if they "flame out" on the test, keep on going. When they do respond nicely, however, it is a good way to follow optic nerve disease.

44. You can even use this as a form of *color comparison* in optic nerve disease. Cover the bad eye, and hold up a red Mydriacyl top before the good eye. Tell them: "This is $1 worth of RED!" Now, cover the good eye, and show that red bottle top to the involved eye and ask—"Now, how much is that amount of red color worth?" This is more difficult for them, but will at least start them describing color comparison in the two eyes, and will remind you to compare the saturation of the red bottle top when presented on the temporal and nasal sides of fixation. This is still a very helpful test in looking for chiasmal disease!

45. There are definitely some *visual* complications to *open heart surgery.* Patients who have been on the heart-lung machine for quite a time may wake up with occipital lobe infarctions—retinal and optic nerve microembolism—and other significant ischemic complications. Dr. Schatz has seen several patients with occipital lobe embolism associated with Barlow's syndrome (floppy mitral valves). We need to be on the lookout for that.

46. Whenever I see a patient with *downbeat* nystagmus, I ask them to walk across the room and turn around. Look at their gait. Test them for the Romberg test, but this is usually negative (it is really a gross test for ataxia). However, if you then ask them to walk *tandem*—i.e., touch the heel of one shoe to the tip of the other and walk—most patients with downbeat nystagmus simply cannot do that. That is a quick screening test even for an ophthalmologist to do!

47. We have encountered a patient with classic *serpiginous choroiditis* who presented with a slowly developing *unilateral basal ganglion syndrome.* We saw a young man also with serpiginous choroiditis who simply didn't swing the arm on one side

while walking while he did on the other. We are going to work these cases up better, and Dr. Katz hopes to report these in detail elsewhere. Please don't scoop us on this, but I do advise that you get a good baseline *neurological exam* on all patients in whom you suspect serpiginous choroiditis from the fundus. Now, if you have sweat popping off your brow wondering down inside—"But . . . but . . . but . . . , what is serpiginous choroiditis?"—then, you should look at Dr. J. Donald M. Gass' *Stereoscopic Atlas at Macular Diseases.* C. V. Mosby Co., St. Louis, 1977, second edition, on pages 112–117. A synonym for serpiginous choroiditis is helicoid peripapillary choroidopathy. Dr. Gass believes these are always the same, but I'm not totally sure of that. However, the differential of this fundus lesion includes peripapillary scarring from ocular histoplasmosis syndrome, posterior multifocal placoid pigment epitheliopathy, senile macular degeneration, and angioid streaks. If you look at the fundus with indirect ophthalmoscopy and use a +14 Nikon lens, however, in a typical case you simply cannot miss the fact that there are lesions extending out from around the disc that look like *propellor* blades or legs. They really look like the old-timey propellors that the Red Baron had on his plane! These can extend along and satellite a bit, but with the +14 lens, those propellor blades are awfully specific, I think.

48. Evidence continues to confirm the fact that *optic glioma* is not really a benign disease in many, many cases. Both optic nerve gliomas and chiasm gliomas may progress, and tissue culture studies made from these tumors have shown growth of typical astrocytic tumor cells. One must individualize the management of each of these patients. I personally believe that optic glioma is a true neoplasm and is not simply a hamartoma. If the lesion progresses significantly in the optic nerve, surgery is advised. If the lesion is in the chiasm, and is significant or progressive, irradiation therapy is advised. See *Surg. Neurol.* **10:** 175, Sept. 1978, for a very interesting case.

49. True unilateral papilledema can occur from intracranial lesions. It is rare but does happen. We need to look more carefully for these cases!

50. If you have a giant carotid aneurysm

that does not respond to ipsilateral carotid ligation and/or a Dandy trapping procedure, consider ligation of the *external* carotid on the opposite side! This was very dramatic in one case that we have seen. This was reported in *Surg. Neurol.* **9:** 382, June 1978. The external carotid is getting more important than had previously been thought. It can even be a cause of amaurosis fugax—see *Arch. Neurol.* **34:** 532, Sept. 1977. This should be remembered, however, in management of some of these large aneurysms!

Finally, doctor, if you have a question or an interesting case or some problem not covered in this book, why not write us about it? We can't always answer all the correspondence quickly, but we do like to keep in touch and will do our best to get back to you in reasonable time. Write to this address—Dr. J. L. Smith, 9820 S. W. 62 Court, Miami, Florida 33156. Thank you so much!

2 Radiology for the Ophthalmologist: Plain Skull Films

John A. Costin, M.D.

INTRODUCTION

The ophthalmologist is often confronted with a situation in which he must have some knowledge of plain skull x-rays. This may be with the trauma patient in the Emergency Room, in the office, or most commonly in front of an x-ray viewer looking over the x-rays with a radiologist. It is the purpose of this chapter to describe the most common views obtained in a routine skull series and provide a simple approach to reading them.

Just as we were taught in medical school to develop a routine when looking at the electrocardiograms, i.e., rate, rhythm, axis, etc., it is necessary to develop a similar routine in looking at x-rays. This will minimize errors and also improve one's efficiency.

APPROACH TO PLAIN SKULL FILMS

Step 1.   Quality of Films

When looking at a skull series, the first decision to make is, are the x-rays of good quality or not? That is, are they overexposed or underexposed (too light or too dark)?

Step 2.   Adequacy of Films

Is the area which is of interest well-demonstrated? For example, if the patient is suspected of having an orbital floor fracture, does the x-ray clearly show the orbital floor? Or if the patient is suspected of having a carotid cavernous fistual, is the superior orbital fissure clearly viewed?

Step 3.   Caldwell View

The P-A view, for practical purposes, has been replaced by the Caldwell view on a routine skull series. On a P-A view, dense bones of the petrous pyramids project into the orbits, thereby obscuring the majority of orbital structures. For this reason, the Caldwell is preferred. The technique of the Caldwell (as seen in Fig. 1) is to place the patient facing the film plate with the nose and forehead touching the plate. The x-ray beam is angulated approximately 25°, thereby projecting most of the petrous pyramids into the maxillary sinus.

When presented with a Caldwell view (Fig. 2), a good way to begin the routine of evaluation is to compare the size of the orbits. There is much variation in orbital size from one individual to another, but there is remarkably little variation in the same individual when comparing right to left. There should not be more than 2 mm of difference in orbital size.[1] If a difference is found, the next question that must be addressed is, which is the abnormal side? Is the smaller orbit abnormal or is the larger one abnormal? One helpful clue is to look at the sinuses, especially the ethmoid and maxillary. If the small orbit is the abnormal one, many times the ethmoid and maxillary sinus will "invade" the orbit. That is, asymmetry of the sinuses will be present with the sinuses extending into the smaller, ab-

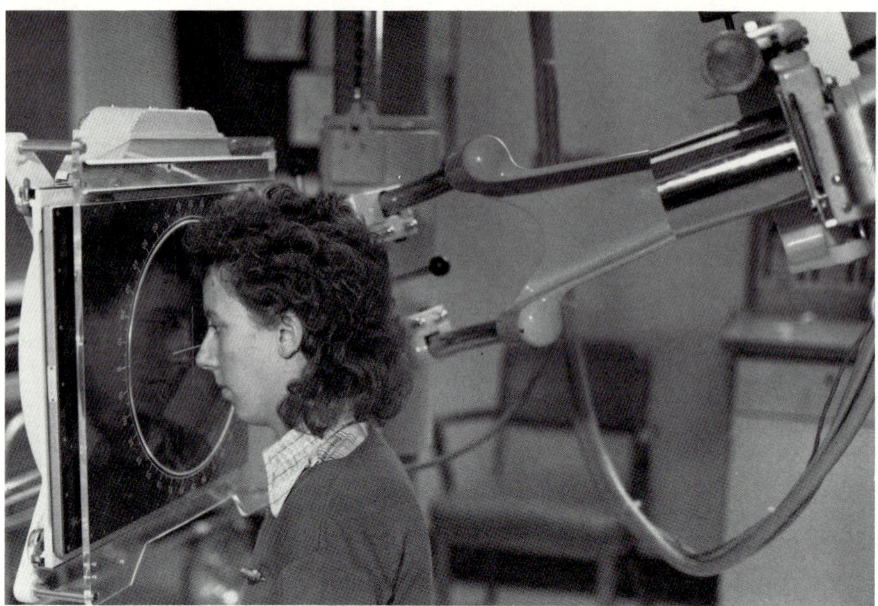

Fig. 1. Caldwell view—technique.

normal orbit. A mucocele can do the same thing. Slow, chronic accumulation of fluid in the sinuses can cause thinning of the sinus walls with extension or encroachment on the orbit. This will give the appearance of a small orbit. The key here is to inspect the sinuses, especially the frontal sinus for opacification.

There are many causes for a small orbit with early enucleation surely leading the list (see Table I).

Enlargement of the orbit similarly can be caused by a number of processes. It is said that tumors within the muscle cone give a diffuse enlargement and that tumors outside the muscle cone tend to give asymmetric enlargement.[3]

The orbits reach their adult size at approximately 9–12 years of age with 50% growth in the first 6–9 years.[4,5] The sinuses do not develop fully until the patient is in the twenties. Any lesion, therefore, which has produced orbital enlargement in a patient whose orbit has already reached adult size (9–12 years of age) must have been present for several years to do so.

Step 4.   Sclerosis (Hyperostosis)

After judging orbital symmetry, one should look for sclerosis of the orbital bones. Here the bony margins will be better defined and denser or more radio-opaque.

Meningiomas are classically thought of as a cause of sclerosis. They can be intraorbital and cause bony sclerosis of the orbital walls. More commonly, however, they involve the greater and lesser wings of the sphenoid to produce sclerosis. An example of a meningioma involving the sphenoid wings and producing sclerosis can be seen in Figure 3.

Step 5.   "Lines"

The next step is the identification of "lines." Follow through this section with Figure 2, which has many of these "lines" marked.

The innominate line runs obliquely through the lateral part of the orbit. It probably corresponds to the medial wall of the temporal fossa. This line can be used very quickly to tell if the patient has been rotated. The distance from the lateral orbital wall to the innominate line should be equal on each side if there is no rotation.

The orbits are shaped somewhat like pears, with the stem being the orbital apex. By using this analogy, the pear is tilted or directed upward with the stem higher than the base. Because of this, one will often see

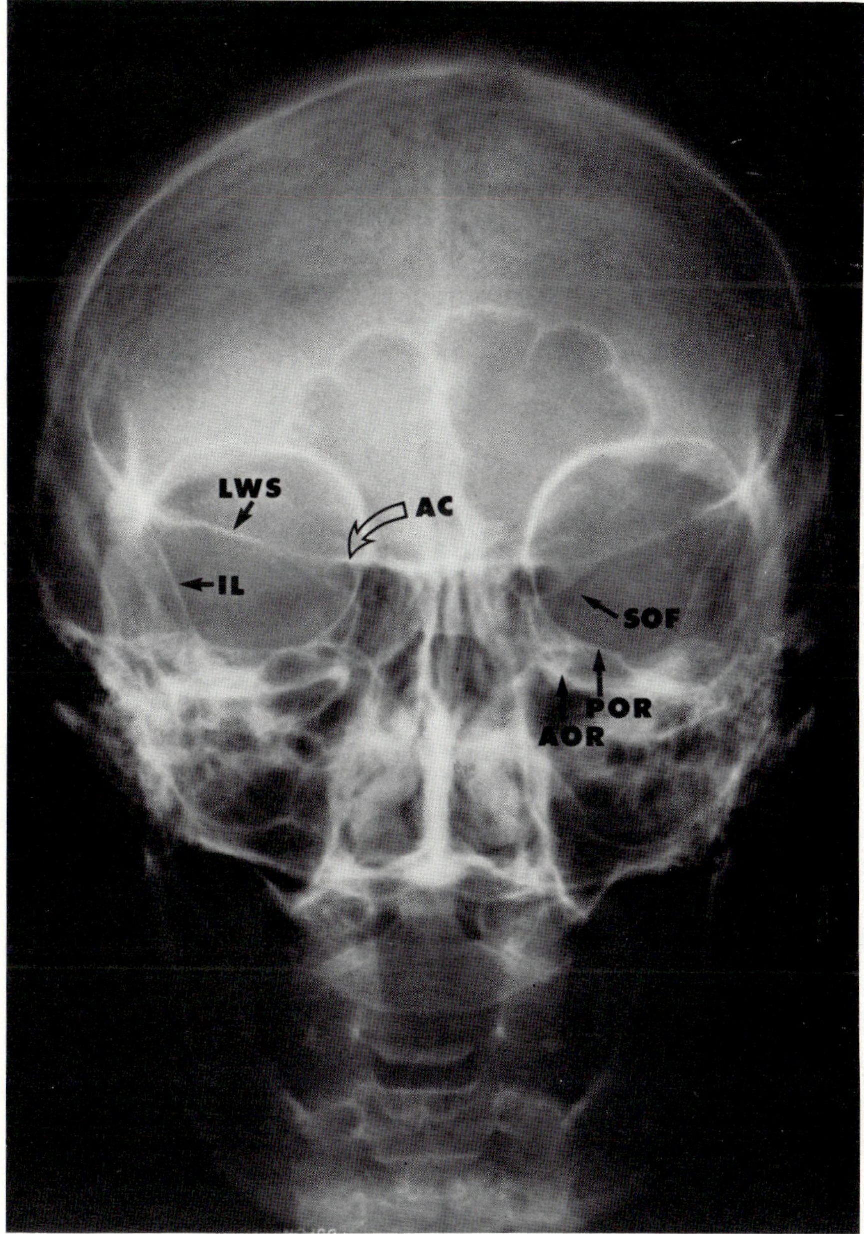

Fig. 2. Caldwell view: LWS—lesser wing of the sphenoid; AC—anterior clinoid; IL—innominate line; SOF—superior orbital fissure; AOR—anterior orbital rim; POR—posterior orbital rim.

two orbital floors and two medial orbital walls. The lower most orbital line corresponds to the anterior orbital rim. The same is true of the medial most line. The higher orbital line corresponds to a more posterior part of the orbital floor. When looking at the medial wall, the more lateral line corresponds to a more posterior part of the wall. The orbital roof and lateral walls are seen as one line.

A line runs almost horizontally through the upper roof of the orbits in a Caldwell projection. This corresponds to the sphenoid ridge and is produced by the lesser wing of the sphenoid. As this line proceeds medially, it eventually terminates in a round,

TABLE I. *Small orbit*
1. Early enucleation
2. Paget's disease
3. Trisomy 13–15
4. Crouzon's disease
5. Fibrous dysplasia
6. Osteogenesis imperfecta
7. Apert's syndrome
8. Radiation—It is of interest that early enucleation, say for retinoblastoma, plus radiation therapy, will give a smaller and more irregular orbit than just early enucleation.[2]

TABLE II. *Large orbit*
1. Tumors
2. Congenital glaucoma with buphthalmus
3. Neurofibromatosis—usually seen as dysplasia for the orbital bones
4. Orbital venous malformtion
5. Meningoencephaloceles

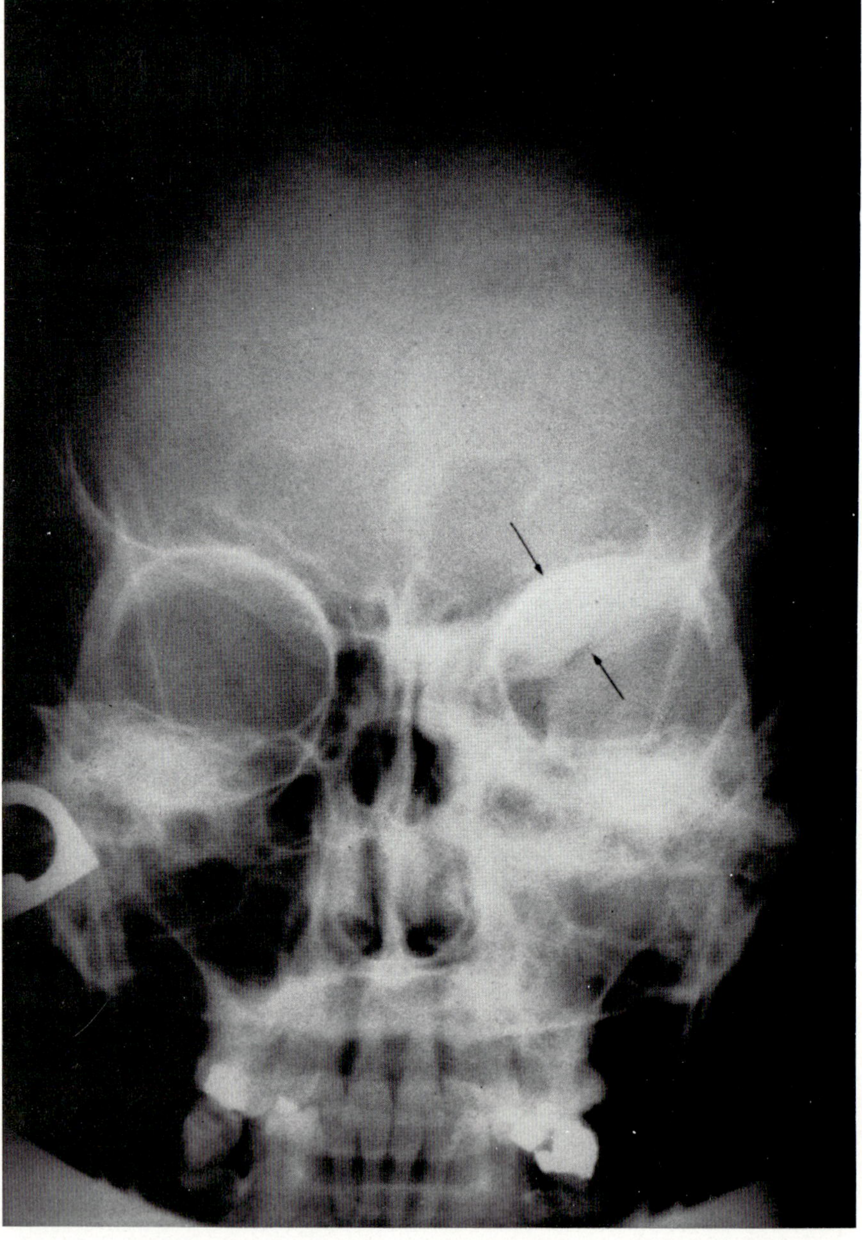

Fig. 3. Sclerosis—meningioma of the greater and lesser wings of the sphenoid.

pneumatized structure, the anterior clinoid. This is most often confused for the optic canal by the ophthalmologist. *This brings up a fundamental rule: the optic canals cannot be seen on routine orbital or skull views.*

The superior orbital fissure appears as a dark (radiolucent) wide line and can best be seen on the Caldwell view. It lies between the lesser wing of the sphenoid above and the greater wing of the sphenoid below. It is approximately 22 mm long, and unfortunately does tend to show variation in some individuals when comparing right to left.[6] This can be seen in Figure 4, where the right superior orbital fissure appears narrowed as compared to the left side. Tomography of the region can usually differentiate normal variations from pathological process. Several other important structures here are clearly seen and labeled.

TABLE III. *Sclerosis*

1. Meningioma
2. Fibrous dysplasia—again look for thickening of the sphenoid wings and body
3. Sinusitis—usually frontal sinus
4. Paget's disease of bone—late in the disease
5. Lacrimal gland tumors and dermoids

There are many causes for enlargement of the superior orbital fissure. Some are seen in Table IV.

Step 6.   Basal Foramina

Just as the anterior clinoids are frequently mistaken for the optic canals on plain views by the inexperienced observer, so is the foramen rotundum. Remember, the second division of the trigeminal nerve (the maxillary division) courses through this opening. Although the foramen rotundum is not seen well in Figure 2, it can be seen in Figure 4, especially on the left. On the Caldwell projection, it usually lies at the level of the orbital floor or just below. On the Water's projection, it is projected in the maxillary sinus as in Figure 10. Again, remember that the optic canals are not seen on routine posterior–anterior views.

Step 7.   Water's View

Having just covered the Caldwell projection, attention is now shifted to the Water's projection. Here, the x-ray beam is held horizontal, and the patient's head is tipped back as in Figure 8. The chin and the nose touch the plate. A simple way to remember this is to associate the Water's view with

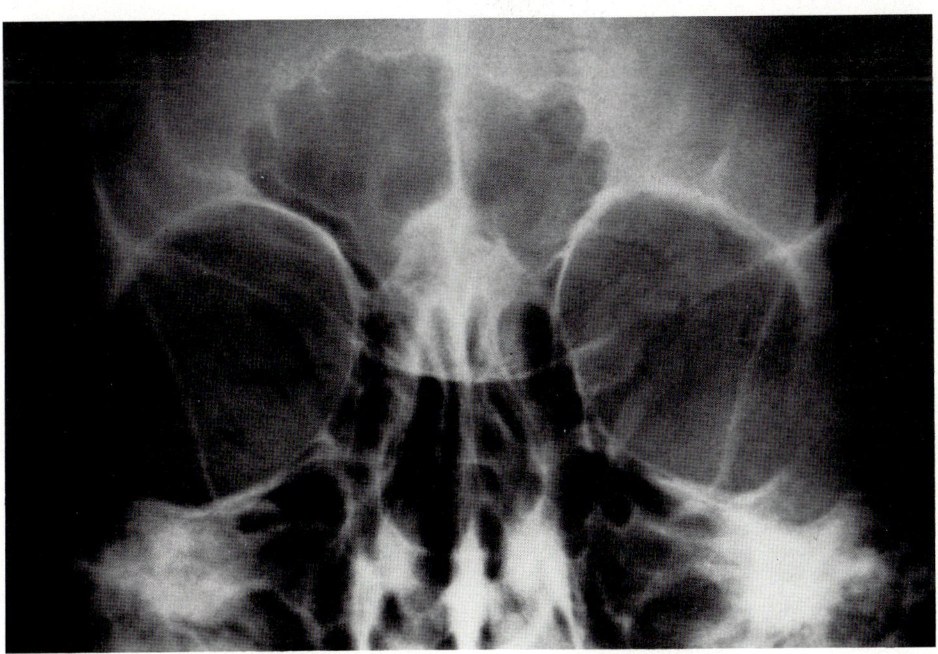

Fig. 4. Caldwell views showing asymmetry of the superior orbital fissures.

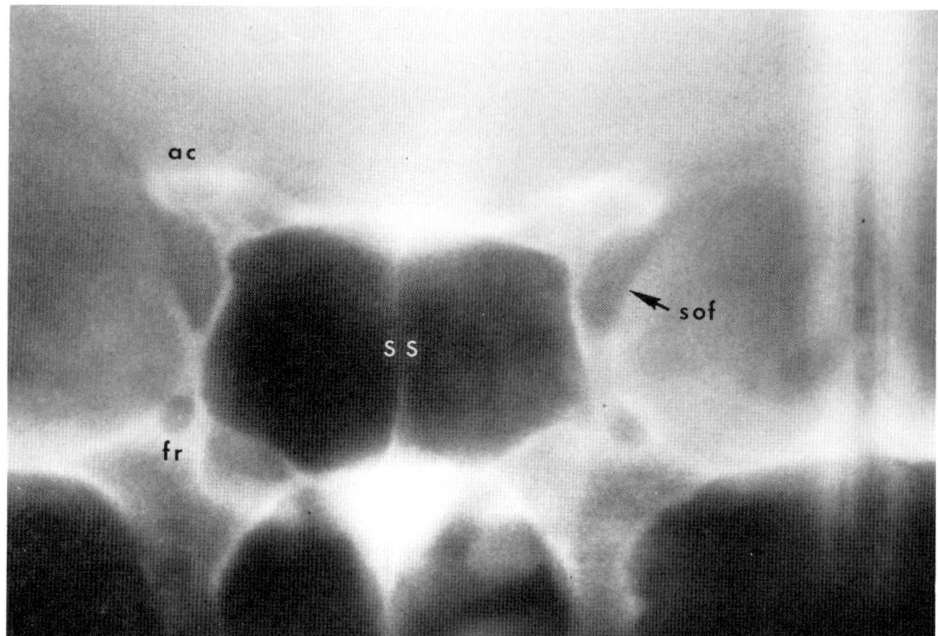

Fig. 5. Tomography of the superior orbital fissures: ac—anterior clinoid; fr—foramen rotundum; sof—superior orbital fissure; SS—sphenoid sinus.

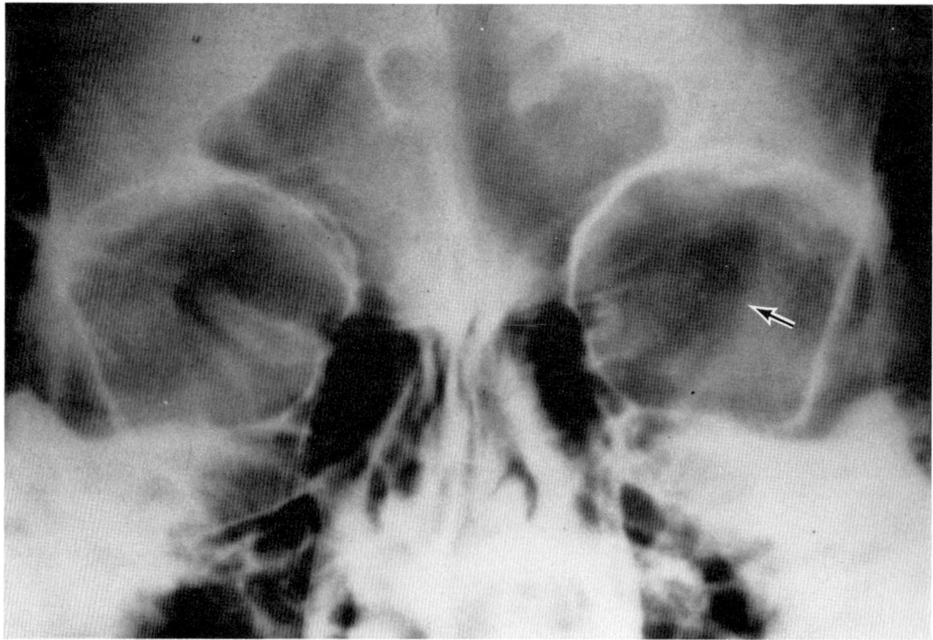

Fig. 6. Widening of the superior orbital fissure in the left orbit (see arrow).

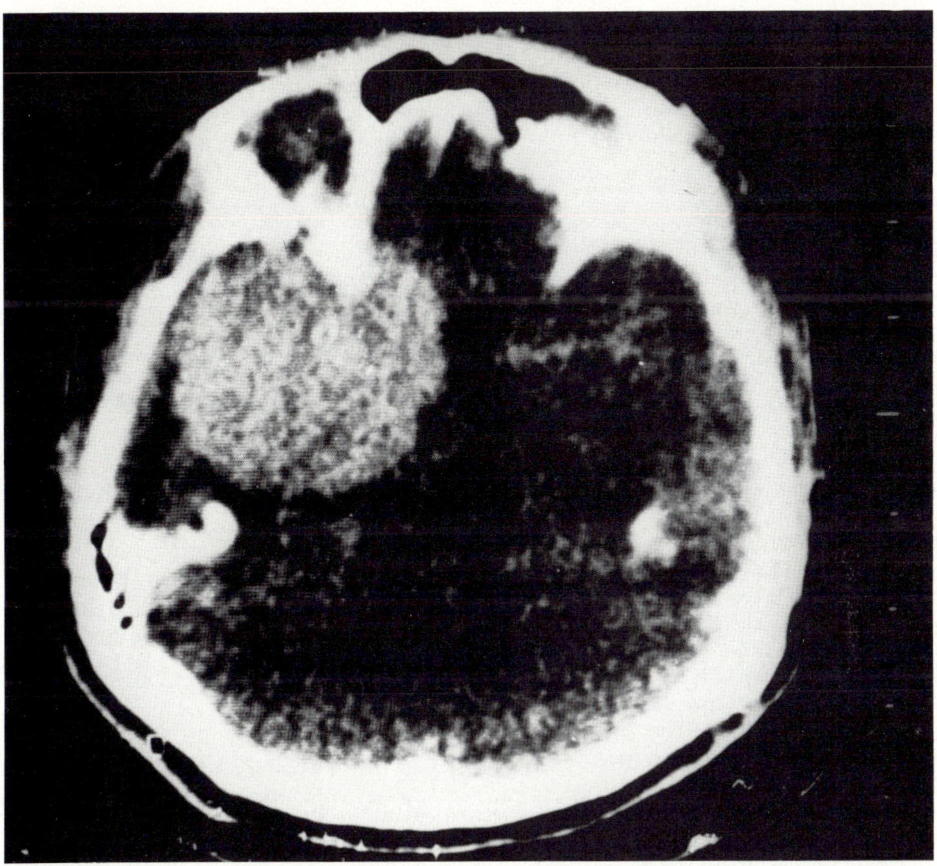

Fig. 7. Computerized tomography in the patient with a widened superior orbital fissure.

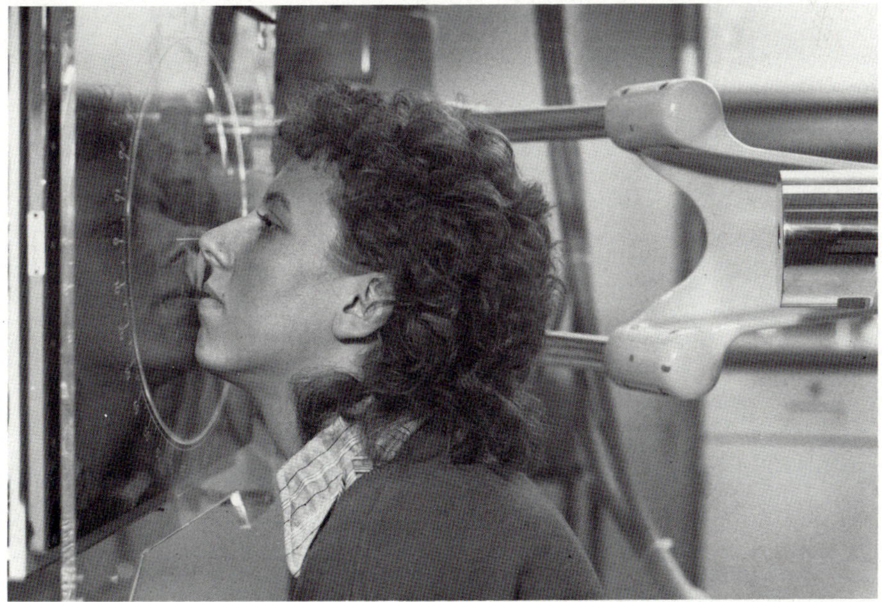

Fig. 8. Water's view—technique.

drinking water (Fig. 9). This is just about the exact position used for the view.

Since the petrous pyramids are projected

TABLE IV. *Enlarged superior orbital fissure*

1. Pituitary adenoma—usually with anterior extension
2. Carotid cavernous fistula—presumably due to the high pressure and high antegrade flow into the ophthalamic veins
3. Intracavernous carotid aneurysm—according to one study, superior orbital fissure enlargement was the most common radiographic finding. This was present in 73% of their cases with intracavernous carotid aneurysms
4. Varix—enlargement of the fissure is only present in a small percentage
5. Meningioma—as mentioned previously, meningiomas of the greater and lesser wings of the sphenoid are likely to produce "meningioma bone" and thereby sclerosis. This will narrow the fissure rather than widen it (Fig. 3). Meningiomas, however, of the middle cranial fossa can cause enlargement of the superior orbital fissure, but also show sclerosis. Figure 6 shows enlargement with some sclerosis of the greater wing of the sphenoid. A CT scan (Fig. 7) confirmed a large mass in the middle cranial fossa. It proved to be a meningioma at surgery.
6. Neurofibromatosis—neurofibromas involving any of the nerves coursing through the superior orbital fissure can lead to widening
7. Chronic increased intracranial pressure

below the maxillary antra in this view, a good look at the orbital floors is possible as well as the maxillary sinuses. It is the preferred view for trauma cases with suspected orbital floor fractures. Figure 10 shows a Water's projection. On the left, the foramen rotundum is well seen in the maxillary sinus. The floor of the orbit is intact, and the infraorbital canal is nicely demonstrated. On the right side, however, there is a so-called blow-out fracture of the floor. The periosteum is thickened and there is prolapse of tissue through the fracture site into the maxillary sinus. A fluid level in the sinus can also be seen—probably blood in this case. A discussion of orbital fractures is beyond the scope of this chapter, except to say that when a question of a fracture exists and the plain views are normal, tomography is the last word. Figure 11 shows a case of suspected orbital floor fracture with normal Water's view. The tomographic section clearly shows the fracture site.

Step 8.   Lateral View

Much can be gained from the lateral view. The procedure is simply seen in Figure 12. A properly done lateral will not only show the orbits, but also the sellar region,

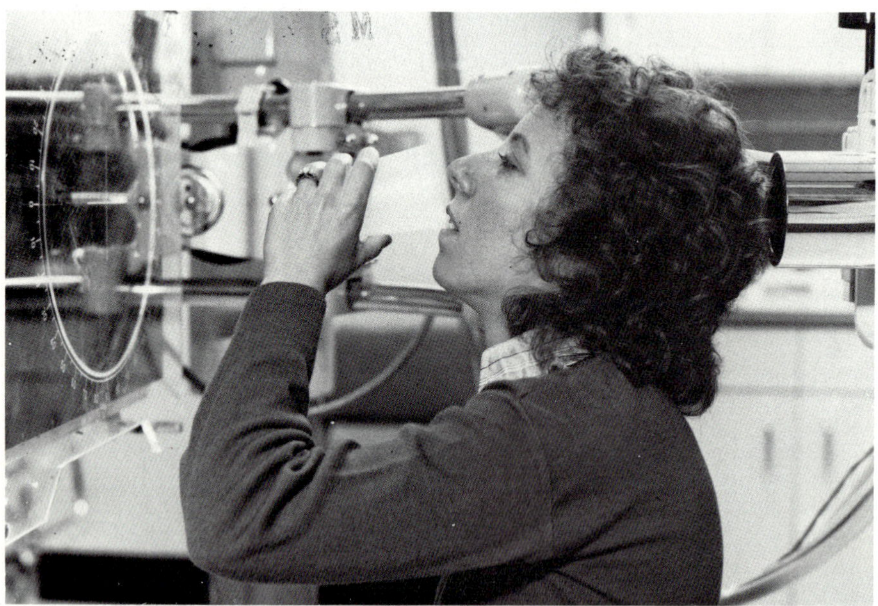

Fig. 9. Drinking water and the Water's view.

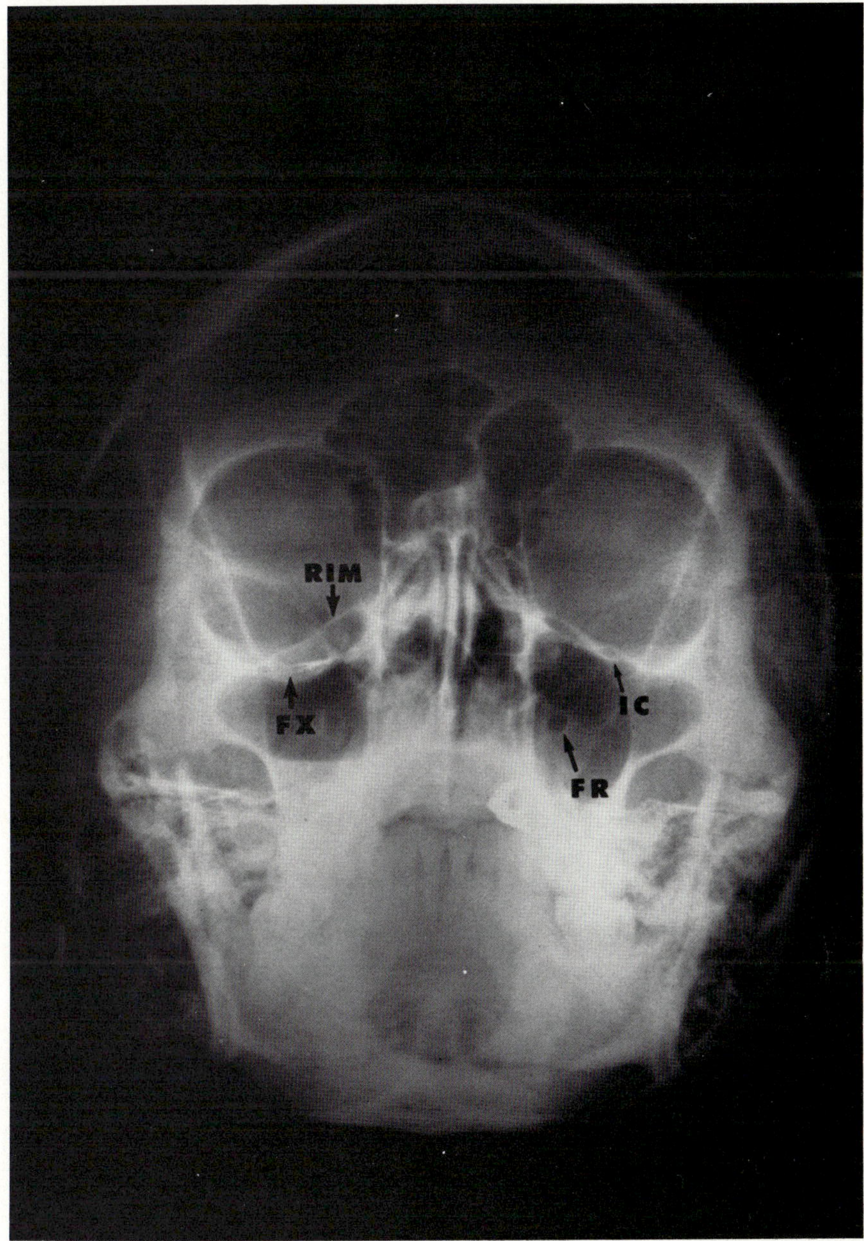

Fig. 10. Water's view; RIM—inferior orbital rim; FX—floor fracture; IC—infraorbital canal; FR—foramen rotundum.

which is very important to the practicing ophthalmologist.

The roof of the orbit as seen in Figure 13 is irregular. Remember that the frontal lobe lies on the roof and its convolutions account for the wavy pattern on the roof. A horizontal line lies just below and almost parallel to the roof. This corresponds to the superior margin of the ethmoid bone. The posterior wall of the orbit is also well visualized and is largely due to the greater wing of the sphenoid. The orbital floors are superimposed and give a rather diffuse, faint line. Air in the nasopharynx acts to nicely outline this structure also.

To appreciate the sellar region, it is best

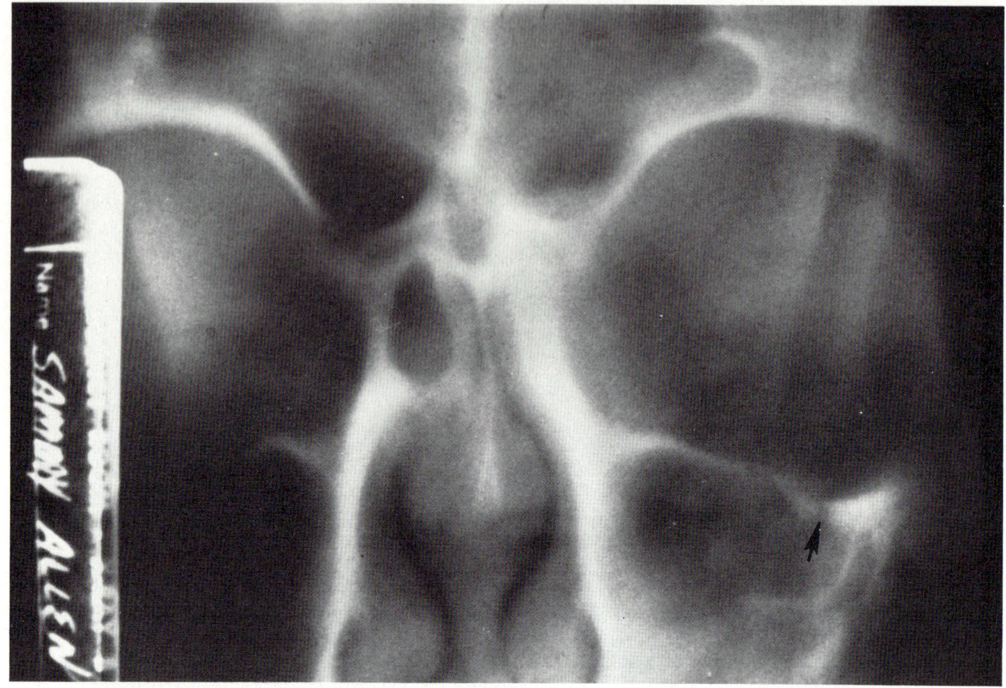

Fig. 11. Tomography of the orbits demonstrating a floor fracture on the left side (see arrow).

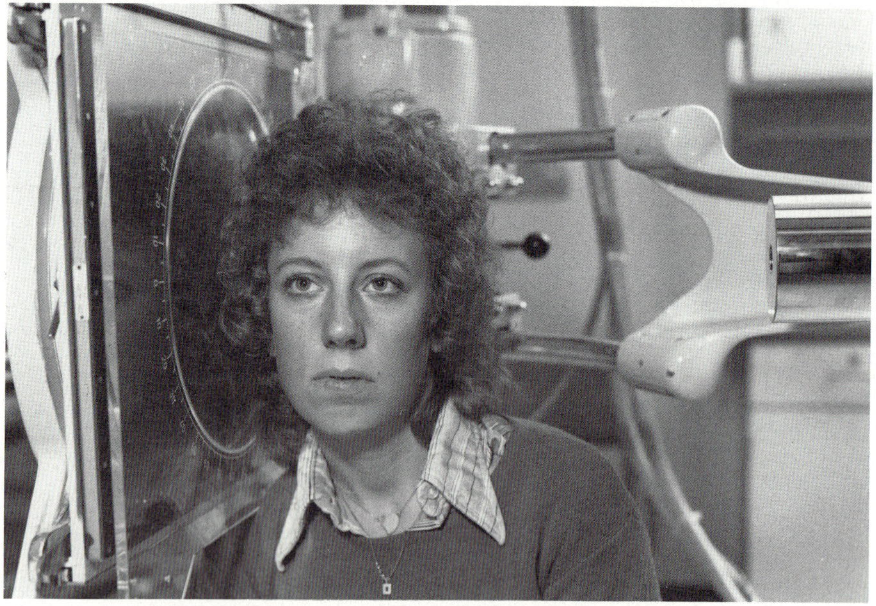

Fig. 12. Lateral view—technique.

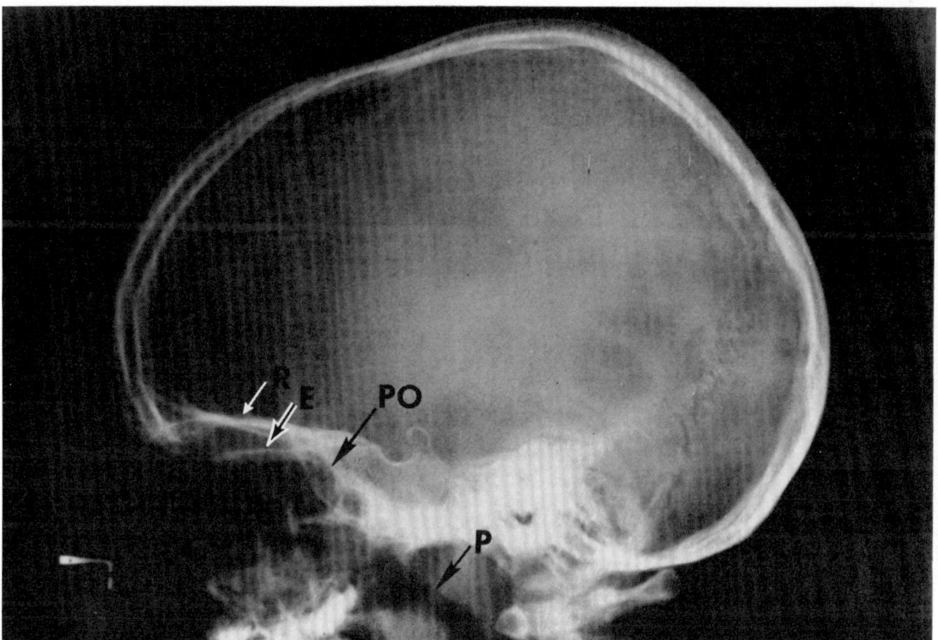

Fig. 13. Lateral view: R—orbital roof; E—ethmoid bone; PO—posterior orbit; P—nasopharynx.

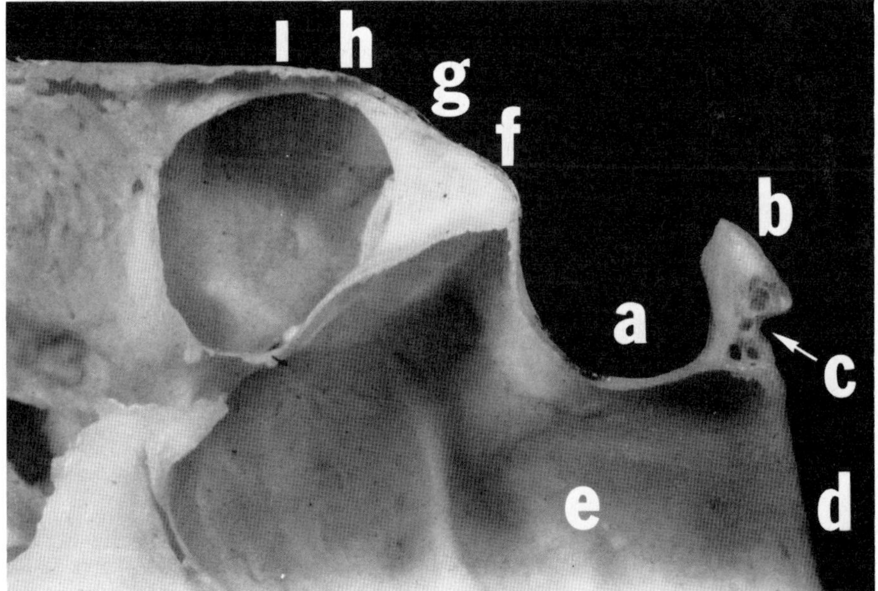

Fig. 14. Anatomy of the sellar region: a. sella turcica; b. posterior clinoid; c. dorsum sellae; d. clivus; e. sphenoid sinus; f. tuberculum sella; g. chiasmatic sulcus; h. limbus sphenoidale; i. planum sphenoidale.

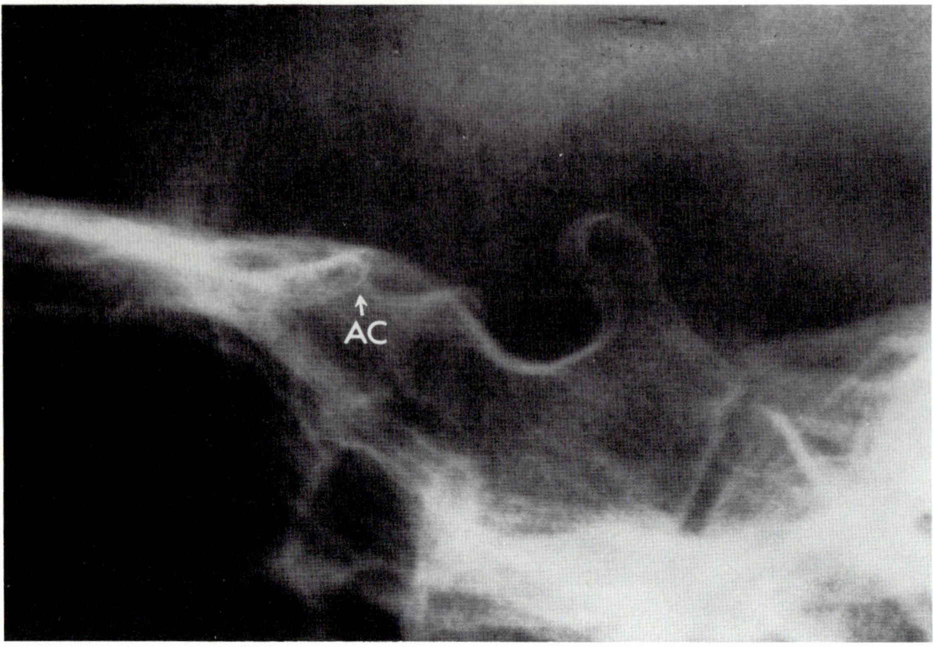

Fig. 15. Blow up of Figure 13: AC—anterior clinoid.

to have an understanding of the anatomy. Figure 14 is a sagittal section through the midline of a cadaver skull. The important structures are labeled. After reviewing this section, go to Figure 13 and systematically identify the corresponding radiographic areas. A blow-up of the sellar region (Fig. 15) is included for further study. Since the anatomic section does not contain the anterior clinoid, it is labeled in Figure 15.

CONCLUSION

It is the purpose of this chapter to make the reviewing of orbital x-rays not only more rewarding but also enjoyable. An eight-step approach is offered to systematically begin examining plain orbital x-rays.

1. Quality of films
2. Adequacy of films
3. Caldwell view
4. Sclerosis (hyperostosis)
5. "Lines"
6. Basal foramina
7. Water's view
8. Lateral view

With this foundation, further appreciation and understanding of x-rays can be obtained for the practicing ophthalmologist or resident in training.

REFERENCES

1. Potter, G. The Orbit: Refresher Course of the American Roentgen Ray Society, September, 1969.
2. Kennedy, R. E. The effect of early enucleation on the orbit in animals and humans. Am. J. Ophthal. *60*:277–306 (1965).
3. Newton, T. H., Potts, D. G., Evans, R. A., *et al.* Radiologic diagnosis in pediatric ophthalmology. Radiol. Clin. North Am. *1*:459–495 (1963).
4. Whitnall, S. E. *Anatomy of the Human Orbit and Accessory Organs.* Henry Frowde and Hodder and Stoughton, London, England, 1921.
5. Wolff, E. *The Anatomy of the Eye and Orbit,* 3rd ed. The Blakiston Company, Philadelphia, Pa., 1948.
6. Kornblum, K. and Kennedy, G. R. Sphenoidal fissure: anatomic, radiographic, and clinical study. Am. J. Roentgenol. *47*:845–858 (1942).
7. Rischbieth, R. H. C. and Bull, J. W. D. Significance of enlargement of the superior orbital fissures. Br. J. Radiol. *31*:125–135 (1958).
8. Zizmor, J. and Lombardi, G. *Atlas of Orbital Radiography.* Aesculapius Publishing Co., Birmingham, Ala., 1973.
9. Newton, T. H. and Potts, D. G. Radiology of the Skull and Brain. *The Skull,* Vol. 1, Book 2. C. V. Mosby Co., St. Louis, 1971.

3 Quantitation of the Afferent Pupillary Defect

Edward Fineberg, M.D.
H. Stanley Thompson, M.D.

INTRODUCTION

The afferent pupillary defect (Gunn pupil) is a well-established sign of optic nerve and retinal disease. There has been no standard method for quantitating this clinical sign. The purpose of this paper is to present a technique of measuring afferent pupillary defects, which we have developed and applied over the past several years.

BACKGROUND

For more than a century the diminished pupillary response on the side of an organic lesion of the optic nerve has been well recognized.[1] Lowenstein, in his pupillographic studies, called it a "low intensity reaction," since the reduced pupillary response on the side of an optic nerve lesion could be closely matched by the response of the normal eye to reduced illumination.[2] The principle of balancing the afferent pupillary defect with neutral density filters has also been demonstrated pupillographically (see Fig. 1). The swinging flashlight technique of Levatin makes the afferent pupil defect easier to recognize by calling the attention to the *direction* of movement rather than the final pupil size.[3] Our clinical method for neutralizing the afferent pupillary defect combines the swinging flashlight technique with the use of a neutral density filter in front of the intact eye (see Fig. 2). The amount of filter needed to balance the pupillary abnormality is reported in log units.

EQUIPMENT

The equipment required for this test is simple. It consists of a bright, focal light source (either an indirect ophthalmoscope or a hand light) and a set of neutral density filters. These filters can be purchased from most photographic catalogs. The list in Table I is extracted from the Kodak catalog. Each 3-in. square Wratten gelatin filter costs $6.30. These filters when used singly or in combination will give a filter range of 4.0 log units in 0.1-log-unit steps. The filters can be mounted between two glass lantern slides and then taped at the edges (see Fig. 3). The light filtering effect of each glass lantern slide is 0.03 log. A filter holder (Kodak catalog #1486638) may be purchased at $3.75 each.

A filter card has been developed which might prove more convenient than loose filters (see Fig. 4).

METHODS

Reliable measurements can be obtained by adhering to the following steps:

1. Avoid prolonged bright light examinations just before the test.

2. Keep the room lights dim (for larger pupillary excursion).

3. Have the patient fix his or her gaze on a distant target (to eliminate near response).

4. Swing the light from eye to eye in a symmetrical fashion and allow 2–4 seconds light exposure to each eye.

5. Observe the initial response of each pupil to the light stimulus.

(a) Equal constriction of each pupil is the normal response.

(b) Dilation of one pupil and constriction of the other pupil as each is exposed to the

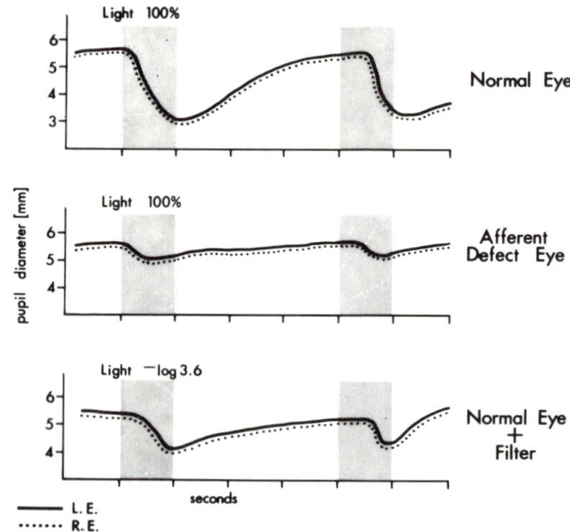

Fig. 1. Placing a 3.6 log filter over the normal eye (bottom graph) produces a tracing which closely resembles the tracing seen when the defective eye receives 100% light stimulation. [Redrawn from Am. J. Ophthalmol. *61*:863 (1966).]

swinging light indicates a relative afferent pupillary defect in the eye with the dilating pupil.

6. Balance the relative afferent pupillary defect by adding neutral density filters in 0.3 logarithmic steps over the *good* eye while swinging the light.

7. After determining the rough end point, it is often possible to refine it, using a 0.1–0.2-log filter (see Fig. 5)

8. Record the measurement of the relative afferent pupillary defect as precisely as possible. For example, if there is a defect in the left eye neutralized by placing 1.1-log neutral density filter over the right eye during the test, then this part of the pupil examination might be recorded thus: Pupils: left eye, 1.1-log afferent pupillary defect.

COMMENT ON TECHNIQUE

The principle of the technique is to reduce the light intensity over the intact eye until each pupil constricts equally during the swinging flashlight maneuver; that is, until the afferent pupillary defect disappears and the pupillary responses appear normal. For this reason, care must be taken to deliver the same light exposure to each eye. Attention to certain details will nearly eliminate this source of problems.

a. The light must not be held closer to one eye than the other.

b. The light must not be held longer over one eye than the other.

c. The light should not be directed

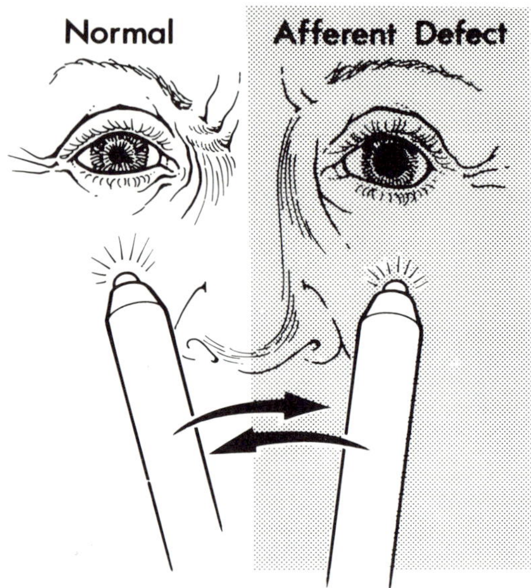

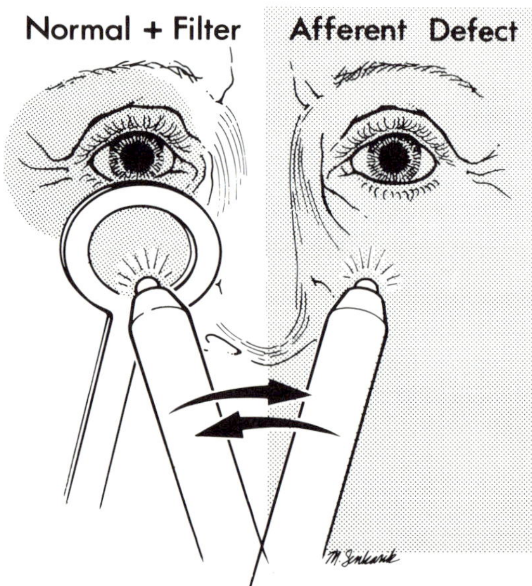

Fig. 2. (a) An afferent pupillary defect in the left eye is present when, during a swinging light maneuver, the left pupil dilates and the right pupil constricts. (b) After screening for an afferent pupillary defect (OS) by the swinging light technique the filter is placed before the intact eye (OD). By choosing the appropriate amount of filter one can neutralize the afferent pupillary defect so that the pupils constrict equally and reach the same final resting size.

TABLE I

Neutral density (log units)	Percent transmission	Kodak Co. Catalog #
0.1	80	149-6314
0.2	63	149-6322
0.3	50	149-6330
0.6	25	149-6363
1.0	10	149-6045
2.0	1	149-6413

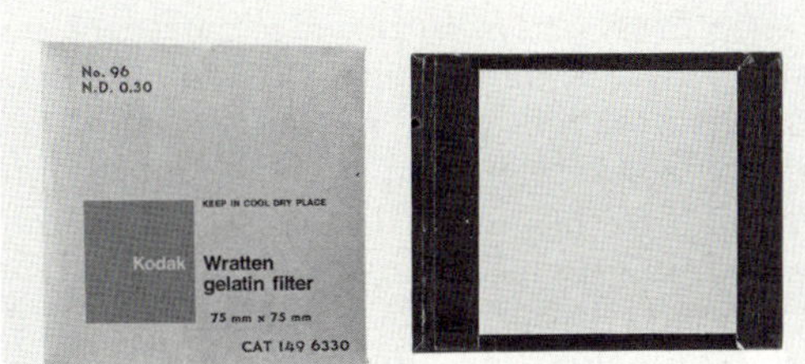

Fig. 3. The 3-in. square filters may be mounted between glass slides and then taped at the edges. These may then be added one to another in combination.

obliquely through one pupil and directly at the macula in the other eye. If the two eyes are not pointing in the same direction, then care should be taken to shine the light along the visual axis in each eye.

d. It should be recognized that a difference in pupil size can significantly affect that amount of light entering each eye. When the pupil is 8 mm on one side and 1.5 mm on the other, 30 times more light (equivalent to 1 log unit) will enter the side with the dilated pupil. Thus, a small pupil tends to shade the retina on that side. This is analogous to the concept used in photography in which each "f stop" setting represents a change in the area of the aperture by a factor of 2 or 0.3 logarithmic units (see Fig. 6). To compensate for the unequal retinal illumination due to unequal pupil size, one can place a neutral density filter in front of the eye with the larger pupil (0.1 log for every millimeter of anisocoria).[4]

e. Asymmetric bleaching of the retinas, which may occur inadvertently prior to or during the test, may invalidate the results. It is important to realize that asymmetric bleaching may occur during the neutralization test itself as the balancing filter shades the retina of the intact eye. With prolonged testing the defective eye will thus be relatively unprotected and may be ov-

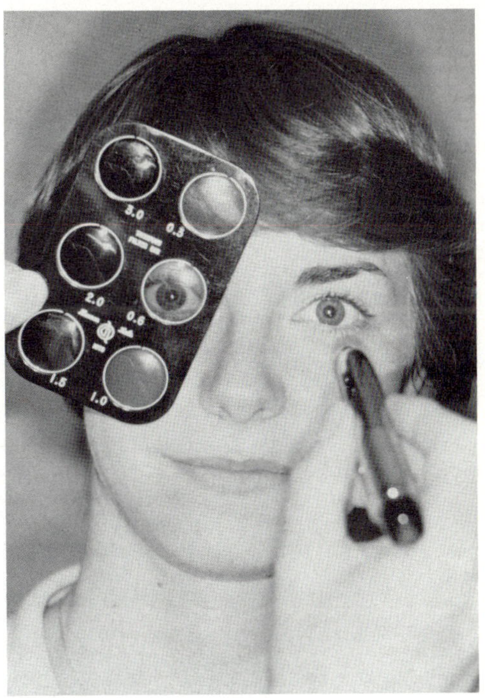

Fig. 4. Pocket filter card with six clinically useful filters (0.3, 0.6, 1.0, 1.5, 2.0, and 3.0 log units). These filters divide the range of possible afferent pupil defects into seven categories:

Grade	Log units	Description of afferent pupil defect
"Mini"	0.1–0.2	Equivocal, hard to measure
1+	0.3–0.5	Small, but definite
2+	0.6–0.9	Moderate
3+	1.0–1.4	Marked
4+	1.5–1.9	Large
5+	2.0–2.9	Enormous
6+	3.0–	Amaurotic pupil

Refinement of the measurement to the nearest 0.1 log unit is not possible with this filter card. This filter card is being made by Hansen Ophthalmic Development Labs, P.O. Box 613, Iowa City, Iowa 52240.

erbleached. This can result in a falsely high end point. To avoid this, shorter testing runs should be used. If this is not possible, one should remove the filter after every two to four passes and try to balance the bleach by exposing both eyes to the light.

ENHANCEMENT OF THE RELATIVE AFFERENT PUPILLARY DEFECT

Below a value of 0.2–0.3 log filter units,

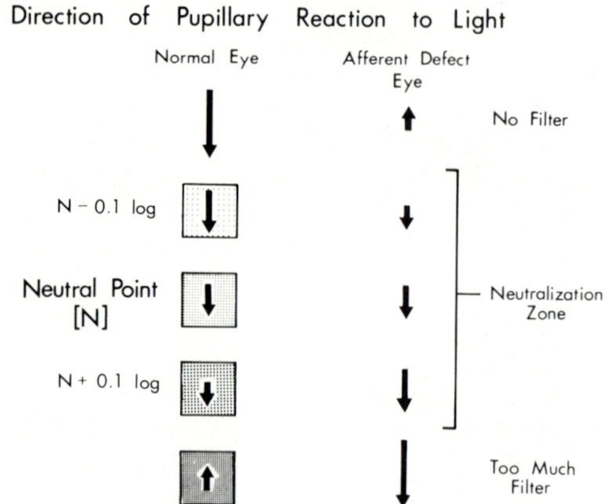

Fig. 5. Arrows indicate the direction of pupil reaction during swinging light test: (↓) pupil constriction; (↑) pupil dilatation. By over- and under-correcting the afferent defect (as with retinoscopy or the cover test) it is possible to more clearly define the neutral point.

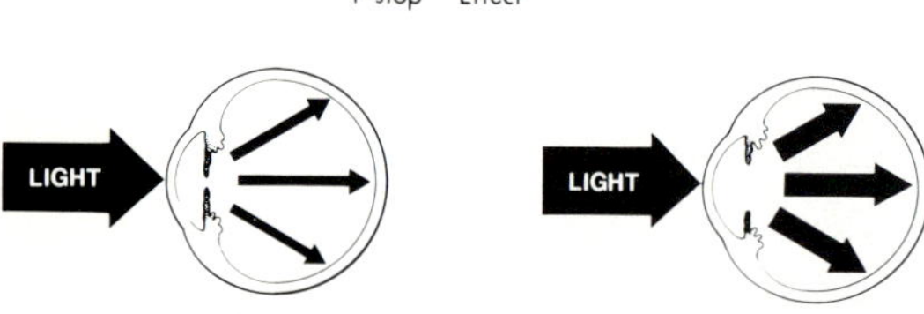

Fig. 6. A significant difference in pupil size may significantly affect the amount of light entering the eye. This "f stop" effect is not entirely corrected by using a supramaximal stimulus, and should be recognized as an aggravating or balancing factor in an uncorrected afferent pupillary defect.

many afferent pupil defects may be undetected or equivocal. In such cases, a 0.1-log filter placed over the suspected abnormal eye may enhance the pupillary sign. Thus, it may be possible to reach a decision in some doubtful situations.

SUMMARY

We have presented a means of quantitating the afferent pupillary defect. The principle of the technique is to balance the pupillary reactions of the two eyes by reducing the light response of the good eye to a point where it matches that of the abnormal eye and both pupils appear to react equally. This is accomplished by placing a neutral density over the intact side and then performing the swinging flashlight maneuver. The technique is objective and re-

producible. With little time added to the routine pupil examination, it is possible to extract more useful information. In future publications, we hope to correlate the quantitated afferent pupillary defect with retinal lesions or visual field defects of known size and location.

EDITOR'S NOTE

The Marcus Gunn pupil, or afferent pupillary defect, or "swinging flashlight test," has been called *THE most important* pupillary abnormality in clinical neuro-ophthalmology by Dr. Glaser, and I cannot agree more with that statement. Therefore, it bears repetition and emphasis—*the Marcus Gunn pupil* or afferent pupil defect *is THE MOST IMPORTANT pupillary abnormality in medicine!* Drs. Fineberg and Thompson have written an important paper showing that one can not only detect such a pupillary abnormality but can quantitate it. I have graded the Marcus Gunn pupil from 1+ to 4+ for years and have found that extremely helpful. A few points should be emphasized: (1) There are important points in technique in doing the test—(a) have the patient fix on a specific target at distance, (b) use a semidarkened room, (c) hold the indirect ophthalmoscope light wide open in your hand as an excellent stimulus, (d) test each pupil for the direct response at least three times and grade this 1-4+, (e) move this from one eye to the other at a moderate rate of speed and leave it on the second eye long enough to assess accurately what is happening (too rapid and too slow movements from eye to eye BOTH are wrong!). The first movement of the pupil should be DOWN (i.e., a bit of constriction) in the normal patient. If the first movement of the pupil is UP (i.e., a bit of "slip" or dilatation), you have an afferent pupil defect. Remember, you get MORE Marcus Gunn pupil out of a 20/40 optic neuritis than out of a 20/200 macular lesion! You CAN get an afferent pupil with retinomacular disease, but it is a poor one—all the Marcus Gunn pupil tells you is a conduction defect in the eye on that side—primarily of optic nerve, and to a lesser degree of retinomacular fibers that will pass in the optic nerve. This is another reason why it is helpful to quantitate the Marcus Gunn pupil. If you have 20/30–3 best corrected vision in the right eye and 20/15 best corrected vision in the left eye, yet you have a definite 2–2.5+ Marcus Gunn pupil in that right eye, you are going to be confident that this is on an optic nerve basis. There will be considerable involvement of the visual field in that eye—more than you would have expected from the acuity! On the other hand, if you have 20/100 best corrected acuity in the left eye and 20/15 in the right eye, but there is only an equivocal (0.5+) Marcus Gunn pupil in left eye, you have either something like cystoid macular edema in that eye, or some functional visual loss, or you need to check that vision more carefully! You may find that with a pinhole in a trial frame, head holder, and 10 more minutes, that the 20/100 in left eye turns out to be 1 on the 20/25 line!

Another practical point to mention is that when you move the light from one eye to the other, if the patient shifts fixation (i.e., you see the eyes themselves move due to a tropia or a large phoria), you should go slow in interpreting that pupil. You often will get a "bounce" of the pupil with each shift of the eye, so if the patient shifts fixation with the light, go SLOW on calling that pupil—you may be getting an artefact!

Another pearl is the "reverse Marcus Gunn pupil." We have described this in a little book "The Pupil"—if you are interested. This lets you assess the optic nerve function in an eye WITHOUT a pupil! In other words, aniridia, occlusio or seclusio pupillae, a dilated and fixed pupil—any or all of these in the RIGHT eye—still will not slow you down on assessing optic nerve function in the right eye (even when you can't see the fundus with indirect!)—if you read the LEFT (good) pupil carefully! Finally, remember that there is NO SUCH ANIMAL as a BILATERAL Marcus Gunn pupil. Anyone using that term is probably trying to describe "light-near dissociation" of the pupils (i.e., the pupils are reacting poorly to light but more crisply to near in both eyes). However, anyone talking about a bilateral Marcus Gunn pupil is using the term inaccurately and is tipping you off to the fact that he really is not too familiar or comfortable with the test—for the point is that ONE eye is the control that is telling you about the other eye in this test. Dr. Fineberg also has some other "pearls" about the amount of afferent pupil defect you get with various size retinal detachments, but he is holding that off for later publication. In the meantime, I think it is very important that you learn to quantitate the Marcus Gunn pupil, and with practice you can call it 1–4+ and won't even have to use his "spiffy" filters. The important point of this paper, however, is that we need to quantitate the Marcus Gunn pupil in the office, and that it is not really too hard to do!

JLS

REFERENCES

1. Thompson, H. S. Afferent Pupillary Defects. Pupillary Findings Associated with Defects of the Afferent Arm of the Pupillary Light Reflex. Am. J. Ophthalmol. *62*:860 (1966).
2. Lowenstein, O. Clinical Pupillary Symptoms in Lesions of the Optic Nerve, Optic Chiasm and Optic Tract. Arch. Ophthalmol. *52*:385–403 (1954).
3. Levatin, P. Pupillary Escape in Disease of the Retina or Optic Nerve. Arch. Ophthalmol. *62*:768 (1959).
4. Thompson, H. S. Pupillary Signs in the Diagnosis of Optic Nerve Disease. Trans. Ophthalmol. Soc. UK *96*:279 (1976).

4 Choroidal Osteoma. A New Clinicopathologic Syndrome

Patrick S. O'Connor, Major, USAF, MC

INTRODUCTION

Choroidal osteoma is a newly recognized clinicopathologic syndrome first described by Gass *et al.*[1] While characteristic in its clinical appearance, this benign tumor may be mistaken for choroidal hemangioma, leukemia, metastasic carcinoma, or an amelanotic melanoma of the choroid. Such misdiagnosis has led to unnecessary enucleation for this lesion.[2, 3] Computerized tomography in this clinical setting is diagnostic.

CASE REPORT

A 31-year-old, right-handed, white female was seen in October 1978 through the courtesy of Dr. Ansell. She complained of right-sided periorbital and ocular pain with poor vision, since July 1973. At that time following a bout of vomiting, the patient developed sudden visual loss and ocular pain. She was hospitalized and an EEG, lumbar puncture, brain scan, and neurologic examination were felt to be normal. Fluorescein angiography revealed a "detachment of the retinal pigment epithelium" and a diagnosis of macular pigment epitheliopathy was made. After discharge her vision remained stable, but recent increasing pain raised the question of tic doloureux. The patient denied diplopia, muscular weakness, incoordination or other neurologic symptoms, and except for some "colitis" in the past was in good health.

Examination revealed a best corrected vision of 20/100 OD and 20/15 OS. External, ocular motility, pupillary, and slit-lamp examinations were all normal. The blood pressure was 110/70 (both arms sitting), and no carotid, cranial, or ocular bruits were heard. Amsler grid testing of the right eye showed a large temporal paracentral scotoma while Goldmann visual fields revealed a central scotoma with nasal and temporal paracentral scotomas of varying density. On dilated fundus examination, an elevated yellow-white juxtapapillary tumor was seen extending through the macula of the right eye (Fig. 1). Its scalloped margins were orange-red in color. On the tumor surface there was a mottled pattern of orange pigment clumping and multiple small branching vascular tufts. In the macula there was a grey plaque with pigment clumping. The left eye was normal. Computerized tomography of the orbits revealed a choroidal mass in the right eye (Fig. 2a) that when enlarged and compared to a standard had the same density as bone (Fig. 2b). Further neurologic evaluation with four-vessel angiography and pneumoencephalography was normal. Laboratory evaluation including a CBC, urinalysis, FTA-ABS, serum calcium, phosphorus, alkaline phosphatase, and thyroid function studies were normal. Fluorescein angiography failed to show evidence of any abnormality in the retinal circulation. However, a large portion of the mass demonstrated early hyperfluorescence probably caused by perfusion of the capillary network on the inner surface of the tumor (Fig. 3). Although there was some fading of the fluo-

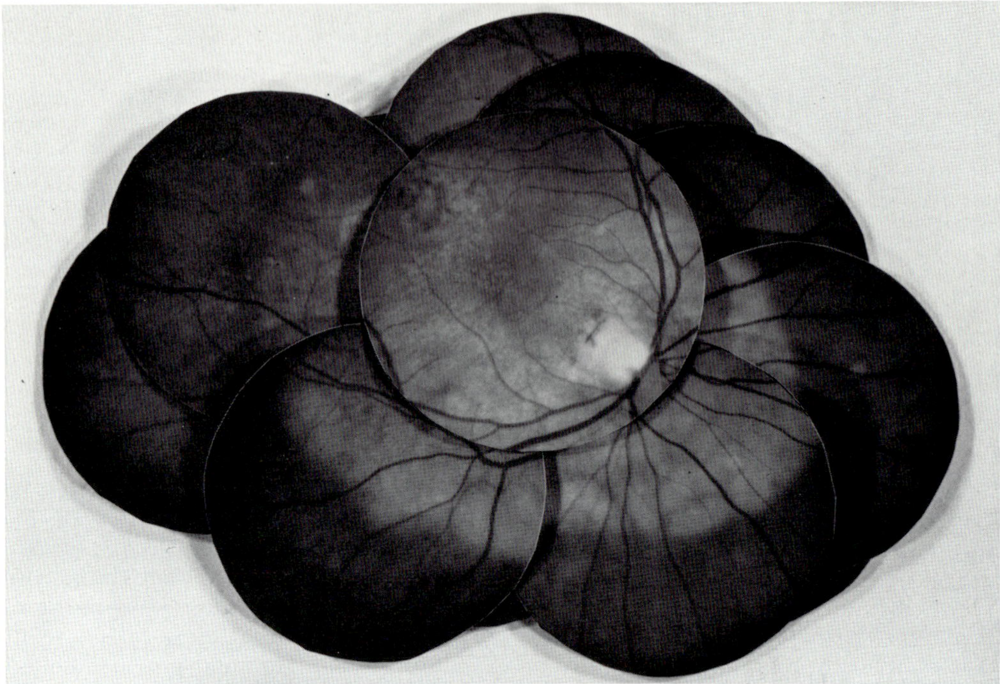

Fig. 1. Composite fundus photograph of the right eye showing extent of osteoma.

rescence, staining was significant in the late stages of angiography (Fig. 4). Old fundus photographs from 1969 and 1973 were reviewed and showed unquestionable enlargement of the choroidal mass. A diagnosis of choroidal osteoma with unrelated atypical facial pain was made.

DISCUSSION

Choroidal osteomas typically occur in young Caucasian females who present with blurred vision, paracentral scotomata, or metamorphopsia. Both eyes were involved initially in three patients and another developed a tumor in the previously unaffected eye during follow-up.[4] The majority of reported cases have had 20/30 or better vision with a field defect that was smaller than the tumor. A few have had no field loss. Tumors have varied in size from 1.5 to 2 to 9 × 15 disc diameters (dd).[4] In all patients studied the past medical history, family history, and laboratory studies have been negative. Our patient is the only case reported with neurologic symptoms, but these appear unrelated to the ocular findings. Gass[4] found that orbital roentgeno-

grams demonstrated the presence of a radiodensity in all but one eye studied. Initially, however, this density was missed in 10 eyes and polytomography was necessary to visualize the tumor in seven eyes. Computerized tomography of the orbits easily demonstrated this radiodensity in all patients examined. These tumors also caused a characteristic ultrasonographic picture showing an acoustically dense and irregularly elevated posterior polar mass.

Old photos of our patient taken in 1969 clearly documented that significant growth had taken place. Ophthalmoscopic evidence of growth has been reported in eight other patients.[4] Of particular interest in this regard was one such patient who had a markedly positive P-32 test (270%). This in the presence of documented growth led to enucleation.[2] The histologic features of this tumor easily explain the positive P-32 test.

Heterotopic bone formation commonly occurs around the optic disc and at the ora serrata in degenerating eyes following inflammation, trauma, and long standing retinal detachment.[5] Identical ossification may occur overlying the surface of solitary choroidal cavernous hemangiomas in 20% of cases.[6] Typically such changes occur in association with extensive evidence of hyperplasia of the pigment epithelium and rarely involve ossification within the depth of the choroid.

Histopathologic examination of a choroidal osteoma shows the tumor arising from the inner ⅓ of the choroid (Fig. 5). The tumor is "composed solely of mature bone with numerous interconnecting marrow spaces filled with loose connective tissue and some dilated thin-walled blood vessels."[1] Some feel this, like certain isolated lid tumors,[7] represents an osseous choristoma (choristoma being defined as a congenital tumorlike malformation made of elements not normally present in the involved tissue).[8] Features of choroidal osteomas which are atypical for a developmental tumor include their predilection for females (all but one case), exclusive location in the juxtapapillary choroid, and their growth pattern during adulthood. Gass believes that these are "probably not choristomas but acquired tumors caused by one or more as yet unidentified stimuli that may be significantly influenced by sex hormones."[4]

SUMMARY

A case of choroidal osteoma with documented growth is presented. This newly described clinicopathologic syndrome is reviewed. The problem of misdiagnosis and false positive P-32 testing leading to unnecessary enucleation is stressed. In such a

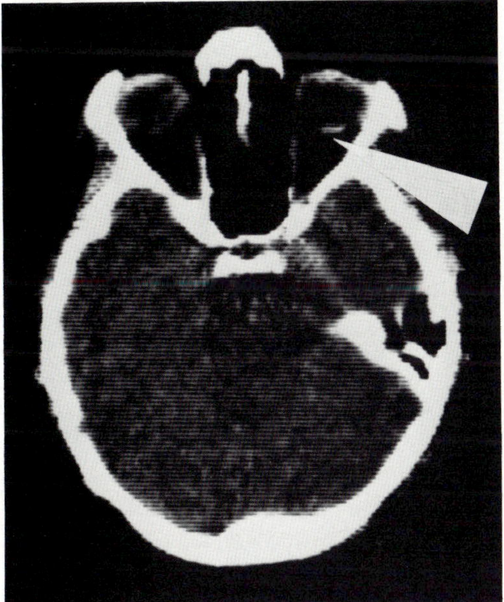

Fig. 2a. Computerized axial tomography scan showing presence of bony plaque in posterior pole of the right eye.

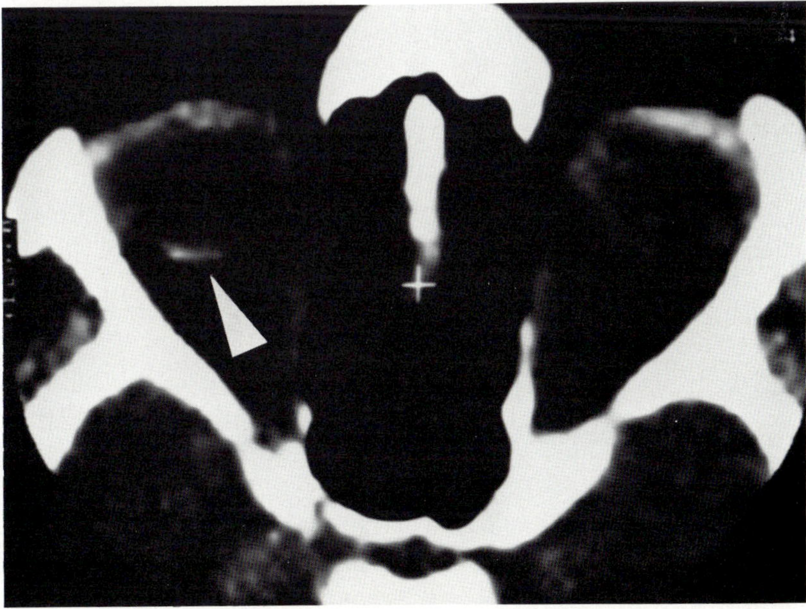

Fig. 2b. Enlargement of orbital area in 2a demonstrating the bony density of choroidal osteoma.

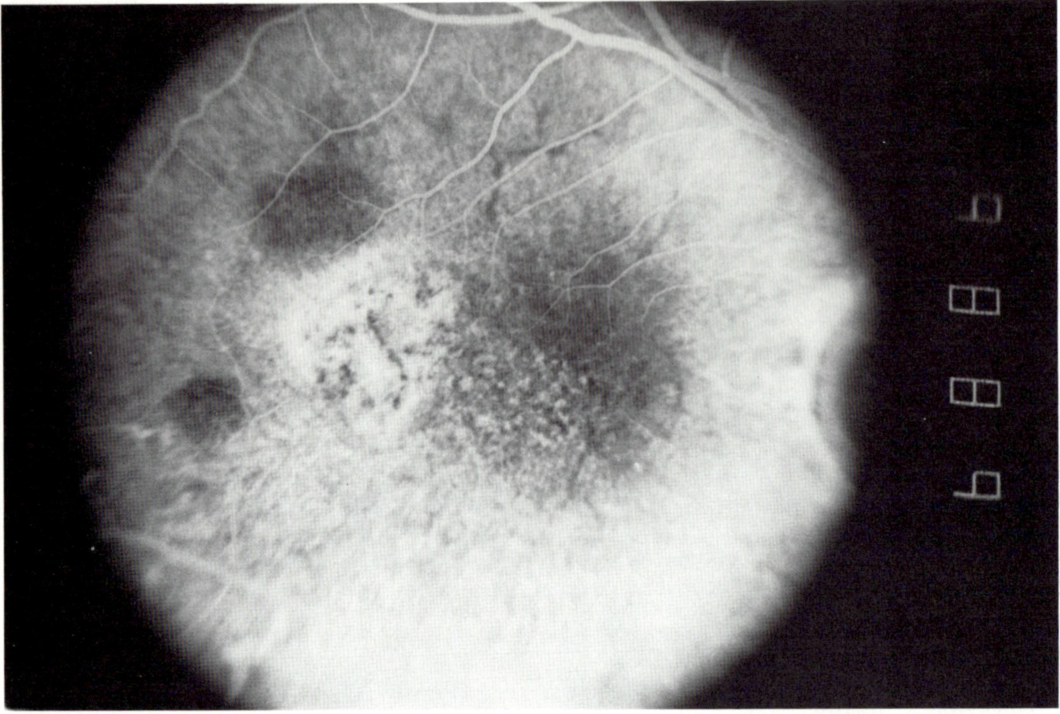

Fig. 3. Early angiogram. Note fine capillary pattern on tumor surface.

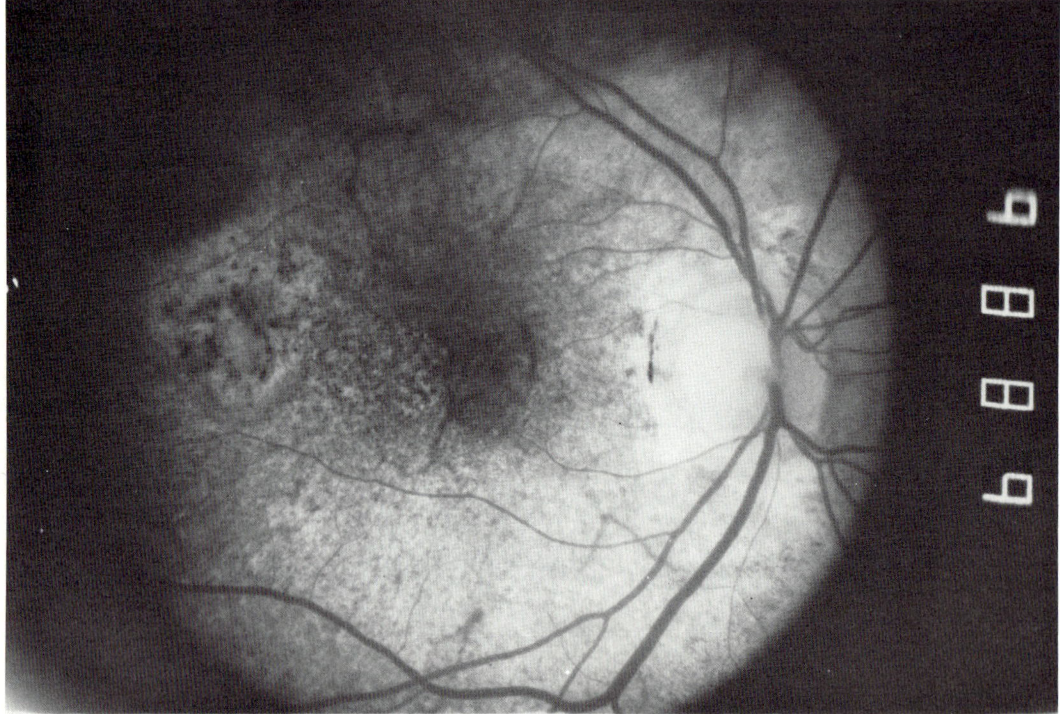

Fig. 4. Late angiogram. Note late staining of tumor.

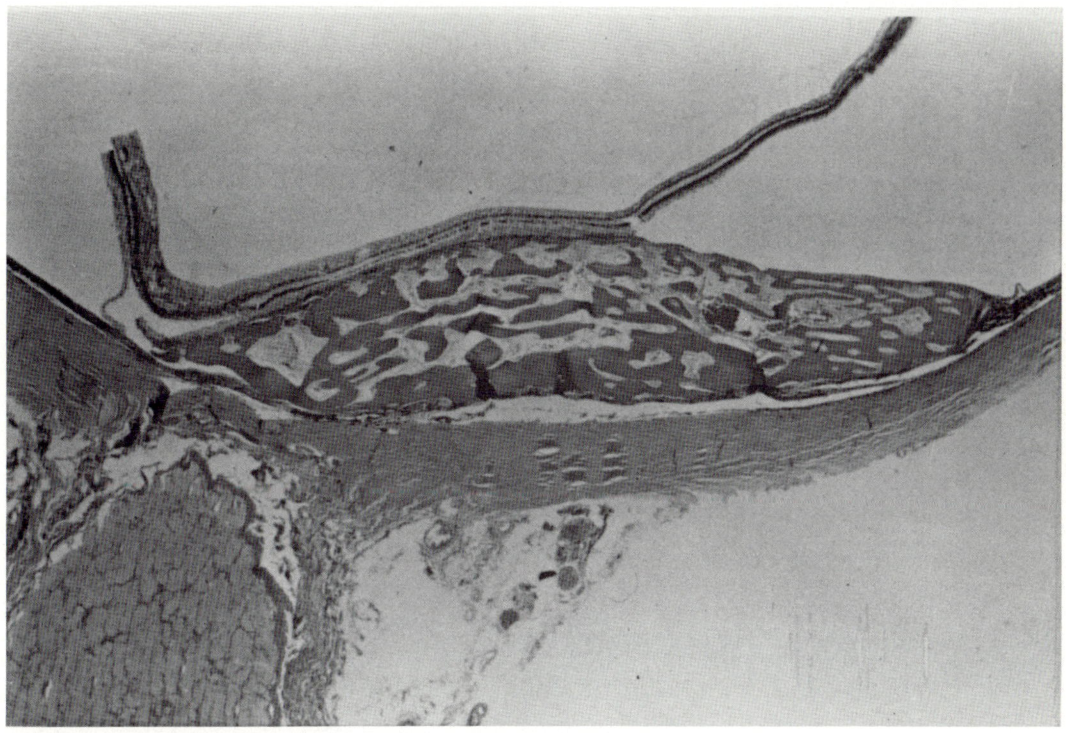

Fig. 5. Photomicrograph showing osseous choroidal tumor (PAS, original magnification × 19) (courtesy, of J. D. M. Gass, M.D.)

clinical situation computerized orbital tomography is diagnostic.

EDITOR'S NOTE

Dr. Gass strikes again! He has knocked another new syndrome out of the ball park! The *choroidal osteoma* can be diagnosed by simply knowing that, in a young white woman presenting with blurred vision in one eye but with reasonably good acuity, there is a posterior pole lesion with scalloped margins and a typical orange-red color that makes it confused with hemangioma of the choroid. The tip off, however, is that you can find this lesion on plain skull x-rays (if you look for it, and know that it is present!) and also on CT scan. Note that Figure 2a in this paper shows the lesion in the back of the right eye, but that Figure 2b has been reversed so that the patient's right eye is on your left. Don't let that confuse you—and in fact, I put a nice big fat white arrow on each of his pictures of the CT scan to show you the "bone" in the

eye. Also see the next paper by Dr. Laibovitz in the following chapter!

JLS

REFERENCES

1. Gass, J. D. M., Guerry, R. K., Jack, R. L., and Harris, G. Choroidal Osteoma. Arch. Ophthalmol. *96:*428–435 (1978).
2. Williams, A. T., Font, R. L., Van Dyk, H. J. L., and Riekhof, T. Osseous Choristoma of the Choroid Simulating a Choroidal Melanoma. Arch. Ophthalmol. *96:*1874–1877 (1978).
3. Reese, A. B. *Tumors of the Eye,* 2nd ed. Harper and Row, New York, 1963, p. 394.
4. Gass, J. D. M. New Observations Concerning Choroidal Osteomas. Arch. Ophthalmol. (in press)
5. Duke-Elder, S. and Perkins, E. S. *System of Ophthalmology. Vol. IX. Diseases of the Uveal Track.* C. V. Mosby Co., St Louis, 1966, pp. 740–748.
6. Witschel, H. and Font, R. L. Hemangioma of the Choroid: A Clinicopathologic Study of 71 Cases and a Review of the Literature. Survey Ophthalmol. *20:*415–431 (1976).
7. Boniuk, M. and Zimmerman, L. E. Epibulbar Choristoma (Episcleral Osseous Choristoma). Am. J. Ophthalmol. *53:*290–296 (1962).
8. Joffe, L., Shields, J. A., and Fitzgerald, J. R. Osseous Choristoma of the Choroid. Arch. Ophthalmol. *96:*1809–1812 (1978).

5 Choroidal Osteoma

Robert A. Laibovitz, M.D.

Gass and others have recently focused attention on a new diagnostic entity called choroidal osteoma.[1-4] First mentioned by Reese,[5] this choroidal tumor apparently represents a primary osseous choristoma. This article will outline the clinical, angiographic, radiographic, and ultrasonographic characteristics that help define this unusual lesion. Important points in differential diagnosis and the characteristic histopathology will also be outlined.

Reese described the eye from a nineteen-year-old female apparently removed because of suspicion of choroidal malignant melanoma. The lesion was primarily osteoid histopathologically, and he labelled the tumor as an osteoma of the choroid, but believed this was actually secondary ossification of a choroidal hemangioma. In a landmark paper, Gass described in detail the case histories of four young females with choroidal osteoma. Subsequent contributions have confirmed and expanded his findings. Basically this unique lesion occurs in one eye of an otherwise healthy young female. The chief complaint is usually progressive loss of vision in one eye. It must, however, be emphasized that the lesion can be bilateral and can effect males.

The ophthalmoscopic picture is very similar in all cases reported. In the posterior pole, typically adjacent to the disc, a yellowish-white or cream-colored mass is seen (Fig. 1). The lesion is typically flat or only slightly elevated at most. Commonly there is marked depigmentation of the retinal pigment epithelium, and prominent vascular spaces may be seen on the surface of the tumor. Not uncommonly, subretinal fluid or blood may be seen along with clinically apparent choroidal neovascularization. The tumor is generally static without rapid growth, but occasionally some increase in size may be documented. In most cases the osteoma is juxtapapillary with well-defined and smooth borders and small pseudopod or finger-like projections (Fig. 2). Without exception, the remainder of the ophthalmological examination and general physical examination is totally normal.

The laboratory diagnosis of choroidal osteoma is quite dramatic and characteristic. Fluorescein angiography shows early hyperfluorescence with late staining without any suggestion of tumor vessels or double circulation (Fig. 3). Choroidal neovascularization can be documented, and this may be quite helpful should photocoagulation be considered (Fig. 4). Conventional radiographs often show a characteristic orbital ossification but can be negative even in the face of rather dramatic ossification as shown on computerized tomography (Fig. 5). Ultrasound can be used to show the acoustically dense nature of the intraocular lesion with marked attenuation of the immediate retrobulbar structures. Of all the laboratory studies described, it must be remembered that the most dramatic and characteristic picture is obtained with computerized tomography, and this test should never be omitted in the evaluation of a patient with a suspected primary osseous choristoma of the choroid (Fig. 6).

The diagnosis of choroidal osteoma is really quite easy in the typical clinical setting, but occasionally points of confusion can arise. The most important consideration to the patient is the differentiation from amelanotic malignant melanoma.

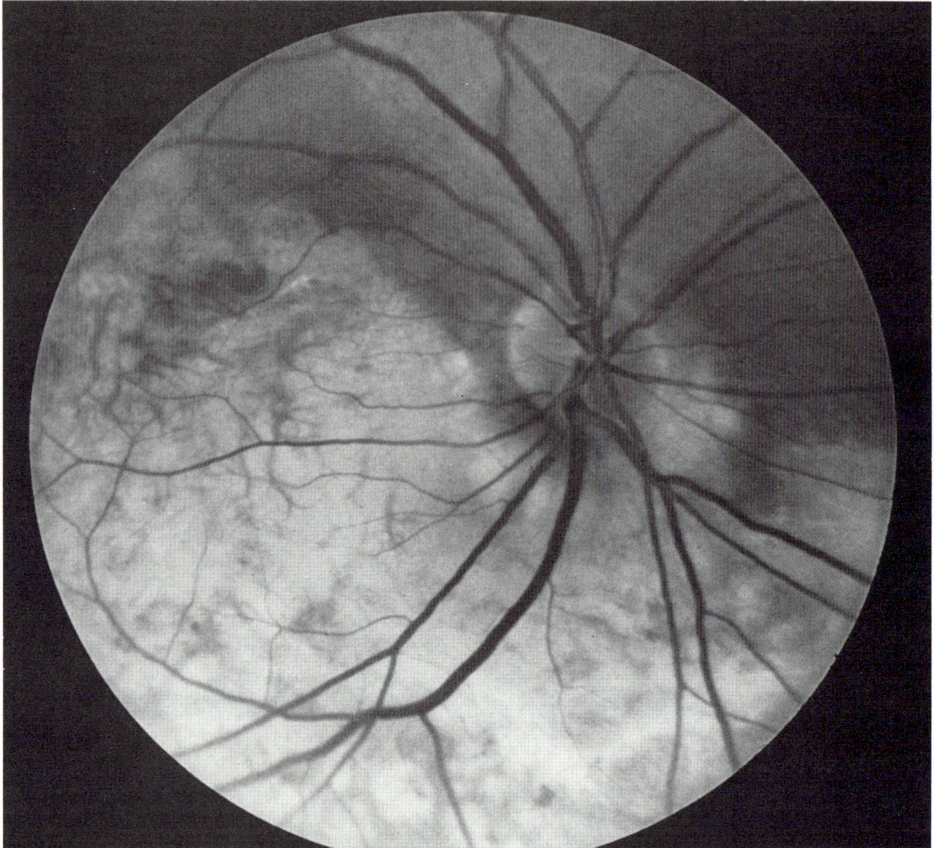

Fig. 1. Osteoma with choroidal neovascularization.

This distinction is extremely important because the P-32 test will be markedly positive in choroidal osteoma since the intraocular bone will avidly take up the phosphorous. The P-32 test will be falsely positive and could easily result in enucleation for a benign lesion. For this reason, the P-32 test is contraindicated in the evaluation of a suspected choroidal osteoma. Other diagnostic possibilities include metastatic tumor, leukemic or lymphomatous invasion of the choroid, atypical hemangioma, serpiginous choroidopathy, or even possibly an exophytic retinoblastoma. All of these lesions are usually removed from consideration by history, physical examination, and appropriate and well-chosen laboratory tests.

The histopathology of choroidal osteoma is exceptionally unique and easily distinguished from other primary choroidal lesions including hemangioma. Not uncommonly, a choroidal hemangioma will show ossification of an epichoroidal membrane.[6] This membrane is presumably derived from metaplasia of the retinal pigment epithelium. Moreover, the retina overlying choroidal hemangioma is usually cystic from long standing or recurrent serous detachment of the retina, and secondly choroidal neovascularization is almost never seen with choroidal hemangioma.[7] In addition, no other choroidal lesion has the deep, full-thickness mature bone of choroidal osteoma.

The treatment of choroidal osteoma is essentially passive on the part of the ophthalmologist. Careful follow-up is mandatory, and the documentation of choroidal neovascularization with fluorescein angiography is essential. Although never applied in the past, the possibility of using photocoagulation must be remembered for the treatment of choroidal neovascularization

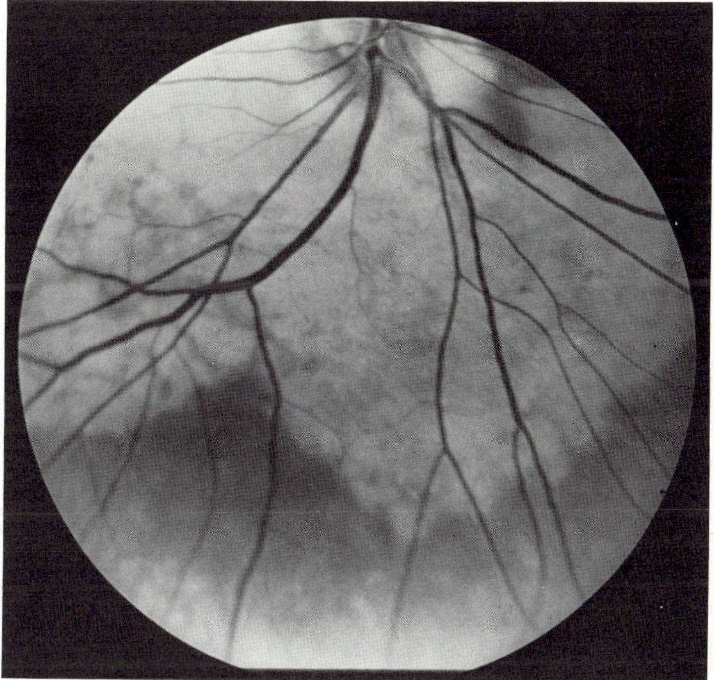

Fig. 2. Osteoma with well-defined borders and small pseudopodic projections.

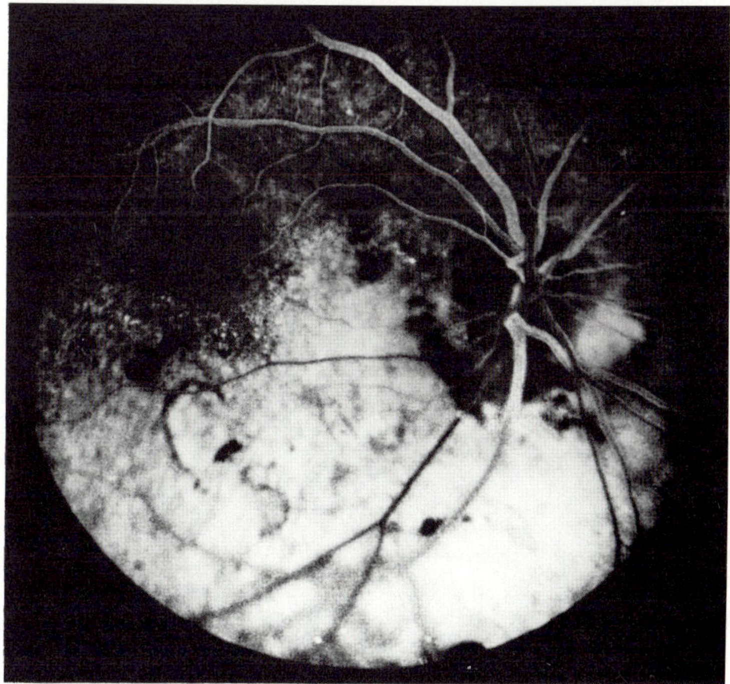

Fig. 3. Fluorescein angiogram showing irregular hyperfluorescence.

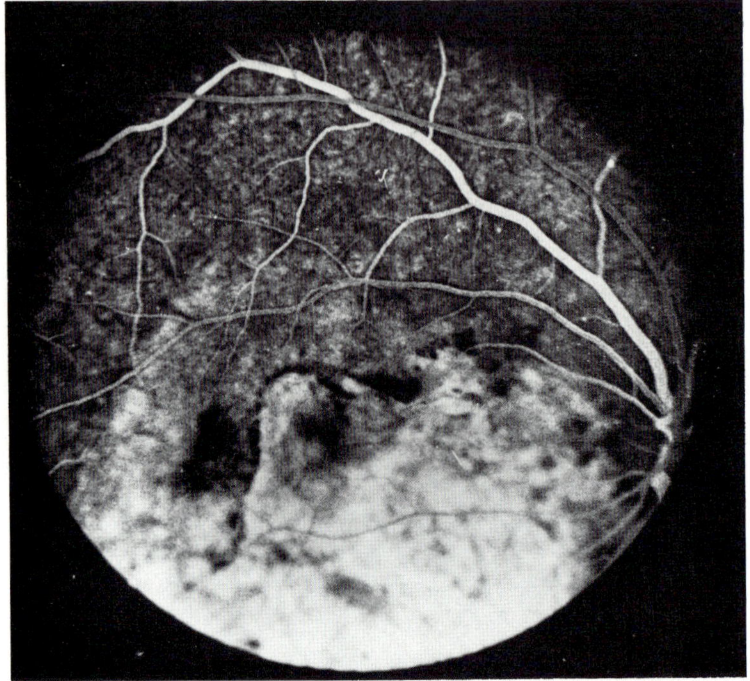

Fig. 4. Choroidal neovascularization involving the capillary-free zone.

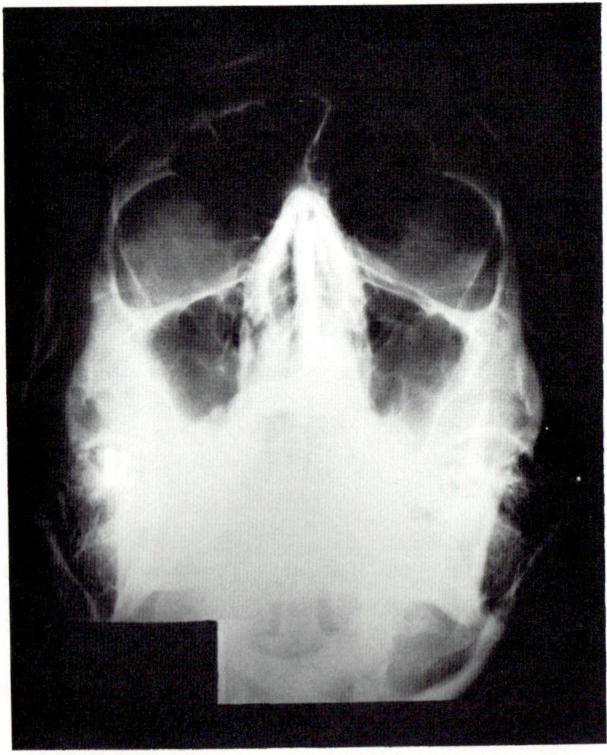

Fig. 5. Skull film negative for orbital calcification.

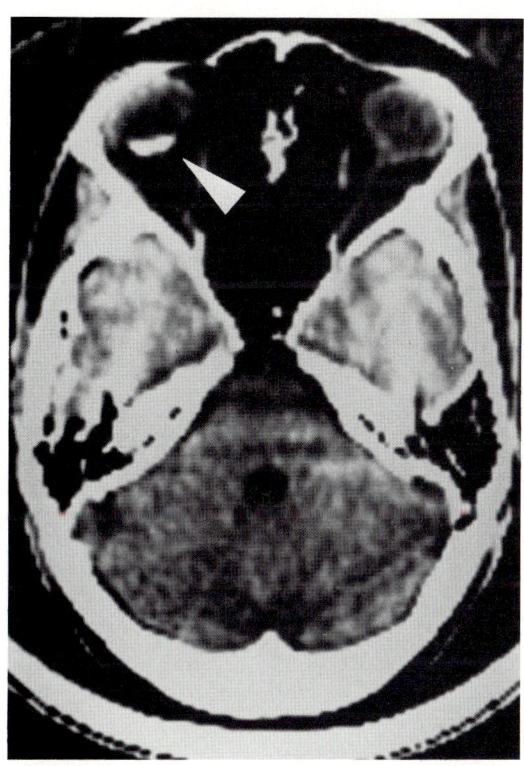

Fig. 6. CT scan with choroidal ossification in same patient as in Figure 4.

induced by an osteoma. It is the responsibility of the ophthalmologist to maintain a high level of suspicion when confronted with an unusual choroidal tumor and to include choroidal osteoma in his differential diagnosis in order to insure the most appropriate diagnostic and treatment regimen for his patient.

EDITOR'S NOTE

Again note that the fundus appearance is very similar in the cases of choroidal osteoma—or as Dr. Gass calls it—the "bone in the eye." This chapter emphasizes that you can miss the calcium on plain skull films, so that you may want to get a good CT scan of the orbit for confirmation. The typical clinical features and the characteristic fundus appearance should allow you to make the diagnosis at a good office visit, however. The reason for diagnosing this "bone" in the patient's eye is obvious—so that you will *NOT* remove such an eye. Again note that the P-32 test "goes down in flames" with this lesion. I feel that the P-32 test is worse than of little value—in other words, it has led to enucleation of some eyes which should not have been removed, and may therefore lead the physician to dangerous conclusions. I'd like to cast a vote against the P-32 test. If one would ask me when a P-32 test would be of help in practice, I'd say—"Never!" It is even less helpful than tonography.

JLS

REFERENCES

1. Gass, J. D. M., Gverry, R. K., Jack, R. L. and Harris, G. Choroidal Osteoma. Arch. Ophthalmol. *96*:428–435 (1978).
2. Coston, T. O. and Wilkinson, C. P. Choroidal Osteoma. Am. J. Ophthalmol. *86*:368–372 (1978).
3. Williams, A. T., Font, R. L., VanDyk, H. J. L., and Riekhof, F. T. Osseous Choristoma of the Choroid Simulating a Choroidal Melanoma. Arch. Ophthalmol. *96*:1874–1877 (1978).
4. Joffe, L., Shields, J. A. and Fitzgerald, J. R. Osseous Choristoma of the Choroid. Arch. Ophthalmol. *96*:1809–1812 (1978).
5. Reese, A. B. *Tumors of the Eye*, 2nd ed. Harper and Row, New York, 1963, pp. 392–394.
6. Witschel, H. and Font, R. L. Hemangioma of the Choroid: A clinicopathologic study of 71 cases and a review of the literature. Surv. Ophthalmol. *20*: 422–423 (1976).
7. Gass, J. D. M. Pathogenesis of Disciform Detachment of the Neuroepithium. Am. J. Ophthalmol. *63*:689–711 (1967).
8. Laibovitz, R. A. An Unusual Cause of Intraocular Calcification: Choroidal Osteoma. Ann. Ophthalmol. (in press).

6 Monochromatic (Red-Free) Photography and Ophthalmoscopy of the Peripapillary Retinal Nerve Fiber Layer

Neil R. Miller, M.D.
Terry W. George, R.B.P., F.B.P.A.

Summary

The appearance of the peripapillary retinal nerve fiber layer is crucial in the evaluation of patients with presumed optic neuropathies as well as in the differentiation of true optic disc edema from pseudopapilledema. Monochromatic (red-free) photography performed at 2× magnification using a Zeiss fundus camera, a filter with maximum transmission at 540 nm, and Kodak Plus X black and white film, provides excellent nerve fiber layer detail. Since direct ophthalmoscopy depends upon maximum illumination which in turn depends upon increased color temperature of the light source, use of a direct ophthalmoscope with a gas-surrounded, tungsten filament light source driven at 4.5 V raises color temperature sufficiently to allow practical use of monochromatic, red-free filters for optimum peripapillary retinal nerve fiber layer evaluation.

The use of monochromatic light for ophthalmoscopic examination of the ocular fundus was first suggested by Ginestous in 1911,[1] and a practical means to accomplish it was demonstrated by Vogt[2-4] several years later. Although other investigators also advocated the use of various filters and light sources for observation of the fundus, their results were inconsistent and seemed impractical for clinical application. Subsequently, Behrendt and Wilson[5] found that the spectral reflectance (the amount of light reflected vs. the amount of light absorbed) of specific fundus components differed depending on the wavelength of light used to optimally illuminate specific fundus elements. Nevertheless, the practical advantage of such an approach was ignored until Hoyt and co-workers[6-8] published a series of articles stressing the clinical usefulness of red-free illumination of the peripapillary retinal nerve fiber layer in the evaluation of patients with suspected optic neuropathies. We have evaluated the efficacy of the monochromatic filter systems for both photography and direct ophthalmoscopy of the nerve fiber layer and have identified an optimum filter system for both.

Fundus Photography. A Zeiss fundus camera with a high-intensity xenon arc bulb was modified to permit placement of narrow bandpass and neutral density filters, 10 nm wide at 50% transmission, in the pathway of light from the camera's lamp. Fundus photographs of individuals with varying skin and intraocular pigmentation were made at 10 nm intervals from 400 nm to 900 nm, using Kodak Plus X black and white film developed in Kodak D-11 (diluted 1:1 with water) for six minutes at 70°F. Based on data from these experiments, commercial filters with maximum transmission from 450 nm to 600 nm were used in an unmodified Zeiss fundus camera using the same film and developing technique.

Optimum visualization of the nerve fiber layer was obtained with a 540 nm filter (Spectrotech Corporation, Lincoln, Mass.). We find that this filter, when used in an unmodified Zeiss fundus camera, highlights the fine, radially-oriented striations, superficial light reflexes, and capillaries of the normal peripapillary retinal nerve fiber layer (Figs. 1 and 2). The filter system also enhances the distortion or loss of these features in patients with various optic neuropathies (Figs. 3–10).

Direct Ophthalmoscopy. A variety of commercial filters with maximum transmissions ranging from 450 nm to 600 nm were used in several direct ophthalmoscopes with various light and power sources. Independent observers compared their abilities to evaluate the nerve fiber layer in individuals with varying skin and intraocular pigmentation.

In individuals with heavy pigment epithelial and choroidal pigmentation, a number of filters that transmit maximally in the range of 520 nm to 560 nm permit excellent observation of the nerve fiber layer when combined with the increased illumination provided by a 4.5 V ophthalmoscope with a light source consisting of a tungsten filament surrounded by either an inert (krypton, xenon) or halogen (iodine) gas. Ophthalmoscopes with weaker power sources provided inadequate illumination as did tungsten filament vacuum type bulbs.

In patients with lightly pigmented choroid and pigment epithelium, Kodak Wratten filters #57 and #60 provided excellent contrast and detail in observation of the nerve fiber layer. Both filters have a domi-

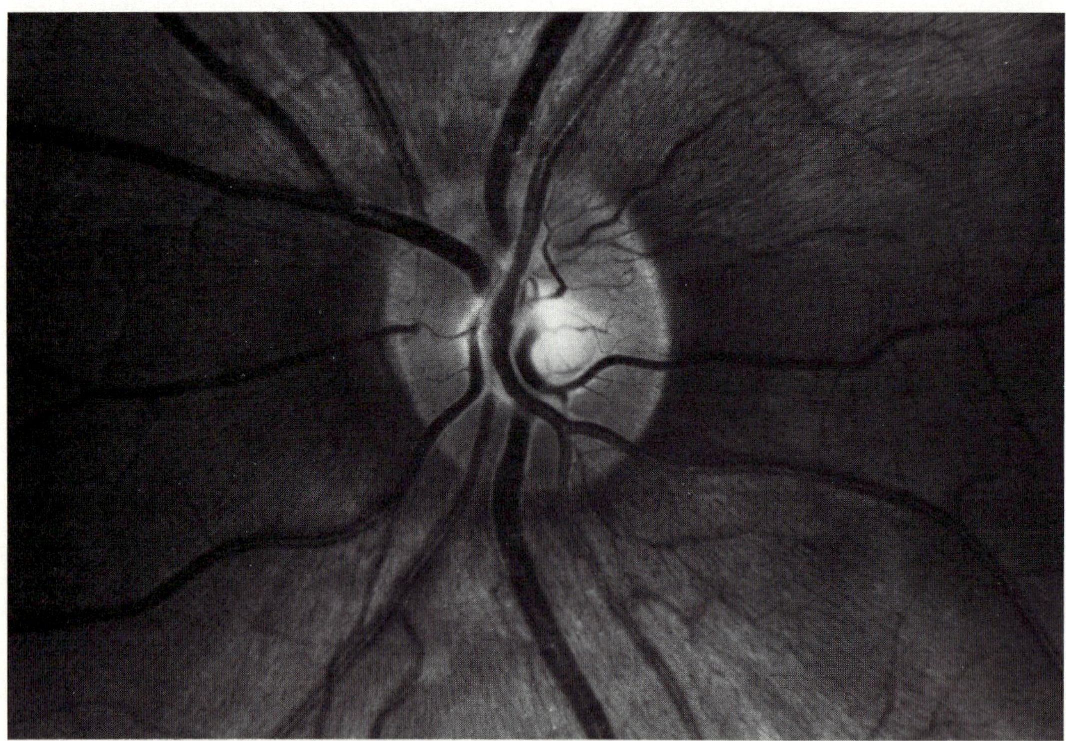

Fig. 1. Normal optic disc and nerve fiber layer. Note fine linear striations representing nerve fiber layer axons. The striations begin at the disc margin. Striations are more easily seen in the superior and inferior arcuate bundles but can also be seen nasal to the optic disc and in the papillomacular bundle. Small disc vessels are easily visible as are numerous peripapillary capillaries.

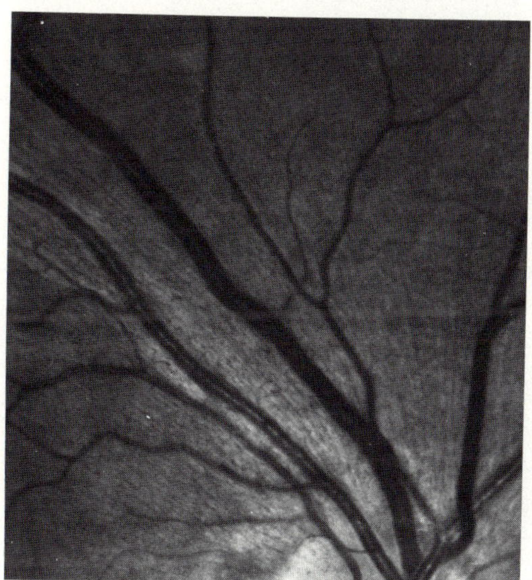

Fig. 2. Normal arcuate nerve fiber bundle. Fine linear striations are visible beginning at the disc margin.

nant wavelength at 525 nm with a maximum transmittance of 60%.

Using narrow, bandpass filters to examine the ocular fundus, Behrendt and Wilson[5] and, later, Delori and co-workers[9, 10] concluded that monochromatic photography and ophthalmoscopy require a multiple filter system to view optimally each fundus component in any given individual. In addition, these authors found that the nerve fiber layer was optimally visualized at wavelengths between 470 nm and 530 nm. However, Flower and co-workers[11] have recently found that for wavelengths from 400 nm to 900 nm, at each wavelength, all structures in the fundus have spectral reflectances in a relatively narrow region. Differences in spectral reflectance therefore occur among different individuals, not among different fundus components in a single individual. Moreover, they found that, in individuals with varying skin and intraocular pigmentation, the "envelopes" of spectral reflectance were quite close in the 520–560-nm range. We agree with Flower that the use of filters transmitting in this range facilitates observation not only of the nerve fiber layer but also of the macula, arteries, veins, and capillaries.

Hoyt and Knight[7] originally produced red-free photographs by using color transparencies from which black and white neg-

atives were made using a Kodak Wratten #65 filter. These in turn were printed on Kodak Ektomatic SC-F paper. We believe that sharper photographs can be produced using our filter system in an unmodified Zeiss fundus camera with Kodak black and white Plus X film. All photographs are made at 2X magnification, thereby eliminating the need for secondary magnification techniques. Finally, all observations are made from the black and white transparencies rather than from black and white prints.

Optimum observation of the ocular fundus depends upon the contrast that is produced when maximum illumination is combined with an optimum filter. The tungsten filament vacuum lamps used in most older, less powerful direct ophthalmoscopes produce uneven illumination across the visible spectrum, with significantly reduced luminance in the lower end of the spectrum (400–550 nm) than in the higher end (Fig. 11). For this reason, light produced by these lamps appears more yellow than true white light (sunlight), and filters that absorb light in the red spectral region cause a marked reduction in total fundus illumination, making observation of critical fundus impossible. Since the luminance of any bulb is dependent upon its color temperature, raising the color temperature of the bulb will increase its total luminance, particularly across the lower end of the visible spectrum.

Color temperature, defined as the absolute temperature of a blackbody that has the same chromaticity as that of the light source under consideration, can be raised by either increasing the voltage used to power the light source or changing the nature of the light source itself. Recently, halogen (iodine) and inert (krypton, xenon) gases have been used in the tungsten filament ophthalmoscope bulbs, replacing the previous vacuum type bulb. The color temperature of these bulbs is significantly higher than that of the vacuum bulb, resulting in an increased luminance across the entire visible spectrum, particularly in the lower end (Fig. 11). Increasing the power source of the ophthalmoscope to 4.5 V raises the color temperature of the gas-filled bulbs even higher, providing increased illumination and permitting opti-

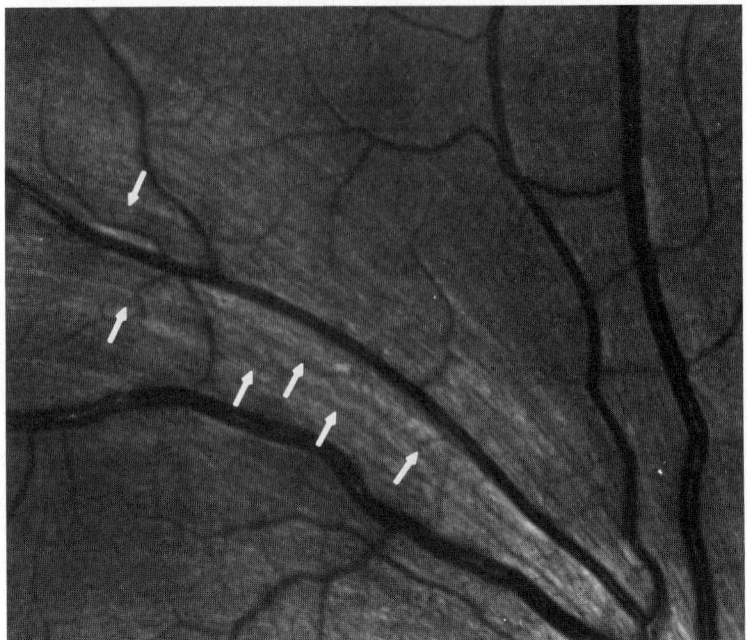

Fig. 3. Arcuate nerve fiber bundle defects. In this patient with presumed multiple sclerosis and a history of retrobulbar optic neuritis, defects in the peripapillary retinal nerve fiber layer appear as dark lines (arrows) within the arcuate bundle. Note that these lines begin just beyond the optic disc and can be seen at least two to three disc diameters away from the disc margin.

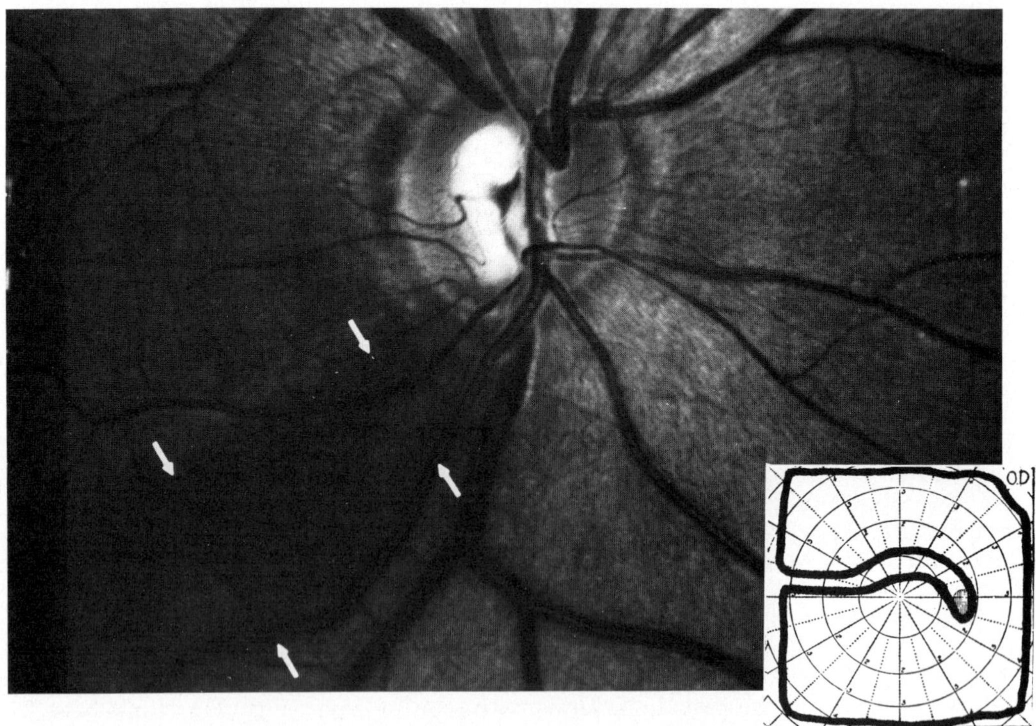

Fig. 4. Arcuate nerve fiber bundle loss. In this patient with secondary glaucoma after trauma, the optic cup can be seen to be elongated in the inferior vertical direction. Linear striations representing a normal nerve fiber bundle surround the disc except in the region of the inferior arcuate nerve fibers. In this region, no striations are seen and the area appears dark and granular (arrows). The corresponding superior arcuate visual field defect is seen in the inset.

46

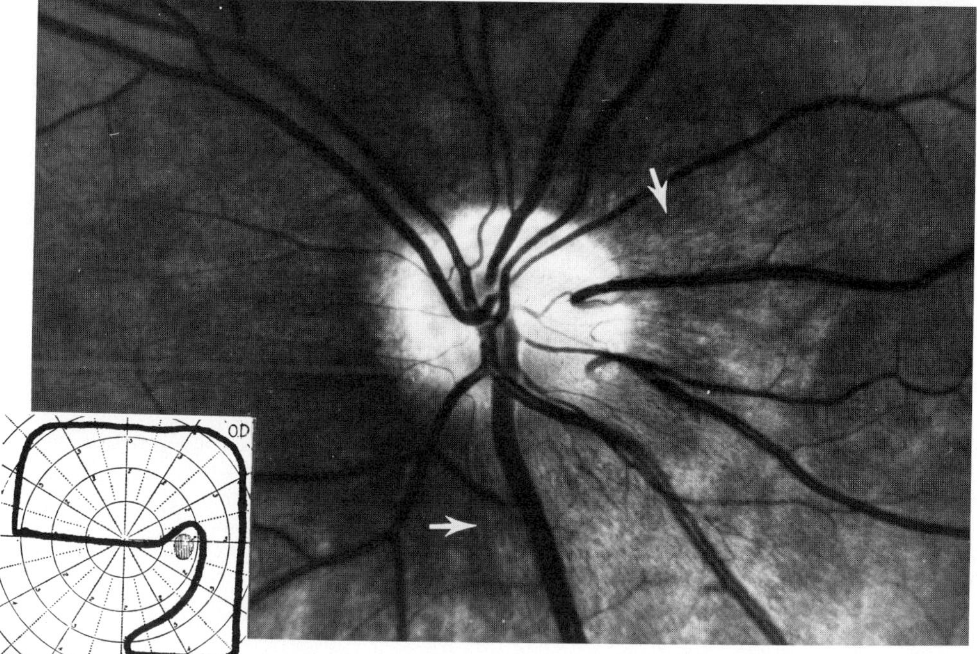

Fig. 5. Optic nerve hypoplasia. This patient, the daughter of a diabetic mother, was found on routine examination to have bilateral optic nerve hypoplasia, normal visual acuity, and bilateral inferior arcuate (quadrantic) visual field defects. Red-free photograph shows nerve fiber striations from two o'clock to six o'clock (arrows). The remainder of the peripapillary region appeared granular and devoid of striations. In that region, the retinal vessels are seen with more clarity because of the absence of overlying nerve fiber layer. The apparent absence of superior and temporal nerve fiber accounts for the large inferior arcuate defect in the visual field (inset). It is interesting that the patient sees 20/20 despite the apparent absence of nerve fibers in the papillomacular bundle.

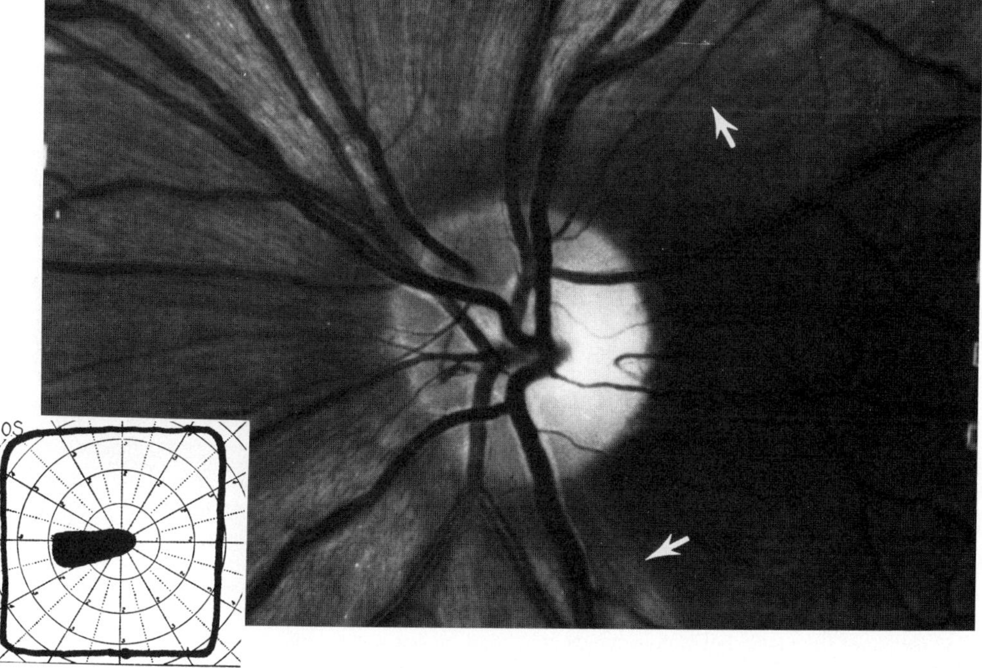

Fig. 6. The patient is a 35-year-old man with severe nutritional amblyopia. Visual acuity was 20/400 with a large cecocentral defect (inset). Note normal appearing disc and nerve fiber layer except in the region of the

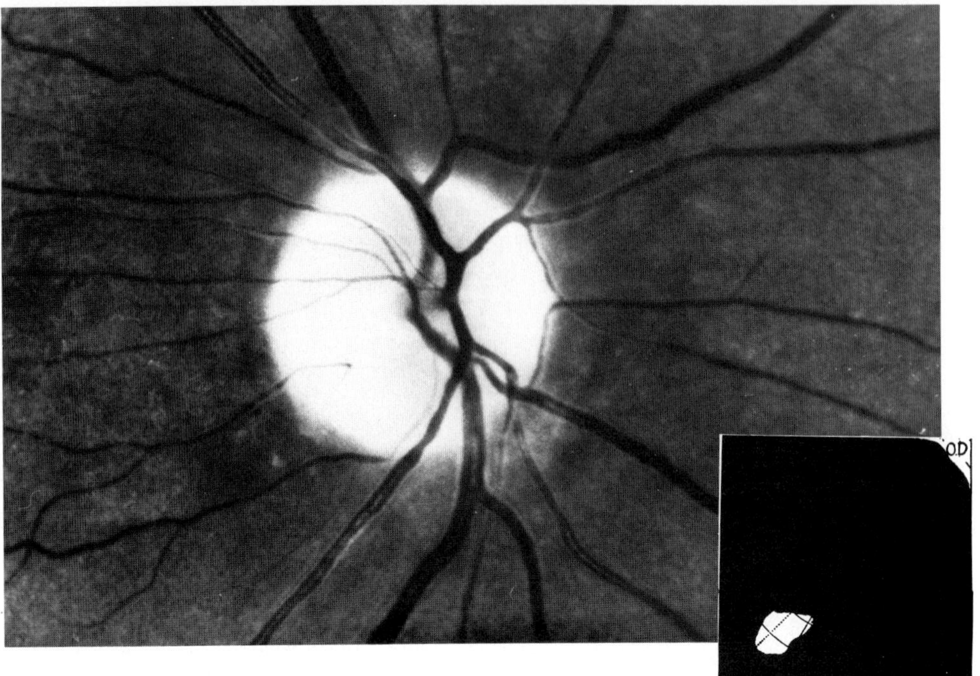

Fig. 7. Optic atrophy. The patient is a 75-year-old male who was examined six months after a central retinal artery occlusion. Visual acuity is hand motions with a small inferior temporal field. Note that the peripapillary region is devoid of visible nerve fibers and has a marked granular appearance. The retinal arteries are narrowed and sheathed. The disc is pale with loss of visible capillaries.

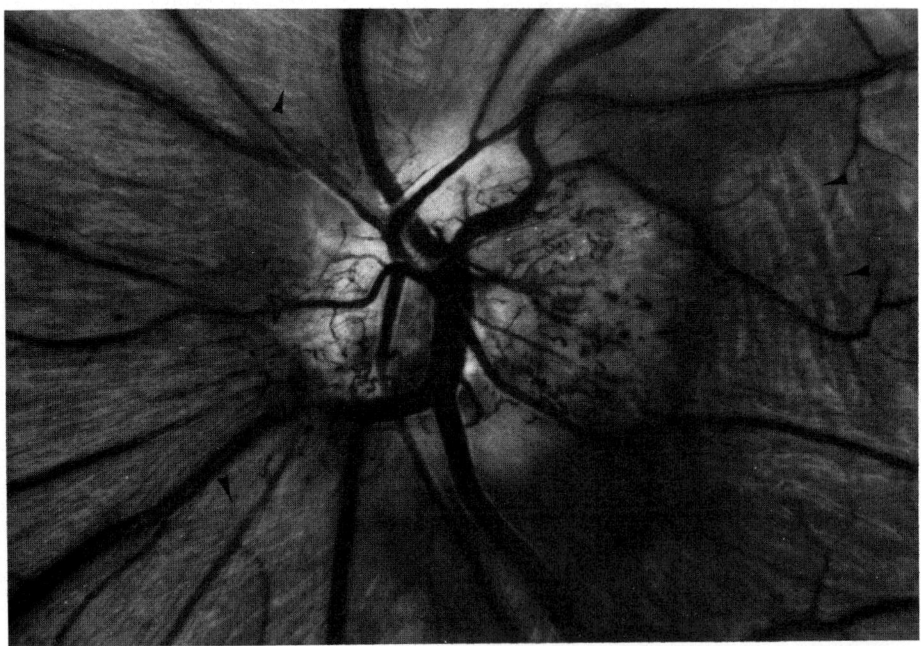

Fig. 8. Anterior optic neuritis. This 35-year-old patient had the sudden onset of visual blurring in the left eye associated with pain on eye movement. The left visual field showed a central scotoma. Red-free photograph shows obvious edema and elevation of the disc. In addition, the normal disc capillaries are markedly enlarged and are easily visible. The normal linear striations in the peripapillary nerve fiber layer are no longer visible due to the disc edema. Instead, superficial light reflexes (arrows) appear obliquely due to alteration of the normal nerve fiber layer pattern.

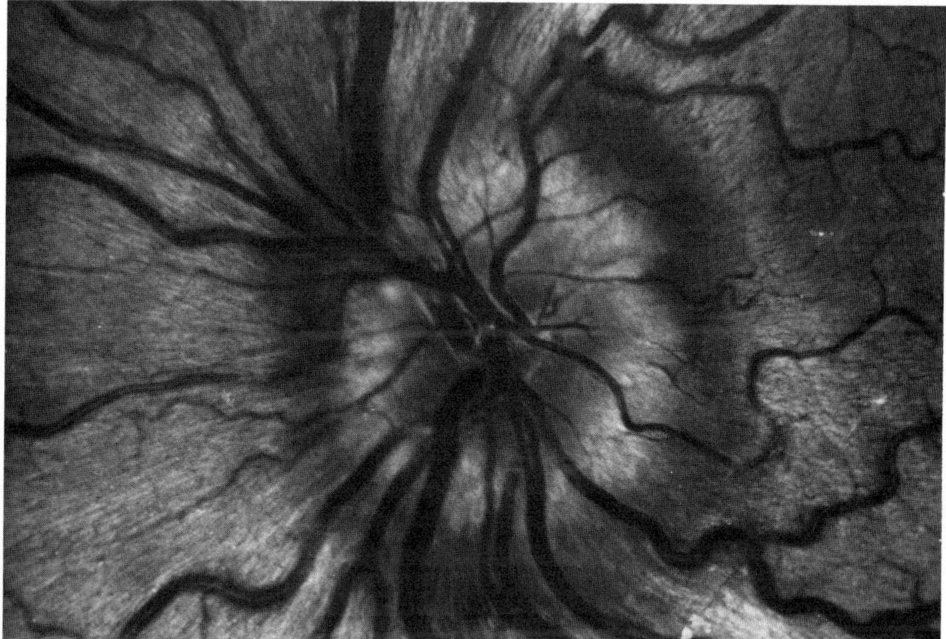

Fig. 9. Pseudopapilledema. This 23-year-old female had no visual complaints. In contrast to the previous photograph (Fig. 8), note that, despite obvious elevation of the disc with blurred margins, the nerve fiber layer striations are easily visible in the peripapillary region. In addition, red-free photography emphasizes the abnormal disc vasculature characteristic of pseudopapilledema from buried drusen.

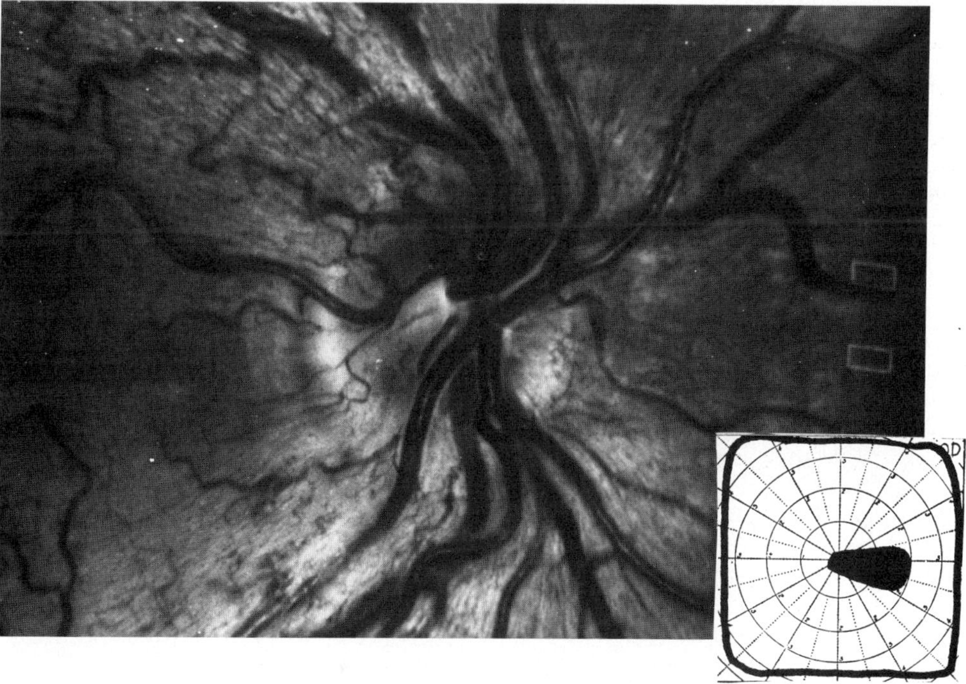

Fig. 10. Leber's optic neuropathy. This 30-year-old male developed loss of vision in the right eye over a six-week period. Visual acuity in the right eye was 20/400 with a cecocentral scotoma (inset). The visual acuity in the left eye is 20/20 with a cecocentral scotoma to red only. In this photograph, the nerve fiber bundle striations can be seen surrounding the disc. However, particularly in the superior and inferior arcuate region, numerous telangiectatic vessels can be seen. Note that these abnormal vessels are also present on the disc surface.

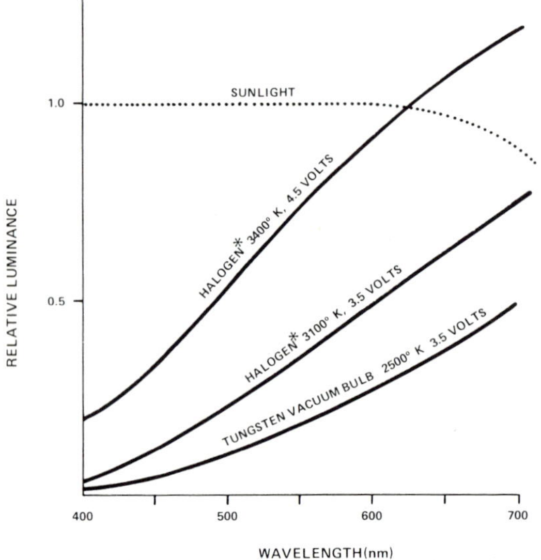

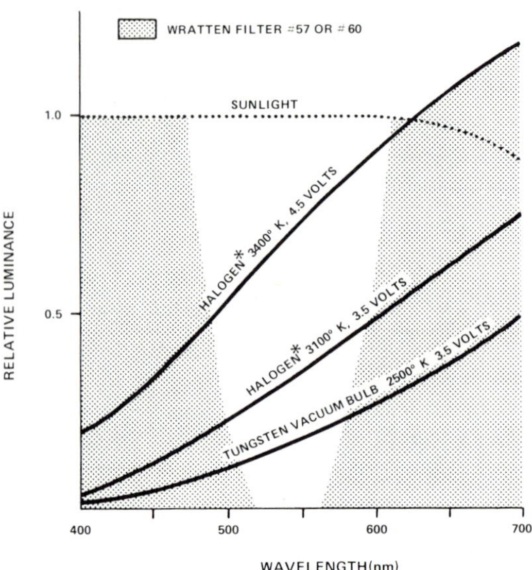

Fig. 11. Relative luminance of various light sources with different color temperatures. Note marked increase in relative luminance in the lower (blue-green) end of the visible spectrum with light sources having higher color temperatures. *Similar curves apply to krypton- and xenon-filled tungsten bulbs.

Fig. 12. Effect of monochromatic (red-free) filter on relative luminance of various light sources with different color temperatures. Note marked increase in luminance when gas-filled, tungsten filament light source is combined with increased power source. *Similar curves apply to krypton- and xenon-filled tungsten bulbs.

mum use of a monochromatic filter (Fig. 12). At present, we prefer a gas-filled (halogen or krypton) tungsten bulb in a direct ophthalmoscope with a 4.5-V power source; however, a different light source with an intrinsically higher color temperature rather than a power boost may ultimately provide optimum observation of the peripapillary retinal nerve fiber layer in the future.

EDITOR'S NOTE

Dr. Miller used the abbreviation "PRNFL" for peripapillary retinal nerve fiber layer throughout this paper. Since I personally find that these observations make reading medical literature more difficult (and things are tough enough as is!), I simply changed it to "nerve fiber layer" when he used the abbreviation in the text. I hope this is alright with him, as I am trying to keep all "DKA's" ("doctor killin' abbreviations") out of this book.

With regards to the nerve fiber layer pictures, a little bit of history might be helpful to the reader. When Dr. Hoyt first started showing these pictures, there were many skeptics of their real clinical value. I remember several years ago when Dr. Hoyt gave a paper on this at the Neuro-ophthalmology Course, he remarked that it really required a superb fundus photographer to get pictures good enough to show these nerve fiber defects and that a particularly good photographer who had worked with him at Cal was now gone. Dr. Noble David teasingly made the comment off the cuff that—"It wasn't the photographic work that got to him out there—it was all that brush work it required!"

The moral of the story, however, is that this emphasis HAS made us look more closely not only at the disc but at its adnexae—i.e., the immediately adjacent retina—more carefully. I use the Hruby lens and a thin beam and walk around the disc looking at the upper temporal and lower temporal arcades of the nerve fiber layer, and also like to put the green light on the slit lamp and fatten the beam up a bit and look around the disc margin this way as well. I believe you can tell most of these findings from really carefully looking at the disc itself with the Hruby lens, but the pictures Dr. Miller provides are really good and I believe we should continue to expand looking at the nerve fiber layer. In the following chapter, Dr. Frisen reports on this same point but he uses line drawings to show the points that were made on fundus photographs in this chapter. Obviously, some of the quality of the photographs doesn't reproduce perfectly in printing a book, but we have tried to do the best we can with these.

JLS

REFERENCES

1. Ginestous, E. La lumièreen ophthalmologie, examen du fond de l'oeil en lumière colorée. J. Med. Bordeaux *4*:24 (1911).
2. Vogt, A. Herstellung eines gelbblauen Lichtfiltrates in welchem die Macula centralis in vivo in gelber Farbung erscheint, die Nervenfasern der Netzhaut und andere feine Einzelheiten derselben sichtbar werden und der Grad der Gelbfarfund der Linse ophthalmoskopisch nachweisbar ist. Graefes Arch. Ophthalmol. *84:*293 (1913).
3. Vogt, A. Die Nervenfaserstreifung der menschlichen Netahaut mit besonderer Beruchsichtigung der Differentialdiagnose gegenuber pathologischen streifenformigen Reflexen (praretinalen Faltelungen). Klin. Monatsbl. Augenheilkd. *58:*399 (1917).
4. Vogt, A. Die Ophthalmoskopie im rotfreien Light. In: Handbuch der gesamten Augenheilk. unde. Graefe-Saemisch (Ed.), Bergmann, Munich, 1925, Vol. 3, No. 3, pp. 1–118.
5. Behrendt, T. and Wilson, L. A. Spectral reflectance photography of the retina. Am. J. Ophthalmol. *59:*1079 (1965).
6. Hoyt, W. F., Schlicke, B., and Eckelhoff, R. J. Funduscopic appearance of a nerve fibre bundle defect. Br. J. Ophthalmol. *56:*577 (1972).
7. Hoyt, W. F. and Knight, C. L. Comparison of congenital disc blurring and incipient papilledema in red-free light—a photographic study. Invest. Ophthalmol. *12:*241 (1973).
8. Hoyt, W. F. Ophthalmoscopy of the retinal nerve fiber layer in neuro-ophthalmologic diagnosis. Aust. J. Ophthalmol. *4:*14 (1976).
9. Delori, F. C. and Gragoudas, E. S. Examination of the ocular fundus with monochromatic light. Ann. Ophthalmol. *8:*703 (1976).
10. Delori, F. C., Gragoudas, E. S., Francisco, R., and Pruett, R. C. Monochromatic ophthalmoscopy and fundus photography. The normal fundus. Arch. Ophthalmol. *95:*861 (1977).
11. Flower, R. S., McLeod, S., and Pitts, S. M. Reflection of light by small areas of the ocular fundus. Invest. Ophthalmol. *16:*981 (1977).

7 Ophthalmoscopic Evaluation of the Retinal Nerve Fiber Layer in Neuro-ophthalmologic Disease

Lars Frisén, M.D.

One of the most exciting recent discoveries in the field of ophthalmoscopy was made by William F. Hoyt at the University of California at San Francisco, when he in 1972 observed and photographed focal gaps in the retinal nerve fiber layer in patients with visual field defects due to glaucoma.[20, 23, 25] This discovery initiated a series of studies by several investigators on abnormalities of the retinal nerve fiber layer in various conditions. By now, so much information has been collected, and its value so well established, that examination of the retinal nerve fiber layer by ophthalmoscopy (or fundus photography) has become a remarkably useful component of the neuro-ophthalmologic work-up.

It is legitimate to ask why this important aspect of ophthalmoscopy has escaped attention for such a long time: after all, the ophthalmoscope was described more than one hundred years ago. As a matter of fact, the discovery is not all new. The appearance of the retinal nerve fiber layer in health and disease was given careful attention already in the early part of this century. In particular, Alfred Vogt of Zürich made important studies that were published in the German literature.[49] His findings attracted little interest at that time and over the following years, and the subject was more or less forgotten until rediscovered by Dr. Hoyt. Why, then, has development in this field proceeded so slowly? First, it must be recognized that the retinal

nerve fiber layer has to be translucent. This has to do with its position in relation to the photoreceptors: the lesser the reflection or absorption of light in pre-receptoral layers of the retina, the more light is able to reach the photoreceptors. The poor reflection of light from the retinal nerve fiber layer causes this layer to appear with rather poor visibility under ordinary circumstances. Its contrast against background retino-choroidal structures can be enhanced by using so-called red-free (green) light: this suppresses the normal dominance of the retino-choroidal background. Although this was well known already by Dr. Vogt, it was not until his unwieldy light source could be replaced with modern high output ophthalmoscopes that examination of the retinal nerve fiber layer became practically feasible. The delayed elimination of technical obstacles is the main factor explaining why nerve fiber diagnosis has been so long in development.

The best conditions for visualizing the retinal nerve fiber layer are created when the examiner has access to an ophthalmoscope with a very bright light and a greenish filter in the illumination beam. The precise characterisics of the filter are not very important.[32] The pupil of the eye to be examined should be widely dilated. Nerve fiber bundles are best seen when the optical media of the eye are perfectly clear and non-astigmatic, when the ophthalmoscope is carefully focused on the retinal surface, and when the retino-choroidal background is deeply pigmented. However, with training, the retinal nerve fiber layer can be examined in considerable detail also in patients with moderate imperfections in the optical media and an ordinary or even poor background pigmentation.[31] Increased ophthalmoscopic magnification,[9] or secondary enlargement of carefully focused fundus photographs,[8, 26, 38] are often helpful. The photographic approach also allows additional processing, e.g., color subtraction and unsharp masking,[14, 27] that may further enhance the visibility of nerve fiber bundles.

Another way of enhancing important features of the retinal nerve fiber layer is to represent findings graphically.[20] This technique has been used for most of the illustrations in this chapter. Although naturally occurring abnormalities are most often less distinct than they appear in the drawings, our approach allows overemphasis of important features, and may so facilitate the introduction to ordinary ophthalmoscopic evaluation.

CLINICAL ANATOMY OF THE RETINAL NERVE FIBER LAYER

Each retinal ganglion cell, and there are more than one million in each eye, sends its axon towards the optic disc, where it turns 90° backwards and contributes to the optic nerve. The single axon has too small a diameter to allow resolution *in vivo* by presently available optical techniques.[8] The convergence of axons on the optic disc fortunately causes the formation of increasingly thick bundles, and bundles of nerve fibers can normally be easily visualized in the peripapillary area, at least above and below the optic disc (Fig. 1). Normal bundles of retinal nerve fibers appear as superficial, opaque striae of a pale grey color, with very fine radial striations. Minute bright dots may be interspersed in between

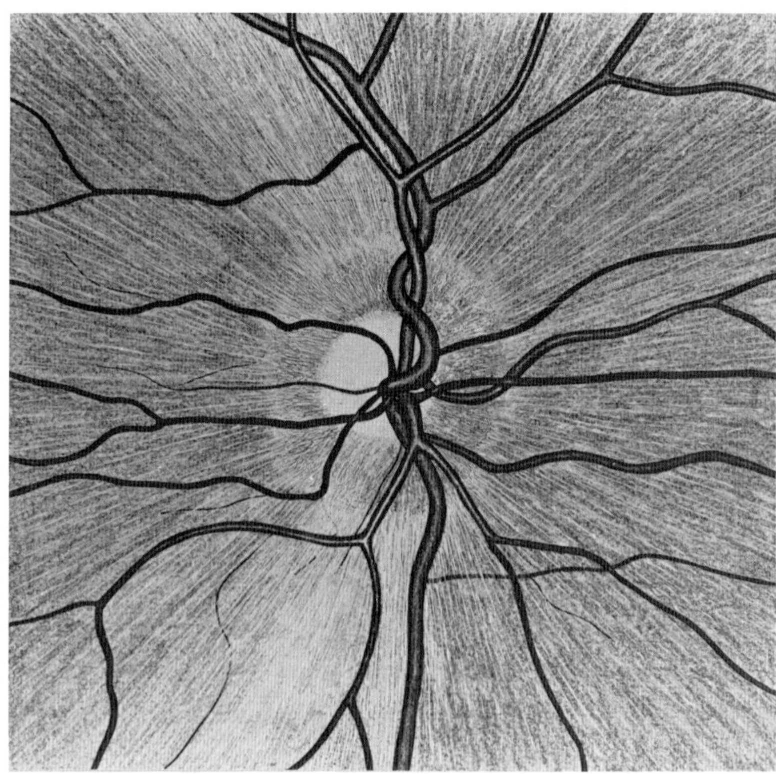

Fig. 1. Normal fundus. The retinal nerve fiber bundles appear as superficial pale gray striae with very fine radial striations. The nerve fiber bundles cause crosshatching and blurring of small retinal vessels. Note the prominence of the arcuate bundles in relation to the nasal and papillo-macular bundles, and the blurring of the disc border by overlying nerve fibers.

the bundles in larger or smaller numbers: these are called Gunn's dots. The nerve fiber bundles obscure detail in the underlying retinal structures and cause cross-hatching and blurring of small retinal vessels. Bundles of retinal nerve fibers are much more difficult to see within the optic disc itself because of the poor contrast against the supporting tissues of the optic nerve head. The fibers forming the *papillo-macular bundles* are particularly thin and are the ones that are most difficult to visualize. Also the bundles approaching the disc on its *nasal side* form a comparatively thin layer with little contrast. The *arcuate bundles*, on the other hand, are normally quite prominent. These bundles, which approach the disc from above and below, serve primarily the temporal retina (the nasal visual field), and the areas above and below the optic disc. There is extensive intermingling of fibers within the arcuate bundles,[39] and little is known about the exact points of origin of these fibers (see Lundström[32] for a recent review). Further detail on nerve fiber topography will be given in subsequent sections.

THE TWO MAIN TYPES OF NERVE FIBER ABNORMALITY: SWELLING AND WASTING

Simple inspection of nerve fiber bundles gives little insight into the complete transport phenomena that occur in normal axons. There is a continuous movement of different axoplasmic constituents at different rates in anterograde (eye to brain) and retrograde (brain to eye) directions.[2, 50] Disturbances of transport mechanisms may result in a local accumulation of axoplasm, with local swelling and tortuosity of axons. So-called cotton-wool spots in the retina are telltale signs of localized blocks of anterograde and retrograde transport.[36, 37] In retrobulbar visual system disease, signs of interrupted axoplasmic flow are conspicuous only when the optic nervehead is the site of interference. This is the case, for instance, in papilledema from increased intracranial pressure. Such a block causes swelling of the axons within the optic disc and in the peripapillary retina (Fig. 2).[17, 47]

The other main type of nerve fiber abnormality is degeneration. Damage to ax-ons within the anterior visual system leads to both anterograde and retrograde axonal degeneration.[1, 2, 42] Damage to axons somewhere posterior to the eye can be visualized from effects of retrograde degeneration: pallor of the optic disc, loss of retinal nerve fiber opacity, and exposure of vascular and retino-choroidal detail (Fig. 3).[4, 33] A circumspect lesion may produce localized disc pallor and localized wasting of retinal nerve fibers. Recent studies suggest that disc pallor primarily is caused by changes in intra-disc light transmission and light reflection properties with loss of nerve fibers.[41] Pallor, therefore, is an indirect sign of loss of nerve fibers. Its rather poor reliability in diagnosis, particularly in cases with epipapillary membranes,[28] requires no comment here. The essential hallmark of optic atrophy, viz. loss of axons, can be better evaluated by ophthalmoscopic examination of the peripapillary retinal nerve fiber layer as the nerve fibers all have to pass through the peripapillary area to reach the optic disc. They are easier to visualize against the background of retina and choroid than against the background of the disc supporting tissues. Retrograde degeneration of axons is characteristic of many types of lesions of the anterior visual pathway. Posterior visual pathway lesions rarely occasion changes in the retinal nerve fiber layer: this requires trans-synaptic degeneration, a phenomenon that appears to occur only in lesions acquired in early life (see further below). Retinal nerve fiber layer atrophy is therefore primarily associated with structural lesions of the anterior visual pathway.

Some clinical conditions of neuro-ophthalmologic interest that are associated with nerve fiber swelling, or nerve fiber degeneration, or both, and their ophthalmoscopic appearances, will be described in the following.

AXONAL SWELLING

Axonal swelling occurs in diseases that block normal axoplasmic transport mechanisms. From a neuro-ophthalmologic point of view, papilledema from increased intracranial pressure may be the most important example. In this condition axonal flow is impaired in the region of the optic disc,[17, 47] with the production of a greyish, reticulated

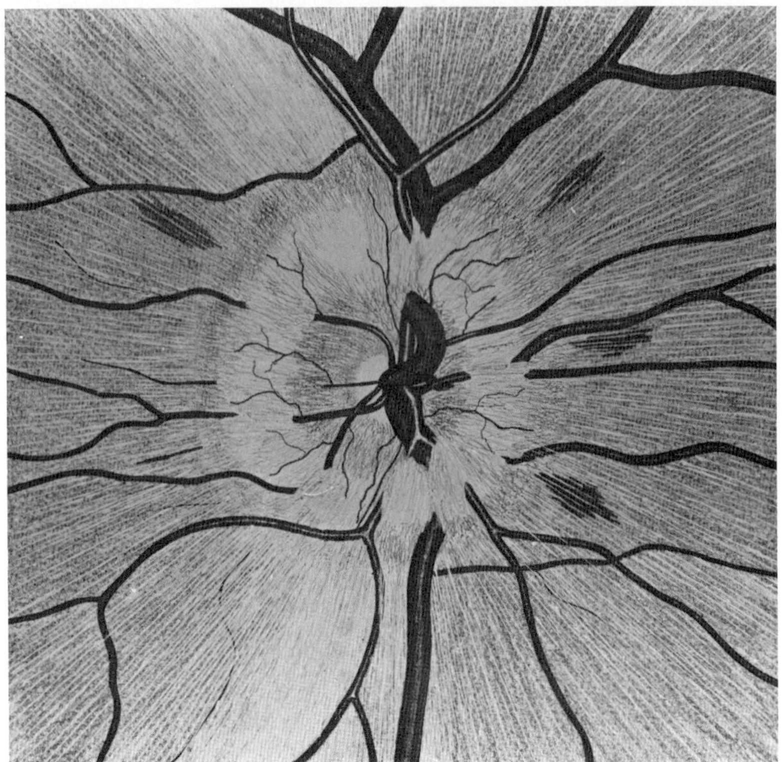

Fig. 2. A moderate degree of papilledema, with broadening and elevation of the optic nerve head due to local swelling and elongation of axons. Signs of circulatory disturbances appear as secondary phenomena. Compare with Figure 1.

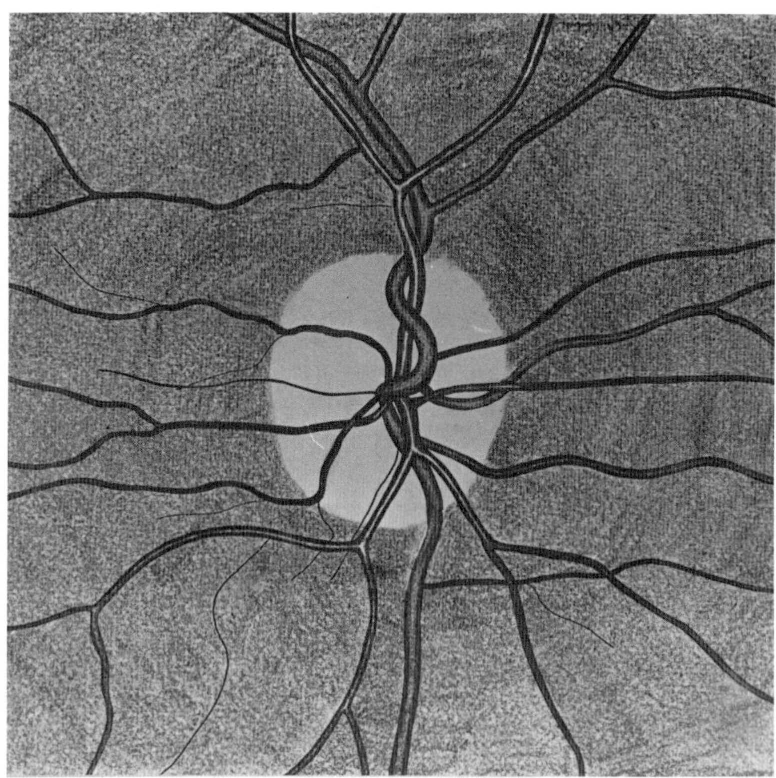

Fig. 3. Complete optic atrophy. Loss of the retinal nerve fiber layer leads to exposure of the disc margin and the retinal vessels. Pallor of the optic disc is a secondary phenomenon. Compare with Figure 1.

halo at the disc border, and swelling of the nerve head itself. The main component of these abnormalities appears to be local swelling and elongation of axons (Figs. 2 and 4).[17, 19, 21] These changes lead to a breakup of the normal, strictly radial arrangement of nerve fiber bundles in the peripapillary area, with increased reflection of light and impaired visualization of deeper fundus structures. The crowding of swollen axons within the unyielding scleral opening causes hyperemia and venous dilatation. Hemorrhages and yellowish spots appear as secondary phenomena.[17] Stasis of axonal flow does not necessary impair axonal conduction. The increased size of the blind spot in papilledema is probably primarily a reflection of a pre-receptor absorption of light in the masses of thickened axons, in combination with disalignment of photoreceptors. The brief obscurations of vision that patients with increased intracranial pressure may experience are more likely to be reflections of conduction disturbances. Their cause is not known.

Axoplasmic transport is a many-faceted phenomenon both in terms of direction of transport and in terms of rates of trans-

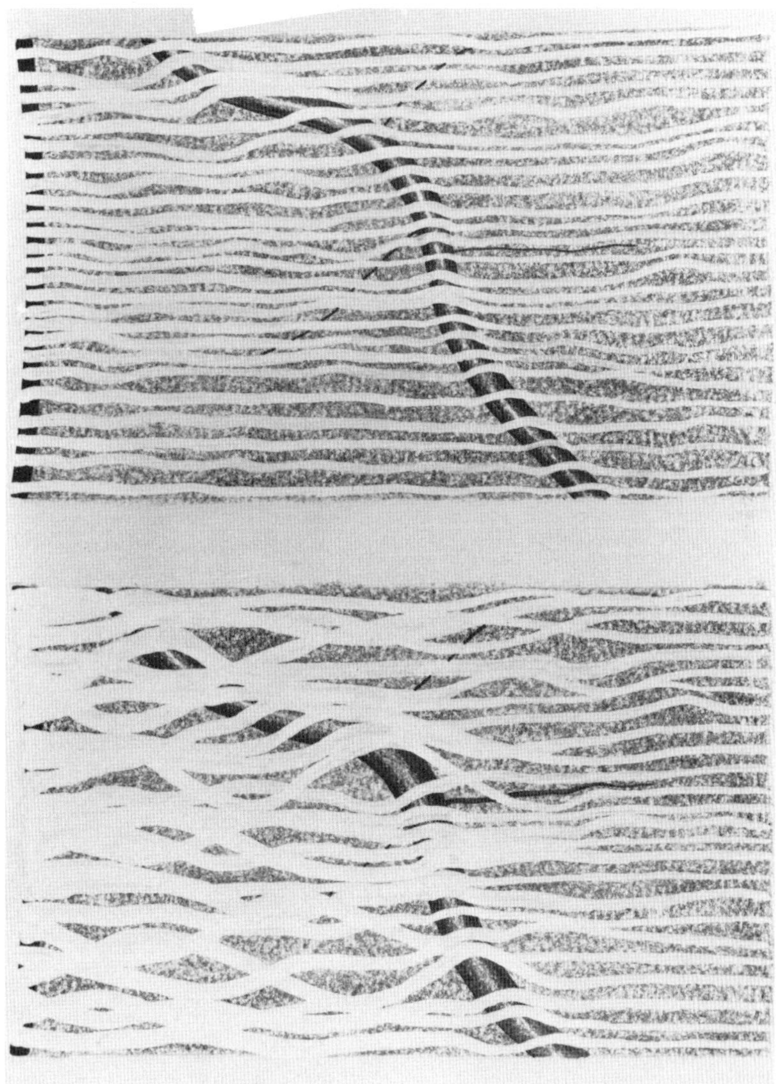

Fig. 4. Schematic drawings visualizing how axonal swelling and elongation breaks up the radial arrangement of nerve fibers and produces a grayish, reticulated halo that blurs out the disc border.

port.[2, 50] The bulk of axonal constituents appear to move at a rate of a few millimeters per 24 hours in anterograde direction. The tardiness of axoplasmic transport explains why papilledema is so slow in appearance even after an abrupt rise in intracranial pressure. Most patients that acquire papilledema on this basis require several days or even weeks to reach the full-blown stage. Axonal atrophy may ensue if intracranial pressure remains elevated for long periods: as axons die off, vascular obstruction is decreased, with loss of hyperemia, and loss of disc swelling. The ophthalmoscopic signs of atrophy will be further described below.

Axonal distension is also characteristic of the early phases of many optic neuropathies, for example papillitis, and hypertensive, anterior ischemic, and constrictive optic neuropathies.[19] The three latter conditions are often associated with a peculiarly glassy pallor of the swollen masses of axons, undoubtedly related to subnormal perfusion of the tissues. Axonal distension is also seen in the early phase of Leber's acute optic neuropathy, together with striking hyperemia of the retinal nerve fiber layer.[44] The same clinical picture with central scotomata and hyperemic axonal swelling is characteristic also of the acute phase of so-called tobacco-alcohol amblyopia (unpublished observations). Most optic neuropathies show signs of nerve fiber wasting in later stages. A complete loss of nerve fibers prevents recurrence of disc swelling.

Ophthalmoscopic evaluation of the peripapillary retinal nerve fiber layer may assist not only in correct recognition of early disc abnormality, but may also aid in the differ-

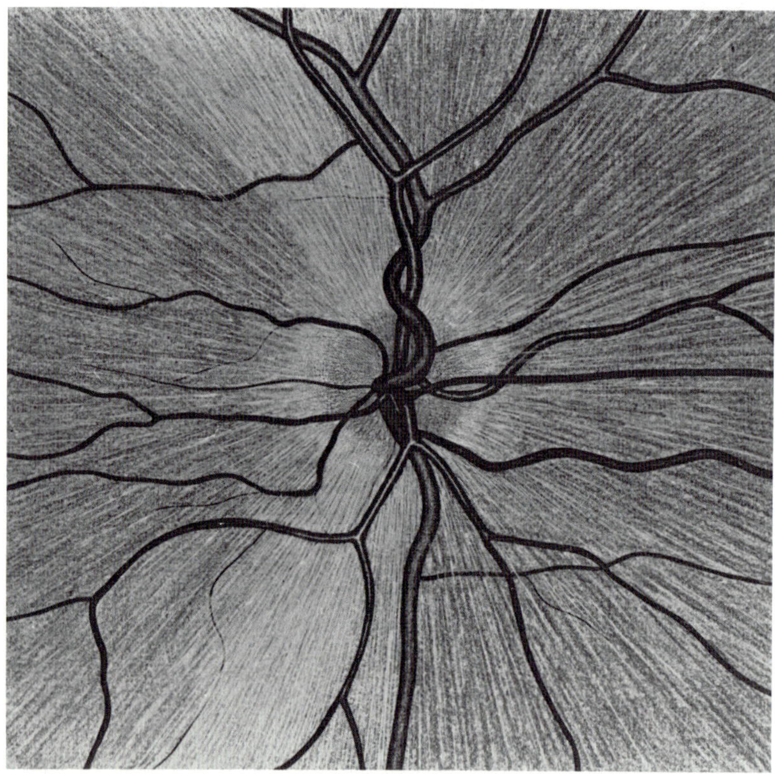

Fig. 5A

Fig. 5. The diameter of the scleral opening influences on the appearance of the optic disc. A. A small scleral opening forces crowding of nerve fibers. Note the pronounced blurring of the disc border and the lack of an optic cup. The radial arrangement of nerve fibers is retained in this normal variant. Compare with Figures 1 and 2. B. A large scleral opening gives abundant space for nerve fibers, with the formation of a well-defined disc border and a large optic cup. This normal variant may mimic an atrophic optic disc. Compare with Figures 1 and 3.

ential diagnosis against normal variants.[12, 19, 21] One of the most important differential diagnoses to true papilledema is what may be called the "crowded disc." This is a normal variant associated with a smaller than average scleral opening for the optic nerve. The small area of the scleral opening forces a crowding of nerve fiber bundles, with the formation of a smaller than average optic cup, a higher than average nerve fiber rim at the disc border, and a thicker than average nerve fiber layer at the border of the scleral opening. The latter factor explains the pronounced blurring of the disc border that the unwary observer easily misinterprets as acquired papilledema (Fig. 5A). This congenital variant further differs from acquired disease in that it retains a regular radial arrangement of nerve fibers at the disc border and lacks a reticulated halo of swollen and tortuous axons. Conversely, an unusually large scleral opening occasions the formation of a larger than average optic disc cup (that often is quite pale in appearance), a thinner than average optic disc rim, and a thinner than average peripapillary nerve fiber layer (Fig. 5B). This normal variant may cause confusion with acquired optic atrophy unless the large size of the disc is recognized.[12]

Another cause of disc swelling that may be confused with papilledema is so-called buried drusen of the optic nerve head (Fig. 6). Buried drusen characteristically cause a crowding of axons within the disc area with the formation of an irregularly prominent nerve head with scalloped and poorly defined margins. The nerve head often protrudes like a somewhat irregular cupola, with a very small cup. The slope between the disc tissue and the surrounding retina is often quite steep. Although drusen may be associated with axonal stasis within the optic nerve head,[45] the stasis rarely extends into the peripapillary area. Therefore, there is once again lack of a greyish, reticulated halo of swollen and elongated axons: the axons can be followed across the disc border in a permanently radial course. Also, there is no hyperemia within the peripapillary

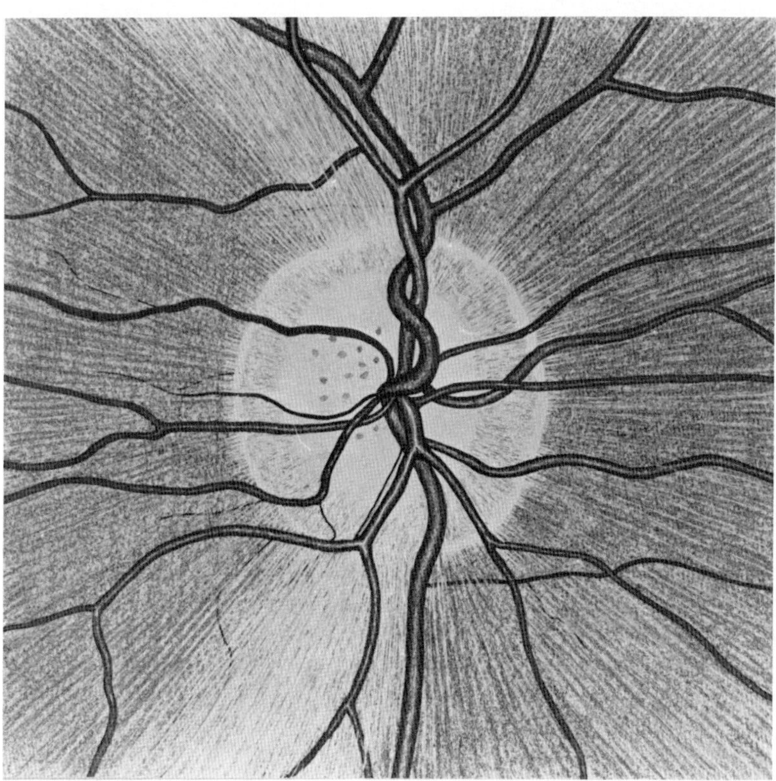

Fig. 5B

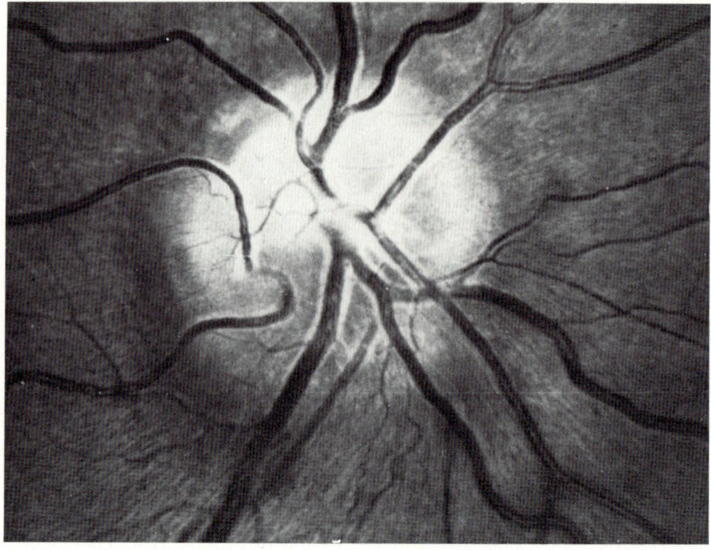

Fig. 6. Appearance of buried drusen of the optic disc (the presence of drusen was confirmed by computed tomography). Note preservation of a radial arrangement of nerve fiber bundles, allowing differentiation from papilledema (compare with Figs. 2, 4, and 11). There is complete loss of nerve fibers in a broad sector above, exposing the disc border and the retina. The patient had an absolute lower arcuate scotoma breaking out to the periphery.

retinal nerve fiber layer. Another characteristic feature of drusen that aids differentiation against papilledema is the formation of bright peripapillary, ring-like reflexes. In cases of doubt computerized tomography offers the ultimate means of identification of buried drusen[16]: they show up as bright dots of abnormally high attenuation in computed tomograms of the optic nerve head, by virtue of their calcification.

Drusen that are superficial enough to be visualized directly with the ophthalmoscope are regularly associated with signs of both diffuse and localized wasting of retinal nerve fiber bundles.

DIFFUSE AND FOCAL LOSS OF AXONS

Complete loss of the retinal nerve fiber layer is easily recognized, not only because of the loss of nerve fiber opacity, but also because of the resulting exposure of retinal and choroidal detail (Figs. 3 and 7): small vessels can be seen unobscured by overlying nerve fiber bundles throughout their course, and minute detail characterizes also other retinal and choroidal structures. The optic disc margin, of course, becomes very sharply defined with loss of overlying nerve fibers. Major vessels often appear sheathed,

and they may acquire broad, bright paravascular reflexes. These latter phenomena may be attributed to loss of paravascular nerve fiber bundles that normally prevent vascular indentations of the posterior vitreous. The denuded retina has a finely mottled appearance.[4, 33] Any ectopic patches of myelin will also disappear.[43]

A partial loss of retinal nerve fibers, uniformly distributed across the optic nerve, is much more difficult to identify with present techniques, particularly if it is bilateral. Cases with unilateral lesions, or asymmetrical bilateral lesions, are best identified by juxtapositioning well-focused fundus photographs, and looking for differences between the two eyes with regard to the relative prominence of nerve fiber opacity and the definition of small detail. The optic neuropathies associated with compression, chronic demyelinating disease, chronically elevated intracranial pressure, drusen, and glaucoma are examples of disorders that appear prone to produce a predominantly diffuse loss of retinal nerve fibers.

Focal loss denotes loss of nerve fibers within a circumscript region of the anterior visual pathway and the corresponding circumscript part of the retinal nerve fiber layer (Figs. 7 and 8). The appearance of

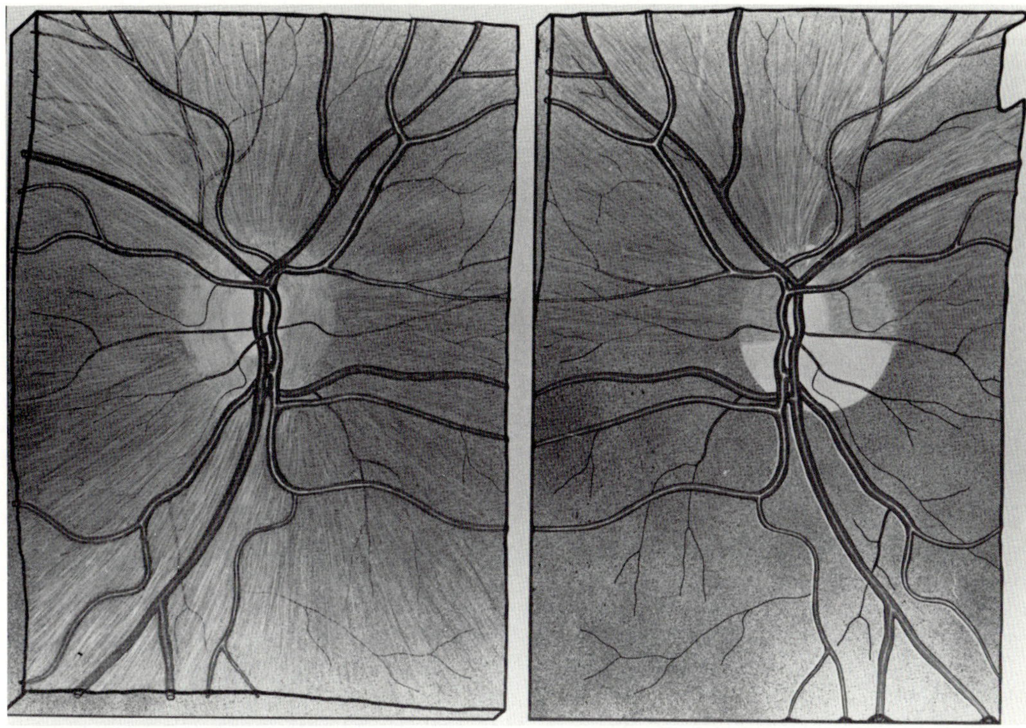

Fig. 7A   Fig. 7B

Fig. 7. Schematic representation of normal (A) and abnormal (B) retinal nerve fiber layers. In B, there is complete loss of nerve fiber bundles in an upper temporal wedge and in the lower half of the fundus. The denuded retina lacks nerve fiber opacity and striations. It is therefore dark in appearance and finely mottled. Vascular detail is clearly exposed within atrophic areas.

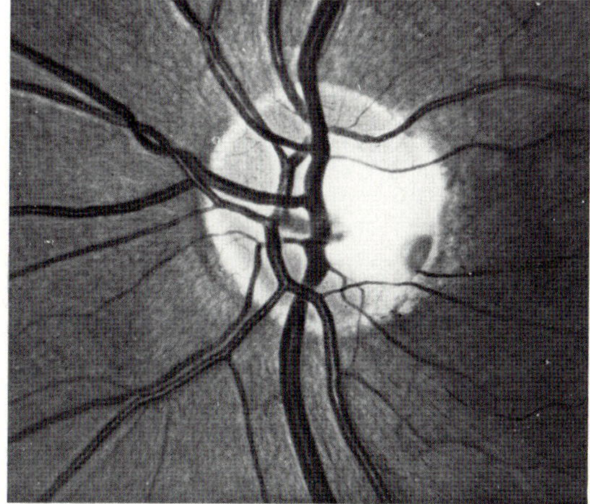

Fig. 8. Absence of retinal nerve fiber bundles in a sector abutting on an optic nerve pit. The nerve fiber layer appears normal outside this sector. The patient had an absolute ceco-central scotoma.

such defects depend on their depth, width, and position in relation to the circumference of the optic disc.[20] Full thickness defects are easiest to recognize, particularly within the arcuate bundles. Partial thickness defects are more difficult to define but shallow grooves are often multiple, and tend to give the nerve fiber layer a raked appearance. Focal defects are always bounded by curves conforming with the curvilinear arrangement of the nerve fiber bundles, and they always taper towards the optic disc. Narrow defects are usually best seen about one to three disc diameters from the disc margin and fade from view both more peripherally, with decreasing thickness of the nerve fiber layer, and more centripetally, in the crowding of bundles at the disc margin. Broader, wedge-shaped defects may be followed for longer distances, sometimes all the way down to the disc margin. Focal defects are perhaps easiest to visualize in the atrophic stage of focal ischemic optic neuropathy, and in so-called low-tension glaucoma.[19, 30] Chronic glaucoma is considerably more difficult to evaluate as this appears to be a disease with a pronounced component of diffuse loss of retinal nerve fibers: any focal defects are hard to appreciate ophthalmoscopically because of the poor contrast against the surrounding, diffusely wasted areas of the retinal nerve fiber layer.

The distribution of focal nerve fiber lesions depends on the site of the lesion within the anterior visual pathway, and it is practical to subdivide the subject into optic nerve, chiasmal, and retrochiasmal lesions.

Optic Nerve Lesions

Focal nerve fiber defects are often encountered in optic nerve lesions of various types, although a majority of such lesions certainly may be capable of producing also a diffuse attrition of axons. Irrespective of the actual mechanism of axonal damage, it will result in descending degeneration of axons. The appearance of the nerve fiber layer therefore cannot inform on the nature of the lesions. By analyzing the distribution of the defects in the nerve fiber layer the prospects of obtaining diagnostic informations become somewhat brighter. Toxic, acute demyelinating, and heredo-degenerative lesions apparently favor the papillo-macular bundle in the optic nerve, with the production of a central scotoma with a more or less well-conserved peripheral visual field. The papillo-macular bundle is usually involved also in compressive lesions, although these lesions rarely save other bundles completely. Traumatic and vascular lesions often favor other bundles within the optic nerve, in keeping with their tendency to produce altitudinal visual field defects.

The correlation between the distribution of focal damage in the retinal nerve fiber layer, and the visual field defect, is generally very good in patients with substantial optic nerve lesions.[10, 19, 20] Smaller lesions may be better identified by ophthalmoscopy than by routine visual field examinations. Chronic demyelinating optic neuropathy is an example in point.[15] This disease has a tendency, at least in the relatively early stages, to destroy quite small bundles of adjacent nerve fibers. The resulting scotomata are narrow and slit-like, and they have the same orientation as the nerve fiber bundles. Such field defects are easiest to demonstrate in the arcuate areas, but they can occur also in other locations. However, current perimetric procedures are not very sensitive to narrow, elongated field defects outside the arcuate areas. They are also surprisingly insensitive to a diffusely distributed wasting of nerve fibers.[10]

Chiasmal Lesions

Chiasmal lesions are regularly associated with localized wasting of retinal nerve fibers in both eyes.[34, 35, 48] Cases with extensive mid-chiasmal lesions affecting crossing nerve fibers, with complete bitemporal hemianopia, usually present very distinctive changes in the peripapillary retinal nerve fiber layer (Fig. 9). The crossing nerve fibers, which have their cell bodies in the nasal hemi-retina,* are then lost. This has the effect of enhancing the apparent contrast of the arcuate bundles. Sometimes there is also a horizontal band of pallor across the optic disc. This picture, of course, suggests a very poor prognosis for recovery of vision upon removal of the responsible lesion. Less pronounced degrees of damage, as shown by incomplete loss of nerve fibers in nasal and papillo-macular areas, and relative visual field defects, naturally indicate a better prognosis. It has been shown that there is a good correlation between the appearance of the retinal nerve fiber layer with lesions of the chiasm due to pituitary adenoma, and the visual field defects, once the patient has reached a steady state stage after successful surgery.[34] Prior to surgery, many patients show field defects that are excessive in relation to the degree of atrophy. Such excessive functional loss points to the operation of potentially reversible mechanisms for defective conduction. The extent of recovery that is possible is naturally limited by the degree of structural damage.[35] A similar relationship between damage and function has recently been demonstrated also for the papillo-macular bundle in optic neuropathies.[46]

Importantly, many patients with seemingly pure temporal visual field defects also show distinctive signs of wasting of nerve fibers coming from the temporal hemi-ret-

* In this context, the dividing line between nasal and temporal halves of the retina is taken to run vertically through the fovea.

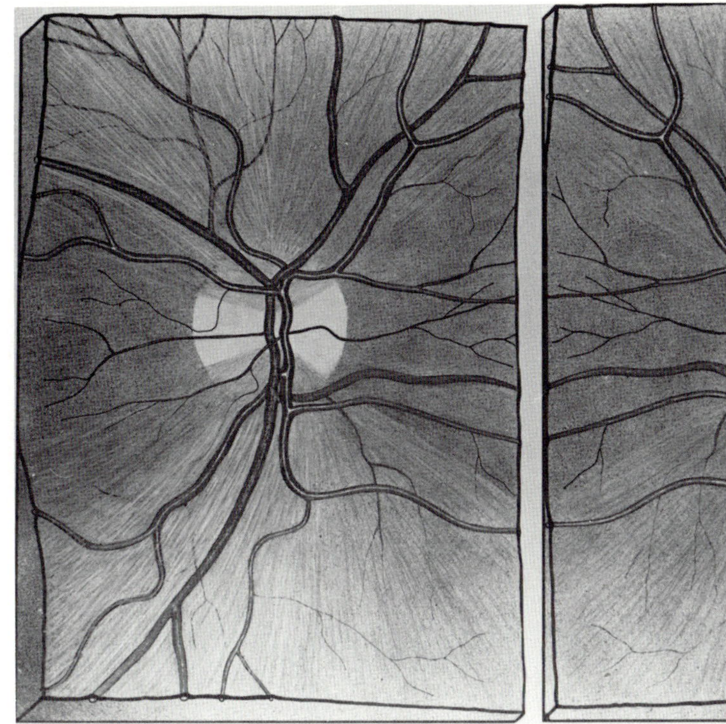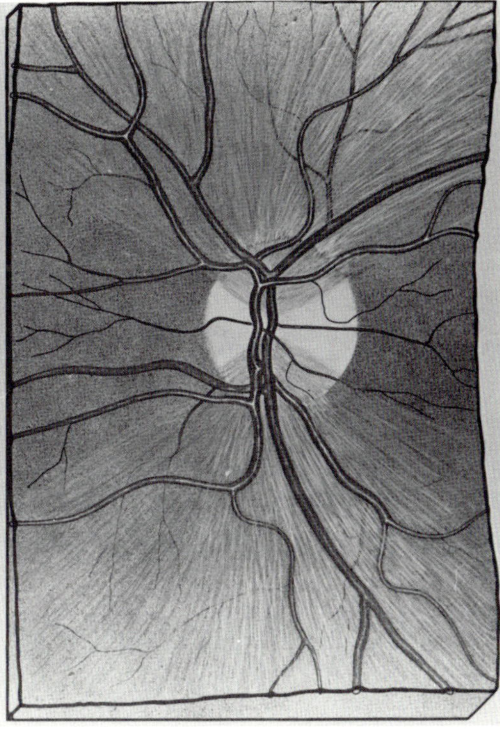

Fig. 9. Representation of loss of nerve fiber bundles within horizontal sectors of the nerve fiber layer in irreversible bitemporal hemianopia. Note the horizontal strip of pallor across the optic disc. Compare with Figure 7A.

ina. This indicates that anatomical damage in the chiasm often is more extensive than taught previously, an observation that correlates well with the usual appearance at surgery, with stretching of the whole chiasm over the tumor dome. This explains the sometime absence of focal visual field defects in patients with large suprasellar lesions.[10]

Although bitemporal hemianopia is a classical hallmark of chiasmal damage, asymmetric syndromes appear to be still more common. Again, ophthalmoscopic evaluation of the retinal nerve fiber layer improves insight into these phenomena. Take the patient with a unilateral temporal field defect and a contralateral normal field, for instance. Such a patient typically shows diffuse wasting of nerve fibers in the perimetrically normal eye. The problem of explaining unilateral visual field defects in patients with chiasmal disorders is therefore not an anatomical problem, but an instrumental problem.

Also homonymous visual field defects are encountered now and then with suprasellar lesions. Clinical differentiation against tract lesions is often difficult,* and the fundus changes associated with homonymous visual field defects with anterior visual pathway lesions are better treated under a separate heading.

Optic Tract and Lateral Geniculate Lesions

Complete tract lesions, with complete homonymous hemianopia, produce distinctive changes in the ocular fundus (Fig. 10).[22, 24, 29] In the eye contralateral to the lesion, the eye with the temporal field defect, the nerve fiber layer presents abnormalities that are indistinguishable from those produced by pure mid-chiasmal lesions. Abnormalities are more difficult to detect in the ipsilateral eye, the eye with the nasal hemianopia.

* Recent observations suggest that coexisting impairment of visual acuity points to chiasmal damage. Acuity seems to remain normal in patients with pure tract lesions (Frisén, in preparation).

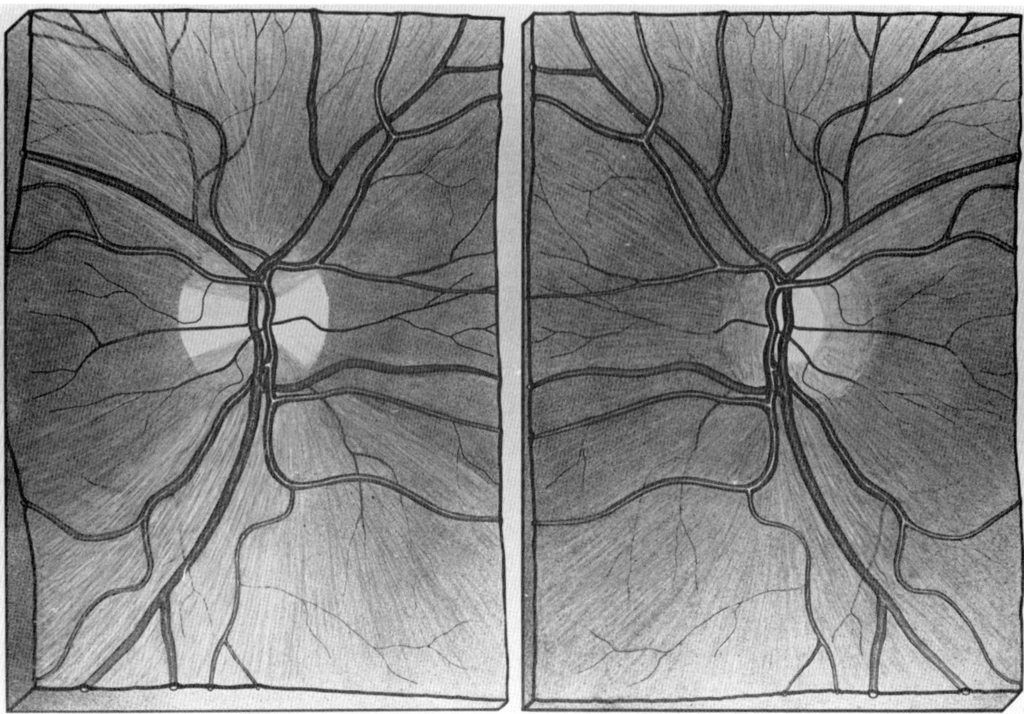

Fig. 10. Representation of nerve fiber layer defects in right homonymous hemianopia due to an irreversible optic tract or lateral geniculate lesion on the left. The nerve fiber layer in the eye contralateral to the lesion is atrophic within horizontal sectors. The ipsilateral eye shows only a reduced prominence of the arcuate bundles.

Nasal hemianopia signifies impaired conduction from the temporal hemi-retina. This is served by fibers occupying parts of the arcuate bundles. These fibers intermingle with other fibers in the arcuate bundles, fibers that serve the *nasal* hemi-retina. Temporal hemi-retinal atrophy therefore does not produce complete loss of nerve fibers within the peripapillary area but only thinning of the arcuate bundles. Smaller degrees of damage, with relative visual field defects, are difficult to detect ophthalmoscopically.

Tract lesions are generally impossible to distinguish from lateral geniculate lesions from the appearance of the retinal nerve fiber layer or the visual field defects. Homonymous sectorial defects, with corresponding sectorial optic atrophy, constitute exceptions indicative of partial lateral geniculate damage.[11, 13, 18]

Superposition of papilledema upon homonymous hemi-optic atrophy produces striking signs in the eye with temporal hemianopia:[7, 40] here the axonal swelling is limited to the upper and lower poles of the optic nerve head ("twin-peak papilledema"). The other eye shows a more regular distribution of swelling by virtue of the lack of completely denuded sectors (Fig. 11).

TIME COURSE OF OPTIC ATROPHY

A cross-sectional lesion of the optic nerve results in loss of retinal nerve fiber about six weeks after the lesion.[4, 6, 33] Experimental studies show that degeneration does not occur step by step along the axon, but all of the axon anterior to the lesion degenerates at the same time.[1, 42] This observation suggests that the time course of fundus changes with anterior visual pathway lesions should be independent of the actual site of the lesion. The delay must be kept in mind when evaluating the nerve fiber layer in patients with acute impairment of vision due to retrobulbar disease: the nerve fiber

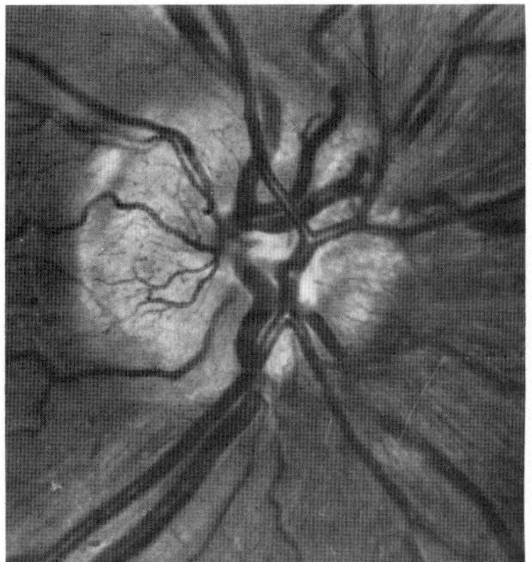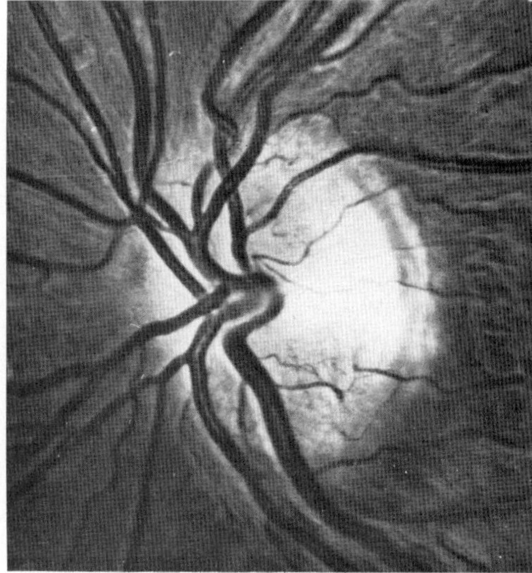

Fig. 11. Papilledema due to increased intracranial pressure superposed upon homonymous, hemioptic atrophy caused by a right optic tract lesion. The patient had a left homonymous hemianopia. Note the production of a blurred, reticulated halo at the disc border, with loss of normal radial striations (compare with Figs. 6 and 8). Atrophy of horizontal sectors of the retinal nerve fiber layer in the left eye (the eye with the temporal hemianopia) explains the twin-peak distribution of disc swelling.

bundles usually appear perfectly normal for several weeks following the debut of visual loss. Disc pallor is a still more protracted sign.[33] The same delay occurs with slowly progressive lesions, so prudence must always be exercised when prognosticating the degree of recovery that may be possible. Further, the delayed appearance of retinal nerve fiber atrophy may explain many instances of progression of optic atrophy following successful surgical treatment of the responsible lesion: the surgeon is not always to blame if atrophy progresses. Progression that occurs more than two months after surgery obviously must have another explanation, however.[35]

CONGENITAL VS. ACQUIRED OPTIC ATROPHY

The sequence of events outlined above is characteristic of lesions that damage the fully developed visual system. Lesions operating before complete development has occurred regularly seem to activate mechanisms that adjust the size of the optic nerve head to the remaining mass of axons. Hence lesions acquired before full development of the visual system has taken place are characterized not only by retinal nerve fiber abnormalities and corollary visual field defects as described above, but also by remodelling of the optic disc. So-called hypoplasia of the optic nerve can be distinguished from acquired atrophy primarily by signs of disc modelling and lack of progression.[12] Remodelling occurs also in de Morsier's syndrome (bitemporal visual field defects due to septo-optic dysplasia)[5] and in retro-chiasmal lesions acquired early in life (homonymous hemianopia with so-called homonymous hemioptic hypoplasia).[3, 19, 24]

The same type of funduscopic correlates of homonymous visual field defects that was described above is sometimes seen also in patients who have acquired a *suprageniculate* lesion at an early age.[24] This points to the possibility of trans-synaptic degeneration, at least in the immature visual system. At what age trans-synaptic degeneration no longer occurs is not yet known, but there is no indication that substantial degeneration of this type occurs in adults.

EDITOR'S NOTE

The syndrome of *congenital homonymous hemianopia* is not terribly rare in neuro-ophthalmologic practice. It seems to be unappreciated by many neurologists, however, and they often admit such patients to the hospital for an extensive, expensive, and, in my opinion, unnecessary work-up. Helpful features are as follows: (1) the patient often may not know that he or she has a hemianopia, and it may be found simply on a routine field examination done for some other reason; (2) even after it has been pointed out to the patient, it doesn't bother them in the least (quite different from an acquired hemianopia in an adult!); (3) a careful look at the optic discs and adjacent nerve fiber layer shows the telltale appropriate changes; (4) the thumb nail will often be just a bit smaller on the side of the hemianopia as an additional "tip" that this was present in early development; (5) the optokinetic responses are usually symmetrical (i.e., there is a "negative ON sign" or a normal optokinetic response, consistent with an occipital lobe origin to the field defect); (6) there is no other neurologic complaint at this time, and (7) the CT scan of the brain now provides a good outpatient confirmation showing often an occipital lobe lesion that is old, does not change with enhancement, and often is due to occipital porencephaly which occurred during development. All that one should do is make the diagnosis, reassure the patient, and follow them on occasion. I recall the first case of this that I saw was a young football player from Oklahoma who received a nasty bump on the head after a tackle during a college football game. He was stunned, and the attending physician did a confrontation field on the boy as he regained consciousness. Everyone was immediately concerned when a total left homonymous hemianopia was consistently obtained. The young man was referred to Dr. Frank Walsh and I saw him with Dr. Walsh around 1956–1957. Dr. Walsh immediately recognized this as a congenital hemianopia which was simply detected with that confrontation field, for the boy did not know he had it, and still didn't know it after it was brought to his attention. All of the other points on history and examination were otherwise normal. The additional evidence of the nerve fiber layer pattern is also of great help in making this diagnosis! A reference on congenital homonymous hemianopia is by Dr. F. B. Bajandas *et al.* in *Am. J. Ophth.* **82**:498–500, Sept. 1976.

JLS

ACKNOWLEDGMENT

Peter Hansson's assistance in producing the illustrations is gratefully acknowledged.

REFERENCES

1. Anderson, D. R. Ascending and descending optic atrophy produced experimentally in squirrel monkeys. Am. J. Ophthalmol. *76*:693–711 (1973).
2. Anderson, D. R. Axonal transport in the retina and optic nerve. In: *Neuro-ophthalmology.* J. S. Glaser (Ed.), C. V. Mosby, St. Louis, 1977, Vol. IX, pp. 140–153.
3. Bajandas, F. J., McBeath, J. B., and Smith, J. L. Congenital homonymous hemianopia. Am. J. Ophthalmol. *82*:498–500 (1975).
4. Bell, F. C. and Behrens, M. M. Observation of retinal nerve fiber degeneration after optic nerve injury. In: *Neuro-ophthalmology.* J. S. Glaser (Ed.), C. V. Mosby, St. Louis, 1977, Vol. IX, pp. 207–214.
5. Davis, G. V. and Shock, J. P. Septo-optic dysplasia associated with see-saw nystagmus. Arch. Ophthalmol. *93*:137–139 (1975).
6. Enoksson, P. and Johansson, J. O. Altitudinal field defects and retinal nerve fiber degeneration in optic nerve lesions. Acta Ophthalmol. *56*:957–968 (1978).
7. Freusberg, O. Halbteilige homonyme Stauungspapille bei partieller Optikusatrophie nach einseitiger Traktusläsion. Klin. Monatsbl. Augenheilkd. *101*:494–507 (1938).
8. Frisén, L. Resolution at low contrast with a fundus camera. Comparison of various photographic films. Invest. Ophthalmol. *12*:865–869 (1973).
9. Frisén, L. High magnification ophthalmoscopy. Am. J. Ophthalmol. *86*:272–273 (1978).
10. Frisén, L. Funduscopic correlates of visual field defects in lesions of the anterior visual pathway. Doc. Ophthalmol. Proc. Ser., in press.
11. Frisén, L. Quadruple sectoranopia and sectorial optic atrophy: a syndrome of the distal anterior choroidal artery. J. Neurol. Neurosurg. Psychiatr., in press.
12. Frisén, L. and Holmegaard, L. Spectrum of optic nerve hypoplasia. Br. J. Ophthalmol. *62*:7–15 (1978).
13. Frisén, L., Holmegaard, L., and Rosencrantz, M. Sectorial optic atrophy and homonymous, horizontal sectoranopia: a lateral choroidal artery syndrome? J. Neurol. Neurosurg. Psychiatr. *41*:374–380 (1978).
14. Frisén, L. and Hoyt, W. F. Unsharp masking in fundus photography. Invest. Ophthalmol. *12*:461–464 (1973).
15. Frisén, L., and Hoyt, W. F. Insidious atrophy of retinal nerve fibers in multiple sclerosis. Funduscopic identification in patients with and without

visual complaints. Arch. Ophthalmol. *92:*91–97 (1974).

16. Frisén, L., Schöldström, G., and Svendsen, P. Drusen in the optic nerve head. Verification by computerized tomography. Arch. Ophthalmol. *96:* 1611–1614 (1978).

17. Hayreh, S. S. Optic disc edema in raised intracranial pressure. V. Pathogenesis. Arch. Ophthalmol. *95:*1553–1565 (1977).

18. Hoyt, W. F. Geniculate hemianopia: incongruous visual defects from involvement of the lateral geniculate nucleus. Proc. Aust. Assoc. Neurol. *12:*7–16 (1975).

19. Hoyt, W. F. Ophthalmoscopy of the retinal nerve fiber layer in neuro-ophthalmologic diagnosis. Aust. J. Ophthalmol. *4:*13–34 (1976).

20. Hoyt, W. F., Frisén, L., and Newman, N. M. Funduscopy of nerve fiber layer defects in glaucoma. Invest. Ophthalmol. *12:*814–829 (1973).

21. Hoyt, W. F. and Knight, C. L. Comparison of congenital disc blurring and incipient papilledema in red-free light—a photographic study. Invest. Ophthalmol. *12:*241–247 (1973).

22. Hoyt, W. F. and Kommerell, G. Der Fundus oculi bei homonymer Hemianopie. Klin. Monatsbl. Augenheilkd. *162:*456–464 (1973).

23. Hoyt, W. F. and Newman, N. M. The earliest observable defect in glaucoma? Lancet *1:*692–693 (1972).

24. Hoyt, W. F., Rios-Montenegro, E. N., Behrens, M. M., and Eckelhoff, R. J. Homonymous hemioptic hypoplasia. Funduscopic features in standard and red-free illumination in three patients with congenital hemiplegia. Br. J. Ophthalmol. *56:*537–545 (1972).

25. Hoyt, W. F., Schlicke, B., and Ecklehoff, R. J. Funduscopic appearance of a nerve-fibre-bundle defect. Br. J. Ophthalmol. *56:*577–583 (1972).

26. Ito, H., Ozawa, K., Suga, S., and Mizuno, K. Red-free light magnifying photography in neuritis and some retinal vascular lesions. Folia Ophthalmol. Jp. *20:*282–287 (1969).

27. Iwata, K., Yaoeda, H., and Sofue, K. Changes of retinal nerve fiber layer in glaucoma. I. Methodology of investigations in vivo. Acta Soc. Ophthalmol. Jpn. *79:*1062–1066 (1975).

28. Jerndal, T. The epipapillary membrane and the glaucomatous disc. Acta Ophthalmol. *54:*185–192 (1976).

29. Lauber, H. Die ophthalmoskopische Differentialdiagnose der infra- und supranukleären Hemianopsie, zugleich ein Beitrag zur Topographie der Faserverteilung in der Netzhaut. Ber. Dtsch Ophthalmol. Ges. *46:*89–94 (1927).

30. Lundström, M. Wasting of nerve fibers in the retina. Photographic documentation. Acta Ophthalmol. *52:*872–880 (1974).

31. Lundström, M. Atrophy of optic nerve fibres in compression of the chiasm. Observer variation in assessment of atrophy. Acta Ophthalmol. *55:*217–226 (1977).

32. Lundström, M. Optic atrophy in compression of the chiasm. A funduscopic study of the human retinal nerve fiber layer. Thesis, University of Göteborg, 1977.

33. Lundström, M. and Frisén, L. Evolution of descending optic atrophy. A case report. Acta Ophthalmol. *53:*738–746, (1975).

34. Lundström, M. and Frisén, L. Atrophy of optic nerve fibers in compression of the chiasm. Degree and distribution of ophthalmoscopic changes. Acta Ophthalmol. *54:*623–640 (1976).

35. Lundström, M. and Frisén, L. Atrophy of optic nerve fibers in compression of the chiasm. Prognostic implications. Acta Ophthalmol. *55:*208–216 (1977).

36. McLeod, D. Ophthalmoscopic signs of obstructed axoplasmic transport after ocular vascular occlusion. Br. J. Ophthalmol. *58:*551–556 (1976).

37. McLeod, D., Marshall, J., Kohner, E. M., and Bird, A. C. The role of axoplasmic transport in the pathogenesis of retinal cotton-wool spots. Br. J. Ophthalmol. *61:*177–191 (1977).

38. Mizuno, K., Ozawa, K., and Ito, H. High magnification red-free light fundus photography. Mod. Probl. Ophthalmol. *9:*50–54 (1971).

39. Ogden, T. E. The nerve-fiber layer of the primate retina: an autoradiographic study. Invest. Ophthalmol. *13:*95–100 (1974).

40. Paul, T. O. and Hoyt, W. F. Funduscopic appearance of papilledema with optic tract atrophy. Arch. Ophthalmol. *94:*467–468 (1976).

41. Quigley, H. A. and Anderson, D. R. The histologic basis of optic disk pallor in experimental optic atrophy. Am. J. Ophthalmol. *83:*709–717 (1977).

42. Quigley, H. A., David, E. B., and Anderson, R. A. Descending optic nerve degeneration in primates. Invest. Ophthalmol. Visual Sci. *16:*841–849 (1977).

43. Sharpe, J. A. and Sanders, M. D. Atrophy of myelinated nerve fibers in the retina in optic neuritis. Br. J. Ophthalmol. *59:*229–232 (1975).

44. Smith, J. L., Hoyt, W. F., and Susac, J. O. Ocular fundus in acute Leber optic neuropathy. Arch. Ophthalmol. *90:*349–354 (1973).

45. Spencer, W. H. Drusen of the optic disk and aberrant axoplasmic transport. Am. J. Ophthalmol. *85:*1–12 (1978).

46. Tagami, Y. Correlations between atrophy of maculopapillar bundles and visual functions in cases of optic neuropathies. Doc. Ophthalmol. Proc. Ser., in press.

47. Tso, M. O. M. and Fine, B. S. Electron microscopic study of human papilledema. Am. J. Ophthalmol. *82:*424–434 (1976).

48. Vannas, A., Raitta, C., and Lemberg, S. Photography of the nerve fiber layer in retinal disturbances. Acta Ophthalmol. *55:*79–87 (1977).

49. Vogt, A. Die Ophthalmoskopie im rotfreien Licht. In: *Handbuch der gesamten Augenheilkunde.* 3rd ed. Graefe-Saemisch (Ed.), Julius Springer, Berlin, 1925, Vol. III, pp. 1–118.

50. Wirtschafter, J. D., Rizzo, F. J., and Smiley, B. C. Optic nerve axoplasm and papilledema. Surv. Ophthalmol. *20:*157–189 (1975).

8 Papillophlebitis Causing Cilioretinal Artery Occlusion

Raananah S. Katz, M.D.
J. Lawton Smith, M.D.

Papillophlebitis is a benign unilateral retinal vasculitis occurring in young, otherwise healthy adults. Clinically, it closely resembles a central retinal vein occlusion, but has a different pathogenesis and prognosis. The disc is swollen and the veins are engorged and tortuous. In addition there are peripapillary and diffuse flame-shaped retinal hemorrhages scattered throughout the fundus. The fellow eye is usually normal with no evidence of vascular disease. In most cases excellent visual acuity is maintained. The single most important feature of the disease is the recognition that papillophlebitis is a benign condition with a good long-range prognosis and should simply be followed clinically. Two cases are here described. The first is typical of the entity. The second concerns a patient we have recently encountered with papillophlebitis accompanied by an occlusion of the cilioretinal artery. To our knowledge this association has not been previously described, and this combination in a healthy 26-year-old female is the subject of this report.

CASE I

This healthy 30-year-old white female was seen through the courtesy of Dr. Davidson. She recently noted the sudden onset of blurred central vision in her left eye. This resolved within several hours but was followed by similar transient episodes over the next three days. However, on the fourth day central dimness recurred and persisted. She was not taking birth control pills at the time.

Neuro-ophthalmologic examination on January 14, 1972 revealed a visual acuity of 20/15−1 in both eyes. There was a very slight Marcus Gunn pupil on the left. Amsler grid testing showed an oval defect inferior to fixation in the left eye. Central field testing confirmed this inferior arcuate scotoma. The peripheral fields were normal in both eyes. Ophthalmoscopic examination of the right eye was unremarkable. In the left eye the disc was swollen, with several areas of white exudative material overlying the distended disc vessels. There was prominent venous dilatation, and small superficial retinal hemorrhages were scattered throughout the peripheral fundus. The arterial system was normal. The clinical impression was papillophlebitis.

General medical evaluation including routine blood tests, ANA fixation, and chest x-rays were all within normal limits. She was treated with sub-Tenon's injection of aqueous Triamcinalone and was started on a six-week course of anticoagulation therapy. Two months later her ophthalmoscopic picture had completely resolved. The patient remains asymptomatic with no ocular complications at a five-year follow-up.

CASE II

This healthy 26-year-old white female was seen July 5, 1977 through the courtesy of Dr. B. Bercaw. She first noted the sudden onset of a "spot" in the central vision of her left eye in June 1977. This was not associated with any ocular pain or tenderness. The symptoms cleared within an hour. The following day she had multiple recurrences of the same complaint. When seen by her ophthalmologist the visual acuity was 20/20 in the right eye and 20/25 in the left eye. A mild afferent pupillary defect was observed in the left eye. There were no cells or flare in the anterior chamber. Ophthalmoscopic examination of the right eye was normal. The left eye disclosed dilated tortuous veins with multiple superficial and deep retinal hemorrhages scattered throughout the posterior pole and peripheral retina. Exudates were present near the disc extending into the macular area.

Her symptoms progressed, and three days later the central defect became permanent. The patient was started on 60 mg of Prednisone daily for eight days. Neurologic evaluation including skull x-rays, CAT scan, and routine blood tests were all normal. She was referred to the Bascom Palmer Eye Institute with a tentative diagnosis of papillophlebitis.

Neuro-ophthalmologic examination one month after the onset of symptoms revealed a visual acuity of 20/15 in the right

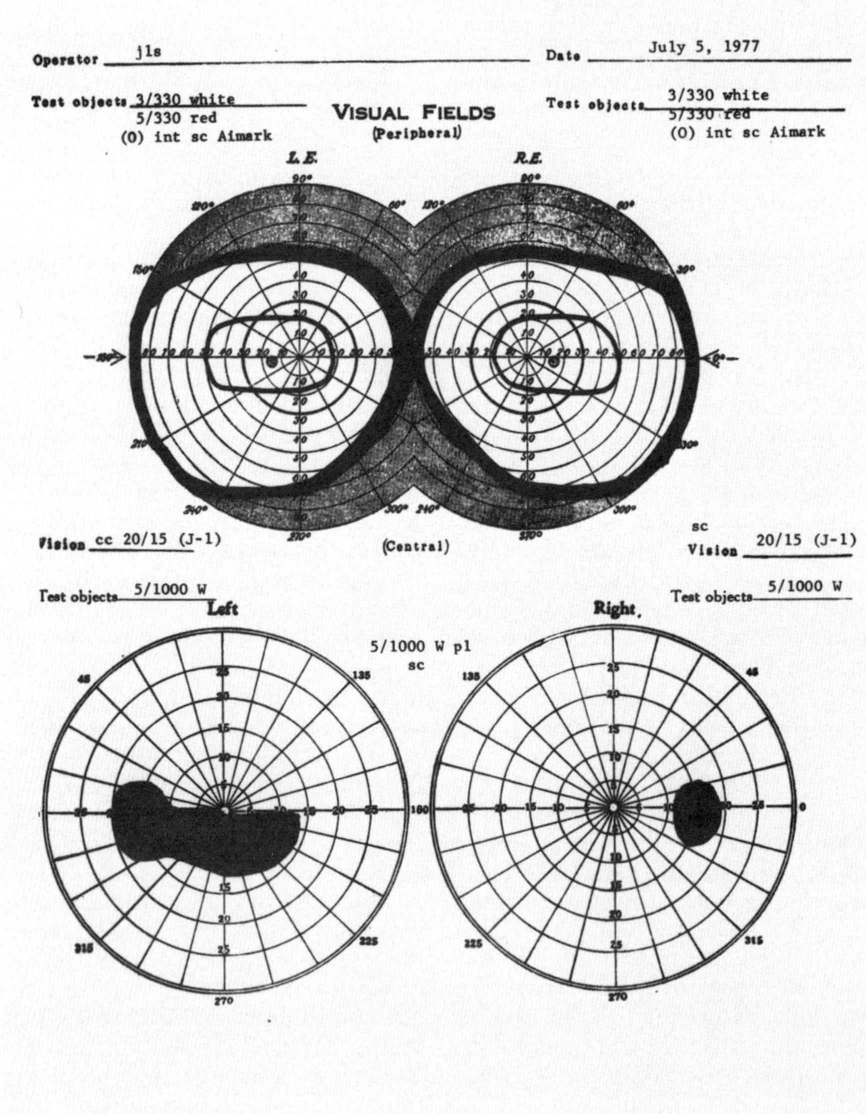

Fig. 1. Case 2. Peripheral fields are full. An inferior cecocentral scotoma is present in the central field of the left eye.

eye and 20/20+1 in the left eye. A 1+ Marcus Gunn pupil was observed on the left. A horizontal oval-shaped scotoma was noted inferiorly on the Amsler grid in her left eye. Central fields in the left eye demonstrated a lower altitudinal cecocentral scotoma extending from the disc to a point just inferior to fixation (Fig. 1). Peripheral fields were normal in both eyes. Ophthalmoscopic examination of the right eye was within normal limits. The left disc (Fig. 2) was swollen and hyperemic with indistinct edges; exudates with overlying fluffy deposits were present on the disc. The retinal veins were markedly dilated and tortuous in all quadrants; small dot and blot hemorrhages were scattered throughout the posterior pole. A scimitar shaped area of hemorrhage extended from the disc between 3:00 and 5:00, passing temporally towards the fovea. The macular area superiorly was pale white in color. The cilio-retinal artery was attenuated as it emerged from the disc at 2:00. The diagnosis of papillophlebitis with occlusion of the cilioretinal artery in the left eye was made.

The fluorescein angiogram was abnormal. There was delayed filling of the cilioretinal artery—it did not fill before the central retinal artery—and there was late staining of the disc (Figs. 3, 4, 5).

The patient was tapered off steroid medication. Her symptoms abated, but a small residual scotoma persists.

DISCUSSION

Papillophlebitis is a benign retinal vasculitis occurring in young, otherwise healthy adults.[1-3] It is almost always a unilateral process. Clinically papillophlebitis resembles an impending central retinal vein occlusion; the disc is swollen and the veins are engorged and tortuous. In addition

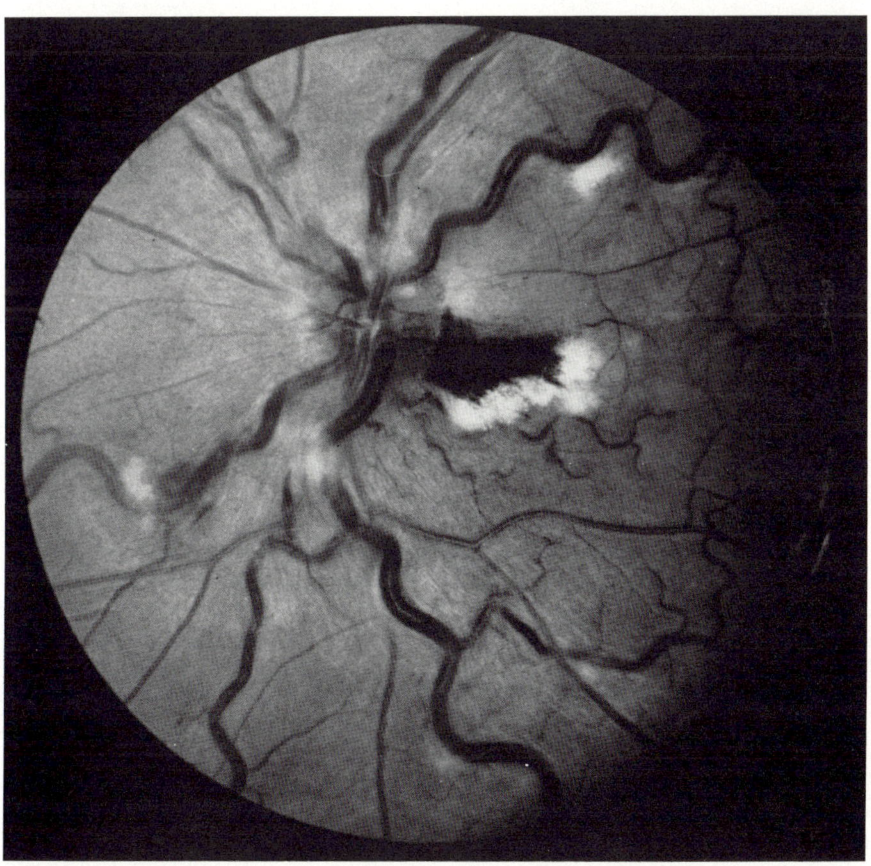

Fig. 2. Case 2. Fundus photograph of the left eye. A large intraretinal flame shaped hemorrhage extends temporally from the disc. Note the attenuation of the cilioretinal artery as it emerges from the disc at 2 o'clock.

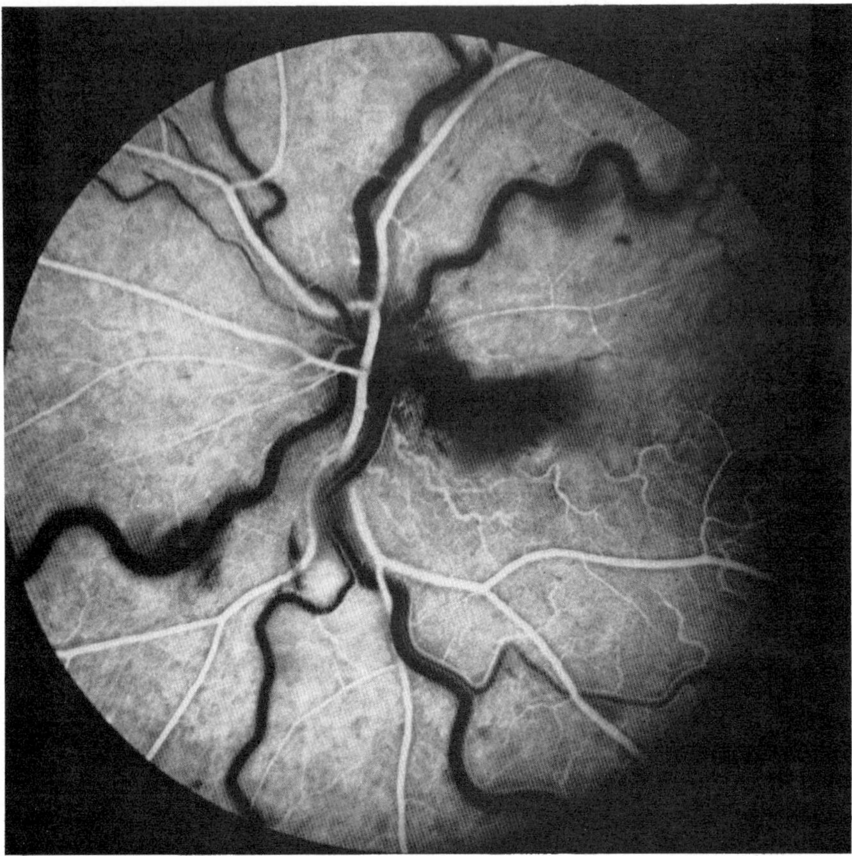

Fig. 3. Case 2. Fluorescein angiogram of the left eye. *Arterial* phase. Note that the cilioretinal artery has not filled temporally indicating delay in flow. Veins are dilated and scattered hemorrhages are seen.

there are peripapillary and diffuse flame-shaped retinal hemorrhages scattered throughout the fundus. The fellow eye is usually normal with no evidence of vascular disease. In most cases excellent visual acuity is maintained. The patient's complaints are those of foggy vision in one eye. Visual field testing may demonstrate an enlarged blind spot. The course of the disease runs from six to eighteen months, and its sequelae are confined to retinal sheathing and mild mottling of the pigment epithelium in the macular area. In addition, papillophlebitis may present as unilateral disc edema which clinically is similar to papilledema from other causes[4]; however, the presence of spontaneous venous pulsations in the unaffected fellow eye rules out increased intracranial pressure.

The pathogenesis of this disease remains uncertain. Cogan[5] and others[3, 6] have pos-tulated that papillophlebitis may be due to a mild retinal phlebitis leading to obstruction of the central retinal vein in or around the optic nerve head. The benign course of this disease in young individuals is thought in part to be due to the development of compensatory retino-ciliary shunt vessels.

Papillophlebitis belongs to a wide spectrum of retinal vasculitis. Cogan[5] divided retinal vasculitis into three groups: mild, moderate, and severe. Papillophlebitis represents the mild form, which is characterized by its occurrence in young adults with signs of partial venous occlusion. It involves only the venous side of the retinal circulation. Three of the ten patients in his series had signs of a systemic vasculitis (i.e., Systemic Lupus, cerebral vasculitis, and a superficial skin vasculitis). Characteristically there is total resolution of the symptoms; venous sheathing and mottling of the pig-

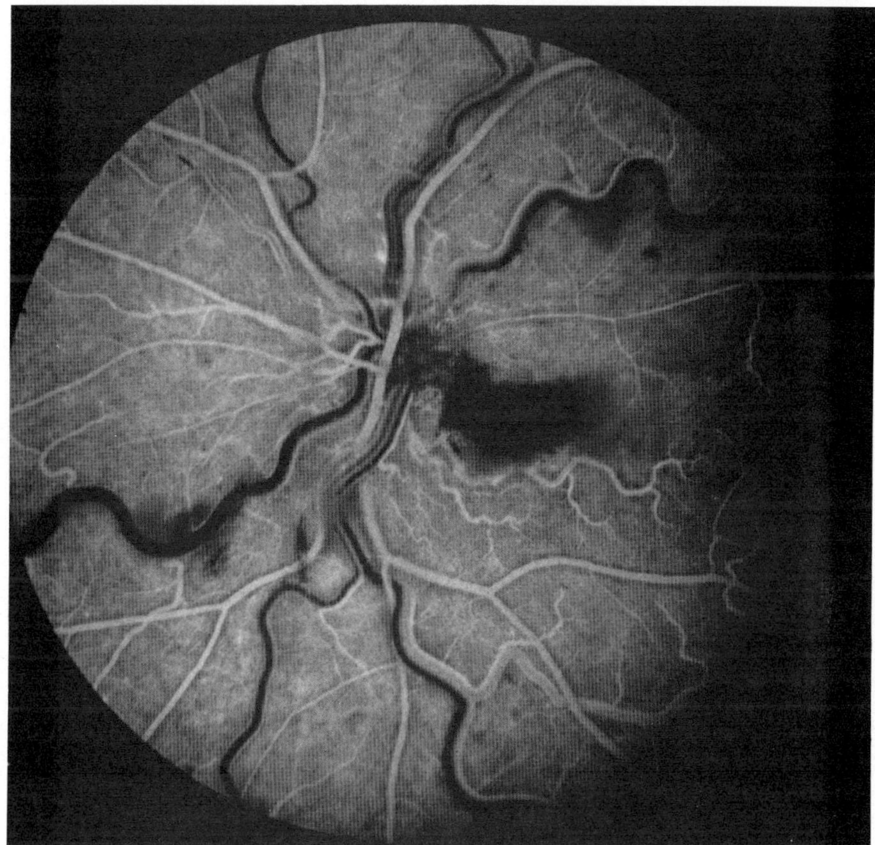

Fig. 4. Case 2. Fluorescein angiogram of the left eye. *Early venous* phase.

ment epithelium are the usual ophthalmo-scopic residua. It does not recur. Because of its benign course no pathologic specimens are available.

Moderate vasculitis is a more serious condition which is often bilateral and involves both the arteries and the veins of the retinal circulation. It is not confined to young adults; patients range in age from 14 to 62 years of age. In Cogan's[5] series permanent visual loss was encountered in several of these patients.

At the far end of the spectrum is severe vasculitis. It occurs more commonly in males over a wide range of ages. It tends to be bilateral and involves both the arteries and the veins in the retina. The visual prognosis is guarded with visual loss due to arterial occlusion, retinal detachment, and absolute glaucoma which are frequently encountered in this group of patients. It should be emphasized that moderate and severe vasculitis are distinctly different disease states than simple benign papillophlebitis.

While the first case presented in this report illustrates the typical presentation and course of papillophlebitis, the second is unique and provides us with the opportunity to study the pathophysiology of the disease. It is most likely that the papillophlebitis caused the occlusion of the cilioretinal artery on a mechanical basis. The marked edema of the optic nerve head may have caused compression of the cilioretinal artery on the disc with resultant ischemia in its distribution. Alternatively it is possible that the marked rise in the central venous pressure may have caused a decrease in the perfusion pressure in the cilioretinal artery circulation to a point of ischemia. The perfusion pressure of the retinal circulation is determined by the difference between two factors: the pressure in

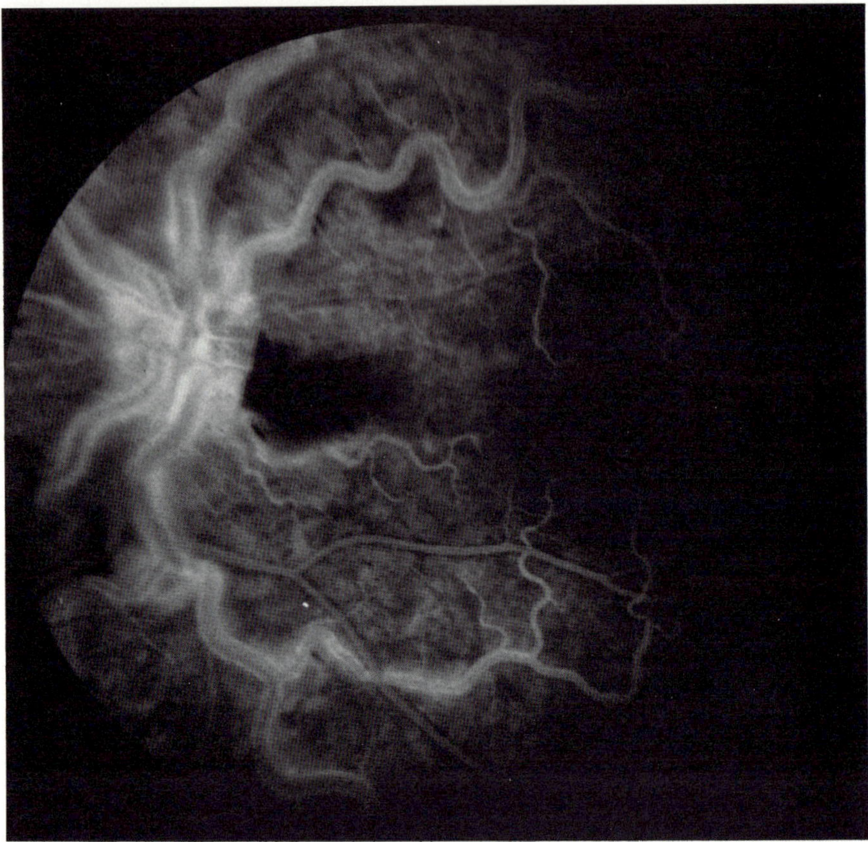

Fig. 5. Case 2. Fluorescein angiogram of the left eye. *Late phase.* Note the perivascular staining and hyperfluorescence of the disc.

the arterial system minus the pressure in the venous system.[7] In papillophlebitis, Hart, Sanders, and Miller[1] have shown that the arterial pressure is normal in both the affected and the normal eye, but the venous pressure is markedly elevated, approaching the diastolic arterial pressure. The retinal ischemia in our second case is most likely due to a decrease in the perfusion pressure in the cilioretinal artery circulation.

Fluorescein angiography demonstrates abnormalities confined to the dilated retinal veins. Areas of perivenous fluorescence suggesting a localized vasculitis are seen. Capillary dilatation and micro-aneurysms occur in more severe cases. Cystoid macular edema may be present and can account for a more pronounced visual loss than is usually associated with this disease. The arterial phase of the angiogram is normal.

The role of corticosteroids in the treatment of this disorder remains controversial as the disease appears self-limited. While several studies have employed large doses of oral steroids,[4] we have used sub-Tenon's injections of steroids to avoid the hazards of systemic therapy.

The single most important feature of papillophlebitis is its benign course. Visual deficits are usually minimal despite the florid ophthalmoscopic picture. The patients are typically young healthy adults with no evidence of hypertensive or atherosclerotic vascular disease. The patient should be followed closely. Extensive invasive procedures are not indicated.

EDITOR'S NOTE

Several years ago, when a young physician's wife was referred down to see me, and the question of "papillophlebitis" was raised in the differential diagnosis, I really did not know how to differentiate a central retinal vein occlusion from papillophlebitis. Indeed, that patient (Case I in this chapter) was the first instance of this specific diagnosis that I recall having encountered. Since my friend, Dr. William F. Hoyt, had originally described papillophlebitis, I decided to call him up on the telephone and get the differentiating features straight "from the horse's mouth." I called Dr. Hoyt in San Francisco and asked—"Bill, how do *you really* differentiate a central vein occlusion from papillophlebitis?" He promptly replied—"I can't! That's why we put it in the journal that we did." I am quoting him from memory to the best of my ability, but he went on to say that he simply thought papillophlebitis was a form of vein occlusion that usually occurred in younger patients—without glaucoma—without diabetes—without hypertension—without systemic vascular disease—and that it appeared to have more likely an inflammatory etiology and a better prognosis. Therefore, he thought that steroids might be more logical in its treatment (than in the usual central vein occlusion) and that the chance of hemorrhagic glaucoma later might be less. This really helped me because if Dr. Hoyt really couldn't necessarily differentiate these ophthalmoscopically, that was of great help to someone out in the office! I believe knowing that historical point will help you, too! When you see one of these—

see if she has been on "the pill" and try to get her off, if she has. Then use subtenon's steroids and, if you like, anticoagulate her for six weeks. The prognosis should be good. Note that McLeod and Ring reported cilioretinal occlusion complicating a central vein occlusion, and, therefore, our case of cilioretinal occlusing complicating papillophlebitis would not be that unexpected. At any rate, here is a case of that, and this may help to point out the practical office aspects of this syndrome!

JLS

REFERENCES

1. Hart, C. D., Sanders, M. D. and Miller, S. J. H. Benign retinal vasculitis. Br. J. Ophthal. *55:*721 (1971).
2. Lonn, L. L. and Hoyt, W. F. Papillophlebitis. A course of protracted yet benign optic disc edema. Eye Ear Nose Throat Mon. *45:*77 (1966).
3. Lyle, T. K. and Wybar, K. Retinal vasculitis. Br. J. Ophthal. *45:*77 (1961).
4. Hayreh, S. S. Optic disc vasculitis. Br. J. Ophthal. *56:*652 (1972).
5. Cogan, D. G. Retinal and papillary vasculitis. In: *The William MacKenzie Centenary Symposium on Ocular Circulation in Health and Disease.* C. V. Mosby Co., St. Louis, 1969, pp. 249–270.
6. Vandervliet, S. K. Papillophlebitis associated with systemic thrombophlebitis. Ann. Ophthalmol. *9:* 171 (1977).
7. McLeod, D. and Ring, C. P. Cilio-retinal infarction after retinal vein occlusion. Br. J. Ophthalmol. *60:* 419 (1976).

9 Syphilitic Optic Perineuritis and Uveitis

Lanning B. Kline, M.D.
W. Bruce Jackson, M.D.

SUMMARY

A 51-year-old male presenting with normal visual acuity and swollen optic discs was admitted to hospital with the diagnosis of papilledema. During his neurological evaluation he developed uveitis, visual field nerve fiber bundle defects, and was subsequently found to have a reactive FTA-ABS serology in his serum, cerebrospinal fluid, and aqueous. This patient had optic perineuritis secondary to syphilis, and this rarely recognized clinical entity is discussed.

PERINEURITIS AND UVEITIS

Optic perineuritis is an inflammation of the meningeal sheaths of the optic nerve presenting as optic disc edema with essentially normal visual function.[1] As a unique clinical entity it has rarely been recognized. Recently we had the opportunity to study a patient who presented with optic perineuritis and then developed a uveitis. He was subsequently found to have active syphilis. We report this case to review the criteria for the diagnosis of optic perineuritis, to describe its resolution with appropriate therapy, and to emphasize syphilis in the differential diagnosis when dealing with ocular inflammation.

CASE REPORT

A 51-year-old male presented complaining of bilateral leg pains, decreased hearing, and black spots with blurred vision in both eyes of seven days duration. He denied previous systemic, venereal, or ocular disease. The visual acuity was 20/20 in both eyes. The pupillary reactions were normal, and the fields were full to confrontation. The extraocular movements were normal, and the optokinetic responses were symmetrical. Slit-lamp examination was normal in both eyes. Ophthalmoscopy revealed bilaterally swollen discs with engorged veins, dilated capillaries, a feathery dilatation of the peripapillary capillary plexus, and multiple infarcts on both nerve heads (Fig. 1). Apart from the venous dilatation, the retinal vessels were normal as was the rest of the retinal examination. The admitting diagnosis was bilateral papilledema. Complete medical and neurological examinations were normal except for evidence of previous cleft palate surgery and a maculopapular pruritic rash on the scrotum and penis which had been present for approximately ten days. The skin lesions were round and oval, 0.3–0.6 cm in diameter, appearing atrophic and whitish in some areas with a reddish border.

A complete blood count, serum chemistry, urinalysis, chest x-ray, skull x-ray, and brain scan were all normal. A Westergren erythrocyte sedimentation rate was elevated at 44 mm/hr. An EEG revealed a mild diffuse nonspecific disturbance. A computerized tomographic scan showed ventricular dilatation with moderate diffuse cortical atrophy.

Five days after admission, the visual acuity was still 20/20 in both eyes, but the slit lamp examination revealed mild bilateral conjunctival hyperemia. Numerous fine keratic precipitates with one plus cells and

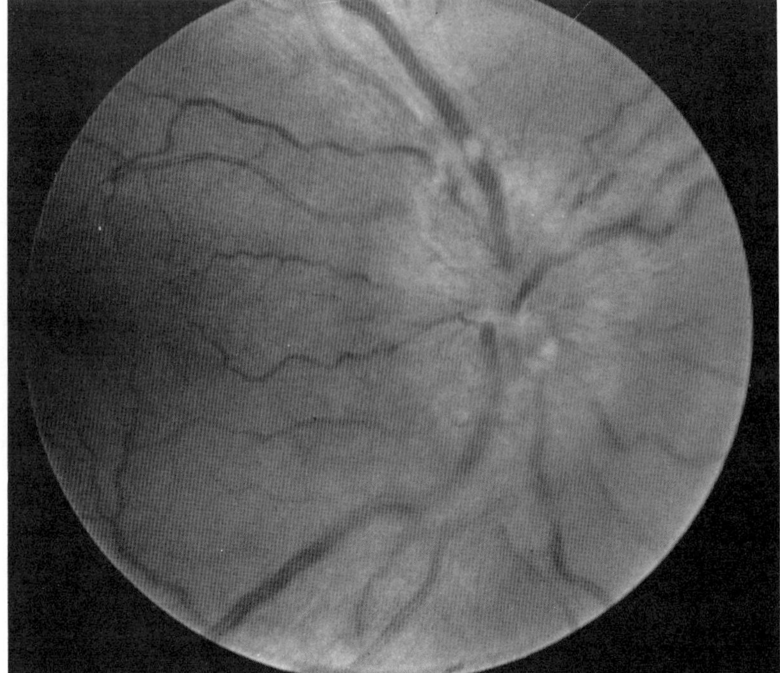

Fig. 1A

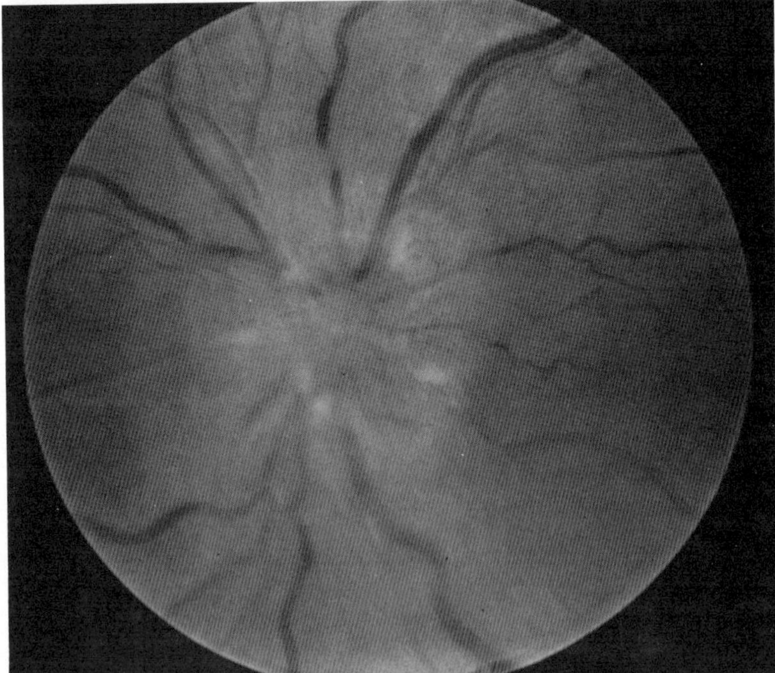

Fig. 1B

Fig. 1. Bilateral optic disc edema at the time of initial ophthalmological examination.

flare were noted in both eyes. The vitreous now revealed a two plus cellular reaction in both eyes. No snow balls or evidence of a focal chorioretinitis were noted. The appearance of the discs remained unchanged, and visual fields showed enlarged blind spots in both eyes. Additional laboratory investigations disclosed one positive and one negative antinuclear antibody, negative rheumatoid factor, and an elevated gamma globulin at 2.01 g% (normal 0.85–1.80 g%). Immunoelectrophoresis revealed normal IgG, IgA, and C3 serum levels, while the IgM level was elevated at 570 g% (normal, 50–150 g%). Fluorescent antibody titer for toxoplasmosis was negative as were skin tests for mumps, candida, trichophytin, varidase, and intermediate strength PPD. A temporal artery biopsy was performed which was normal.

The dermatologist performed a biopsy of his skin rash and labeled the lesions lichenoid sclerosis and atrophicus. A bilateral sensory neural hearing loss was confirmed by the otolaryngologist.

Two weeks following admission the visual acuity decreased to 20/50 in the right eye and 20/25 in the left eye. The anterior chamber reaction in both eyes was unchanged, but the right vitreous had become more hazy. Bilateral arcuate scotomas and nasal steps were now detected in both eyes by Goldmann field examination (Fig. 2). The neurological examination remained normal but lumbar puncture revealed an opening pressure of 200 mm of water (normal, 70–200 mm of water). There were 11 cells/mm^3, mainly monocytes and neutrophilis with a few lymphocytes and plasma cells. The protein was elevated at 82 mg%

(20–50 mg%) with an increased IgG at 16% of the total protein (normal up to 10.5%). The CSF sugar was normal at 55 mg% (50–80 mg%).

Although an etiologic diagnosis could not be made, the patient was started on Prednisone 60 mg a day because of the increasing vitreous reaction in the right eye and the progressive visual field changes suggestive of ischemic involvement at the nerve head.

Two days after commencing steroid therapy, the blood serology results returned from the Provincial laboratory indicating that the VDRL was reactive as was the FTA-ABS in both the serum and the cerebral spinal fluid. The VDRL titer in the serum was 1:32. An aqueous tap was performed revealing numerous spirochetes with the motility and morphology of *Treponema pallidum* as well as a positive FTA-ABS. On careful questioning the patient admitted to being a practicing homosexual. He was started immediately on a course of intramuscular Penicillin receiving 9.6 million units over four weeks while the systemic steroids were gradually tapered over this period.

One month after starting Penicillin and Prednisone therapy the visual acuity had improved in the right eye to 20/30 and in the left eye to 20/25. The anterior chamber

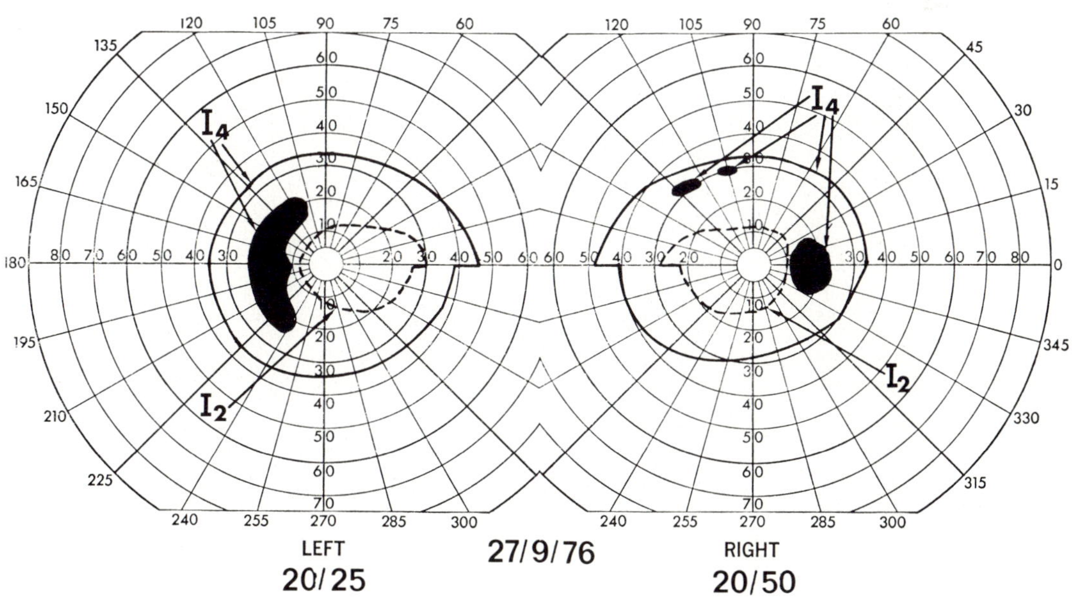

Fig. 2. Visual fields two weeks after initial exam showing bilateral nerve fiber bundle defects.

reaction had completely cleared and the disc edema and the vitreous haze were resolving. A flame shaped hemorrhage was present in the 8:00 position on the right disc (Fig. 3). The arcuate field defects cleared in both eyes leaving only a small nasal step in

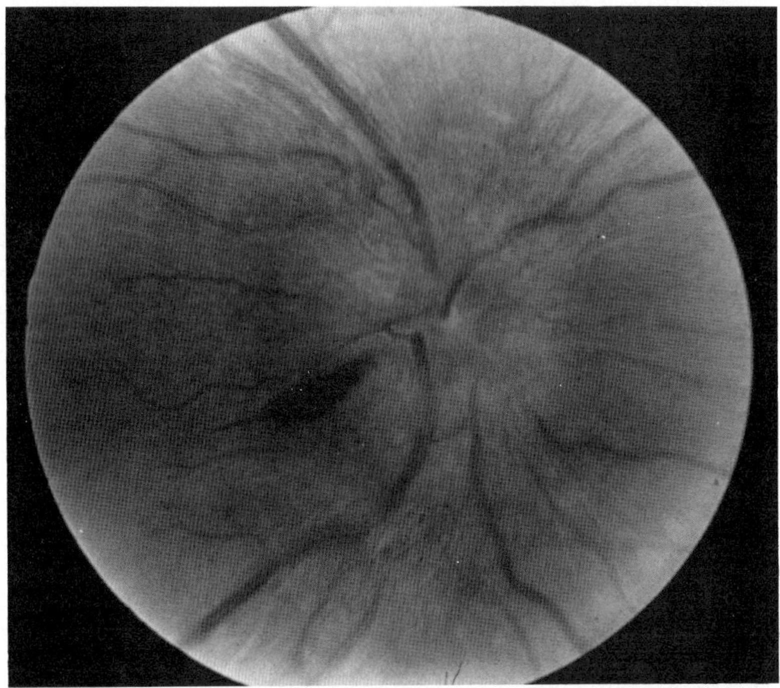

Fig. 3A

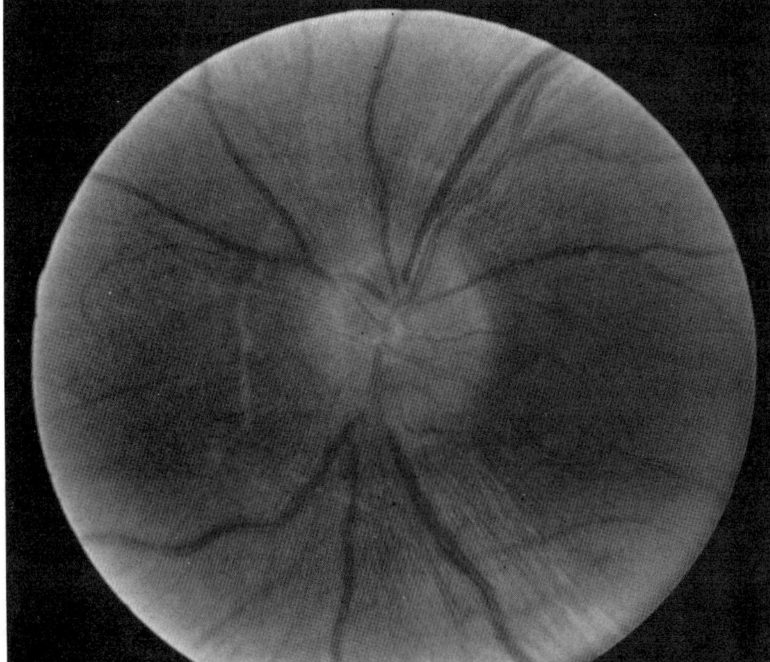

Fig. 3B

Fig. 3. Appearance of the optic discs six weeks after presentation and four weeks after commencement of penicillin therapy.

the RE, which finally disappeared on retesting four months later. Two months following therapy the visual acuity was 20/20 in both eyes and the ocular examination was felt to be entirely normal (Fig. 4). The serum VDRL was now reactive at a titer of 1:8, and when checked six months later was positive in undiluted serum only. The FTA-ABS remained weakly positive. Examination of the cerebral spinal fluid five months later revealed an opening pressure of 190 mm of water with normal protein and sugar. Cytologic examination showed 2 lymphocytes/mm[3]. The VDRL on the CSF was negative, but the FTA-ABS remained weakly positive.

DISCUSSION

Optic perineuritis is an infrequent clinical diagnosis and not well documented as a complication of ocular syphilis. Edmunds[2] pointed out the possibility of intracranial meningeal inflammation leading to optic disc edema and this was shown pathologically in a variety of diseases but not syphilis.[3] Cone and MacMillan[4] also discussed the pathology of optic perineuritis but did not describe its clinical course. Woods[5] reviewed the many possible manifestations of optic nerve involvement in syphilis, including this entity, but did not use the term optic perineuritis. Walsh and Hoyt[6] specifically discuss syphilitic optic perineuritis, and they suggest that infiltrative diseases of the meninges can also produce this clinical picture.

In discussing the pathogenesis of optic perineuritis, Edmunds and Lawford[3] pointed out that both tumors and infections of the central nervous system could cause meningeal inflammation with direct extension along the optic nerves producing optic disc edema. In our case, as evidence of widespread meningeal inflammation, there was diminished hearing, bilateral leg pains, pleocytosis and elevated protein in the cerebrospinal fluid, and electroencephalographic and CAT scan abnormalities.

The pathology of optic perineuritis[3, 4, 7] is one of a leptomeningitis with invasion of the optic nerve septa by inflammatory cells. The peripheral portions of the nerve are contiguous with the inflammatory process while the axial portions are spared. The progression and resolution of the visual field changes in our case correlates with the pathology of optic perineuritis. Nerve fiber bundle defects were observed, and this could be explained by peripheral optic nerve inflammation. At no time was a central scotoma noted, indicating that the axial regions of the optic nerves remained essentially uninvolved.

It is important to distinguish optic perineuritis from other causes of optic disc edema with essentially normal visual function, including papillophlebitis, papillitis with normal visual acuity, and papilledema. Papillophlebitis or benign retinal vasculitis[8, 9] is characterized by minimally reduced visual acuity, no relative afferent pupillary defect, optic disc edema, and strikingly engorged and tortuous retinal veins. It is this last feature, along with its unilaterality, that differentiates papillophlebitis from optic perineuritis. Papillitis with normal visual acuity presents as a swollen optic disc, with an afferent pupillary defect, cells in the vitreous, and a visual field nerve fiber bundle defect.[10] The fact that it is unilateral with a pupillary defect and has cells in the vitreous distinguishes it from optic perineuritis. As Walsh and Hoyt[11] have noted, papilledema is very difficult to differentiate from optic perineuritis. The clinical appearance may be identical and the differentiation can only be made by measuring the cerebrospinal fluid pressure. In papilledema this is elevated while in optic perineuritis it is within normal limits. Therefore, accurate measurement of intracranial pressure is essential in order to make the diagnosis of optic perineuritis. However, a lumbar puncture should only be done after an appropriate neurological evaluation has been completed.

It is difficult to state with certainty the precise stage of our patient's syphilitic infection. The EEG abnormalities reflect diffuse central nervous system involvement while the CAT scan revealed cortical atrophy. These findings suggest the late or tertiary stage—symptomatic neurosyphilis. However, the maculopapular skin rash occurs rarely in late syphilis,[12] being more commonly observed in the secondary stage.[13] Also, uveitis is most frequently seen

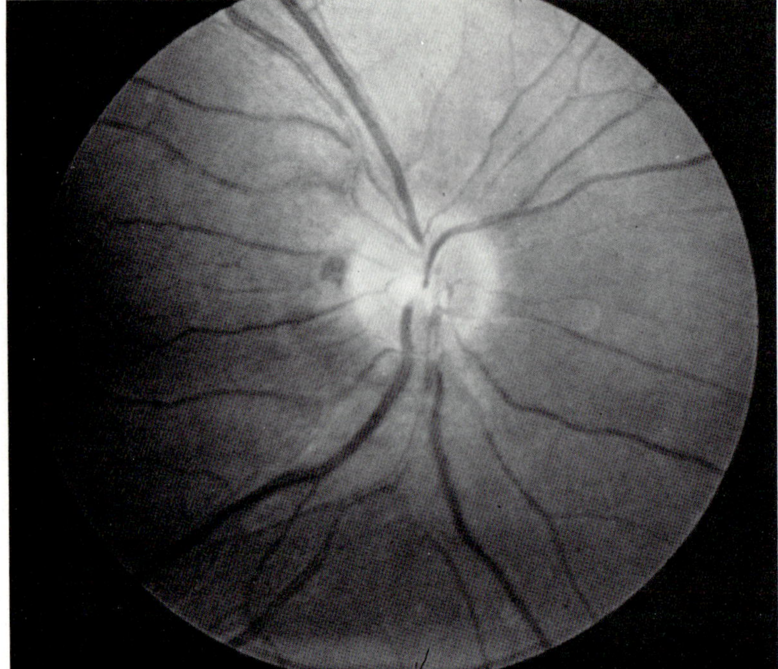

Fig. 4A

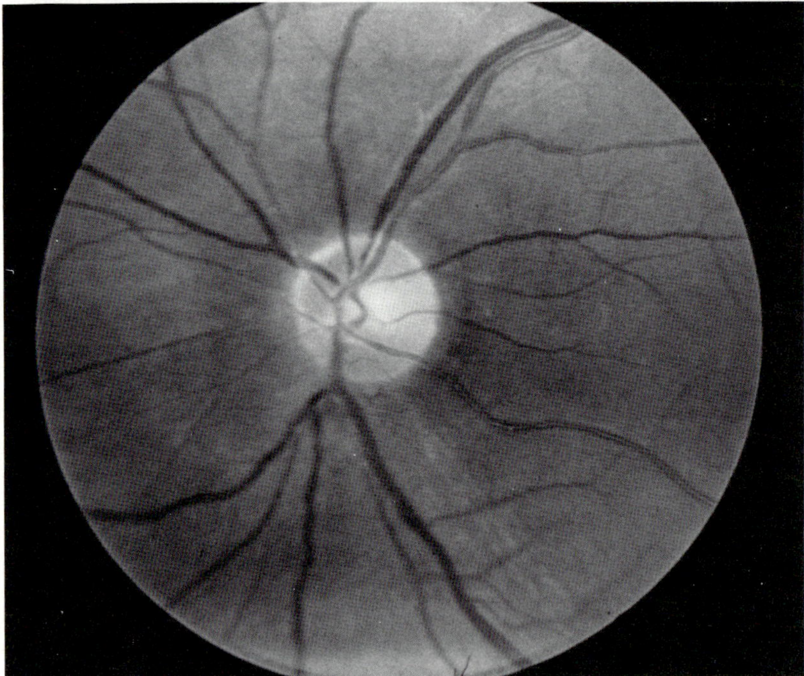

Fig. 4B

Fig. 4. Two months after completion of penicillin therapy, the optic discs have returned to normal. There is a focal area of disturbance of temporal peripapillary pigment epithelium of the right eye.

during secondary stage,[14] but certainly occurs in late syphilis.[15] Although it is known that a uveitis can cause disc edema,[16] the sequence of events in our case report demonstrates that the uveitis followed the disc edema. Presumably the syphilitic inflammatory process became more widespread and involved the uveal tract. It is our opinion this case represents late secondary syphilis.

The patient underwent extensive investigations for his uveitis; only the abnormal serology and aqueous studies revealed the etiologic agent. Although spiral forms were seen in the aqueous of our patient, it has been shown that these treponemes are not necessarily *T. pallidum*, even if a fluorescent antibody technique is employed.[17, 18] The major investigative effort in the diagnosis of ocular syphilis has been an attempt to identify *T. pallidum* in the aqueous. With the recognized problems of the fluorescent antibody technique,[19] possibly the detection of specific anti-*T. pallidum* antibody in the aqueous using the FTA-ABS technique would be more reliable. In our patient the aqueous FTA-ABS was strongly reactive, and other reports of ocular syphilis have mentioned a reactive aqueous serology.[20, 21] Just as the blood-brain barrier may allow the serum serology to be reactive and that of the cerebrospinal fluid to be nonreactive, so the blood-aqueous barrier might play a similar role. Thus, in a patient with uveitis a reactive FTA-ABS aqueous serology would support the diagnosis of ocular inflammation secondary to syphilis while a nonreactive FTA-ABS aqueous serology would make this diagnosis less likely.

Our patient was treated as a case of symptomatic neurosyphilis. Recent literature has cautioned about the difficulty in treating both ocular and neurosyphilis.[22-25] The prompt clinical improvement seen in our patient, along with falling VDRL titers and return of the cerebrospinal fluid to normal, all point to adequate antibiotic therapy for the present time. However, long-term follow-up is necessary by both the ophthalmologist and neurologist, for *T. pallidum* has been shown to survive for long periods of time in both ocular and nervous tissue even after large doses of penicillin.[23] Currently two explanations have been presented to account for this difficulty with therapy.[26] First, penicillin being a bactericidal antibiotic is effective against growing organisms and would allow nonreplicating *T. pallidum* to survive. Second, the possibility also exists that spirochetal *L*-forms may be present, and penicillin is ineffective against organisms lacking a cell wall.

EDITOR'S NOTE

It is important to emphasize to the clinician that syphilis is still around—that it is still causing active eye and neurologic disease—and that the only way to make the diagnosis is to have a high index of suspicion. It may be worthwhile to emphasize the five commonest ocular indications for a serum FTA-ABS test. These are—interstitial keratitis, light-near dissociation of the pupil, uveitis, optic atrophy, and a retinitis pigmentosa like fundus. The five commonest neurologic syndromes pointing for a serum FTA-ABS test are: asymptomatic neurosyphilis, meningeal neurosyphilis, vascular neurosyphilis, tabes, and paresis. It is *inadequate* to get *only* a serum *VDRL* test in a patient in whom you suspect late ocular or neurosyphilis—you should *ALSO get* a *serum FTA-ABS* test. Several state health departments are not really cognizant of the frequence of late ocular and neurosyphilis and make it difficult for the clinician to get a serum FTA-ABS test. The problem is NOT getting an FTA-ABS test when you have a reactive VDRL to diagnose a biologic false positive. The *problem* is making the diagnosis of late syphilis when the patient has a nonreactive serum VDRL, but a reactive serum FTA-ABS test! Finally, when you see an eye patient with a reactive serum FTA-ABS test, you do *NOT* have to rush in and do a *lumbar puncture* simply on that fact alone. An important paper in this regard was by *Traviesa, D. C. et al.* in *Ann. Neurol.* 4 (6): 524–530, Dec. 1978. It is entitled "Cerebrospinal Fluid Findings in Asymptomatic Patients with Reactive Serum Fluorescent Treponemal Antibody Absorption Tests." He studied 39 patients with reactive serum FTA-ABS tests, and he was talking about syphilis alright, because the TPI was also reactive in 30 (77%). The TPI test is known to be less sensitive than the FTA-ABS. It is held in very high repute for specificity, however (although it is so difficult for you to obtain one that you can just about forget it!). The thing to do is: (1) have a high index of suspicion, (2) get a serum FTA-ABS test, (3) if the latter is reactive, take a *tight history*, and (4) when in doubt, treat the patient. I frequently give an eye patient erythromycin 1 g/day for 20 days or 750 mg/day for six weeks. That is helpful in a private patient who does not want to come back frequently for penicillin injections and who is cooperative. Finally, the patient reported in this chapter was said to be a practicing homosexual and that should be remembered in the increasing incidence of venereal diseases.

JLS

REFERENCES

1. Walsh, F. B. *Clinical Neuro-ophthalmology.* Williams and Wilkins, Baltimore, 1947, p. 666.
2. Edmunds, W. Optic neuritis in intra-cranial disease. Trans. Ophthalmol. Soc. UK *1:*115 (1881).
3. Edmunds, W. and Lawford, J. B. Examination of the optic nerves in cases of intra-cranial disease, with remarks on the immediate causation of optic neuritis. Trans. Ophthalmol. Soc. UK *3:*138 (1883).
4. Cone, W. and MacMillan, J. A. The optic nerve and papilla. In *Cytology and Cellular Pathology of the Nervous System.* W. Penfield (Ed.), Paul B. Hoeber Inc., New York, 1932, p. 852.
5. Woods, A. C. Syphilis of the eye. Am. J. Syph. Gon. Ven. Dis. *27:*133 (1943).
6. Walsh, F. B. and Hoyt, W. F. *Clinical Neuro-ophthalmology.* Williams and Wilkins, Baltimore, 1969, p. 1581.
7. Lindenberg, R., Walsh, F. B., and Sacles, J. G. *Neuro-pathology of Vision: An Atlas.* Lea and Febiger, Philadelphia, 1973, p. 106.
8. Lonn, L. and Hoyt, W. F. Papillophlebitis. A case of protracted benign optic disc edema. Eye Ear Nose Throat Mon. *45:*62 (1966).
9. Hart, C. D., Sanders, B. D., and Miller, S. J. H. Benign retinal vasculitis. Br. J. Ophthalmol. *55:* 721 (1971).
10. Daroff, R. B. and Smith, J. L. Intraocular optic neuritis with normal visual acuity. Neurology *15:* 409 (1965).
11. Walsh, F. B. and Hoyt, W. F. *Clinical Neuro-ophthalmology.* Williams and Wilkins, Baltimore, 1969, p. 609.
12. Domonkos, A. N. *Andrews' Diseases of the Skin.* W. B. Saunders Co., Toronto, 1971, p. 420.
13. Olansky, S. and Norins, L. C. Syphilis and other trepanematoses. In: *Dermatology in General Medicine.* T. B. Fitzpatrick (Ed.), McGraw-Hill, Toronto, 1971, p. 1960.
14. Duke-Elder, S. and Perkins, E. S. Diseases of the uveal tract. In: *System of Ophthalmology.* S. Duke-Elder (Ed.), C. V. Mosby Co., St. Louis, 1966, Vol. 9, p. 297.
15. Moore, J. E. and Gieske, M. Syphilitic iritis: a study of 249 patients. Am. J. Ophthalmol. *14:*110 (1931).
16. Kimura, S. J., Thygeson, P. and Hogan, M. J. Signs and symptoms of uveitis. Am. J. Ophthalmol. *47:*171 (1959).
17. Golden, B. and Thompson, H. S. Implications of spiral forms in the eye. Surv. Ophthalmol. *14:*179 (1969).
18. Ryan, S. J., Nell, E. E. and Hardy, P. H. A study of aqueous humor for the presence of spirochetes. Am. J. Ophthalmol. *73:*250 (1972).
19. Rios Montenegro, E. N., Nicol, W. G. and Smith, J. L. Treponemalike forms and artifacts. Am. J. Ophthalmol. *68:*197 (1969).
20. Smith, J. L. Acute blindness in early syphilis. Arch. Ophthalmol. *90:*256 (1973).
21. Crouch, E. R. and Goldberg, M. F. Retinal periarteritis secondary to syphilis. Arch. Ophthalmol. *93:*384 (1975).
22. Smith, J. L. *Spirochetes in Late Seronegative Syphilis, Penicillin Not Withstanding.* Charles C Thomas, Springfield, 1969.
23. Ryan, S. J., Hardy, P. H., Hardy, J. W. and Oppenheim, E. H. Persistence of virulent Treponema pallidum despite penicillin therapy in congenital syphilis. Am. J. Ophthalmol. *73:*258 (1972).
24. Mohr, J. A., Griffiths, W., Jackson, R., Saddah, H., Bird, P. and Riddle, J. Neurosyphilis and penicillin levels in cerebrospinal fluid. J. Am. Med. Assoc. *236:*2208 (1976).
25. Tramont, E. C. The case against benzathine penicillin as the treatment for neurosyphilis. In: *Neuro-ophthalmology Update.* J. L. Smith (Ed.), Masson, New York, 1977, p. 325.
26. Schlaegel, T. F. and O'Connor, G. R. Metastatic nonsuppurative uveitis. Int. Ophthalmol. Clin. *17*(3):87 (1977).

Hypoplasia of the Optic Nerve and Disc

Lois Lloyd, M.D., F.R.C.S.(C)
J. Raymond Buncic, M.D., F.R.C.S.(C)

Optic nerve hypoplasia presents a challenge to all ophthalmologists. Its early detection and differentiation from optic atrophy permits more accurate prognosis and may avoid unnecessary, painful, expensive investigations. Furthermore, by indicating a need for neurologic and endocrinologic investigation for associated anomalies,[11, 23, 25, 31] accurate diagnosis permits better over-all management of the patient and informed counseling of his family.

Optic nerve hypoplasia is a congenital, nonprogressive condition characterized by a paucity of axons within the optic nerve. It was first reported in 1863 by Newman,[20] who diagnosed the condition in two sisters. For many years, optic nerve hypoplasia was considered a rarity, but now it is recognized as fairly common and more than 100 cases have been reported in the English literature.[1, 8, 11, 22] The clinical spectrum is large[11] and in many cases can be correlated with clinically measurable defects in visual function (i.e., decreased visual acuity and visual field loss). If extreme, the hypoplasia is easily recognizable by smallness of the optic-nerve head, a white peripapillary scleral band surrounding it, and in some cases pigmented mottling; the retinal vessels are relatively normal in size. Mild optic nerve hypoplasia may be more difficult to identify.

Differentiation from Aplasia. Optic-nerve aplasia is defined as complete absence of both optic-nerve axons and retinal vessels[7, 27]; the view of the choroidal pattern of the fundus at the posterior pole is uninterrupted. Studies of cats, blind because of aplasia, showed integrity of the sensory ret-

ina, retinal pigment epithelium and choroid over the posterior pole, but absence of the retinal nerve-fiber layer, optic nerve, and chiasm.[30] Optic-nerve aplasia in humans is unilateral in the vast majority of cases. It is associated with microphthalmia in some, and one case has been described[29] of bilateral aplasia of the optic-nerve, chiasm, and optic tracts, in an infant whose eyes appeared clinically normal but who had gross CNS abnormalities.

EMBRYOLOGY

It is thought that optic nerve hypoplasia results from a primary defect in differentiation of the retinal ganglion cell axons that grow toward the optic nerve and, eventually, the lateral geniculate body. The prosencephalon and its optic vesicles, the mesencephalon, and the rhombencephalon are evident at 28 days (4 mm). The anterior part of the forebrain forms the telencephalon and cerebral hemispheres, and the posterior part forms the diencephalon (including the optic vesicles), by the 9-mm stage.

Axons of the retinal ganglion cells reach the optic stalk by 19 mm and the lateral geniculate body by 25 mm; failure of the retinal ganglion cells to differentiate at the 13–15 mm stage, or of their processes to travel to the optic stalk by 19 mm, results in hypoplasia. The fissure of the optic stalk closes at the 19–20 mm stage and the optic stalk is completely filled with nerve fibers by eight weeks (30 mm), after which the optic nerve increases by glial proliferation and axonal myelination. A mesodermal sheath condenses around the optic nerve in the 27–31 mm stage.

The anterior wall of the diencephalon forms the lamina reunions when the anterior visual system is developing (16–22 mm). Damage in this area results in anomalies of the corpus callosum and septum pellucidum, which occur in some cases of optic nerve hypoplasia.[7, 16, 17]

ETIOLOGY AND PATHOLOGY

The exact cause of optic nerve hypoplasia remains unknown. The anomaly apparently represents a primary developmental failure due to some embryonic insult after six weeks' gestation, while the retinal ganglion cells and septum pellucidum are developing and the diencephalon is differentiating. Several etiologic factors have been suggested, most notably the mother's ingestion of drugs during the first trimester. For example, optic nerve hypoplasia has been reported in infants of mothers who had ingested toxic doses of quinine for its supposed abortifacient effect,[18] seven children (the optic nerve hypoplasia was bilateral in six) of epileptic mothers who were being treated with known teratogenic agents,[13] and in 17 children of severely diabetic mothers.[21] A few bilateral cases suggestive of autosomal dominant or recessive inheritance have been reported.[12, 29]

Hypoplasia of the optic nerve is due to deficiency of retinal ganglion cell axons. Histology shows partial or complete deficiency of the optic nerve axonal fibers, an appearance described in standard pathology texts as "atrophic" (Fig. 1).[28] In fact, clinical optic nerve hypoplasia may be pathologically a mixture of hypoplasia and atrophy, particularly in bilateral severe cases. The so-called homonymous hemioptic hypoplasia associated with congenital hemianopia is thought to result from intrauterine damage to the suprageniculate visual system, which produces descending, transynaptic optic atrophy evident at the optic disc. Frisén and Holmegaard[11] suggested that minimal optic nerve hypoplasia is the result of insult(s) that occurred during early embryologic development and allowed filling of the scleral opening, producing the classic double-ring sign. Injuries later during development might produce more severe optic nerve hypoplasia: failure of the residual nerve tissue to fill in the scleral opening results in a small nerve head with a large surrounding scleral rim. They further suggest that clinical optic nerve hypoplasia represents descending transynaptic atrophy, pathologically true hypoplasia, or both.[11] Although this hypothesis does not correspond to the strict definition of the term "hypoplasia," clinically it has merit.

CLINICAL DIAGNOSIS

The commonest clinical indication of optic nerve hypoplasia is unilateral blindness with severe optic hypoplasia and secondary strabismus. We have diagnosed optic nerve hypoplasia in some patients referred to us for investigation of optic atrophy. A blind child who has roving eye movements, loosely referred to as nystagmus, may have severe bilateral optic nerve hypoplasia. Persons with less severe unilateral optic nerve hypoplasia may remark that their vision in one eye has been slightly "lazy" for years, and many of those with mild optic nerve hypoplasia have no symptoms related to vision.

Severe optic nerve anomaly is readily recognizable. The nerve head is small, pale, and surrounded by a wide corona of white sclera, with pigmentation in the form of stippling or of a border outlining the scleral rim. The large retinal vessels may appear relatively normal. Examination of the nerve-fiber layer shows clear-cut hypoplastic changes: as expected, the layer is thin (diffusely or segmentally, depending on the pattern of hypoplasia at the nerve head), and retinal vessels that normally are buried within the thick nerve-fiber layer are exposed. The superficial retinal vessels are highlighted by "flat" light reflexes from the retinal/vitreous interface that stop abruptly along the vessel wall and give undue prominence to the retinal vessel network. Scrutiny of the retina in the peripapillary area reveals deficient opacity and striations of the nerve fiber layer.

Indirect ophthalmoscopy shows intense redness of the fundus; this coloration is due to the thinness of the nerve fiber layer,

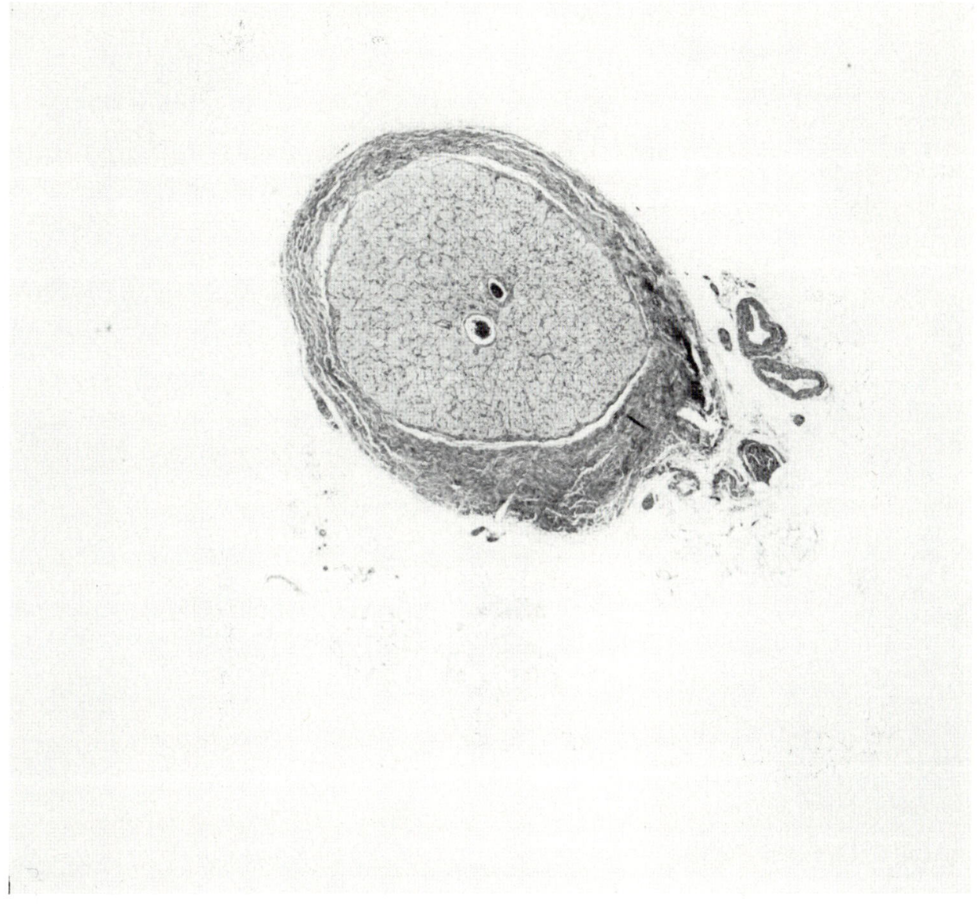

Fig. 1. Case 8: transverse section of hypoplastic optic nerve, demonstrating small diameter, paucity of myelinated axonal fibers, and prominent glial component (Luxol fast blue stain, magnification × 35). (Courtesy of Dr. W. Hunter, Department of Ophthalmology, University of Toronto.)

resulting in absence of the opalescent nerve fiber layer reflexes, superficiality of the retinal blood vessels, and flattening of the macular mound. These abnormalities are most readily appreciable in children and young adults, because of the greater prominence of their superficial retinal light reflexes. Detailed examination of the optic disc is best achieved through a widely dilated pupil, by direct ophthalmoscopy with a red-free light.

Diagnosis is difficult if the size of the optic disc is within normal limits; helpful clues are a fine peripapillary double ring and thinness of the peripapillary nerve fiber layers (Fig. 2). It may not be possible to identify mild optic nerve hypoplasia by direct observation of only size and color of the optic disc. Paucity of the disc's nerve substance is a more reliable diagnostic criterion. This is best determined by studying the appearance of the optic disc and peripapillary retina on good-quality photographs of the fundus.[11]

Uncooperative and restive patients (infants, young children, and the mentally retarded) present special problems in diagnosis. A disc that appears white as it flashes by the observer must be reexamined with the child under sedation or general anesthesia.

Associated Ophthalmologic Findings

Loss of vision reflects the degree and pattern on optic nerve hypoplasia. Most case reports are of patients who have severely defective vision, but visual acuity

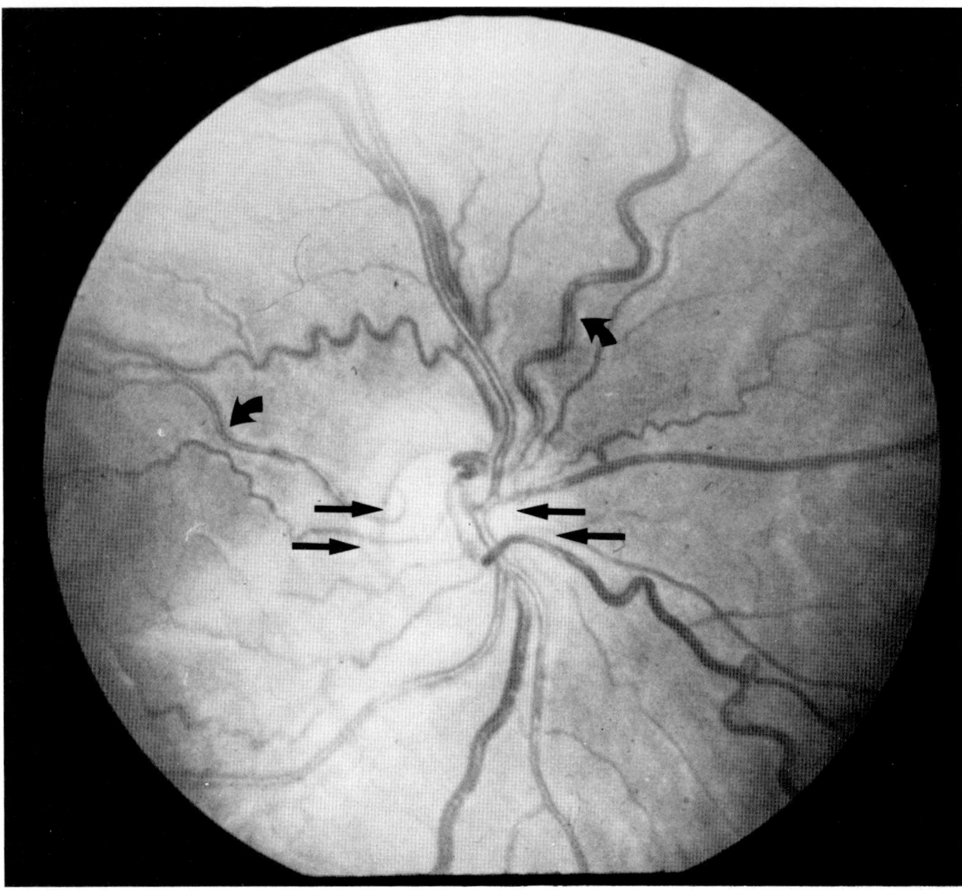

Fig. 2. Mild optic nerve hypoplasia. The optic disc is almost of normal size (inner arrows). Scleral-rim exposure produces a double-ring sign (outer arrows). Retinal light reflexes lying alongside vessels (arrow) demonstrate mild retinal thinness.

may be normal on clinical measurement. Amblyopia resulting from moderate hypoplasia accompanied by strabismus may represent a mixture of organic and strabismic visual loss, and in children this should probably be treated by occlusion therapy.

Severe bilateral optic nerve hypoplasia in infants results in nystagmus and clinical blindness, but unilateral loss of vision may be unsuspected by the parents until secondary strabismus develops; the strabismus responds poorly to surgery and tends to recur. See-saw nystagmus has been reported in a case of optic nerve hypoplasia,[5] but we find this rare form in children most commonly associated with optic atrophy secondary to a large craniopharyngioma. Pupillary testing will reveal afferent defects in severe optic nerve hypoplasia, reflecting the decreased number of optic nerve fibers; Mar-

cus Gunn pupil is usually apparent in unilateral severe cases, but clinical demonstration of afferent pupillary defects may be difficult in mild or symmetric cases.

Visual field defects associated with optic nerve hypoplasia also reflect the severity and pattern of nerve fiber loss.[23] Altitudinal and sector visual field defects may accompany segmental hypoplasia[21] and bitemporal defects; unilateral temporal hemianopia and peripheral visual field constriction have been reported.[14] Bitemporal defects are differentiated from the classical chiasmal variety by their failure to respect the vertical meridian. Hoyt *et al.*[15] described in detail that form of congenital hemianopia which is associated with "homonymous hemioptic hypoplasia"; characteristically it appears as segmental disc hypoplasia, pallor, double-ring sign, and a thin nerve fiber layer in the area that serves the blind portion of the retina. Recognition of this appearance permits diagnosis of hemianopia in a child in whom accurate visual-field testing is not possible. These abnormalities are bilateral but asymmetric: they are more dramatic in the ipsilateral eye (in which the optic disc lies within the blind half of the retina), and only diffuse mild hypoplastic change is evident in the contralateral optic disc (which lies in the seeing retinal tissue).

Other Associated Findings

Optic nerve hypoplasia is usually an isolated anomaly, and ocular manifestations constitute most of the reported associated defects. These include anophthalmos, microphthalmos, coloboma of the choroid and/or optic disc, blepharophimosis, dacryostenosis, ptosis, strabismus, palsy of the third, fourth, or sixth cranial nerve, and paresis of upgaze.

Optic nerve hypoplasia has been reported associated with hypertelorism, midline defects in the palate, lip, and maxilla,[8,26] oxycephaly, facial hemiatrophy, cerebral atrophy, cerebral palsy, epilepsy and gross anomalies involving the medulla, pons, and cerebellum.[8,11] In 1956 de Morsier described a syndrome of septo-optic dysplasia, consisting of absence of the septum pellucidum and bilaterial optic nerve hypoplasia[6] and characterized by growth hormone deficiency and poor vision;[9] the midline defect may involve the pituitary and optic chiasm also. Further, in 1970 Hoyt *et al.*[14] described the association of hypopituitarism with septo-optic dysplasia in children who have visual field defects and stunted growth; these patients, of both sexes, were the first offspring of very young mothers.

Optic nerve hypoplasia has been reported in one case of chondrodysplasia punctata[24] and we have observed another. The chondrodysplasia syndrome, first described by Conradi,[4] is characterized by skeletal dysplasia—stippling of the epiphyseal centers, saddle-nose deformity, hypertelorism, frontal bossing, arched palate, and short neck. The usual associated ocular abnormality is bilateral cataract. In addition, optic nerve hypoplasia has been diagnosed in one patient who had Down's syndrome and one who had died from cardiorenal-dysgenesis.[5]

INVESTIGATIONS

Particularly in children, if vision loss is severe or associated abnormalities are suspected, noninvasive radiologic investigations and, perhaps, neurologic assessment are valuable.

The diagnosis of optic nerve hypoplasia may be confirmed by demonstration of congenitally small optic canals. This is more readily apparent on axial tomograms of the canals than on plain optic foraminal views of the skull (Fig. 3).[19] The normal diameter of the optic foramen has a large variation (4–6 mm), and on optic canal tomograms the lower limit of normal is 5.5 mm diameter.[10] However, normal-sized optic canals may be accompanied by abnormally small optic nerves. B-scan ultrasonography may be useful in demonstrating the optic nerve diameter, which normally is at least 2 mm.[3] Coronal and saggital plane computed tomography (CT scan) of the orbit and cranial contents reveals abnormalities of the midline structure of the brain and the small optic nerves (Figs. 4 and 5)—and may obivate the need for pneumoencephalography (combined with tomography) to outline the optic nerve, chiasm, and third ventricle. Infants in whom hypopituitarism is suspected should be assessed and followed up by an endocrinologist as deficiencies may not become detectable for several years.

CASE REPORTS

The following case reports illustrate severe optic nerve hypoplasia, with and without other anomalies.

Case 1. Left-sided exotropia of 40 prism diopters was noted in a four-year-old boy who was small for his age (third percentile) but intelligent and in whom growth-hormone deficiency and hypothyroidism had been diagnosed.

Visual acuity was 20/20 OD but reduced to counting fingers at 1 ft OS. Examination of the left eye showed a small, pale optic disc and generally thin retinal nerve fiber layer (Fig. 6); OD was normal. Skull roentgenograms in foraminal views confirmed the abnormally small left optic foramen. No further investigations were done, and the amblyopia was not treated, in view of the organic nature of the visual loss.

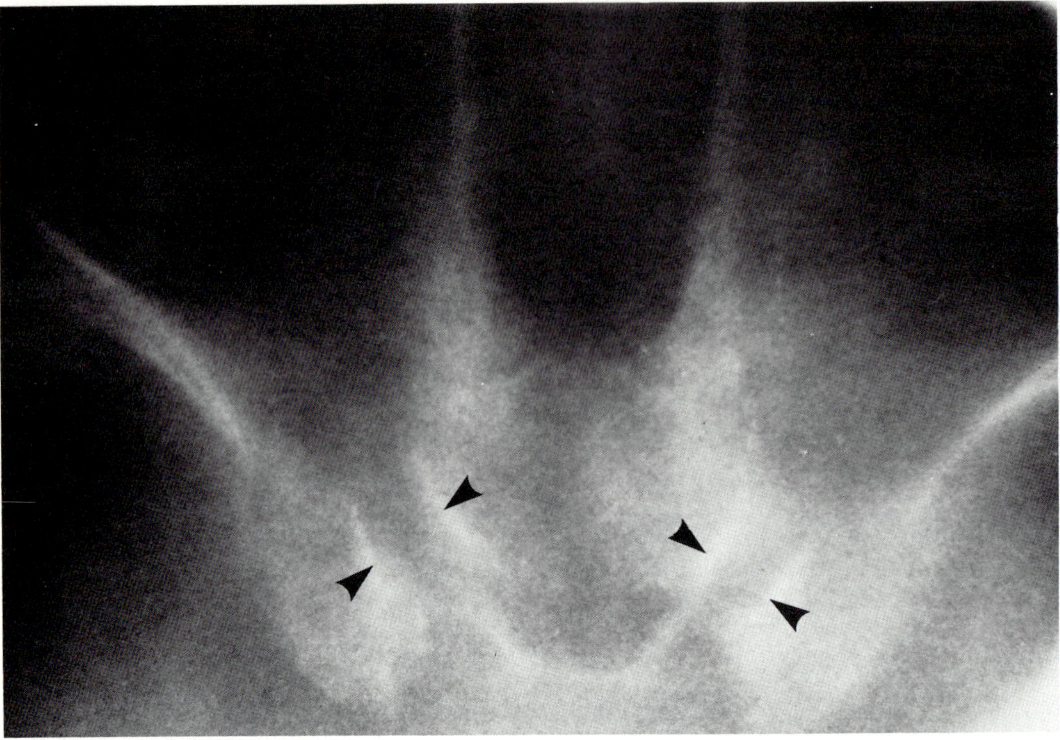

Fig. 3. Axial tomography of the optic canals demonstrates an abnormally small right optic canal and a normal left canal (arrows).

Case 2. Left optic nerve hypoplasia was diagnosed in a 4-year-old girl who had had left-sided exotropia from birth but was otherwise healthy. Her visual acuity was 20/20 OD and no light perception OS. Examination of the left fundus showed the optic nerve to be small and pale, apparently normal large retinal vessels lying superficially in thin nerve fiber layer, and flattened retina; the retinal light reflexes were abnormal, discretely outlining the vessels (Fig. 7). The OD was normal.

Skull roentgenograms were normal, but axial tomography showed a small (5 mm diameter) left optic canal. Severe left-sided optic nerve hypoplasia with secondary strabismus was diagnosed; no further investigations were undertaken, and the amblyopia was not treated.

Case 3. A baby girl, born at term, suffered fetal distress and apneic episodes shortly after birth. Her mother has had two elective abortions and hysterotomy for an ectopic pregnancy, and for six months before delivery of this fourth baby she had

taken phenobarbital and medroxyprogesterone acetate. The child had multiple congenital anomalies, including agenesis of the corpus callosum, hydrocephalus, talipes equinovarus, and bilateral optic-disc and retinal hypoplasia. She had epilepsy and hypotonia, also, and was mentally retarded. The EEG showed epileptiform discharges, and CT scan confirmed agenesis of the corpus callosum and atrophy of the right cerebral hemisphere. Optic canal tomography was not done.

A ventricular peritoneal shunt was inserted to manage the hydrocephalus when the infant was eight months old. Ophthalmologic examination at one year revealed fixation of both eyes in down gaze in an exotropic position of 45° and failure to follow light. Horizontal but not vertical eye movements were present, and no optokinetic response could be elicited. The diagnosis of severe bilateral optic nerve hypoplasia was confirmed.

Case 4. A five-year-old girl who had no family history of ocular disease was referred

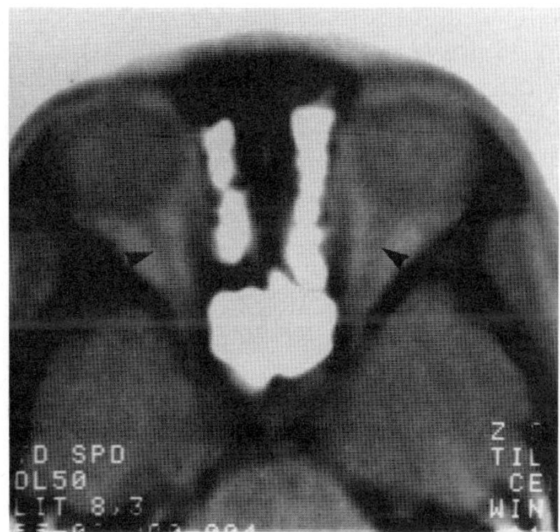

Fig. 4A

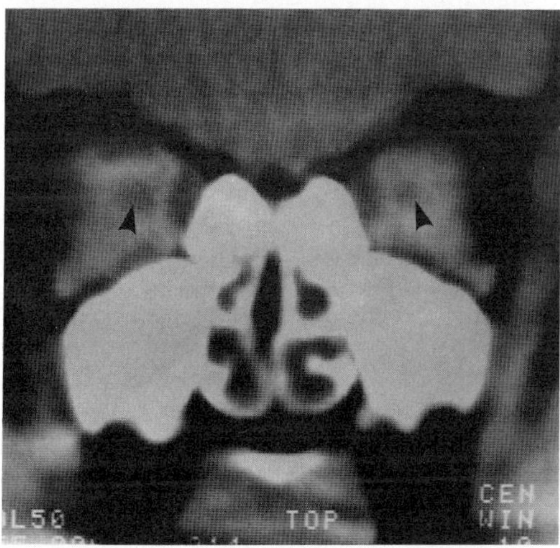

Fig. 4B

Fig. 4. Computed tomography of orbit: A. The left optic nerve is smaller than the (normal-sized) right one, seen in a transverse cut through the orbit. B. In coronal sections through orbits, the left optic nerve is small and the right optic-nerve diameter is normal. (Courtesy of Dr. C. Fitz, Department of Radiology, The Hospital for Sick Children, Toronto.)

for assessment of right esotropia. Vision was normal OS but restricted to identification of hand movement OD. There was an afferent defect of the right pupil, together with moderate hypoplasia of the optic disc; the disc had a double-ring sign, moderate diffuse thinning of the retina in the macular area, and segmental changes (nerve-fiber dropout or "gutters") in the superior and

inferior arcuate bundles (Fig. 8A & B). Latent right-sided nystagmus was present.

Tomography of the optic canals and CT scan of the head and orbits revealed no

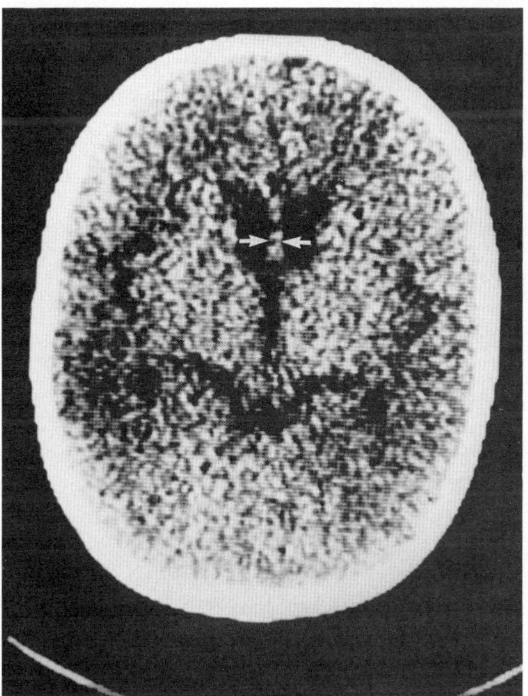

Fig. 5A

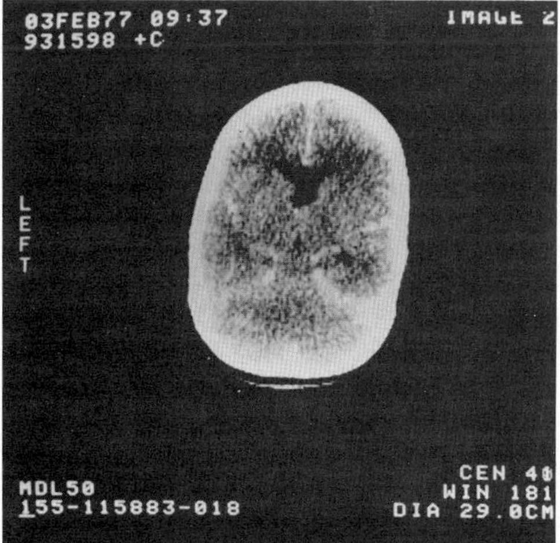

Fig. 5B

Fig. 5. Computed tomography of skull. A. Shows normal septum pellucidum separating the frontal horns (arrow). B. Illustrates absence of septum pellucidum, as in de Morsier's syndrome (e.g., Case 10). (Courtesy of Dr. C. Fitz.)

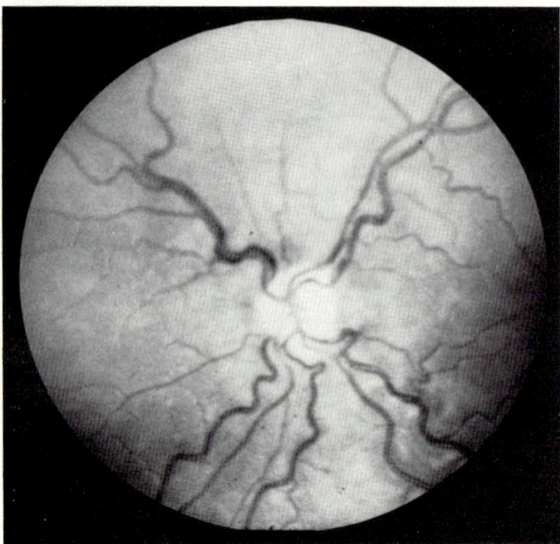

Fig. 6. Case 1: left optic nerve hypoplasia. The optic nerve head is small. Darkening of the fundus, indicating thinness, is most obvious nasal and temporal to the disc. Abnormal superficial light reflexes confirm superficiality of retinal blood vessels.

abnormality. The strabismus was surgically corrected for cosmetic reasons. The child's ocular status has not changed during three years' follow-up.

Case 5. This six-month-old boy had multiple congenital abnormalities (including plagiocephaly, deafness, hemangiomas of the scalp and left eyelid, and clubfeet) and was deaf and mentally retarded. There was a family history of migraine. Ophthalmologic examination revealed wandering, random, conjugate eye movements with occasional nystagmoid jerks on left gaze, anisocoria, and dilation of the right pupil; neither pupil reacted to light stimulation. Funduscopy revealed bilateral small discs, relatively small-caliber retinal vessels, and myopia (OD, −4.00 and OS, −3.50). Skull roentgenography showed severe cranial deformity and right lambdoid synostosis, optic-canal tomography showed a narrow distorted right canal and normal left canal, and ventriculography demonstrated cortical atrophy.

Case 6. A seven-month-old baby girl, the product of an uneventful pregnancy and delivery, appeared to be blind. Her visual fixational reflexes and opticokinetic responses were poor, but she appeared to respond to light shone directly into each eye. The pupils were equal and responded

very sluggishly to light. The eyes were straight but roved continuously. Both optic nerves were severely hypoplastic; the small optic nerve remnants were outlined by prominent white scleral rings. The fundi appeared dark red because of general hypoplasia of the retinal nerve fiber layer, maculae, and retinae. Skull roentgenograms and optic canal tomograms were normal. A CT scan to investigate CNS abnormalities was recommended, but the parents did not agree to further investigation.

Case 7. A 3½-year-old boy was thought by his mother to have poor vision. He had roving, conjugate, occasionally jerking eye movements. There was no visual response when bright lights or large objects were brought close; the pupils reacted minimally to light and much better to convergence. Funduscopy revealed bilateral severe optic nerve and retinal hypoplasia. Optic canal tomography and air encephalography and tomography of the chiasm revealed no CNS abnormality.

Case 8. This infant was born by Cesarean section at 39 weeks' gestation to a 39-year-old primigravida. She weighed 2.78 kg at birth, and head circumference was 34 cm. The pregnancy had been uneventful except for a mild upper respiratory illness in the first trimester, treated with oral antihistamines. Maternal nutrition had been

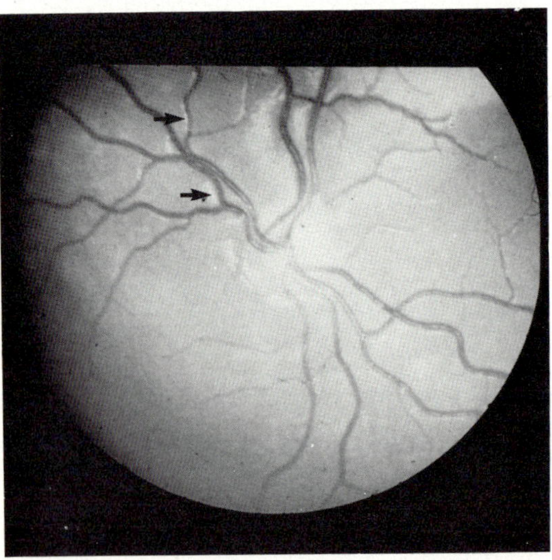

Fig. 7. Case 2: left optic nerve hypoplasia. The optic disc is small and the retina is thin, with light reflexes from the retinal surface coursing along the exposed vasculature (arrows).

good and alcohol intake minimal. The child did poorly from birth; she was lethargic and had a weak abnormal cry. Sucking movements were weak, and the Moro reflex was deficient. She kept her fists clenched but had a good grasp reflex. Her legs were generally hypotonic and response to pain was barely present. Phenobarbital only partly controlled neonatal myoclonic seizures.

Ocular examination revealed bilateral blepharophimosis. The pupils showed some reactivity to light. Both retinae were generally thin and had flat maculae, and the optic nerves were pale, small, and hypoplastic.

The EEG showed slight abnormality and poor organization, with high-amplitude slow activity, and CT scan showed slight dilation of the ventricles and agenesis of the corpus callosum. No specific cause was found for the child's congenital anomalies. She never thrived, and died aged three months of aspiration and respiratory distress. Necropsy showed cerebral dysgenesis, microcephaly and several areas of polymicrogyria, and hypoplasia of the optic and third cranial nerves, and confirmed agenesis of the corpus callosum (Fig. 1).

Case 9. An eight-month-old boy was admitted for investigation of poor vision. He had been born at term. Roving eye move-

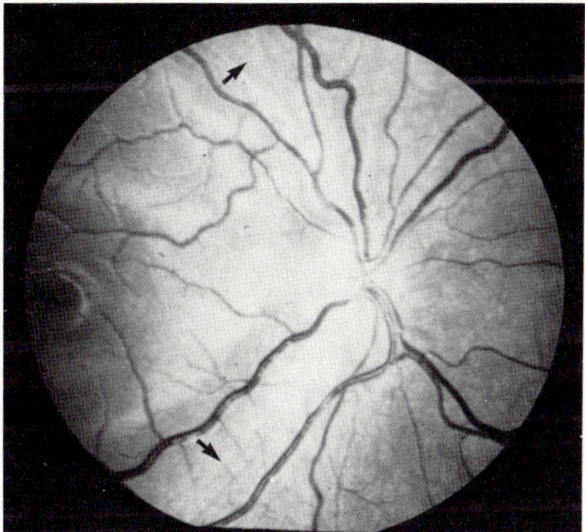

Fig. 8A

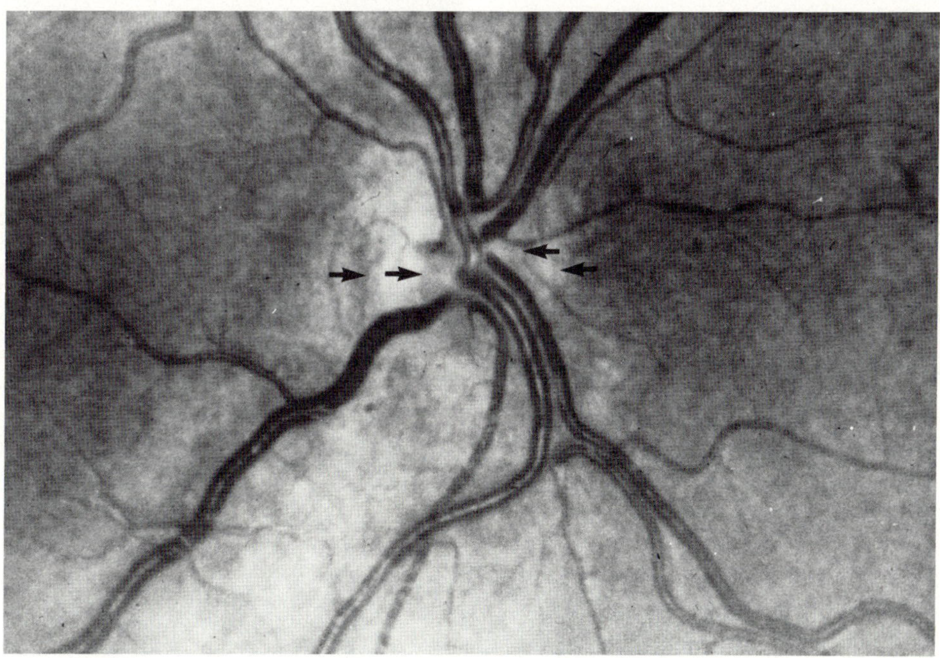

Fig. 8B

Fig. 8. Case 4: right optic nerve hypoplasia. A. The optic disc is small, with moderate thinness of the entire retina and some flattening of the macular mound. The arrows indicate discrete loss of nerve-fiber bundles ("gutters"). B. Three years later: The small optic disc (between inner arrows) is surrounded by a slightly pigmented scleral halo (outer arrows). Thinness of the retina nasally and temporally give these areas a darker, more granular appearance (magnification × 2).

ments were noted at one month, although his eyes were straight, and his mother reported that he had never reached out for toys or food or smiled at her.

Eye movements were slow and roving, with poor fixation, and the infant did not reach out even for large objects. The pupils reacted only sluggishly to light. Funduscopy showed severe thinning of both retinae, flattening of the maculae, and smallness and pallor of both optic nerve heads. No other neurological abnormalities or endocrine deficiencies were clinically apparent, and all other body systems were normal. Skull roentgenograms were normal, and optic-foramen views and axial tomography of the optic canals showed normal size and symmetry. The CT scan showed only mild widening of sulci and ventricles.

This infant is being followed closely, as it is thought that endocrine deficiencies due to a high midline pituitary defect may develop.

Case 10. A six-month-old girl was admitted for investigation of poor vision. Delivery had been normal and the child appeared to be doing well, but from approximately three months of age her parents had noticed that her eyes wandered. She did not react appropriately to smiling faces and objects placed in front of her. Her eyes did not follow objects, and her mother felt that the child could not recognize her face. Her developmental milestones were somewhat delayed, and she was considered mildly retarded.

The girl was placid and had no obvious difficulties except complete unresponsiveness to any visual stimuli. The pupils were equal but did not react directly to light and did not dilate in darkness, although they reacted during spontaneous convergence movements. She had a roving irregular nystagmus of variable pendular conjugate type, with full range of conjugate eye movements. Both optic nerves were severely hypoplastic (Fig. 9). The EEG was normal. Air encephalography showed absence of the septum pellucidum, and four-vessel arteriograms were within normal limits. Tomography of the optic canals showed bilateral small diameters. De Morsier's syndrome was diagnosed (Fig. 4B).

By 5½ years, no endocrine abnormalities

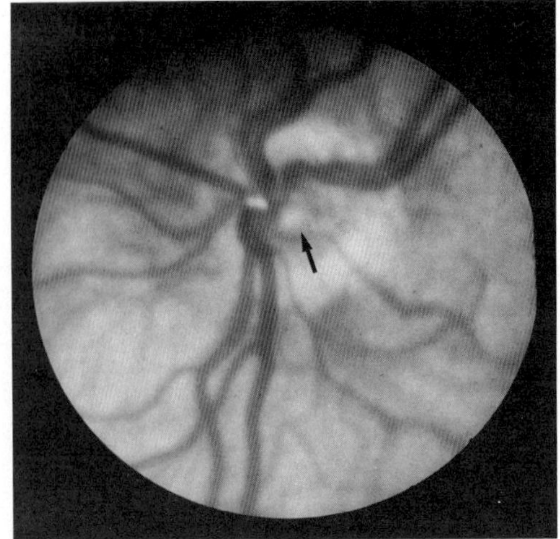

Fig. 9A

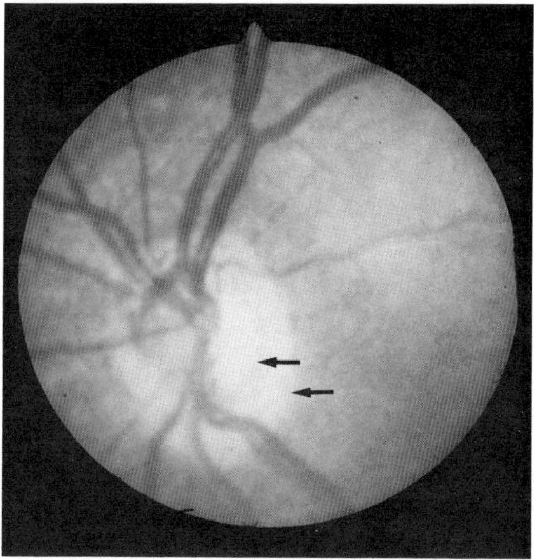

Fig. 9B

Fig. 9. Case 10: bilateral optic nerve hypoplasia. A. The right optic nerve head is very small (arrow); the large retinal vessels are of normal caliber; there is a prominent scleral band. B. Small left optic nerve head surrounded by double halo of sclera (inner arrows) and a band in which retinal pigmentation is absent (outer arrows) (magnification × 2). C. Left optic nerve hypoplasia with nerve head between arrows. The generally thin nerve fiber layer shows diffuse, abnormal, broad, superficial light reflexes which are dissected into geographic pattern by the superficial retinal vascular network.

had developed, and the apparent retardation and slow development seemed based mainly on lack of visual stimulation from

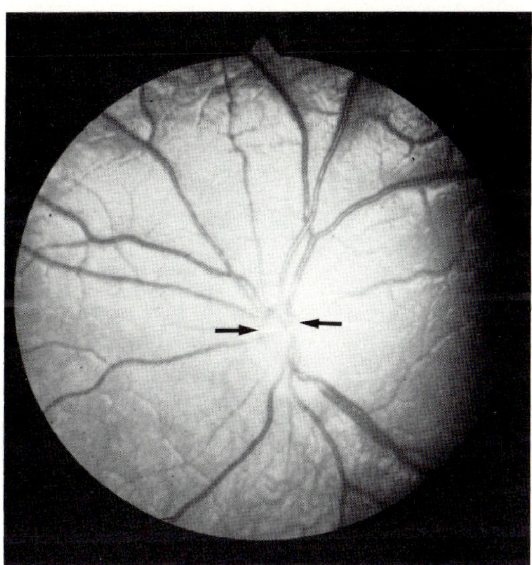

Fig. 9C

birth. The child is coping reasonably well in school and has average verbal and language ability.

SUMMARY

Optic nerve hypoplasia has a wide clinical spectrum. It is a congenital, nonprogressive, unilateral or bilateral anomaly; in some cases it is part of a neurological syndrome (*e.g.*, de Morsier's syndrome). Recognition of minimal optic nerve hypoplasia requires assessment of disc size and color, the peripapillary nerve fiber layer, and detection of the double-ring sign. Although clinicians describe these findings in terms of a spectrum of optic nerve hypoplasia, some cases may represent atrophy (due to late embryonic insult) rather than true hypoplasia.

EDITOR'S NOTE

Optic nerve hypoplasia is a surprisingly frequently encountered finding in small infants in neuro-ophthalmologic practice—particularly so when we didn't even diagnose this entity at all until about 15 years ago. I believe that good fundus photography was the thing that really led to its appreciation because a high quality photograph of the optic disc in an infant really shows more than you can see in the office. The photograph doesn't cry—it doesn't wiggle—and it doesn't squeeze. You can just sit there and relax and look at it to your heart's content. The three commonest causes of optic atrophy in children are: birth trauma, congenital defects, and optic glioma. The three commonest causes of optic atrophy in adults are: brain tumor, glaucoma, and syphilis. Note that these differential diagnoses are quite different in children than in adults. In the congenital optic atrophy group, I'm sure that optic nerve hypoplasia is by far the commonest type seen. The problem is that, in my experience, there really is no good correlation between the appearance of the disc and the visual function in that eye. In other words, there may be only a "nubbin" of disc, and yet the vision may be 20/40 with a surprisingly good field. On the other hand, the disc may be only minimally smaller than its fellow—so much so that you're not really sure it's hypoplastic and you are riding that "double pigment ring sign" as hard as you can—and yet the eye may be amaurotic. I saw two babies the same day brought in with bilateral total blindness, with bilateral amaurotic pupils, and both had hypoplastic discs in both eyes. It is not common for optic nerve hypoplasia to cause total blindness—i.e., no light perception—but it certainly can do so, without any doubt. The 14 diopter Nikon lens is the best way of examining these discs, as well as good 2X disc photos, I believe. Finally, one should ask about diabetes in the family, and particularly any attempt at using quinine or other toxic drugs during the pregnancy by the mother. It is a very important clinical diagnosis because it proves that the visual status will be stable, and is not due to a progressive problem as a craniopharyngioma; but you must be careful of the diagnosis. An excellent photograph of this problem is in Figure 8 and 9 in the chapter by Mr. Alistair R. Fielder.

JLS

REFERENCES

1. Awan, K. J. Ganglionic neuroretinal aplasia and hypoplasia: aplasia and hypoplasia of the optic nerve. Ann. Ophthalmol. *8*:1193–1202 (1976).
2. Billson, F. A. and Hoyt, C. S. Optic nerve hypoplasia in chondrodysplasia punctata. J. Pediatr. Ophthalmol. *14*:144–147 (1977).
3. Boynton, J. R., Pheasant, T. R. and Levine, M. R. Hypoplastic optic nerves studied with B-scan ul-

trasonography and axial tomography of the optic canals. Can. J. Ophthalmol. *10:*473–481 (1975).

4. Conradi, E. Vorzeitges Auftreten von Knochen and eigenartigen Verkalkungskeren bei Chondrodystropia fotalis hypoplastica. Jahrbuch für Kinderheilk. *80:*86–97 (1914).

5. Davis, G. V. and Shock, J. P. Septo-optic dysplasia associated with see-saw nystagmus. Arch. Ophthalmol. *93:*137–139 (1975).

6. de Morsier, G. Etudes sur les dysraphies crânio-encéphaliques; agénésie du septum lucidum avec malformation du tractus optique. La dysplasie septo-optique. Schweiz. Arch. Neurol. Psychiatr. *77:*267–292 (1956).

7. Duke-Elder, S. Aplasia and hypoplasia of the optic nerve. In: *System of Ophthalmology, Vol. 3, Pt. 2: Congenital Deformities.* Kimpton, London, 1964, pp. 668–671.

8. Edwards, W. C. and Layden, W. E. Optic nerve hypoplasia. Am. J. Ophthalmol. *70:*950–959 (1970).

9. Ellenberger, C. and Runyan, T. E. Holoprosencephaly with hypoplasia of the optic nerves, dwarfism and agenesis of the septum pellucidum. Am. J. Ophthalmol. *70:*960–967 (1970).

10. Franceschetti, A. and Bock, R. H. Megalopapilla; a new congenital anomaly. Am. J. Ophthalmol *33:* 227–235 (1950).

11. Frisén, L. and Holmegaard, L. Spectrum of optic nerve hypoplasia. Br. J. Ophthalmol. *62:*7–15 (1978).

12. Hackenbruch, Y., Meerhoff, E., Besio, R. and Cardoso, H. Familial bilateral optic nerve hypoplasia. Am. J. Ophthalmol. *79:*314–320 (1975).

13. Hoyt, C. S. and Billson, F. A. Maternal anticonvulsants and optic nerve hypoplasia. Br. J. Ophthalmol. *62:*3–6 (1978).

14. Hoyt, W. F., Kaplan, S. L., Grumback, M. M. and Glaser, J. S. Septo-optic dysplasia and pituitary dwarfism. Lancet *1:*893–894 (1970).

15. Hoyt, W. F., Rios-Montenegro, E. N., Behrens, M. M. and Eckelhoff, R. J. Homonymous hemioptic hypoplasia. Funduscopic features in standard and red-free illumination in three patients with congenital hemiplegia. Br. J. Ophthalmol. *56:*537–545 (1972).

16. Mann, I. *The Development of the Human Eye.* 3rd ed. British Medical Association, London, 1964, pp. 136–137, 283–286.

17. Martyn, L. J. Disorders of the nervous system in childhood. In: *Pediatric Ophthalmology.* R. D. Harley (Ed.), Saunders, Philadelphia, 1975, pp. 488–546.

18. McKinna, A. J. Quinine induced hypoplasia of the optic nerve. Can. J. Ophthalmol. *1:*261–266 (1966).

19. Merin, S., Harwood-Nash, D. C., Crawford, J. S. Axial tomography of optic canals in diagnosis of children's eye and optic nerve defects. Am. J. Ophthalmol. *72:*1122–1129 (1971).

20. Newman, W. Congenital blindess in two sisters. Ophthalmol. Hosp. *4:*202 (1863–1865).

21. Petersen, R. A. and Walton, D. S. Optic nerve hypoplasia with good visual acuity and visual field defects. A study of children of diabetic mothers. Arch. Ophthalmol. *95:*254–258 (1977).

22. Scheie, H. G. and Adler, F. H. Aplasia of the optic nerve. Arch. Ophthalmol. *26:*61–70 (1941).

23. Seeley, R. L. and Smith, J. L. Visual field defects in optic nerve hypoplasia. Am. J. Ophthalmol. *73:* 882–889 (1972).

24. van Balen, A. and Santens, P. Chondrodystrophia calcificans congenita. J. Pediatr. Ophthalmol. *5:* 151–156 (1968).

25. Walsh, F. B. and Hoyt, W. F. *Clinical Neuro-ophthalmology,* 3rd ed. Williams and Wilkins, Baltimore, 1969, Vol. 6, p. 661.

26. Walton, D. S. and Robb, R. M. Optic nerve hypoplasia, a report of twenty cases. Arch. Ophthalmol. *84:*572–578 (1970).

27. Weiter, J. J., McLean, I. W. and Zimmerman, L. E. Aplasia of the optic nerve and disk. Am. J. Ophthalmol. *83:*569–576 (1977).

28. Yanoff, M. and Fine, B. S. Optic nerve. Congential defects and anatomic variations. In: *Ocular Pathology: A Text and Atlas.* Harper and Row, Hagerstown, Md., 1975, pp. 484–485.

29. Yanoff, M., Rorke, L. B. and Allman, M. I. Bilateral optic system aplasia with relatively normal eyes. Arch. Ophthalmol. *96:*97–101 (1978).

30. Zeeman, W. P. C. and Tumbelaka, R. Das zentrale und periphere optische System bie einer kongenital blinden Katze. Graefes Arch. Ophthal. *91:*242–263 (1916); cited in Duke-Elder, S. *System of Ophthalmology, Vol. 3, Pt. 2: Congenital Deformities.* Kimpton, London, 1964, p. 668.

31. Editorial: Small optic discs. Br. J. Ophthalmol. *62:* 1–2 (1978).

11 The Tilted Disc Syndrome in Craniofacial Diseases

Sheila Margolis, M.D.
Irwin M. Siegel, Ph.D.

Craniofacial anomalies invariably produce malformations of the bony structures of the skull, face, and orbit. It is not surprising that such defects can directly affect the functioning of the eye and visual system in any number of ways. For example, mechanical interference with extraocular muscle movement can result from orbital displacement.[1] Likewise, a stenotic optic foramen may seriously impair development and integrity of the optic nerve. Recently, however, a number of less explicable retinal defects were also found to be associated with craniofacial defects.[2-4] These include situs inversus and tilting of the optic disc, heterotopic maculae, and fundus hypopigmentation. While the rarely occurring abnormal vessel distribution of the optic papilla (situs inversus) and disc orientation have been reported in the literature for some time they have been considered as rare, sporadic occurrences of unknown etiology.[5] The underlying mechanisms, undoubtedly of abnormal embryological and early developmental origins, have not been adequately studied. Investigations of similar defects in patients with craniofacial defects, on the other hand, can provide an organized context within which to pursue systematic study of such ocular anomalies.

Since several of the craniofacial diseases have a known mode of genetic transmission and often affect more than one member of a family, the opportunity for observing seldom seen developmental malformations in a variety of states of expressivity is considerably enhanced. New techniques of plastic reconstructive surgery are now being applied to normalize skull and skeletal structures of such patients. We have now examined, in conjunction with the New York University Medical Center for Craniofacial Anomalies, over 200 patients. Initially, the emphasis was on the strabismic problems naturally arising from the skull and orbit defects. Closer study of this group of patients revealed the presence of optic nerve and retinal abnormalities which were seen only rarely and in isolated circumstances. From this large group, we have chosen only a few of the known craniofacial diseases; admittedly, those which are well defined and understood both in morphological and genetic terms. The skull, face, and skeletal defects of each group will be described and the optic nerve, retina, and associated visual abnormalities associated with the tilted disc syndrome presented.

ORBITAL HYPERTELORISM

As defined by Tessier,[6] hypertelorism is an increase in the interorbital distance and can be subdivided into three grades of severity, depending on the degree of orbital separation. Thus, an interocular distance (measured between the medial orbital walls) of 30–34 mm is labeled a primary hypertelorism; from 34–40 mm, secondary; and a separation greater than 40 mm is tertiary hypertelorism. A number of associated facial anomalies are associated with hypertelorism such as midline cleft, widow's peak, bifid nose, and strabismus. Figure 1 shows a patient with these features. Occasionally ptosis and lacrimal dysfunction may also be present. It should be noted that hypertelorism can be an isolated

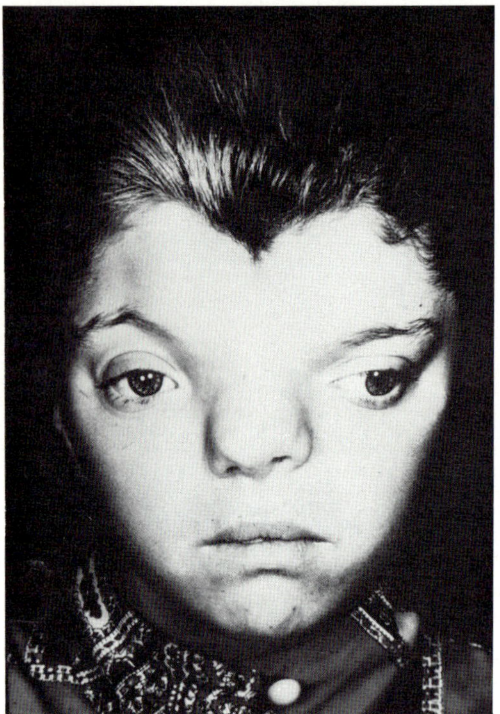

Fig. 1. (Margolis). A patient with orbital hypertelorism with the associated findings of a midline cleft, widow's peak, bifid nose and an exotropia.

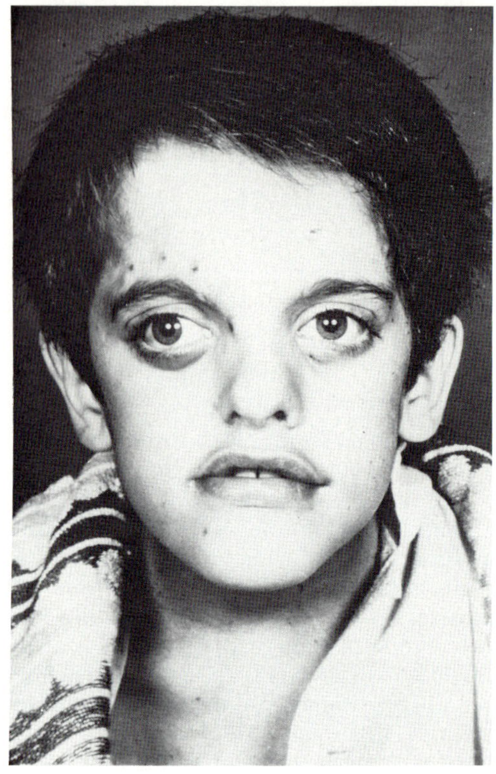

Fig. 2. (Margolis). Case 1: A 10-year-old male with orbital hypertelorism, craniostenosis, and exotropia.

circumstance or, as will be seen in the following sections, as part of more generalized craniofacial syndromes.

Case 1

This 10-year-old white male was born with a rare combination of an immunodeficiency disorder and craniostenosis, the latter due to premature closure of the coronal sutures (see Fig. 2). Prenatal history was noncontributory, and there was a normal, spontaneous, delivery. There were two other siblings, and no other known affected family members. Both mother and father were 38 years old at conception and were alive and well. Three months after birth he began to develop respiratory infections, which have continued as a result of his immune deficiency. At the age of four he underwent a cranial stripping procedure to open the coronal suture.

Ocular Examination. The patient's best corrected visual acuity was RE: counting fingers at two feet; LE: 20/30, pinhole 20/25. Both pupils measured 4 mm in di-

ameter with slower direct responses to light on the right. The interpupillary distance was 67 mm and intercanthal distance 30 mm. There was no nystagmus. There was a V exotropia pattern with bilateral inferior oblique dysfunction. The remainder of the anterior segment and ocular media were normal.

Funduscopic Examination. The right optic disc was chalky white and flat, with anomalous vessel insertion (see Fig. 3).The vessels began at the 10:00 position, very close to the temporal rim, and crossed horizontally leaving the surface of the disc in a nasal direction. The vessels were tortuous, but their caliber was normal. There was a diffuse foveal reflex, but the macula appeared to be in a normal anatomic position. Fundal pigmentation was normal in both eyes. The left optic disc was also pale and flat. The vessels, like those in the right eye were tortuous but followed a normal distribution (see Fig. 4). In this eye, there was a normal foveal reflex and the macular area was in a normal position.

Visual fields for the left eye were performed on a tangent screen at 1 m using 5-, 10-, and 20-mm white test objects and a 20-mm test object on the poorer seeing right eye (see Fig. 5). There was marked peripheral constriction of both fields but more severely reduced for the right eye.

Visual evoked cortical responses (VECP) were performed using a reversing checkerboard stimulus and showed markedly decreased amplitudes for the right eye and normal amplitudes for the left eye. Time to peak of the P1 response of each eye was normal. The electroretinogram showed normal photopic and scotopic b-wave amplitudes in each eye.

Case 2

This 16-year-old white male had second degree orbital hypertelorism (see Fig. 6).

Ocular Examination. The patient's best corrected visual acuity was 20/50 in each eye. Refraction RE: −6.00 DS and LE: −7.00 DS. There was no nystagmus. The pupils measured 4 mm in diameter and reacted slowly to direct light. The interpupillary distance was 70 mm and the intercanthal distance 46 mm. There was a V pattern exotropia with bilateral inferior oblique dysfunction. The remainder of the anterior segment and ocular media were normal.

Funduscopic Examination. Both optic

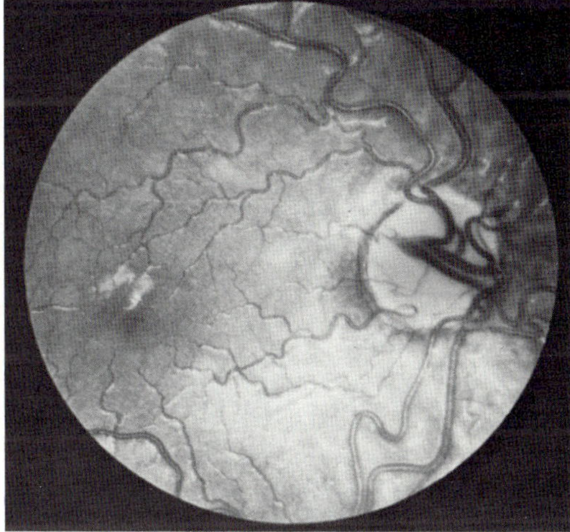

Fig. 3. (Margolis) Case 1: Fundus of the right eye showing a white, flat disc with tortuous vessels inserting temporally and crossing nasally, typical of situs inversus. The macular area is in a normal position with a diffuse foveal reflex.

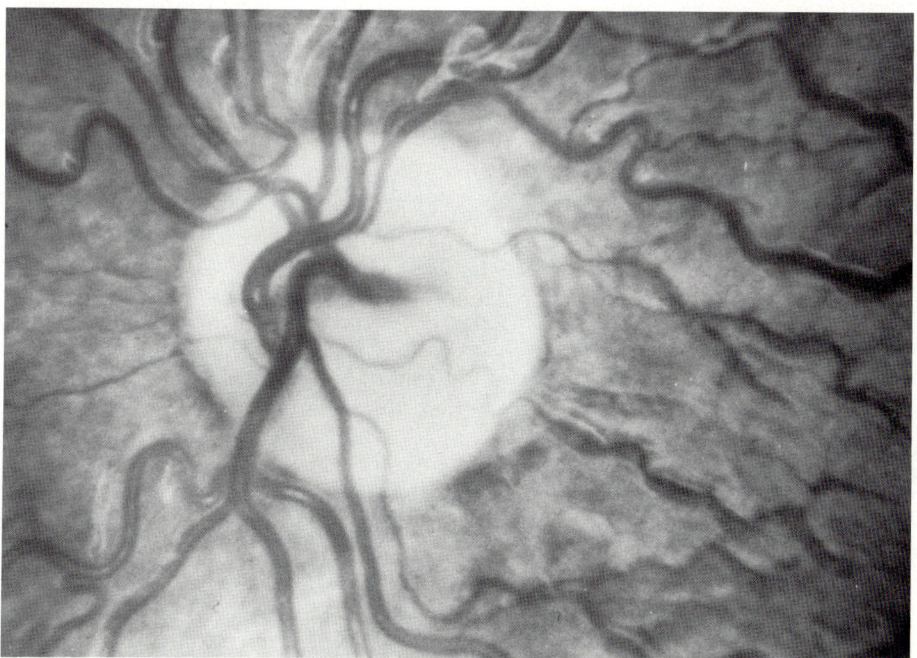

Fig. 4. (Margolis) Case 1: Left eye. The disc was pale and flat with tortuous vessels, but the vessel pattern on the disc was normal. The macular area was also normal and a good foveal reflex is seen.

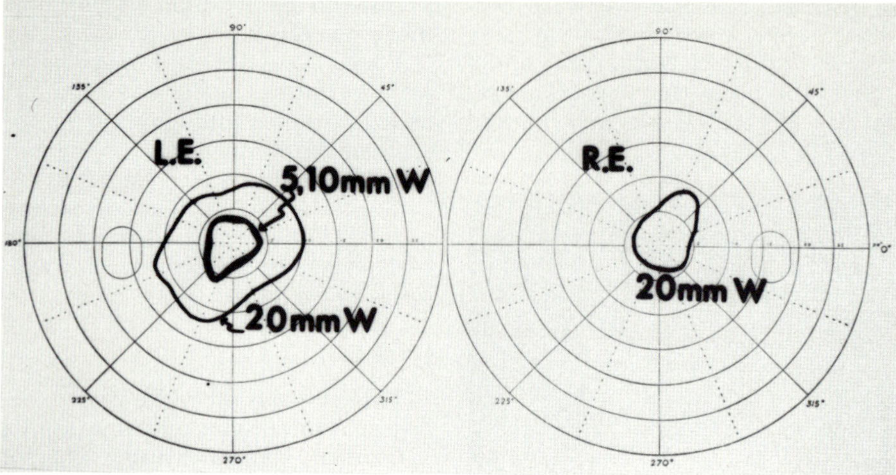

Fig. 5. (Margolis) Case 1: Visual fields done on a tangent screen showed a more severe concentric constriction for the right eye.

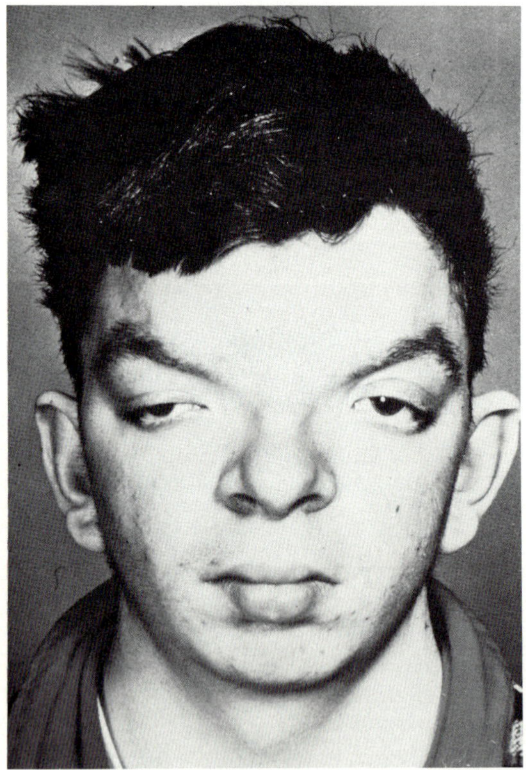

Fig. 6. (Margolis) Case 2: A 16-year-old male with orbital hypertelorism, antimongoloid palpebral fissures, ptosis, and exotropia.

discs were pale and flat with large cups and a circumferential conus more marked inferiorly. Below each disc was a diffuse area of hypopigmentation of the retina with visualization of the underlying choroidal vasculature (see Fig. 7). The retinal vessels were anomalous, suggesting situs inversus or tilting of the disc. The macular areas of each eye showed mild granularity, contained a diffuse foveal reflex, and appeared to be somewhat inferiorly displaced.

Visual fields performed on the Goldmann perimeter using a ¼-mm² white test object at intensity 4 (IV₄) indicated a mild superior bitemporal field defect (see Fig. 8)

Case 3

This is a six-year-old white male with hypertelorism and a bifid nose (see Fig. 9). There was a normal spontaneous delivery and no prenatal complications. The birth weight was 8 lb 3 oz. One other sibling is alive and not affected. The father was 42 years old and the mother 39 years at the time of the birth of the child. Both parents were examined and proved to be normal. No reconstructive surgery has been performed on the patient to date.

Ocular Examination. The patient's best corrected vision was RE: 20/30 and LE: 20/20. Retinoscopy was found to be RE: +4.25, LE: +2.00. The pupils were equal and reacted to light and accommodation. The interpupillary distance was 60 mm and the intercanthal distance was measured at 40 mm. There was no nystagmus. A small V pattern esotropia with bilateral overactions of both inferior obliques and underaction of the superior obliques was noted. The remainder of the anterior segment as well as ocular media were normal.

Funduscopic Examination. Both optic nerve heads were pink and had normal retinal vasculature. There were good foveal reflexes OU. The maculae were normally located. In each inferior nasal quadrant there was deficient fundal pigmentation

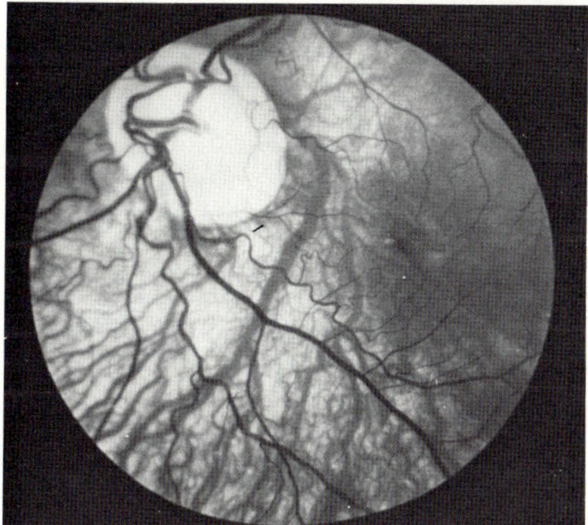

Fig. 7. (Margolis) Case 2: Left eye. The disc is tilted, pale, and flat. Note the large cup and inferior conus suggesting situs inversus. Inferior to the disc there is a large area of hypopigmented retina in which large choroidal vessels are seen. The macular area is inferiorly displaced and in closer proximity to the disc than normal. An identical picture was seen in the right eye.

which allowed easy visualization of the choroidal vasculature (see Fig. 10).

Computerized axial tomography was performed and read as normal. From skull x-rays, the interorbital distance was meas-

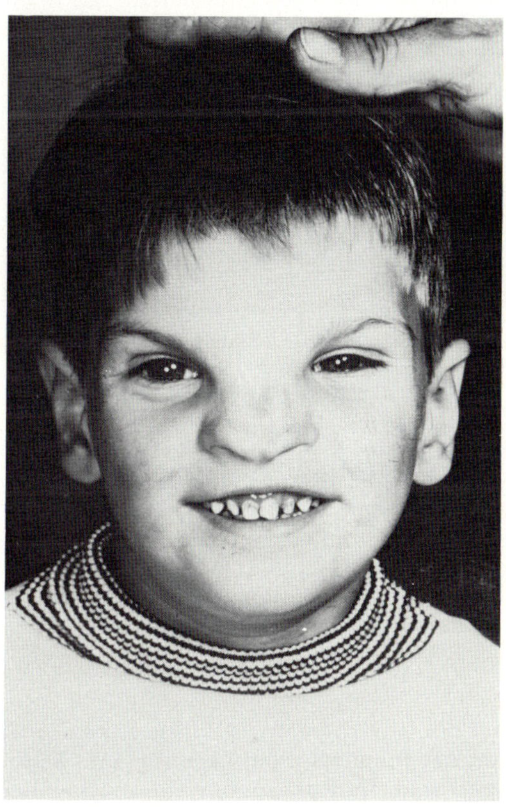

Fig. 9. (Margolis) Case 3: A six-year-old male with orbital hypertelorism, a midline cleft, bifid nose, and strabismus.

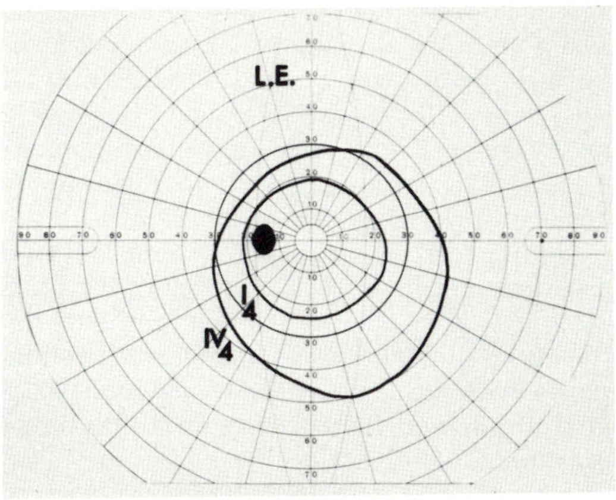

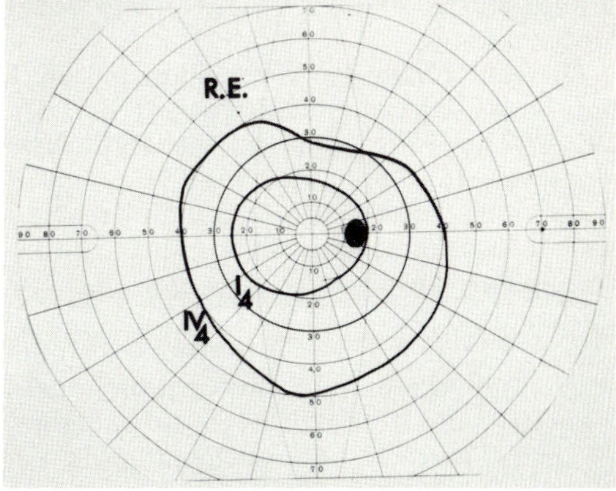

Fig. 8. (Margolis) Case 2: Visual fields performed on a Goldmann perimeter. A mild superior temporal field defect can be seen.

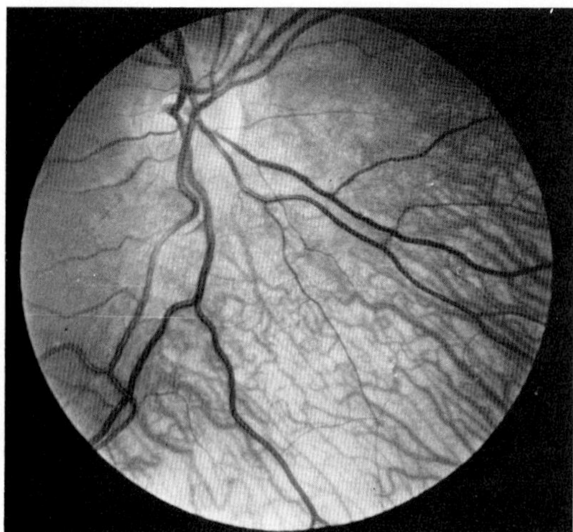

Fig. 10. (Margolis) Case 3: Fundus, left eye. The optic nerve, retinal vasculature, and macula are normal. There is a good foveal reflex (not shown). In the inferior nasal quadrant there is loss of retinal pigment, and the choroidal vessels are easily seen. A comparable picture was seen in the right eye.

ured at 33 mm, the frontal sinuses were small, and the ethmoid cells were enlarged. The nasal bone had an inverted W shape in the area of bifid abnormality.

Case 4

This is a 16-year-old black female with tertiary hypertelorism (see Fig. 11). At the third month of pregnancy the mother had an ovarian cyst removed, but there was a normal spontaneous delivery. The parents were not examined. There were two other siblings who were both normal. There was prior cosmetic surgery, but no orbital translocation done.

Ocular Examination. The patient's best corrected visual acuity was RE: 20/25; LE: 20/40. Refraction in the right eye: $-4.00 = -1.00 \times 90$ and left eye: $-6.50 = -1.00 \times 65$. Pupils were equal and reacted well to light and accommodation. The interpupillary distance was 68 mm and the intercanthal distance was 50 mm. There was no nystagmus. An A-pattern exotropia was found with oblique dysfunction and an associated mongoloid slant to the palpebral fissures. The remainder of the anterior segment as well as ocular media was normal.

Fundscopic Examination. There were large myopic discs in each eye with a cup/

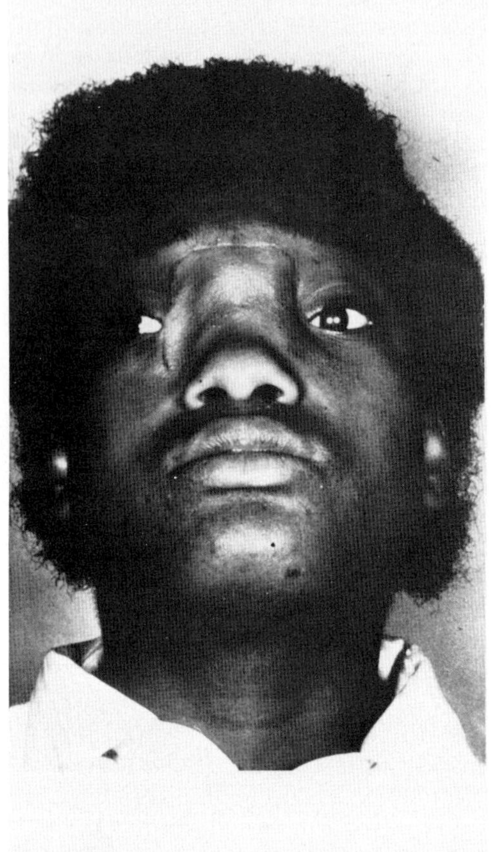

Fig. 11. (Margolis) Case 4: A 16-year-old female shown (postoperatively) with hypertelorism, mongoloid palpebral fissures, and an exotropia.

disc ratio on the left measuring 0.8 and on the right 0.6 (see Figs. 12, 13). The retinal vessel caliber looked generally attenuated and their fundal distribution appeared abnormal. There was a nasal shift of the vessels, especially in the left eye. There were no foveal reflexes seen in either macular region. The fundi showed no pigmentary abnormalities.

Computerized axial tomography showed a widened sphenoid angle to 120°, which is distinctly abnormal. The measurements between the middle and posterior ethmoidal plane were greater than 10.5 which were also abnormal. In the area of the anterior ethmoidal air cells there was a density similar to that of the brain and thought to probably represent an anterior ethmoidal encephalocele. The final impression was or-

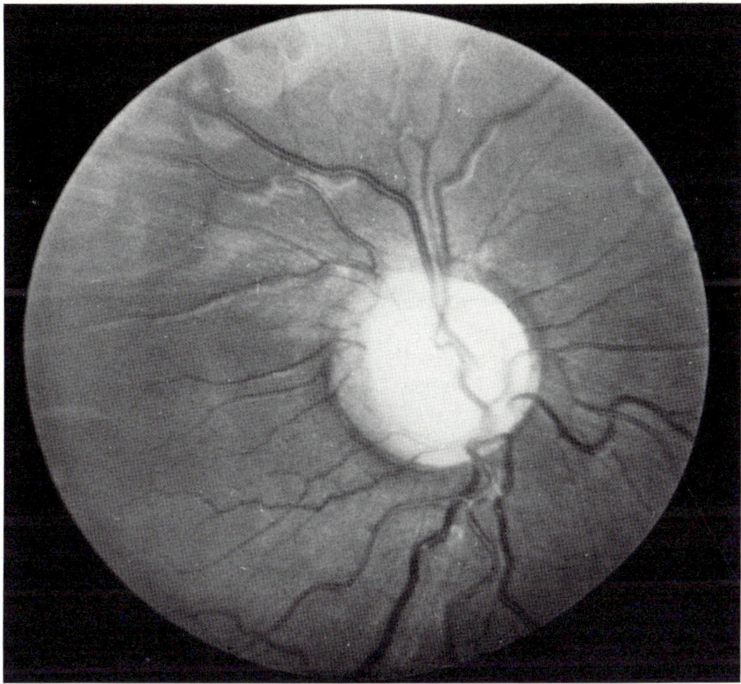

Fig. 12. (Margolis) Case 4: Fundus, right eye. The disc is pale and tilted with a large myopic conus. There is attenuation of the retinal vessels. The macula was in a normal position, but no foveal reflex was seen.

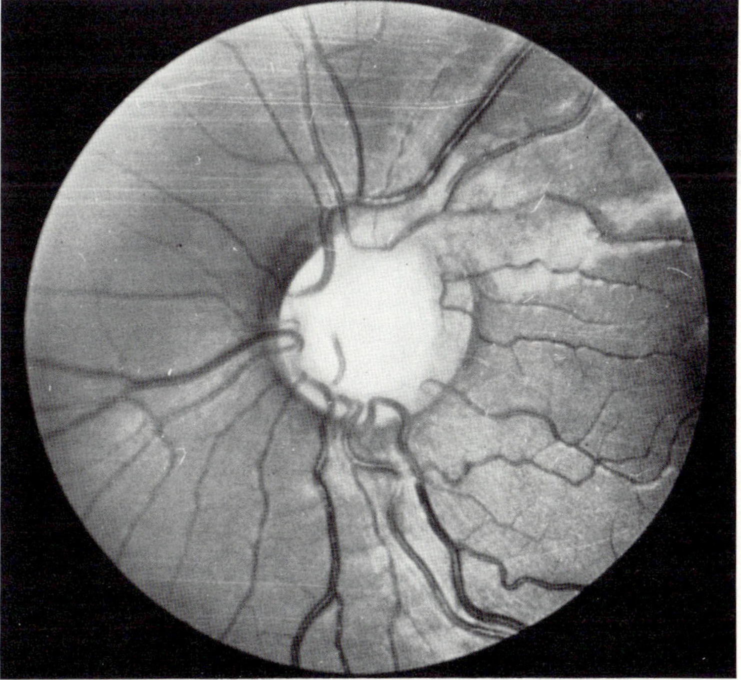

Fig. 13. (Margolis) Case 4: Fundus, left eye. The left disc is pale, with a large cup and myopic conus. There is a nasal shift of the vessels which are attenuated and seem to radiate in an anomalous fashion from the rim of the disc. No foveal reflex was seen.

bital hypertelorism with a midface abnormality and anterior transethmoidal encephalocele.

Case 5

This is a 16-year-old white female with tertiary hypertelorism (see Fig. 14). In addition to hypertelorism there were epicanthal folds, hypoplasia of the frontal bones and supraorbital ridges, coarse heavy eyebrows, widow's peak, low hairline, high arched palate, and a suggestion of a cleft at the tip of the nose. There was also asymmetry of the lengths of the arms and legs. Hers was a full term birth, but trauma was noted over the left eye at the time of delivery. There was a large weight gain during pregnancy of 45 lb, a suggestion of hydramnios. A pelvic x-ray had been done at eight months of pregnancy. There were no previous miscarriages, but two other siblings had club feet. The father was 25 years old and the mother 28 years old at the time of

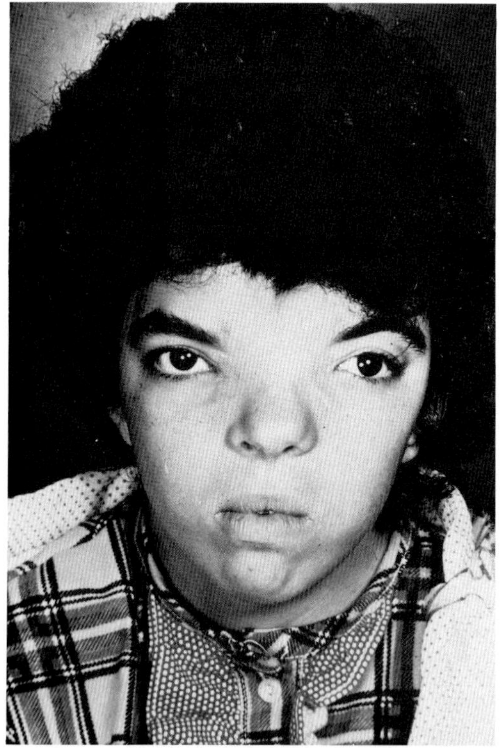

Fig. 14. (Margolis) Case 5: A 16-year-old female with hypertelorism, widow's peak, low hairline, epicanthus, and exotropia.

birth. At age 12 years the patient underwent reconstructive surgery for correction of the hypertelorism.

Ocular Examination. The best corrected visual acuity was RE: 20/25 (6/7) and LE: counting fingers at six feet. Refraction was: RE: +1.25 = −0.50 × 20; and LE: +2.50 = −2.00 × 20. The interpupillary distance was 70 mm and the intercanthal distance was 40 mm. A horizontal jerk nystagmus greater in left gaze was noted since birth. A V-pattern exotropia was present, with overaction of both inferior obliques and underaction of both superior obliques. On visual examination the right eye fixation was central but unsteady, and the left eye was eccentric and near the disc. There were abnormal dermatoglyphics but not specific for any chromosomal syndrome.

Funduscopic Examination. There was a normal pink optic nerve on the right with mild tilting and normal retinal vasculature (see Fig. 15). The macular area appeared to be inferiorly displaced. The left disc (see Fig. 16) had an abnormal vascular insertion in the superior region of the disc, although the retinal vascular caliber looked normal. The general distribution of the retinal vessels coming from the disc was abnormal. The superior temporal vein exited horizontally off the disc just above the normal position of the horizontal raphe. The inferior group of vessels left the disc in a normal position. However, the macular area was inferiorly displaced 1½ disc diameters from its normal position.

CRANIOFACIAL DYSOSTOSES

Crouzon's Disease (Cases 6 and 7)

Figure 17 shows a patient with Crouzon's disease. Typically, such patients manifest a tower skull (oxycephaly) due to premature craniostenosis, maxillary hypoplasia resulting in a flattened midface, and ocular abnormalities. The latter include exophthalmos, orbital hypertelorism, strabismus, antimongoloid palpebral fissures, ptosis, and optic atrophy.[1] Recently an association of oculocutaneous albinism was noted in a high percentage of patients with Crouzon's disease.[4] The syndrome is known to be transmitted by a single autosomal domi-

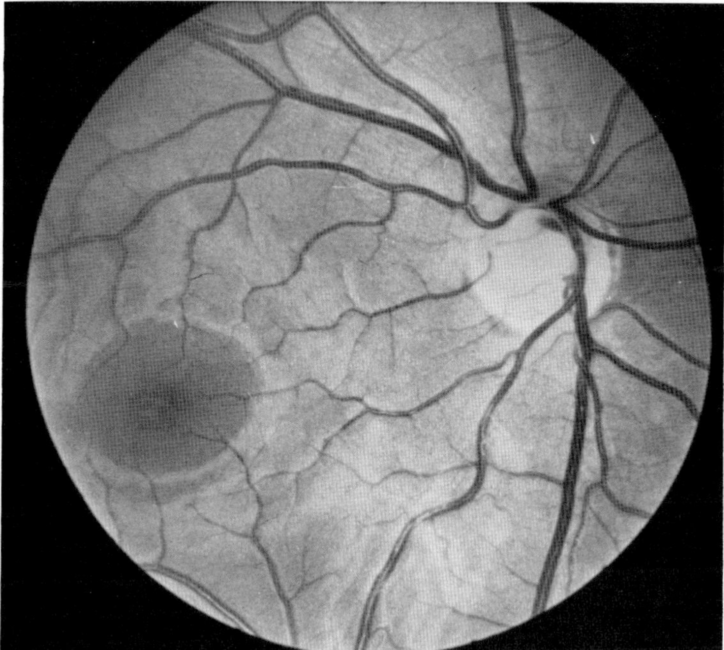

Fig. 15. (Margolis) Case 5: Fundus, right eye. The disc was pink, mildly tilted, with normal retinal vessels. The macular area has a good foveal reflex and is inferiorly displaced.

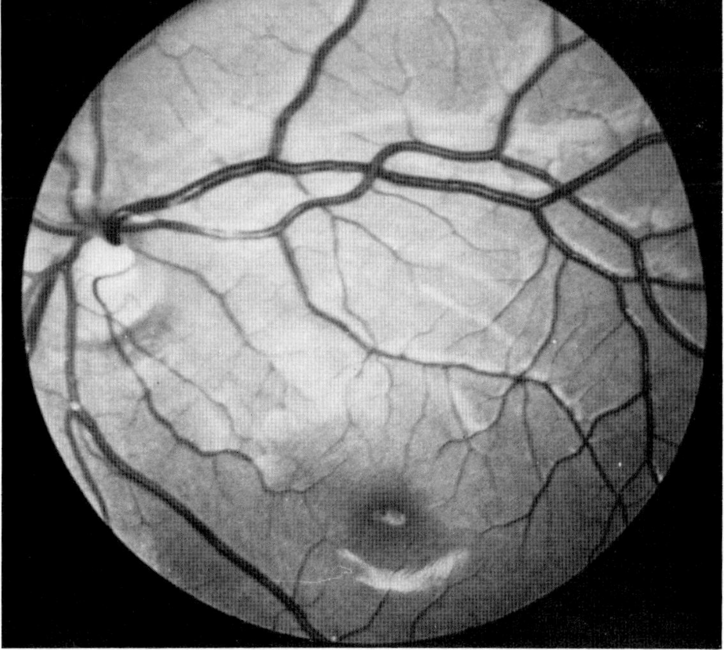

Fig. 16. (Margolis) Case 5: Fundus left eye. The disc has vessels of normal caliber originating from the superior temporal edge of the disc. The vessels cross the posterior pole in nearly horizontal fashion. Note that the macular area was displaced 1½ disc diameters inferiorly.

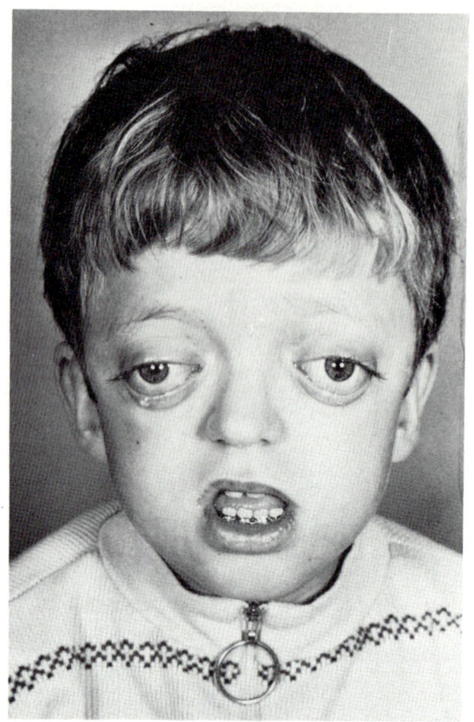

Fig. 17. (Margolis). Patient with Crouzon's disease who manifests oxycephaly (tower skull), maxillary hypoplasia resulting in a flattened midface, exophthalmos, orbital hypertelorism, antimongoloid palpebral fissures, strabismus, and lacrimal dysfunction.

nant gene. Patients with ocular hypopigmentation very often show (as does the true albino) poor vision, photophobia, nystagmus, iris transillumination, and little melaninization of the retinal tissues.

Case 6

A 25-year-old affected white female who has one normal and two affected male offspring (see Fig. 18). The patient's dizygotic twin sister is normal as well as both her parents.There were no complications during her pregnancy or the pregnancy of any of her three children. At the patient's birth her mother was 38 years old and her father 44 years. Permanent lateral tarsorrhaphies have been performed in the past for exposure keratitis secondary to moderately severe exophthalmos.

Ocular Examination. The patient's best corrected visual acuity was RE: 20/400 and LE: 20/200. The refraction was RE:

$-2.75 = 0.5 \times 180$ and LE: $-0.75 = -2.00 \times 45$. The globes were prominent with antimongoloid fissures; exophthalmometer readings were 27 mm RE and 29 mm LE on a base of 115. The interpupillary distance was 61.5 mm and the intercanthal distance measured 32 mm. There was a horizontal pendular nystagmus present. The iris showed a generalized transillumination. Also evident was a V-pattern exotropia with underaction of the superior rectus and superior oblique muscles and overaction of both inferior oblique muscles.

Funduscopy revealed chalk white, flat optic discs. The retinal vessels were of normal caliber and distribution. Below each disc there was a sector of marked hypopigmentation and clear visualization of the choroidal vessels (Fig. 19). However, this pigment deficiency was not sectorial but was generalized and extended to the midperiphery. There were no clearly defined foveal reflexes and the macular areas appeared normally positioned.

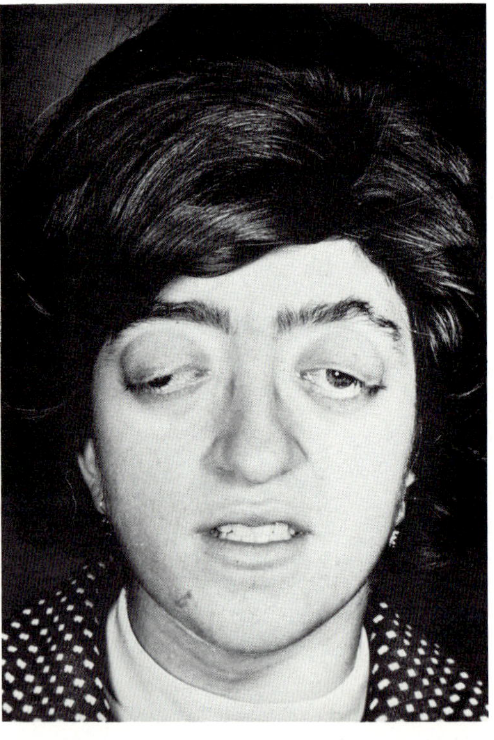

Fig. 18. (Margolis) Case 6: A 25-year-old female with hypertelorism, ptosis, antimongoloid palpebral fissures, exophthalmos, and strabismus.

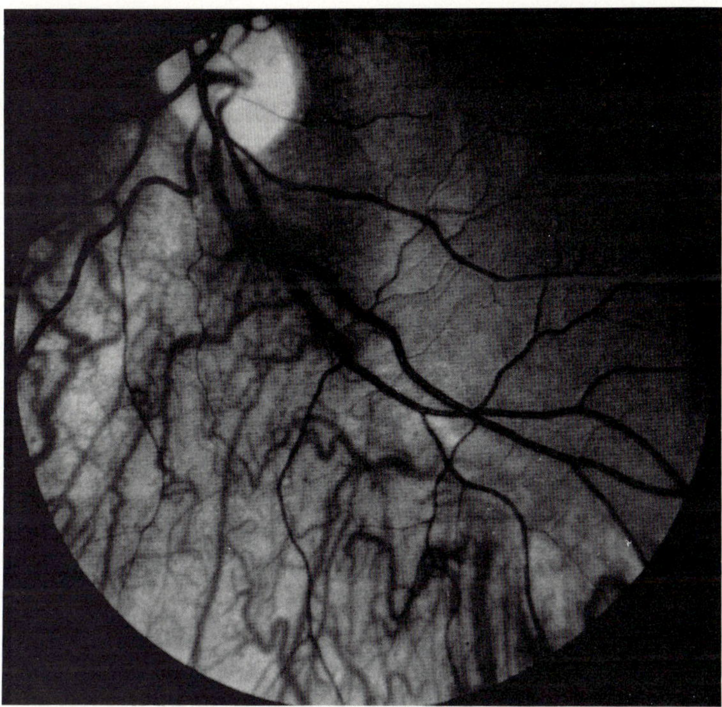

Fig. 19. (Margolis) Case 6: Fundus, left eye. The disc is pale and flat and has a normal distribution of retinal vessels. A well-demarcated hypopigmented area, which extends to the midperiphery, is seen inferior to the disc. The macula is in a normal position with an absent foveal reflex (not shown). An identical fundus picture was seen in the right eye.

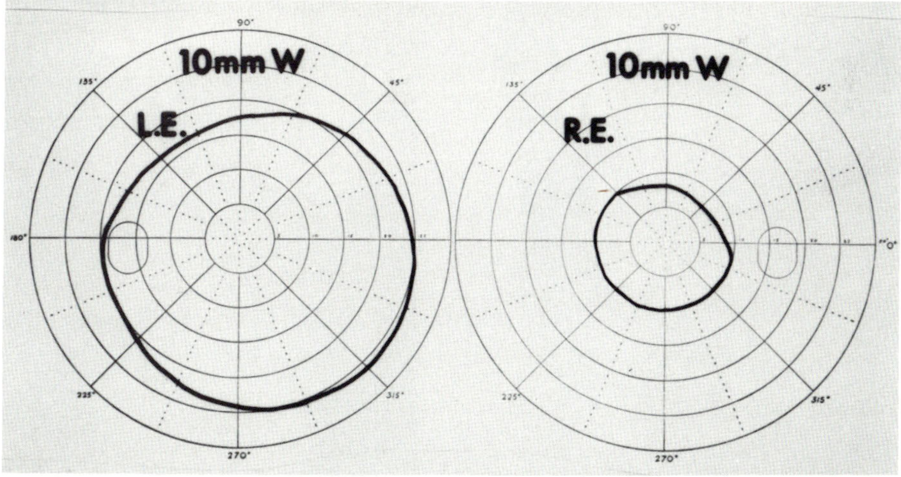

Fig. 20. (Margolis) Case 6: Visual fields performed on a tangent screen using a 10-mm white test object reveals severe concentric constriction of the right eye and a mild superior temporal field defect on the left.

Visual field tests (Fig. 20) were performed on a tangent screen using a 10-mm white test object at 1 m. More severe concentric constriction was seen on the right than the left, and there was a suggestion of a superior temporal field cut crossing the midline in the left eye.

Case 7

This is the son of patient 6. He is a two-year-old white male severely affected with Crouzon's syndrome (see Fig. 21). The delivery of this child was uncomplicated but severe ocular proptosis was noted at birth. The mother was 23 years old and father 26 years at the birth. Before the age of 18 months he underwent four cranial stripping procedures to open the coronal and lambdoidal sutures and decrease intracranial pressure and papilledema. Also, an emergency lateral tarsorrhaphy and decompression of the prolapsed globe was done.

Ocular Examination. An examination under anesthesia revealed the following: retinoscopy with cyclogyl 1%: in the right eye was $-0.50 = -6.00 \times 95$ and left eye, $-0.50 = -3.00 \times 90$. There was no nystagmus present. A V-pattern exotropia with a head turn to the left and right head tilt was noted. The child was markedly photophobic, had a ptosis on the left, and had blue irises that transilluminated.

Funduscopy revealed greyish, full, optic discs with clearly delineated margins without hemorrhages. The retinal veins were tortuous and engorged. The picture was consistent with a chronic papilledema which was recorded on previous examinations. Hypopigmentation was observed in a quadrant below both discs and also in the midperiphery, a pattern similar to that seen in the mother. In each of the areas where deficient retinal pigment was observed both large and small, the choroidal vessels were easily visualized.

Apert's Disease

Patients with Apert's disease have a generally similar appearance to those with Crouzon's disease in that the skull and facial malformations are quite alike. However, Apert's disease is further characterized by the presence of syndactyly defined particularly as the fusion of digits 2 to 4 resulting in a mid-digital hand mass with a common nail (Fig. 22).[7]

Case 8

This 27-year-old white woman had been born with facial and hand deformities typical of Apert's syndrome (Fig. 23). The fig-

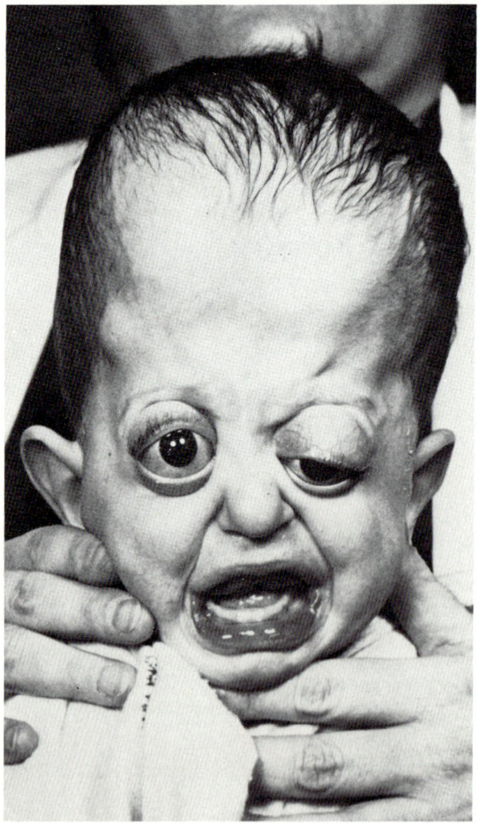

Fig. 21. (Margolis) Case 7: A two-year-old male son of Case 6 who shows severe oxcephaly, ptosis, antimongoloid fissures, exophthalmos, and strabismus.

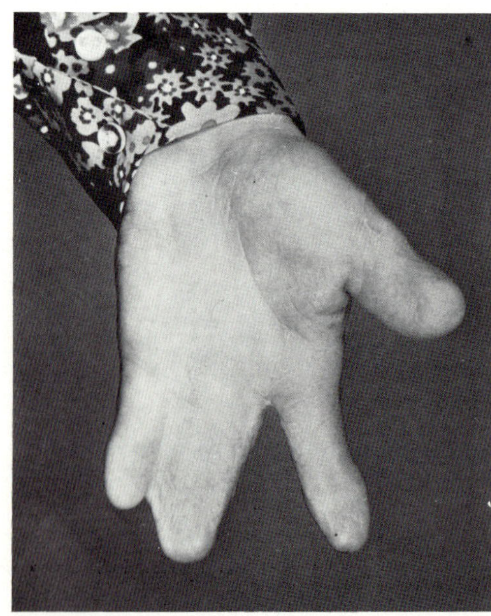

Fig. 22. (Margolis) Case 8: Syndactyly of left hand after the first surgical attempt to separate the digits.

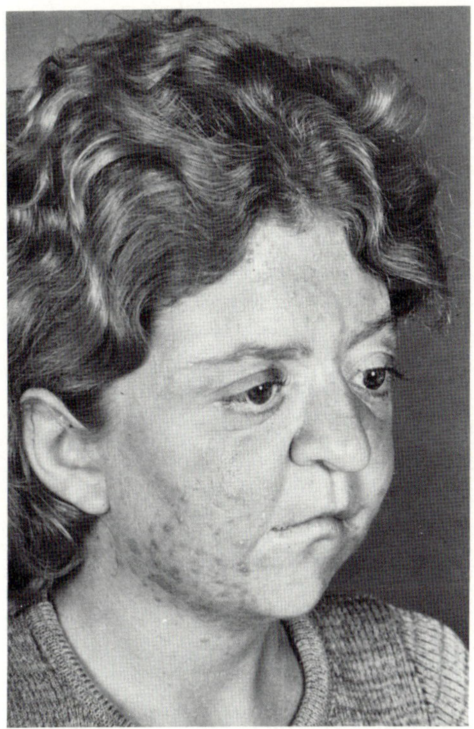

Fig. 23. (Margolis) Case 8: A 27-year-old female who is post-reconstructive surgery for Apert's facial deformities.

ures are post-operative since corrective surgery for syndactyly and strabismus, as well as eight maxillofacial reconstruction procedures, had been performed previously. There was no prenatal complication except for a fall during the third month of the mother's pregnancy. The patient's younger sister was normal. At the birth of the child both parents were 32 years of age.

Ocular Examination. The patient's best corrected visual acuity was RE: 20/50 and LE: 20/40. Refraction was RE: −1.25 = −4.00 × 95 and LE: −1.25 = −0.50 × 125. Single binocular vision was present with a head turn to the right. The globes were prominent with antimongoloid fissures; the exophthalmometer reading was 19 mm and 20 mm on base of 110 mm. The interpupillary distance was 65 mm, and intercanthal distance was 35 mm. There was an occlusion nystagmus in both eyes.

Iris transillumination was noted, but the remainder of the anterior segment was within normal limits. Orientation of the Y sutures in the lens was horizontal instead of the normal vertical position.

There was a V-esotropia pattern and an overaction of both inferior obliques was noted as well as moderate underaction of both superior oblique muscles. There was also marked underaction of the left superior rectus muscle.

Ophthalmoscopic examination of the right eye revealed a pink tilted disc, normal retinal vasculature and a diffuse foveal reflex. The macular area was displaced inferiorly (Fig. 24); pigmentation was reduced in the inferior and nasal quadrants (Fig. 25). The left disc and retinal vasculature appeared normal, but the generalized pigment deficiency made the choroidal vessels visible throughout much of the posterior pole (Fig. 26). The foveal area was diffuse, and the macula was in a normal position.

Case 9

This 10-year-old black female (Fig. 27) had Apert's syndrome and an ocular history of photophobia and tearing. At 10 weeks gestation, the mother had had a pelvic infection and rash which was treated with tetracycline (Achromycin) and until the seventh month of pregnancy she had intermittent vaginal bleeding. The birth was uncomplicated, but the birth weight was reported low at 1.871 kg. Four other siblings were reported to be normal. The mother's sister died one day after birth and reportedly had an "overlapping skull." At the time of our patient's birth, the father was 36 years old and the mother was 31 years old. Both parents were normal. At four months, the patient underwent a cranial stripping procedure and ventricular shunt implantation.

Ocular Examination. The patient's best corrected visual acuity was RE and LE: 20/30. Refraction was not done. The globes were prominent and there were antimongoloid palpebral fissures. The exophthalmometer readings were RE and LE: 23 mm on a base of 110 mm. The interpupillary distance was 70 mm and the intercanthal distance was 40 mm. There was no nystagmus. The pupils were equal and reacted to light and accommodation.

The anterior segment was normal except for absence of all lacrimal puncta. No iris transillumination was noted. There was a V-pattern exotropia with bilateral inferior oblique muscle dysfunction.

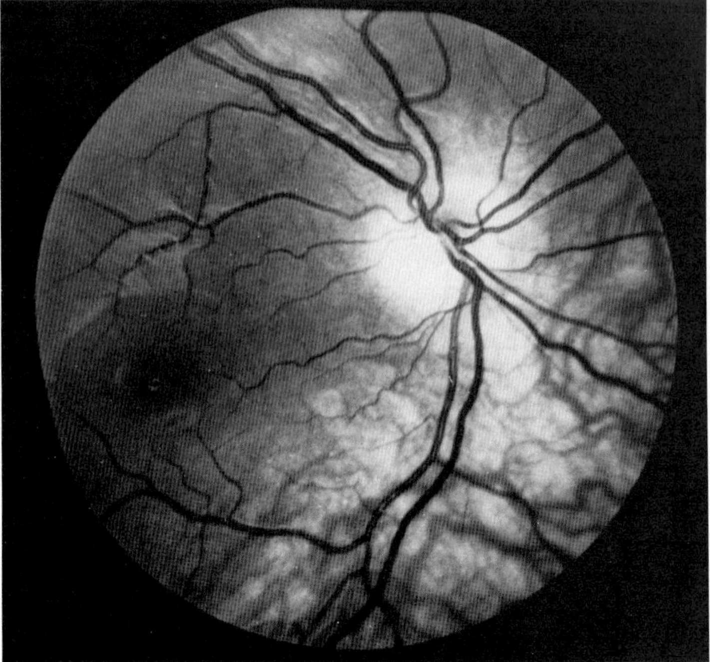

Fig. 24. (Margolis) Case 8: Fundus, right eye. The disc is tilted but shows a normal pattern of retinal vessels. A diffuse foveal reflex is seen in the inferiorly displaced macula. Hypopigmentation can be seen in the inferior nasal quadrant as well as in the midperiphery (see Fig. 25).

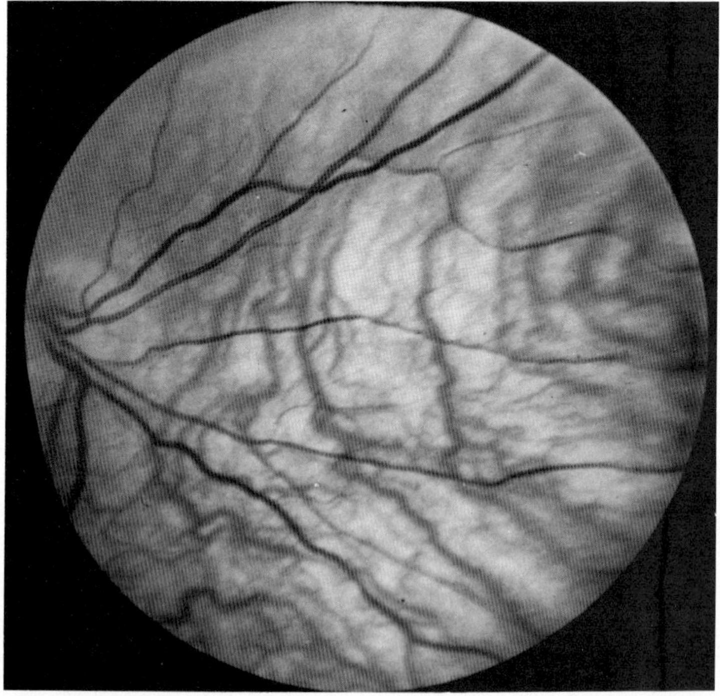

Fig. 25. (Margolis) Case 8: Right eye. Extensive hypopigmentation is seen nasal to the disc.

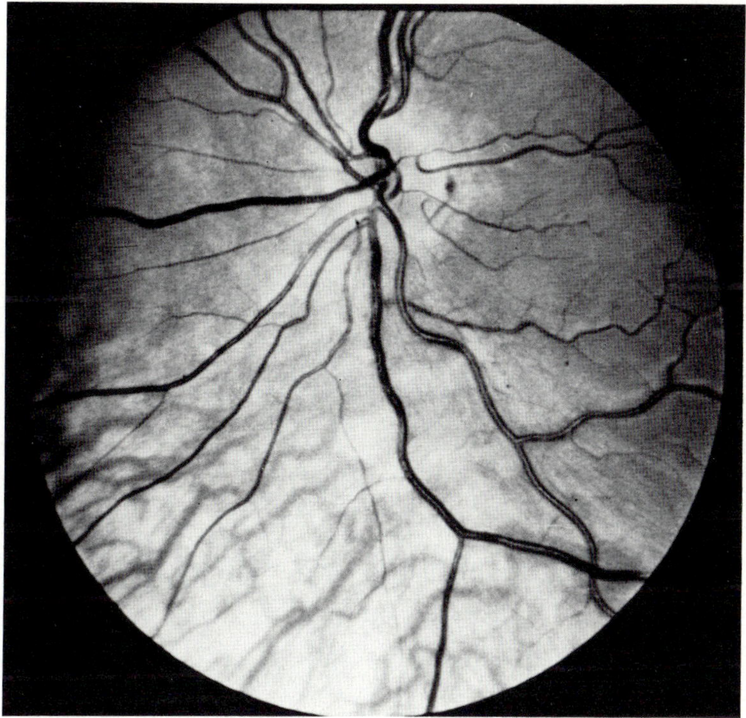

Fig. 26. (Margolis) Case 8: Fundus, left eye. The disc orientation and retinal vasculature appear normal. Marked hypopigmentation is present inferior to the disc and throughout the posterior pole. The macula was in a normal position.

Ophthalmoscopic Examination. There was situs inversus of both discs (Figs. 28, 29). The margins of each disc were well delineated, and there was normal retinal vessel caliber. Pigmentation of the fundus was normal. The foveal reflexes were normal, but the left foveal area appeared to be inferiorly displaced.

Computerized axial tomography revealed mild lateral ventricular dilatation. Electroencephalogram suggested a diffuse bilateral cerebral dysfunction.

DISCUSSION

One of the most striking aspects of the group of patients with craniofacial anomalies is the association of the very rare tilted disc syndrome and the presence in the Crouzon's and Apert's disease of widespread fundal hypopigmentation. Previously, the tilted disc syndrome which incorporates an inferior sector of hypopigmentation was reported as an isolated finding of unknown etiology.[8-13] Apparently a tilted disc is not an unusual finding in craniofacial disease—a condition which may affect to a greater or lesser degree, structure or pigmentation of the eye, skull, face, orbit, and limbs.[3] Furthermore, since the craniofacial dysostoses are transmitted as an autosomal dominant, one could ask whether the "isolated" tilted disc syndrome, for example, is a mild expression of a craniofacial disorder in seemingly normal patients. The lesson is clear. Such patients must have their irises carefully transilluminated and their facial and skull structure examined for any signs of midface hypoplasia, hypertelorism, or other relevant skeletal malformations. Other family members should also be examined if possible in order to judge extreme variations in physiognomy from the norm.

Within the group of craniofacial dysostoses the occurrence of ocular and cutaneous hypopigmentation may at first appear to be inexplicable. The finding is more readily understandable if one considers the chronologic sequence of the pertinent developing systems. The period of skeletal

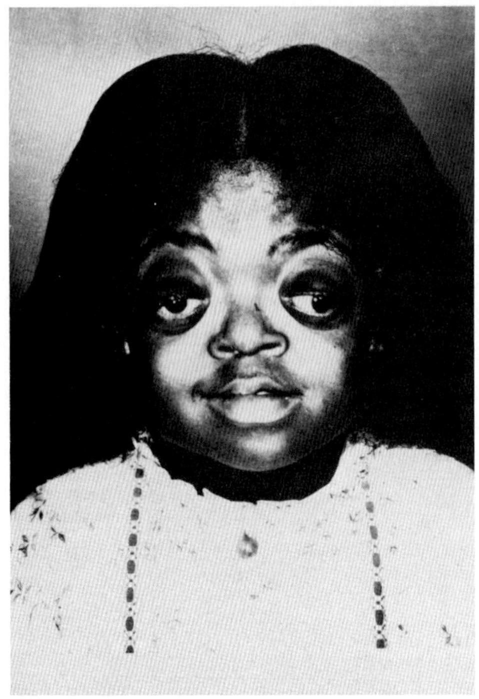

Fig. 27. (Margolis) Case 9: A 10-year-old female with hypertelorism, antimongoloid fissures, exophthalmos, ptosis, absence of all lacrimal puncta, and strabismus.

formation of the skull, face, and limbs overlaps the time of closure of the fetal fissure and disc development. These latter events, which are quite early, coincide quite closely with ocular melanogenesis. It is known from the thalidomide studies, for example, that the critical teratogenic period for differentiation of skull and hand is between the

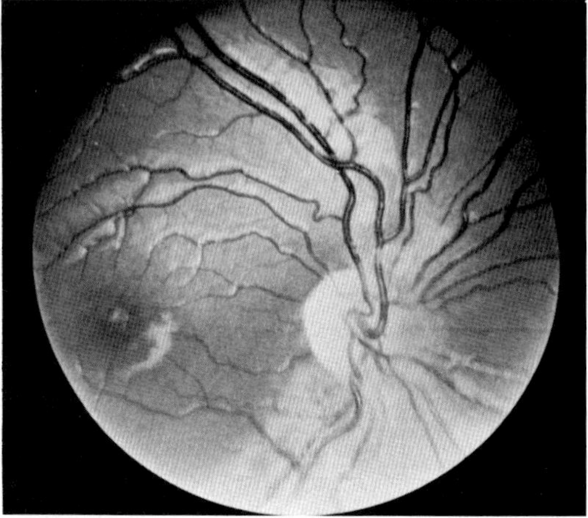

Fig. 28. (Margolis) Case 9: Fundus, right eye. Situs inversus of the disc. The macula positioning is normal.

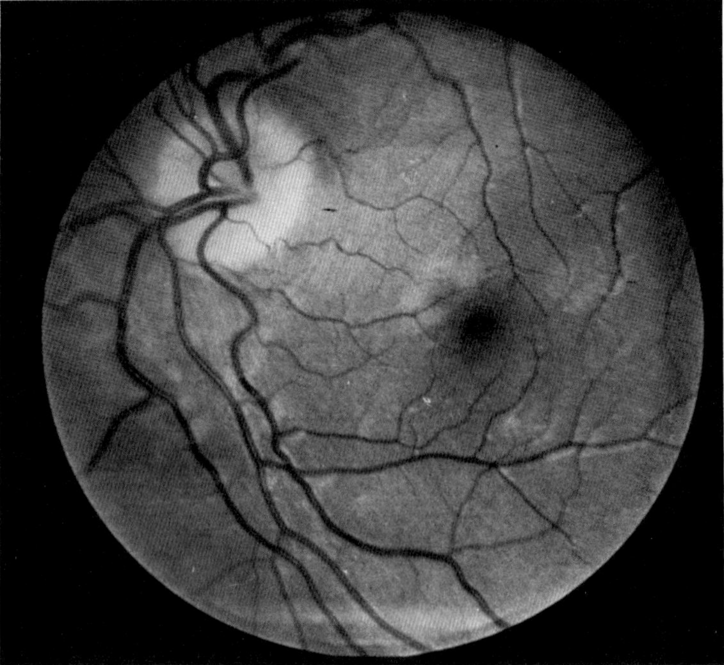

Fig. 29. (Margolis) Case 9: Fundus, left eye. Situs inversus of the left disc, similar to that seen in the right eye (see Fig. 28) was inferiorly displaced.

19th and 35th day of embryonic life.[14] Furthermore, Mann showed that the second phase of retinal differentiation as well as segmentation of the digits normally occurs during the 42nd to 49th days of embryogenesis.[15] The common denominator for these events may be the migration of certain stem lines of the neural crest cells. Caudally moving streams of neural crest cells give rise to primitive melanoblasts which after migration to skin, hair, and iris stroma differentiate to form melanocytes. Other crest cells in this same migration are involved in the formation of the skeletal tissues of the upper face and skull.[16] As the flexure of the head of the embryo is occurring early in development, the neural crest cells are seen to migrate ventrally into the future face, skull, and eye structures. Should any asynchrony in the time of migration occur, or alteration of number of crest cells to designated areas change, then it is likely that the pigment cells of the hair, skin, and iris stroma as well as structures of the skull, face, and orbit would be affected. At the time the embryonic head is flexing, pigmentation of the optic cup, the retinal pigment epithelium and anterior border layer of the iris is also occurring.[17, 18] Taken together, any miscue in this complex series of temporal events could produce the main features of an Apert or Crouzon's disease.

One final point on the retinal hypopigmentation in the patients with craniofacial dysostoses concerns the particular geographical location of the pigment loss. It was noted in several patients (see, for example, Figs. 7, 10, 19, 24, 26) to be almost exclusively localized to the inferior or infero-nasal quadrant—the area corresponding to the embryonic fetal fissure. In fact, this particular sector of depigmented retina was very early on noted to appear below a highly myopic or tilted disc and was termed a Fuch's coloboma.[19] A number of more recent reports describe a tilted disc "syndrome" which may include: an inferior sector of retinal depigmentation below a tilted optic disc, an inferior conus, situs inversus of the disc, and bitemporal field defects.[8–13] It should be recalled that the reversed appearance of the disc in situs inversus is only a consequence of the vessels emerging from the temporal portion of the disc, passing nasally, and then turning back toward the macular region.

But what of the bitemporal field defects themselves? Are they somehow a direct consequence of the tilted discs? Is the hypopigmented sector below the disc a cogent sign of malfunction, perhaps in the nerve fiber layer?

Tilted discs are associated with an inferiorly located conus of tissue. It is believed to have its origin in an anomalous tongue of neural ectoderm resulting from a tilted insertion of the optic stalk into the optic vesicle.[5] Normally, there is a delay in pigmentation of the outer layer of the optic cup in the fetal fissure below the disc. The sequence of these events probably begins in the human at the 8-mm stage when the optic stalk is narrowing down and is fully determined by the 13-mm stage when the fetal fissure has closed and pigmentation of the cup is fully established. Mann[5] refers to a localized failure of pigment epithelium formation with resultant loss of underlying choriocapillaries following faulty insertion of the stalk. It has already been shown that a loop of aberrant nerve fibers were found in conjunction with a superior conus.[17] If a similar association occurred in the inferiorly placed conus, a possible mechanism for the observed field defects can be visualized. The clinician should note that a visual field determination can differentiate ocular from chiasmal lesions, by noting the loss of field relative to the midline.[20] A sharp field cut at the midline implies a chiasmal lesion, in contrast to a defect due to an anomalous disc or retina lesion, which produces a sloping field cut as it crosses the midline. A clinical point of interest here is that the projection of the tilted disc yields, on field testing with small targets, the appearance of a bitemporal hemianopia. It should be kept in mind that an actual loss of retinal tissue corresponding to the depigmented sector would probably not account for the field loss. In fact, histologic study showed an area of retinal ectasia below the disc in such cases, but the underlying retinal pigment epithelium and choriocapillaris were normal.[13] While many mechanisms may exist to account for the temporal field loss in "tilted disc syndrome," two explanations seem particularly relevant.

The first mechanism may involve an abnormality of the optic nerve fiber pathway that is associated with most forms of albinism.[21] It is known that a considerable field loss occurs in albinos because a relatively small portion of temporal optic fibers cross at the chiasm producing serious dislocation within the highly organized lamina of the lateral geniculate body. Such higher center disruption carries on to the next level of visual staging—the occipital cortex—with resulting visual field impairment. A second, simpler, explanation involves the actual loss of those optic fibers from the nasal half of the retina, which cannot cross the chiasm because of the midline cleft.[22, 23] Hypertelorism is known to have associated with it basal encephalocele and midline cleft defects.[20] Such anatomical malformations could certainly interfere with the crossing fibers and thus produce the bitemporal field defects.

The final point to be made about the retinal abnormalities seen in association with tilted discs is the inferiorly displaced foveal areas—heterotopic maculae. Such displacement has been seen in both hypertelorism[11] and situs inversus of the disc.[12] In such instances, it is probably a result of an altered positioned of the macula due to irregularities in maturation and development of the retina.[24] This is in distinction to heterotopias found in association with foci of chorioretinitis, traction bands of the retina, and colobomas of the optic nerve and choroid.[25, 26] The latter heterotopias are obviously produced secondary to mechanical effects.

Considering the severe orbital anomalies that exist in the patients reported here, it could be justifiably asked whether the globe is cyclotorting and all the retinal landmarks merely rotated counterclockwise and clockwise fashion for the right and left eyes, respectively. However, careful fundus and field studies show that not only are the foveal areas inferiorly displaced but are in variable positions in relation to the disc and temporal arcades.[26] This observation would certainly lend weight to the notion of a developmental anomaly affecting the closing of the fetal fissure.

SUMMARY

Optic nerve and retinal findings found in association with craniofacial malformations such as orbital hypertelorism, Apert's, and Crouzon's diseases are presented. Patients with congenital deformities of the skull, face, orbit, and limbs also show optic nerve anomalies, retinal dysfunction, and fundal hypopigmentation. The tilted disc syndrome previously reported in otherwise normal patients is shown to exist in a large group of craniofacial malformations. The diagnostic importance to the clinician is discussed and its relationship to the craniofacial anomalies is delineated. The new associations of hypopigmentation and the tilted disc syndrome with craniofacial malformations is presented in the context of the chronologic sequence of the developing skeletal and ocular structure. The period of (1) skeletal formation of the skull, face, orbits, and limbs, (2) closure of the fetal fissure, and (3) optic disc and pathway development all coincide with ocular melanization. An insult or disturbance in the temporal sequence at a critical point in gestation may affect several seemingly unrelated developing processes.

EDITOR'S NOTE

Dr. Margolis and Dr. Siegel have brought out a very important point here—that of tilted optic discs in craniofacial disease. You may ask—Why is this important? We have been impressed for many years that there is the possibility of optic atrophy developing in patients with Crouzon's disease and other various forms of the craniosynostoses, and many neurosurgeons have done morticillation operations in infancy in an attempt to prevent the later development of optic atrophy in such cases. However, it is now evident that the "plot thickens"! It is now well known that congenital tilting of the optic discs can cause bitemporal visual field defects. A reference to this condition is by Odland, M. in *Acta Neurol. Scand.* **43:**630–639, 1967. There have been several other more recent papers on this, and it is now well appreciated that there is a relative thinning of the pigment epithelium in the lower nasal fundus in this disorder, which can best be appreciated by indirect ophthalmoscopy. This is seen in Dr. Margolis' report. Dr. Y. Goldhammer reported a table listing nonsurgical causes of bitemporal hemianopia in *Neurol.* **24:** 1135–1138, Dec. 1974, which is also helpful for review in that regard. I think it is very important to get a careful look at a good set of skull films including base views and a CT scan in these children with marked hyperteleorism because many of them may be harboring an encephalocele. This was also evident in this chapter. Dr. Goldhammer listed the following ocular anomalies associated with basal encephaloceles: hyperteleorism, exotropia, microphthalmos, cryptophthalmos, peripapillary staphyloma, and the following optic disc anoamlies: pallor, pits, coloboma, dysplasia, megalopapilla, and bitemporal hemianopia in his paper—"Cryptophthalmos Syndrome with Basal Encephaloceles" which appeared in *Am. J. Ophthalmol.* **80**(1):146–149, July 1975. Therefore, if we have to consider these various forms of optic nerve anomalies as well as other defects (situs inversus, displaced maculae, and the like), it is obvious that there are more than a few ways the optic discs can look abnormal in such children. This warrants a much closer neuro-ophthalmologic scrutiny in these children. Congratulations to Dr. Margolis for bringing this to our attention!

JLS

ACKNOWLEDGMENTS

We wish to thank Dr. John M. Converse-Chief of the Institute of Plastic and Reconstructive Surgery and Dr. Joseph G. McCarthy, Associate Director of Craniofacial Anomalies Project for their support and permission to see these patients.

Also we wish to thank Mr. Walter Lentschner for his photographic contributions and Mrs. Sylvia Glasser for her help in the preparation of the manuscript.

This study was supported in part by Grants EY 00213 and EY 00309 from the National Eye Institute, DEO 3568-03 from the National Institute of Dental Research, and a grant to the Ophthalmology Department from Research to Prevent Blindness.

REFERENCES

1. Walsh, F. B. and Hoyt, W. F. *Clinical Neuro-ophthalmology.* 3rd ed. Baltimore, Williams and Wilkins, 1969, Vol. I.
2. Margolis, S., Siegel, I. M., Choy, A., and Breinin, G. M. Oculocutaneous albinism associated with Apert's syndrome. Am. J. Ophthalmol. *84:*830 (1977).
3. Margolis, S., Siegel, I. M., Choy, A., and Breinin, G. M. Depigmentation of hair, skin, and eyes associated with Apert's syndrome. Recent advances in new syndromes. Birth Defects Symposium, March of Dimes Original Articles, Vol. XIV, No. 6B, 1978. pp. 341–360.
4. Margolis, S., Breinin, G. M., and Choy, A. New Retinal Findings in Apert's and Crouzon's Syndromes. *Second International Conference on Craniofacial Deformities. May, 1976.* Mosby, In press.
5. Mann, I. *Developmental Abnormalities of the Eye.* 2nd ed. Lippincott, Philadelphia, 1957, pp. 102–113.
6. Tessier, P., Guiot, G., Delbet, J. P., and Pastoriza, J. Osteotomies cranio-naso-orbito-faciales hypertelorism. Chir. Plast. *12:*103 (1976).
7. Apert, E. De L'acrocephalosyndactylie. Bull. Mem. Soc. Med. Hop. (Paris) *23:*131 (1966).
8. Caccamise, W. C. Situs inversus of the disc with inferior conus and variable myopia. A case report. Am. J. Ophthalmol. *38:*854 (1954).
9. Berry, H. Bitemporal Depression of the visual fields due to an ocular cause. Br. J. Ophthalmol. *47:*441 (1963).
10. Odlund, M. Bitemporal defects of the visual fields due to anomalies of the optic discs. Acta Neurol. Scand. *43:*630 (1967).
11. Graham, M. V. and Wakefield, G. J. Bitemporal visual field defects associated with anomalies of the optic discs. Br. J. Ophthalmol. *57:*307 (1973).
12. Rucker, C. W. Bitemporal defects in the visual fields resulting from developmental anomalies of the optic discs. Arch. Opthalmol. *35:*546 (1946).
13. Young, S. E., Walsh, F., and Knox, D. L. The tilted disc syndrome. Am. J. Ophthalmol. *82:*16 (1976).
14. Degenhardt, K. H. Zum Entwicklungsmenchanischen Problem der Akrocephalo-syndaktylic. Z. Menschl. Vererb. Konstitutionslehre. *29:*791 (1950).
15. Mann, I. *The Development of the Human Eye.* Grune and Stratton, New York, 1964, pp. 282, 288.
16. Johnston, M. C. Neural crest in abnormalities of the face and brain in birth defects. *Original Article Series, March of Dimes.* Liss, New York, 1975, Vol. XI, No. 7, pp. 1–18.
17. Duke-Elder, S. Normal and abnormal development congenital deformities. In *System of Ophthalmology,* C.V. Mosby, St. Louis, 1964, Vol. 3, pt. 2. p. 675–678.
18. Mund, E., Rodriguez, M., and Fine, B. Light and electronmicroscopy on pigmented layers of the human eye. Am. J. Ophthalmol. *73:*167 (1972).
19. Fuchs, E. Über den anatomischen Befund einiger angeborener Anomalien der Netzhaut und des Schnerven. V. Graefes. Arch. Ophthal. *93:*1 (1917).
20. Goldhammer, Y., and Smith, J. L. Bitemporal hemianopia in chloroquine retinopathy. Neurol. *24:*1135 (1974).
21. Creel, D., O'Donnell, F., and Witkop, C. J. Visual system anomalies in human ocular albinos. Science *201:*931 (1978).
22. Francois, J., and DeRouck, A. Electroretino-

graphic study of hypoplasia of the optic nerve. Ophthalmologica, Basel *172*:308 (1976).

23. Gross, H., and Hoff, H. Sur les malformations ventriculaires dépendentes des dysgénésis commissurales; dans Heyer, Teld, and Gruner Malformations Congenitales du cerveau (Masson, Paris, 1959), p. 329.

24. Mann, I. *Developmental Anomalies of the Eye,* Cambridge University Press, London, 1937, p. 157.

25. Bernhard, A. Ein Fall von abnormaler Lage der Makulalutea und partiellen Colobom der Choroidea, Arch. f. Augenh. *37*:51 (1898).

26. Cohen, I., and Weisber, H. Vertical heterotopia of the macula. Arch. Ophthal. *44*:419 (1950).

12 A Sinister Association of the Congenital Tilted Disk Syndrome with Chiasmal Compression

Robert H. Osher, M. D.
Norman J. Schatz, M. D.

"One of the most dependable axioms in ophthalmology is that bitemporal hemianopsia indicates a lesion at the optic chiasm... even to this rule there may be exceptions which can occasionally cause difficulty in diagnosis." C. Wilbur Rucker, M.D., thereby introduced into the English literature the association between bitemporal visual field defects and developmental anomalies of the optic disks.[13] Over 100 subsequent cases have been reported both reemphasizing this benign relationship and providing the literature with the reassuring term "tilted disk syndrome."[1-3, 5, 6, 10-13, 15, 16, 19, 20] While these major features of this syndrome caused significant confusion in the past, they are now recognized as a comforting ocular cause of bitemporal field depression: (1) congenital conus, (2) situs inversus of the optic disk, (3) localized thinning or retinal pigment epithelium, (4) myopic astigmatism, and (5) "temporal hemianopia."

The following case illustrates a different aspect of this syndrome. A 26-year-old man complained of decreased vision over a three-week period. He described a cloud located superotemporally in his left eye and was unaware of any visual difficulty in his right eye. He was otherwise asymptomatic and in excellent health.

Both general and neurological examinations were normal. Best corrected visual acuity was 20/25 in the right eye and 20/70 in the left eye. Ocular motility was unremarkable. Pupillary testing revealed a left afferent defect. A temporal hemianopic field defect was found on tangent screen examination of the left eye. The central field in the right eye showed a temporal hemianopic arcuate scotoma (Fig. 1). Peripheral fields were full in the right eye, while a temporal constriction was present in the left eye. Bitemporal hemianopic defects were conspicuous by confrontation using red colored targets. Ophthalmoscopy revealed an unusual appearance of each optic nerve consistent with the diagnosis of inferior conus (Fig. 2).

In summary, a 26-year-old man with bilateral inferior conus presented with a history of progressive visual disturbance, an afferent pupil, and a bitemporal field defect respecting the vertical meridian. These findings suggested chiasmal compression in addition to coincidental Fuch's colobomas, so a neuroradiologic evaluation was initiated. Plain skull films were normal, while a calcification in the region of the diaphragma sellae was present on polytomography. A brain scan revealed increased uptake in the suprasellar region. Bilateral carotid angiography demonstrated modest elevation of the first portion of the anterior cerebral artery. Pneumoencephalography showed indentation of the third ventricle by a large suprasellar mass. The patient underwent craniotomy, and the surgeon en-

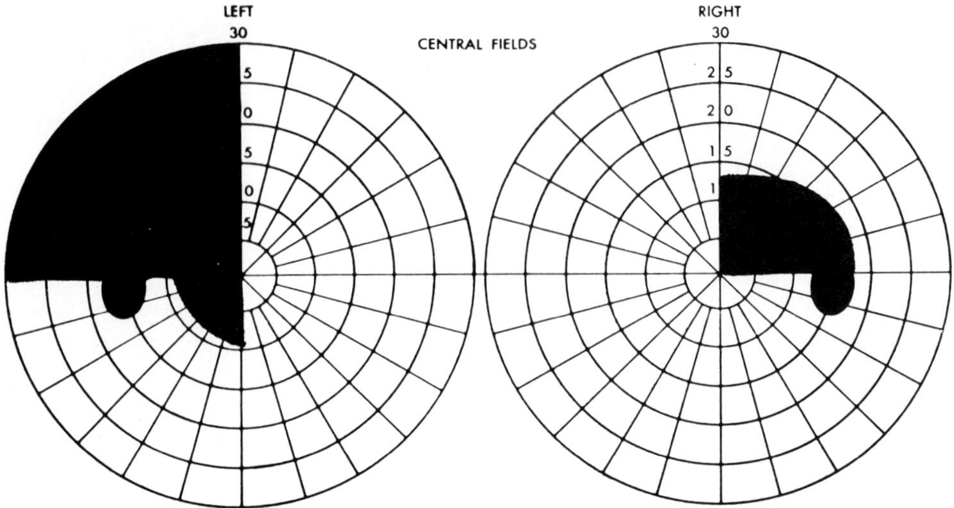

Fig. 1. Central visual field evaluation shows bitemporal hemianopic defects with strict respect for the vertical meridian.

countered a reddish-gray fungating meningioma occupying the area between both optic nerves and extending above the chiasm (Fig. 3). The tumor was resected without complication, and the histologic diagnosis was meningotheliomatous meningioma. The postoperative visual acuity returned to 20/20, and the peripheral fields were normal. Some improvement in the central fields was observed, although a bitemporal depression was still evident.

DISCUSSION

Congenital conus or crescent is a common condition occurring in 3% of all eyes and provides a characteristic ophthalmoscopic appearance.[17] Two-thirds of congenital crescents are located below the disk (Fuch's coloboma) and are frequently associated with bitemporal field defects.[18] The optic disk is horizontally oval and appears to tilt downward toward a white semilunar crescent at its inferior margin. The size of the optic disc is often diminished so that the disk and the crescent together do not amount to more than an ordinary optic disk.[12] The superior rim of the disk appears raised (a source of misinterpretation for papilledema[20]), and the vessels course abruptly over its edge. The inferior rim has a gradual slope separating lamina cribosa from the conus. Usually the width of the crescent is from ⅛ to ½ of the optic disk's diameter and often embraces from ¼ to ½ of the circumference.[12] Crescent has also been described together with pits of the optic disk.[4]

Situs inversus describes the reverse distribution of vessels which emerge nasal to the disk before pursuing their temporal course. This condition frequently accompanies Fuch's coloboma, but may by its own right produce defects in the visual field.[13]

Localized thinning of the retinal pigment epithelium is usually present with inferior conus, extending from the margin of the crescent throughout the inferior fundus. The crescent itself probably results from the failure of pigment epithelium to reach the site of implantation of the optic stalk into the vesicle, while the thinning may be related to the developmental fundus ectasia.[9, 12]

Myopic astigmatism is seen in the majority of these patients. Unusual optical features include an oblique cylindrical axis as well as localized nasal ectasia of the fundus with a difference in refraction between the macula and the ectatic region.[12] Various authors have tested, with variable success, the hypothesis that increasing the myopic correction decreases the temporal field depression.[5, 10–12, 14]

Bitemporal field defects have initiated a

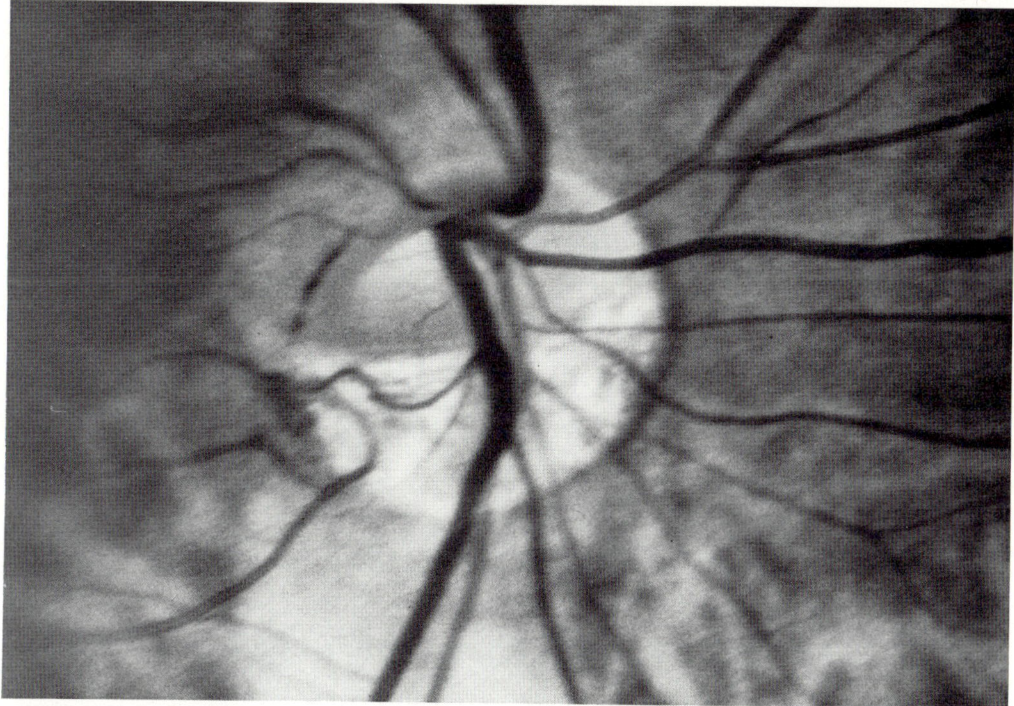

Fig. 2A

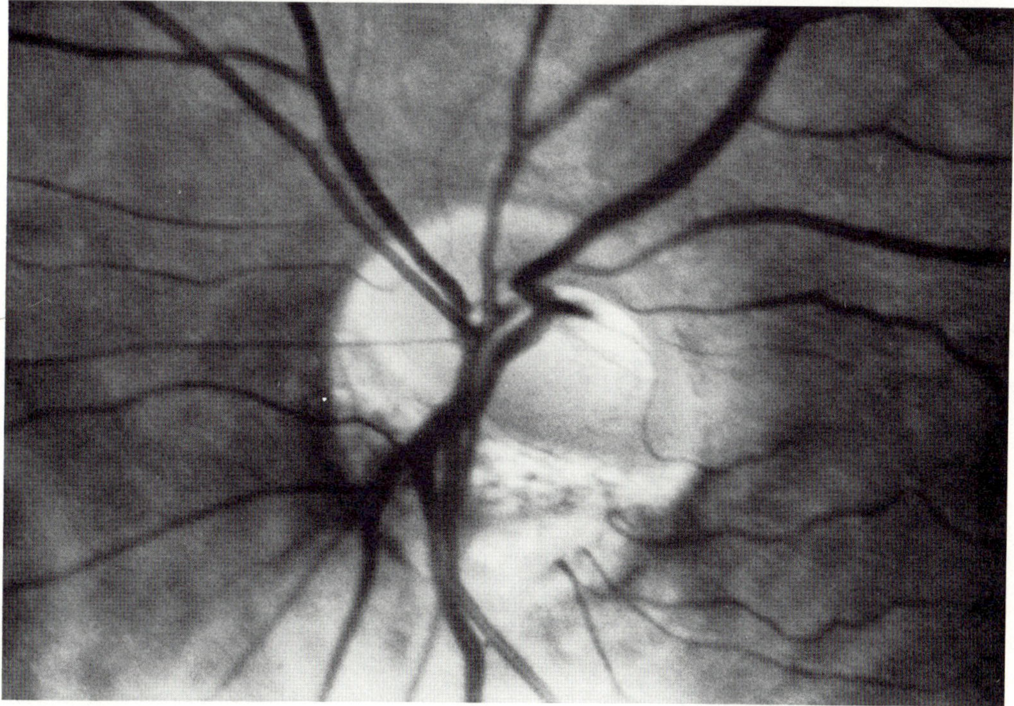

Fig. 2B

Fig. 2. Appearance of optic disks demonstrates features of tilted disk syndrome. Note Fuch's coloboma, situs inversus, and thinning of retinal pigment epithelium below crescent.

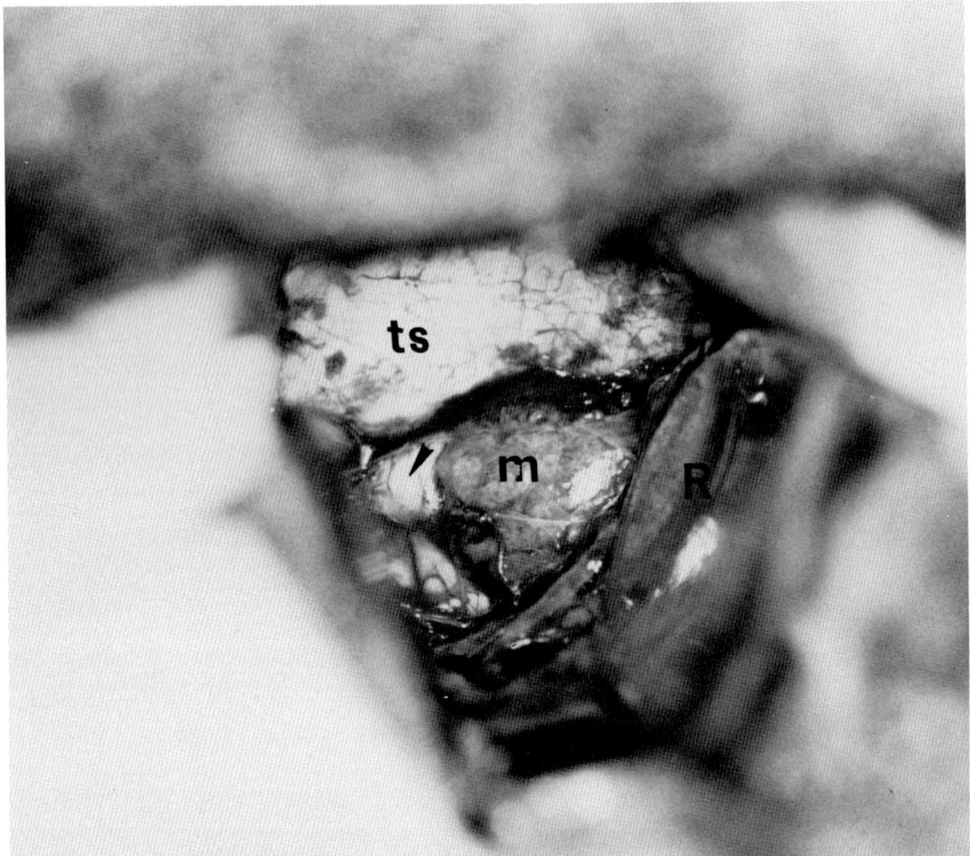

Fig. 3. Surgical exploration. ts = tuberculum sellae, m = meningioma, R = retractor, black arrow = optic nerve.

chain of unnecessary neurodiagnostic studies and even neurosurgical intervention in too many patients with congenital conus. Careful perimetry reveals a bitemporal depression that is not truly hemianopic, since the defect often slopes obliquely across the vertical meridian to involve the superior nasal quadrant. This is best demonstrated with smaller isopters and red targets, while the peripheral fields are invariably normal to larger targets. Local retinal staphylomatous ectasia or local hypoplasia of retina and choroid with fewer receptors per unit are among postulates advanced to explain the field loss.[3]

Color isopters may help the clinician whose visual field has left him unsure of the relationship to the vertical meridian. A chiasmal lesion will produce hemidyschromatopsia in contrast to a refractive field defect. Furthermore, if minus lenses improve the field defect, the diagnosis of

chiasmal syndrome should no longer be entertained.

It is important to emphasize that congenital visual defects are stable, and the patient is unaware of their presence—a fundamental rule in evaluating congenital disk anomalies. *If this rule is violated either by history or by findings derived in the neuro-ophthalmologic assessment of visual acuity, color perception, pupillary function, visual field, or optic disk appearance, then a vigorous neuroradiologic investigation is mandatory.*

Our patient complained of an acquired visual field disturbance with a concomitant reduction in visual acuity. An afferent pupillary defect further helped to clarify the meaning of a bitemporal hemianopia in the presence of bilateral Fuch's colobomas. In conclusion, congenital disk anomalies do not protect against concurrent juxtasellar pathology, and it is hazardous to rely on the diagnosis of benign "tilted disk syndrome" if a true bitemporal hemianopia is present.

EDITOR'S NOTE

The authors have presented another one of Dr. Schatz' typical Wills Eye Hospital cases—namely, not only did the patient truly have congenitally tilted discs with a bitemporal field defect, *BUT* this patient *also* had a suprasellar meningioma as well! They rightly emphasize that if the history or findings are atypical at all that the patient merits further workup. One could spend quite a time discussing this case. To some extent it reminds me of Dr. Walsh's old dictum that "A patient with drusen of the optic nerve can*not* have a brain tumor!" Now, the way that saying got started is simply that for years and years, patients were seen by Dr. Frank B. Walsh with swollen optic discs, which were falsely called papilledema, and the patients were worked up repeatedly and extensively for brain tumors, and yet on a careful Hruby lens exam it was evident that the problem was not papilledema at all, but pseudopapilledema due to buried drusen or hyaline bodies in the nerve. Therefore, as a teaching point, Dr. Walsh began to teach the residents at Wilmer that if you see hyaline bodies in the nerve, the patient simply does *NOT* have a brain tumor! Well one day—it happened!—just as you would guess. Along came a patient (and she happened to be employed by a very distinguished physician in the area!)—who had headaches and funny looking discs and, indeed, when Dr. Walsh examined them, they had drusen in those nerves. However, that lady truly had an intracranial meningioma as well, and to the best of my memory, when the smoke finally cleared, she had THREE meningiomas detected subsequently. The moral of the story is simply this—even though hyaline bodies or drusen of the optic nerve are commonly mistaken for papilledema, they certainly offer no true protection at all from the rare patient who comes along one day and truly develops a brain tumor! Now, that is exactly what happened in the patient presented by Dr. Osher and Dr. Schatz. For years and years, patients were found to have bitemporal visual field defects at times on confrontation fields—the fundus explanation was not detected—and the patients were put through expensive, unpleasant, and frightening neurodiagnostic studies to rule out a parachiasmal tumor. All the time, however, the explanation was right there in the fundus—namely, a congenitally tilted optic disc!

I want to take this a step further. One should also read the comments about tilted discs elsewhere in this book. However, from the strictly *perimetric* point of view there are some important points to make. If one looks at *Figure 2* in this chapter, he will note absolutely classic tilted optic discs with the lower nasal part of the disc looking as if a cat had bitten a big bite out of it. To be sure, the cat crossed the disc on into the lower temporal part as well, but certainly the big sloping bite is out of the lower nasal part of the disc. However, the point I'm trying to emphasize is that the *discs* look very *symmetrical* in appearance in this case. However, if we look at *Figure 1*, it is evident that the *field defects* were *extremely asymmetrical*. Of course, the acuity tells the same thing—the right eye had a good 20/25, but the left eye was down to 20/70. It would have been interesting to have the refractive errors in both eyes recorded in this note, and I should imagine that this showed some modest compound myopic astigmatism in both eyes that again was about the same in degree in both eyes. From the field point of view only, however, one should have been suspicious in this case—because the *discs* were *symmetrical* but the *field* was *asymmetrical*. That should alert you immediately in such a case to promptly get a good set of skull x-rays and look at that sella!

I recall the first case of tilted discs producing a bitemporal field defect I saw. This was a middle-aged pastor's wife who was complaining about her vision and who had a few headaches. I did her central fields before examining her fundi, and—lo-and-behold!—she had upper bitemporal field defects. I said to myself—"Wow! She's going to have a chromophobe adenoma!" I even sent her over to get a set of routine skull films while the drops were working on her pupils before I looked at the fundi.

When she came back, I saw that she had the classic appearance of tilted discs in that a cat had taken a bite out of the lower nasal part of the disc on both eyes, and also there was the typical picture as seen with indirect ophthalmoscopy of thinning of the pigment epithelium over the entire lower nasal quadrant in both eyes. You really need indirect to appreciate the fact that the entire fundus pattern has a normal pinkish color over upper temporal, upper nasal, lower temporal areas—but that lower nasal quadrant suddenly has a demarcation line that is oval in shape and has a light blonde more tessellated appearance in both eyes. This is typically present with the tilted disc syndromes.

Now here are two more pearls —I did her peripheral fields to 3/330 white, and they were perfectly normal in both eyes! Now, many writers like to emphasize that the bitemporal defects in tilted discs are not TRULY bitemporal but they sneak across the midline. They do,—'tis true—but it is interesting to me that they do not sneak across the midline until AFTER you have made the fundus diagnosis! In other words, when you first do that tangent screen exam, they really stop right on that hemianopic line. However, when you push and fight and huff and puff on a repeat exam, you can tease that defect across a bit. They really can look bitemporal, however. You need to go back on the perimeter, after you have found them on the tangent screen, and go into that midzonal field, and you can then find these bitemporal-like defects on the perimeter, and outside the area will be quite normal. I have seen that pattern in several cases and now consider this to be a consistent syndrome. Here it is: (1) upper bitemporal defects on tangent screen—they really look bitemporal!—(2) normal peripheral fields on first run with large isopters; (3) acuity and field defects are symmetrical in both eyes; (4) usually a moderately good amount of compound myopic astigmia (as −5.00 ± 1.75 cylinders in both eyes, for example); (5) the lower nasal disc has been bitten off by a cat bite; (6) there is a more blonde appearance to entire lower nasal quadrant with indirect ophthalmoscopy; (7) you go back now and find that you really CAN tease that central field defect across

the midline a bit; (8) you go back on the perimeter and find that you really CAN find that defect on perimeter but it's close down there to fixation and outside this there is NO hemianopic line or Chamlin's step. Finally, if not sure—get a good set of plain films and you won't miss the next case of the rare concurrence of problems as seen in this case. I thank the authors for providing such a good opportunity to share these little teaching points about this clinical picture!

JLS

ACKNOWLEDGMENT

Barbara Osher and Betsy Barton provided helpful assistance in preparing this manuscript.

REFERENCES

1. Bard, L. A. Tilted disc with inferior conus, a report of 12 cases. Ref. 26th Meeting of the Wilmer Residents Association.
2. Berry, H. Bitemporal depression of the visual fields due to an ocular cause. Br. J. Ophthalmol. 47:441–444 (1963).
3. Caccamise, W. C. Situs inversus of the optic disc with inferior conus and variable myopia. Am. J. Ophthalmol. 38:854–856 (1954).
4. Edmund, C. On congenital colobomatous groove formations in the optic disk. Acta Ophthalmol. 8:56–63 (1930).
5. Enoksson, P. Perimetry in neuro-ophthalmological diagnosis. Acta Ophthalmol. Suppl. 82:5–54 (1965).
6. Graham, M. V. and Wakefield, G. J. Bitemporal visual field defects associated with anomalies of the optic discs. Br. J. Ophthalmol. 57:307–314 (1973).
7. Hoyt, W. F. Personal communication, 1971, cited in Riise, D. The nasal fundus in ectasia. Acta Ophthalmol. Suppl. 126:4–180 (1975).
8. Keane, J. R. Suprasellar tumors and incidental optic disc anomalies. Arch. Ophthalmol. 95:2180–2183 (1977).
9. Mann, I. *Developmental Abnormalities of the Eye.* 2nd ed. Lippincott, London, 1957, p. 101.
10. Manor, R. S. Temporal field defects due to nasal tilting of discs. Ophthalmologica 168:269–281 (1974).
11. Odland, M. Bitemporal defects of the visual fields due to anomalies of the optic discs. Acta Neurol. Scand. 9:630–639 (1967).
12. Riise, D. The nasal fundus ectasia. Acta Ophthalmol. Suppl. 126:4–108 (1975).
13. Rucker, C. W. Bitemporal defects in the visual fields resulting from developmental anomalies of the optic disks. Arch. Ophthalmol. 35:546–554 (1946).

14. Schmidt, T. Perimetric relativer Skotome. Ophthalmologica *129:*303–315 (1955).
15. Smith, J. L. and McCrary, J. A. Recent advances in optic nerve disease. In: *Neuro-ophthalmology Symposium of the University of Miami and the Bascom Palmer Eye Institute.* Huffman Publ., Hallandale, Fla., 1970, pp. 17–22.
16. Veirs, E. R. Inversio papillae with altitudinal fields. Am. J. Ophthalmol. *34:*1596–1597 (1951).
17. von Szily, A. In: *Developmental Abnormalities of the Eye.* 2nd ed. I. Mann (Ed.), Lippincott, London, 1957, p. 101.
18. Vossius, A. In: Ref. 17.
19. Walsh, F. C. and Hoyt, W. F. *Clinical Neuro-ophthalmology.* Williams and Wilkins, Baltimore, 1961, pp 660–661.
20. Young, S. E., Walsh, F. B., and Knox, D. L.: The Tilted disk syndrome. Am. J. Ophthalmol. *82:*16–23 (1976).

13 Optic Neuropathy as Initial Manifestation of Lymphoreticular Diseases. A Report of Five Cases

Tulay Kansu, M.D.,
Linda S. Orr, M.D.,
Peter J. Savino, M.D.,
Norman J. Schatz, M.D.,
and James J. Corbett, M.D.

SUMMARY

Visual loss as the initial manifestation of lymphoreticular disorders is distinctly unusual. Five such patients are presented in this report. Histopathologic diagnosis in these patients include reticulum cell sarcoma, poorly differentiated lymphocytic lymphoma, multiple myeloma (plasmacytoma), lymphomatoid granulomatosis, and eosinophilic granuloma. These cases suggest that lymphoreticular disease may arise primarily in the anterior visual pathway, may be secondary to generalized disease, or may be an expression of multicentricity. Lymphoreticular disorders should be considered in the differential diagnosis of painless progressive loss of vision.

INTRODUCTION

Lymphoreticular diseases rarely affect the anterior visual pathways, and it is particularly unusual for visual loss to be the initial manifestation. Optic nerve or chiasmal involvement has been described in patients with lymphoma,[1-7] multiple myeloma,[8-11] and leukemia.[12-17] The patients reported here all presented initially with visual loss and subsequently the diagnosis of lymphoreticular disease was established.

CASE REPORTS (TABLE I)

Case 1. A 54-year-old man complained of decreased vision in the right eye for nine days. Neuro-ophthalmologic examination revealed a visual acuity of light perception in the right eye and 6/6 in the left eye. Pupils were equal in size with a right relative afferent defect. Ocular motility and funduscopic examination were normal. After treatment for three weeks with systemic corticosteroid vision improved to 6/9 in the right eye, but the optic disc was now pale. Visual field examination revealed a central scotoma in the right eye. The remainder of the neurologic and physical examination was normal. Skull x-ray films revealed a destructive lesion in right sphenoid and posterior ethmoid sinus with enlargement and erosion of the right optic canal (Fig. 1).

A right fronto-ethmo-sphenoidectomy disclosed tumor involving the middle and posterior right ethmoid sinuses and both sphenoid sinuses. The superior and lateral ethmoidal walls were intact. Pathological diagnosis was reticulum cell sarcoma.

TABLE I. *Clinicopathologic data of five patients with lymphoreticular disorders*

Patient no.	Age/ sex	Presenting symptom	Associated symptoms and findings	Interval from onset of symptoms to diagnosis	Histopathology and location	Treatment and follow-up
1	54 M	Sudden decreased vision in right eye	None	Two months	Reticulum cell sarcoma (histiocytic lymphoma) of right sphenoethmoid complex.	4,680 R to tumor. Cyclophosphamide and prednisone; no systemic involvement one year later
2	48 F	Progressive blurred vision in right eye for five months.	None	Five months	Lymphosarcoma of right optic nerve sheath	Total 4,000 R to optic nerve and brain; vincristine, cyclophosphamide, prednisone; no recurrence two years after diagnosis
3	53 F	Sudden blurred vision in right eye	Multiple lytic lesions of spine, pelvis, hips; Bone marrow: 90% plasma cells	One month	Plasmacytoma in right sphenoid sinus, multiple myeloma	4,000 R to skull; L-phenylalanine mustard, prednisone; 6/6 vision in both eyes six months after onset
4	51 M	Blurred vision OD. Progressed to NLP in 3 days.	10 kg weight loss; multiple mass lesions in chest	Three months	Lymphomatoid granulomatosis involving optic nerves in both eyes	2,400 R to orbit; chlorambucil and prednisone; died nine months after onset
5	35 M	Progressive blurred vision in both eyes for 18 months	Right femur fracture following trauma; interstitial pulmonary densities	Eighteen months	Histiocytosis X; eosinophilic; granuloma in suprasellar area	3,000 R to sella; One year later 4,000 R to base of skull and Vinblastine; three years later NLP in both eyes, mental deterioration; expired, six years after onset

Further evaluation including chest x-ray, liver and kidney function studies, liver and spleen scan, intravenous pyelogram, bone marrow aspiration and biopsies, bilateral pedal lymphangiogram, and liver biopsy failed to reveal any evidence of systemic involvement. He was treated with 4,680 rads to the tumor area over 35 days. Chemotherapy included cyclophosphamide and prednisone. He has been followed elsewhere and his physician reported that one year later there was no local recurrence or systemic involvement.

Case 2. A 48-year-old women experienced slowly progressive blurred vision in the right eye for five months. Neuro-ophthalmologic examination revealed visual acuity of finger counting at 1 m in the right eye and 6/6 in the left eye. A relative afferent pupillary defect was present on the right, and the disc was pale. A dense right central scotoma was plotted on the Goldmann perimeter; the left visual field was full. The remainder of the neurologic examination was normal.

Laboratory Studies. Complete blood count, coagulation survey, and liver and kidney functions were within normal limits.

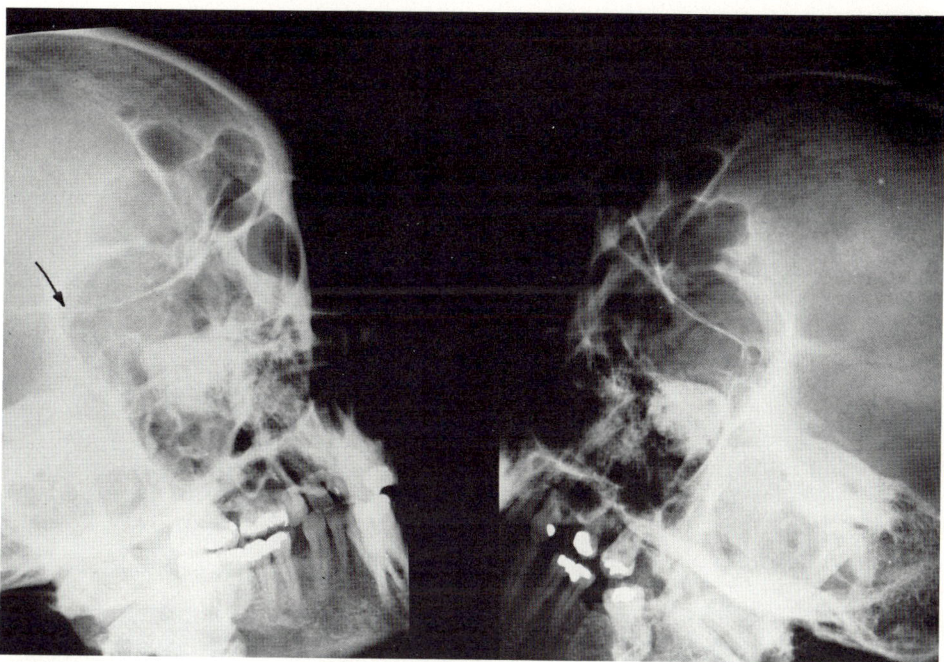

Fig. 1. (Case 1). Margins of right optic canal are indistinct and the canal appears enlarged (arrow); left optic canal is normal.

Lipoprotein electrophoresis was normal. Sedimentation rate was 36 mm/hr (Wintrobe). Serum protein electrophoresis revealed a slight hypoalbuminemia (2.3g%). Immunoglobulin electrophoresis showed a normal pattern with slightly elevated IgM of 195 mg% (N = 50–150). EKG, chest and skull x-rays were normal. Polytomography of the optic canals revealed enlargement on the right with destruction of the cortical boney rim (Fig. 2). Computerized tomographic (CT) scan showed a mass lesion in the region of the right anterior clinoid process. Pancerebral arteriography revealed stretching of the ophthalmic artery on the right.

At craniotomy the right optic nerve was three to four times the diameter of the adjacent carotid artery. Pathologic evaluation revealed poorly differentiated lymphocytic type malignant lymphoma (lymphosarcoma) infiltrating the optic nerve through the septae and to a lesser degree inwards from the piaarachnoid on the surface (Fig. 3). Spinal fluid examination, bone marrow aspiration and biopsy, bone scan, bilateral pedal lymphangiogram, and bone marrow and hepatosplenic scan showed no

evidence of other lymphomatous infiltration.

The patient was treated with radiation (total 4,000 rads to optic nerve and 3,600 rads to whole brain over 28 days) and chemotherapy (vincristine sulfate, cyclophosphamide, prednisone). Postoperatively a superior temporal hemianopic field defect was noted in the left eye which has remained stable for two years. There has been no recurrence or systemic involvement.

Case 3. A 53-year-old woman four weeks prior to admission noted blurred vision in the right eye, which within seven days progressed to inability to read with that eye.

Neuro-ophthalmologic examination revealed visual acuity 6/120 in the right eye and 6/6 in the left eye. The pupils were equal in size, and there was a right relative afferent pupillary defect. The optic discs were normal. Visual fields demonstrated a cecocentral scotoma in the right eye.

Laboratory studies revealed normal CBC, urinalysis, chest x-ray, and SMA-12. The total serum protein was 9.0 g%. Skull and sinus x-rays showed destruction of the right anterior clinoid and increased opacity of the right ethmoid sinus (Fig. 4). Polyto-

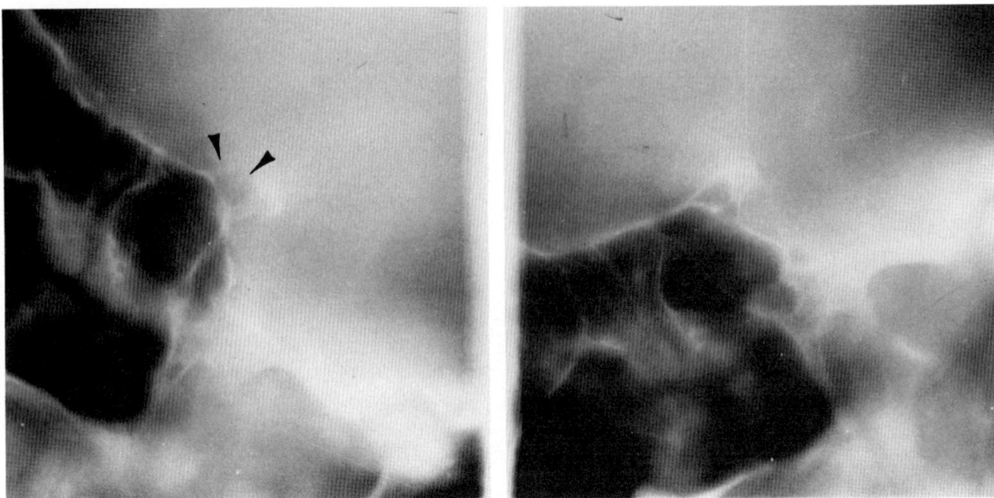

Fig. 2. (Case 2). Enlargement of the right optic canal (left) with destruction of cortical boney rim (arrows). Normal left canal (right).

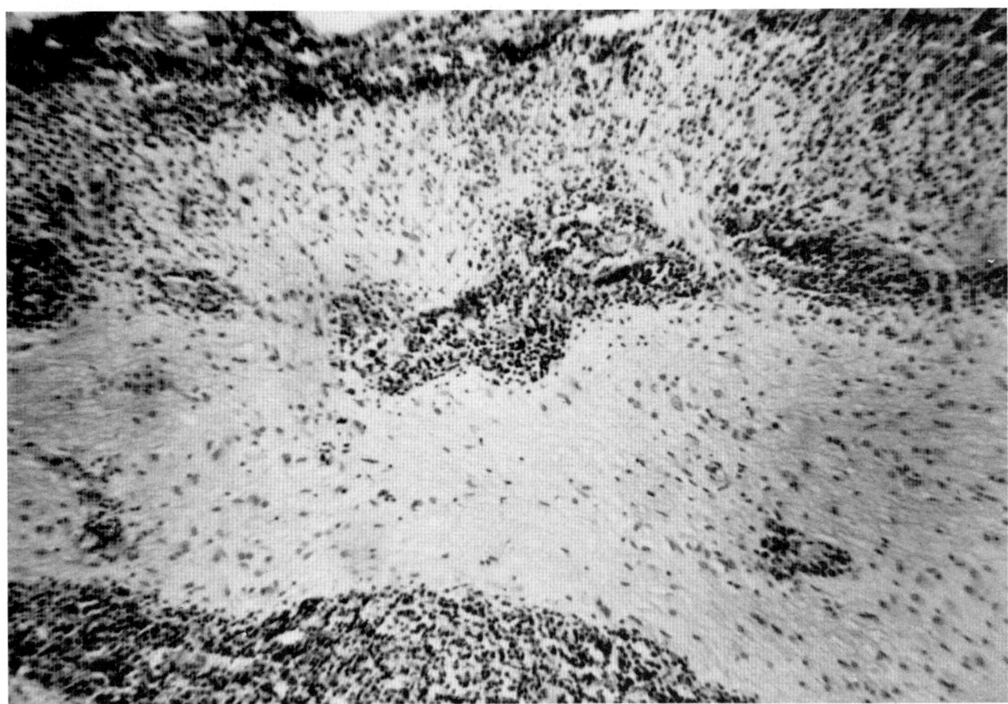

Fig. 3. (Case 2). Histopathologic sections of the optic nerve showing poorly differentiated lymphomatous lymphoma infiltrating the optic nerve.

mography also demonstrated erosion of the anterior clinoid and enlargment of the optic canal. Pancerebral arteriography defined a tumor stain in the region of the right cavernous sinus with segmental narrowing of the carotid siphon. Multiple lytic lesions of the spine, pelvis, and hips were found on a skeletal survey. A monoclonal IgA spike and no free light chains were detected on immunoelectrophoresis. Bone marrow biopsy revealed 90% immature plasma cells consistent with the diagnosis of multiple

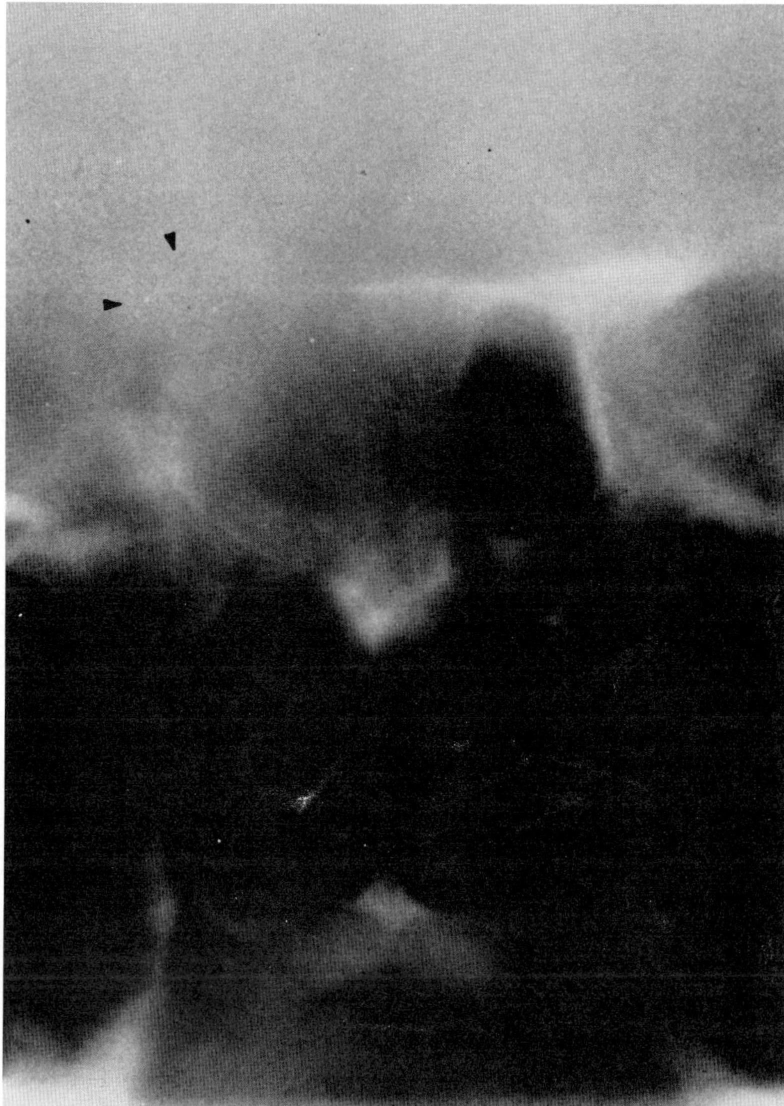

Fig. 4. (Case 3). Anterior-posterior polytomography reveals opacity of the right ethmoid sinus, and arrows indicate erosion of the anterior clinoid. Left ethmoid sinus is clear.

myeloma. Bone scan, liver and spleen scans were normal.

Transethmoidal exploration with biopsy of the sphenoid sinus mass showed a plasmacytoma. Four thousand rads were administered to the brain along with the simultaneous administration of melphalan and prednisone. Vision improved dramatically, and six months following the onset of symptoms was 6/6 in the right eye. There has been no evidence of progression of disease.

Case 4. A 51-year-old man presented with a history of visual loss in the right eye which occurred three months prior to admission. The visual loss was characterized as "a film in front of the eye" which presisted for three days and progressed to total visual loss. The diagnosis of optic neuritis was made elsewhere, and he was treated with systemic prednisone without return of visual function. One month later he developed progressive visual loss and a dull aching pain the left eye. During this time he

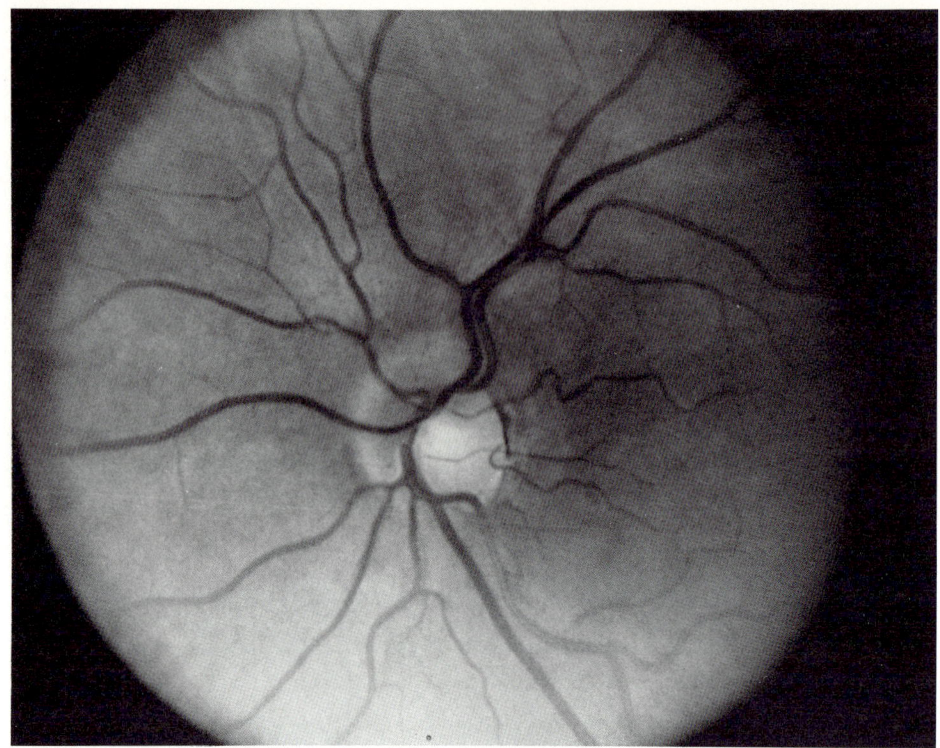

Fig. 5 (*Left optic disc*)

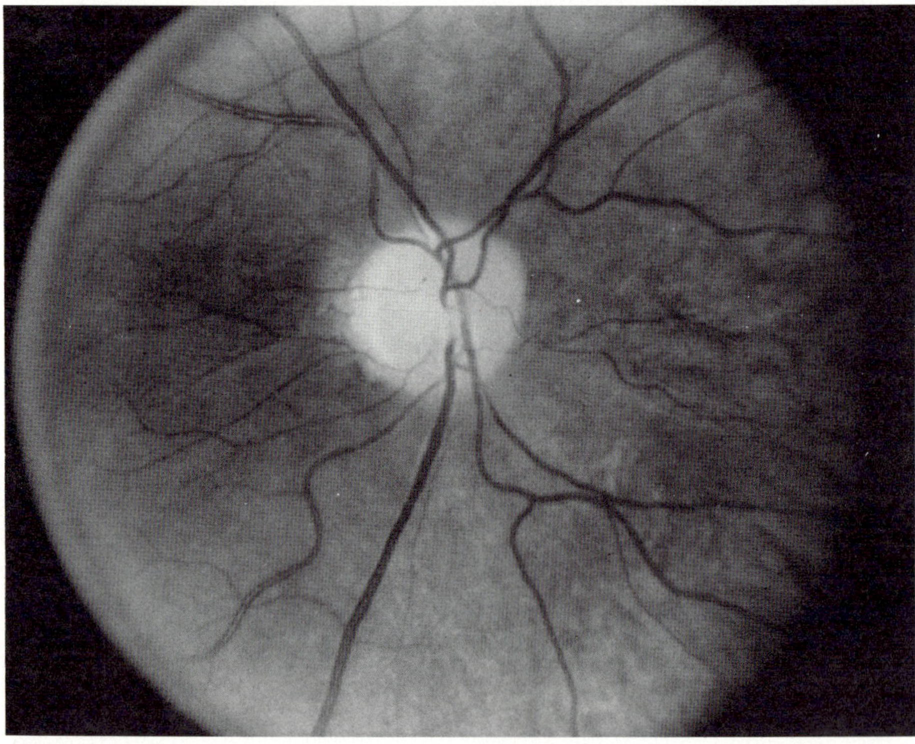

Fig. 5 (*Right optic disc*)

Fig. 5. (Case 4). Right optic disc is pale: there is diffuse drop-out of nerve fiber layer. Left disc is elevated superiorly and nasally with fiber layer edema in the peripapillary area.

complained of poor appetite, a 10-kg weight loss, pain in the left hip, and left chest pain.

Initial neuro-ophthalmologic examination revealed vision of no light perception in the right eye and 6/9-3 in the left eye. There was a right amaurotic pupillary response. Funduscopic examination revealed a pale right disc with marked decrease in the plushness of the nerve fiber layer (Fig. 5). The superior nasal border of the left disc was elevated. Perimetric examination revealed a left central scotoma and enlarged blind spot.

Chest x-ray showed multiple large pulmonary masses. A bronchial biopsy revealed necrosis with vasculitis consistent with lymphomatoid granulomatosis. Abdominal x-ray, upper gastrointestinal series, barium enema, intravenous pyelogram, renal arteriogram, and bone survey were normal. Skull x-rays and tomographic examination of optic canals were normal. Technetium 99 brain scan showed an area of increased uptake in the left orbit. EEG, pancerebral arteriogram, and spinal fluid examination were normal.

Despite combined treatment with radiation and chemotherapy, his condition deteriorated and he died six months later of lung abscess and empyema. Permission for post-mortem examination was denied.

Case 5. A 35-year-old man noted bilat-eral blurring of vision for 18 months. Two years before he sustained an injury to the right leg when he fell from a roof, fracturing the right proximal femur. As a consequence there was a persistent disability in standing and walking.

Neuro-ophthalmologic examination revealed vision of 6/9 in the right eye and 6/6 in the left eye. The pupils were equal in size with a right relative afferent pupillary defect. Both optic discs were pale, more so in the right eye. There was a bitemporal hemianopic visual field defect (Fig. 6). Additional physical findings included prominent xanthelasma of both lower lids.

Laboratory Studies. Hemoglobin and hematocrit were normal. WBC was 7700 with 69% eosinophils. A total eosinophil count was $3500/mm^3$ (normal 150–300/mm^3). Alkaline phosphatase was 102 U (normal 30–85 U). Serum protein electrophoresis showed a slightly decreased total protein of 5.5 g% with a low normal albumin of 3.2 mg%. Cholesterol was 158 mg%; serum lipoprotein electrophoresis showed a type-IV hyperlipidemic pattern. Urine 17-hydrocyclocorticosteroids were 12.6 mg for 24 hours (normal: 2.5–8.5 mg). Serum cortisol, T_3, T_4, and urine 17 ketosteroids were normal.

Bone marrow aspiration showed markedly increased (approximately 50%) eosin-

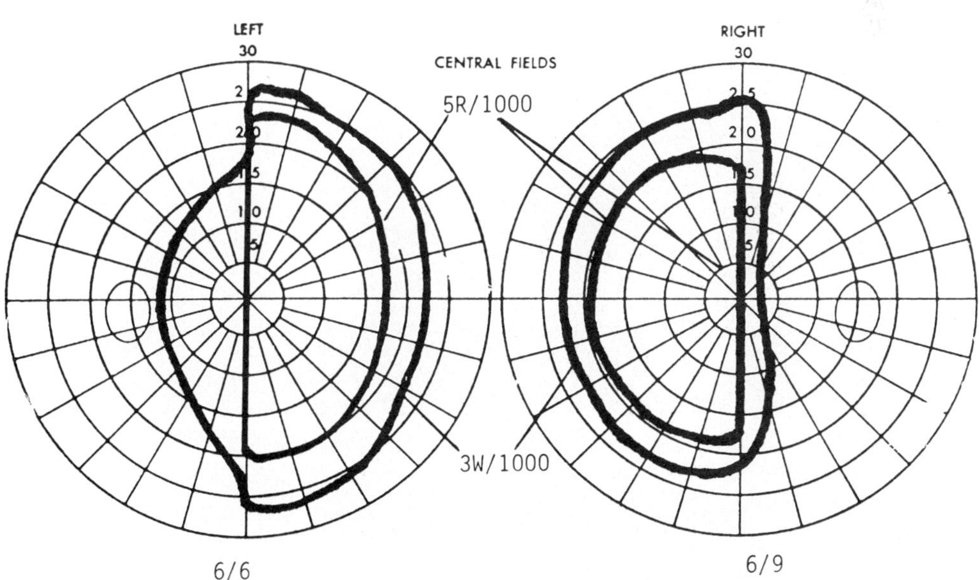

Fig. 6. (Case 5). Bitemporal hemianopia. Relative central scotoma in the right eye accounts for decreased vision. "R, red, W, white, targets."

ophils and eosinophilic precursors with no unusual cells and normal red and white cell precursors. Bone marrow iron stores were diminished.

Chest x-ray revealed increase in interstitial lung markings with diffuse and plate like changes. Lung scan was normal. Skull x-rays revealed bilateral maxillary sinus mucosal thickening. Technetium 99 brain scan, EEG, and spinal fluid examination were normal. Pancerebral arteriography demonstrated elevation of the anterior cerebral arteries suggesting an avascular anterior suprasellar mass. Pneumoencephalogram demonstrated a smooth 2 × 2 cm suprasellar mass with blunting of the rostral third ventricle (Fig. 7).

Right frontal craniotomy was performed with partial removal of the suprasellar mass. The tissue diagnosis was histiocytosis X (eosinophilic granuloma).

The patient was treated with external radiation to the sellar region (3,000 rads in two weeks). Post-operatively there was no light perception in either eye, but eventually the patient began to perceive light

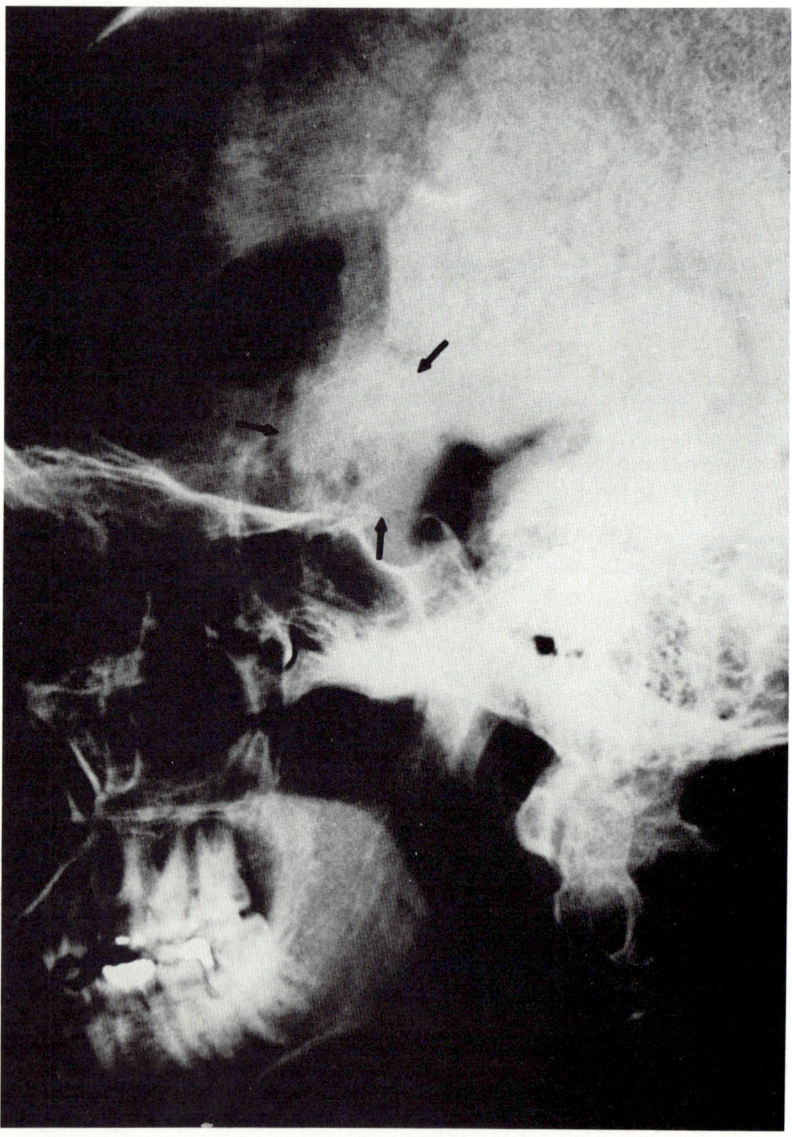

Fig. 7. (Case 5). Pneumoencephalography reveals a suprasellar mass (arrows).

and outlines and was able to count fingers in both eyes.

One year later vison was light perception in the right eye and bare hand motion at 15 cm in the left eye. The rest of the neurologic examination was normal. CT scan revealed an increase in the size of the suprasellar mass. An additional 4,000 rads were administered over 31 days to the base of the skull in combination with chemotherapy. Three years after his initial admission, dementia developed and vision was no light perception in both eyes. He continued to deteriorate and expired six years after the initial diagnosis was established.

COMMENT

The lymphoreticular system in the broadest sense includes all the hematopoietic and reticulo-endothelial tissues. The occurrence of tumor derived from this system with involvement of optic nerves and chiasm is rare.

The terminology and classification of these disorders is complicated. Historically they have been designated under a variety of synonyms: reticulo-endothelial neoplasms, malignant lymphomas, malignant reticulosis, lymphomatous tumors, lymphoid tumors, lymphoproliferative disorders, lymphoreticular disorders, and systemic lymphoma, to mention only a few.[18, 19]

Ocular complications of lymphoreticular disorders include infiltrations of the skin of the eyelids, episclera, conjunctiva, iris, and orbit.[1, 3, 20-26] Intraocular, especially retinal and optic nerve involvement in lymphoma is unusual.[3] Primary intraocular lymphoma is an even rarer occurrence.[1, 24, 27]

Subacute or slowly progressive visual loss in adult life should alert the clinician to the possibility of compression or infiltration of the optic nerves or chiasm. Meningeal tumor cuffing or direct infiltration of the optic nerves causes loss of vision in meningeal carcinomatosis. Visual loss is usually bilateral and progressive and will occur in about one-third of all patients with carcinomatous meningitis.[28, 29] The most common primary sites are breast and lung.[29, 30] Lymphomas accounted for 28% of 50 patients with meningeal cardinomatosis in Olson's review.[31] Four patients in the entire group presented with impaired vision, and 11 patients developed visual loss during the course of the disease. It should be noted that none of our patients had clinical or laboratory evidence of lymphomatous meningitis.

Reticulum cell sarcoma (histiocytic lymphoma) is the most likely systemic lymphoma to invade the brain, usually in the form of a lymphomatous meningitis.[32] It may arise from the meninges of the optic nerve.[33] A few patients with intraocular reticulum cell sarcoma have been reported with primary involvement of the uveal tract, retina, and choroid, clinically resembling uveitis. Neoplastic vitreous seeding may be noted.[1, 25, 34] Optic nerve involvement was present in two of four patients with reticulum cell sarcoma reported by Barr *et al.*[1] Walsh and Shewmake[35] reported a 64-year-old patient with sudden, progressive visual loss in the left eye and subsequent involvement of the cranial nerves III and VI. Reticulum cell sarcoma was diagnosed following exploratory laparotomy for sudden abdominal distress. At necropsy widespread reticulum cell sarcoma was found. The left optic nerve itself was necrotic but not infiltrated by tumor. The dural sheath was involved by tumor. There was also an aneurysm of the left ophthalmic artery.

The term lymphosarcoma has been used to describe many different kinds of malignant lymphoma. The popular terminology at present includes hystiocytic lymphocytic, lymphocytic poorly differentiated and lymphocytic well-differentiated type malignant lymphomas. Optic nerve involvement by lymphosarcoma during the course of disease has been described previously as an extremely rare complication.[3, 26, 37] Kraus and O'Rourke[2] reported a patient with transient unilateral retrobulbar neuritis five years before the diagnosis of lymphosarcoma and another patient with blinding bilateral optic neuritis occuring fifteen years before the detection of Hodgkin's disease. They postulated that optic neuritis associated with malignant lymphoma may be a demyelinative process rather than a direct infiltration of the optic nerve and support this postulate with the wide separation in time of the ocular and systemic manifestations. Our Patient 2 had direct infiltration of the optic nerve by the tumor.

Myeloma may directly involve the optic

nerve by extension from the base of the skull. Clarke[8] reviewed 25 cases of cranial and intracranial myeloma; optic nerve involvement occurred in eight of 25 patients. Langdon[11] reported a patient with bilateral VI nerve paralysis and left retrobulbar neuritis. The retrobulbar neuritis was thought to be on a toxic basis "excreted by the growths," rather than from infiltration or pressure on the nerve. Gudas[9] reported the first histologically proven myeloma of the-nerve in the English literature. Kamin and Hepler[10] described a solitary intracranial plasmacytoma of the sella turcica and optic nerve which was initially mistaken for atypical retrobulbar neuritis.

Lymphomatoid granulomatosis is an angiocentric and angiodestructive lymphoreticular proliferative and granulomatous disease predominantly involving the lungs.[38] It is unclear at present whether lymphoid granulomatosis is a primary atypical lymphoma with secondary granulomatous reaction or a varient of Wegener's granulomatosis. Despite the frequent occurrence of ocular involvement in Wegener's granulomatosis, ocular manifestations in lymphoid granulomatosis are rare.[39] Liebow *et al.*[38] found 20% central nervous system and 15% peripheral nerve involvement in a review of 40 patients with lymphoid granulomatosis. Only one patient in this group had unilateral complete loss of vision and optic atrophy suggestive of optic nerve involvement. Haynes *et al.*[39] reviewed 45 patients with lymphoid granulomatosis. Four had ocular manifestations with only one instance of retinal or optic nerve vasculitis. Although pathologic confirmation is not available in Case #4, the clinical picture leaves little doubt that the site of the visual loss was the anterior visual pathways and almost assuredly both optic nerves.

Eosinophilic granuloma, Hand-Schuller-Christian disease and Letterer-Siwe disease have traditionally been considered as a single group of neoplastic disorders designated histiocytosis X. Eosinophilic granuloma most likely represents a reaction pattern, sharing some histologic features with the other two forms.[19] It usually involves bones, although there are rare instances of soft tissue involvement in the gastrointestinal tract, lymph nodes, and the orbit.[40-42]

Additional changes that have been described include granulomas of the calvaria, anemia, neutropenia, thrombocytopenia, middle ear involvement, and pituitary infiltration. Intraocular involvement is unusual.[43, 44] Visual loss is a rare complaint in eosinophilic granuloma. Enriquez *et al.*[45] reviewed 117 patients with histologically-proven histiocytosis X. The presenting symptoms in this group were palpable or visible masses overlying the osseous lesion, tenderness, rash, enlarged lymph nodes, stomatitis, otitis, diabetes insipidus, exophthalmos, fever, and headache. None of the patients had any symptoms suggestive of optic nerve involvement.

Despite the rarity of visual compromise in lymphoma the patients here reported presented to the ophthalmologists with visual loss as the primary manifestation of a lymphoreticular disorder. The initial impression in Patients 1 and 4 was "optic neuritis" although their ages and the clinical course were atypical. The visual loss responded initially to systemic corticosteroid therapy. As previously described, this does not disprove the presence of tumor.[29]

The optic nerve was examined pathologically only in Patient 1; however, a pathological specimen was obtained in each patient. The clinical course and response to specific therapy leaves little doubt that these patients indeed represent anterior visual pathway involvement from one of the lymphoreticular diseases. These patients serve to remind us that optic nerve or chiasmal involvement may occur in the course of the lymphoreticular disorders, and such involvement may be the initial sign of the disease.

EDITOR'S NOTE

Dr. Kansu and associates have presented five extremely interesting cases of visual loss associated with the lymphomatous diseases. I recall a very interesting patient that I saw briefly several years ago in this regard. This was a middle-aged woman, a patient of Dr. Glaser, who had previously had a bout of optic neuritis in one eye which had progressed to no light perception. She had been seen at the Wilmer Institute in consultation and had been worked up by various consultants with no specific diagnosis having made. When Dr. Glaser was out of town, he asked me to cover for him for 2–3 days, and this particular woman suddenly noted slight blurring in her only remaining eye and came in as an emergency. She had 20/20 minus vision in her only eye with a very subtle lower nasal field defect and a normal disc. The other eye was amaurotic and had notable disc pallor. She gave the interesting history that she had previously had a breast lump removed which histologically turned out to be a plasmacytoma of breast. On that basis, I made the clinical diagnosis of optic neuritis due to plasmacytoma and advised prompt steroids. She declined over the weekend and waited until Dr. Glaser came back. Within three days, the vision had dropped from 20/20 minus down to finger counting in her only eye. She was then hospitalized, treated with steroids and subsequently had the optic nerve irradiated (to the best of my memory) and vision promptly improved to 20/20 in the eye again and remained stable at subsequent follow-ups for well over a year. There was no other evidence of metastatic disease apparent at that time. I personally believe she had optic nerve plasmacytoma.

A review at that time turned up a few other cases, and these have been documented in the bibliography of this paper. I recall that on one of the Audio-Digest of Ophthalmology tapes, an exploration of a suspected chiasmal tumor done in Southern California revealed plasmacytoma involving the optic nerves and chiasm. It is obvious that these cases are around, and Dr. Kansu and associates have done a good job in bringing them to our attention in this paper. The importance of diagnosing them is evident. Finally, Dr. Norton loves to tell the story of the following case. He had a one-eyed patient with a history of myeloma who developed a severe central retinal vein occlusion. I advised that he have this patient's optic nerve irradiated. This was done with about 600–800 roentgens, as I recall, and the distended veins melted away and patient's vision returned to about 20/20 or 20/25 in that eye from a previous level of about 20/200. This was attributed to involvement of optic nerve sheath with plasmacytoma compromising the central vein

in its exit along the vaginal sheath around the nerve, and this showed a nice response to local optic nerve irradiation. This point of therapy may be worth pointing out in other such cases.

JLS

REFERENCES

1. Barr, C. C., Green, W. R. Payne, J. W., *et al.* Intraocular reticulum-cell sarcoma. Surv. Ophthalmol. *19*:224–239 (1975).
2. Kraus, A. M. and O'Rourke, J. Lymphomatous optic neuritis. Arch. Ophthalmol. *70*:173–175 (1963).
3. Lewis, R. A. and Clark, R. B. Infiltrative retinopathy in systemic lymphoma. Am. J. Ophthalmol. *79*:48–52 (1975).
4. Litvak, J., Leder, M. M., and Kauvar, A. J. Hodgkin's disease involving optic nerve and brain. J. Neurosurg. *21*:798–801 (1964).
5. Marshall, G., Roessman, U., and Van Den Noort, U. Invasive Hodgkin's disease of brain. Cancer *22*:621–630 (1968).
6. Miller, N. R. and Iliff, J. Visual loss as the initial symptom in Hodgkin's disease. Arch. Ophthalmol. *93*:1158–1161 (1975).
7. Sohn, D., Valensi, Q., and Miller, S. P. Neurologic manifestations of Hodgkin's disease. Arch. Neurol. *17*:429–436 (1967).
8. Clarke, E. Cranial and intracranial myelomas. Brain *77*:61–79 (1954).
9. Gudas, P. P. Optic nerve myeloma. Am. J. Ophthalmol. *71*:1085–1089 (1971).
10. Kamin, D. F., and Hepler, R. S. Solitary intracranial plasm cytoma mistaken for retrobulbar neuritis. Am. J. Ophthalmol. *73*:584–586 (1972).
11. Langdon, H. M. Multiple myeloma and bilateral sixth nerve paralysis and left retrobulbar neuritis. Trans. Am. Ophthalmol. Soc. *37*:223–229 (1939).
12. Allen, R. A. and Straatsma, B. R. Ocular involvement in leukemia and allied disorders. Arch. Ophthalmol. *66*: 68–86 (1961).
13. Chalfin, A. I., Nash, B. M., and Goldstein, J. H. Optic nerve head involvement in lymphocytic leukemia. J. Pediatr. Ophthalmol. *10*:39–43 (1973).
14. Eichholtz, W. Papillenschwellungen bei Leukamien und verwandten prozessen. Ophthalmologica *170*:494–504 (1975).
15. Ellis, W. and Little, H. L. Leukemic infiltration of the optic nerve head. Am. J. Ophthalmol. *75*:867–871 (1973).
16. Murray, K. H., Paolino, F., Goldman, J. M., *et al.* Ocular involvement in leukemia. Lancet *1*:829–831 (1977).
17. Rosenthal, A. R., Egbert, P. R., Wilbut, J. R., *et al.* Leukemic involvement of the optic nerve. Trans. Pac. Coast Ophthalmol. Soc. *55*:137–158 (1974).
18. Craddock, C. G. In: *Classification of Lymphoreticular Disorders in Hematology.* 2nd ed. W. J. William, E. Butler, A. J. Ersley, and W. Randles (Eds.), McGraw-Hill, New York, pp. 944–946.
19. Jacobiec, F. A., and Jones, I. S. In: *Lymphoma-*

tous, Plasmactyic, Histiocytic and Hematopoietic Tumors in Clinical Ophthalmology. T. D. Duane (Ed.), Harper and Row, New York, 1976, Vol. 2, Chap. 39, pp. 1–45.

20. Baker, T. R. and Spencer, W. H. Ocular findings in multiple myeloma. Arch. Ophthalmol. *91:*110–113 (1974).

21. Leinfelder, P. J. and O'Brien, C. S. Lymphoma of the eye and adnexa. Arch. Ophthalmol. *14:*183–189 (1935).

22. McGavic, J. S. Lymphomatous tumors of the eye. Arch. Ophthalmol. *53:*236–247 (1955).

23. Morgan, G. Lymphocytic tumors of the orbit. Mod. Probl. Ophthalmol. *14:*355–360 (1974).

24. Nevins, R. C., Frey, W. W., and Elliott, J. H. Primary solitary intraocular reticulum cell sarcoma (microgliomatosis). Trans. Am. Acad. Ophthalmol. Otolaryngol. *72:*867–876 (1968).

25. Rodman, H. I. and Font, R. L. Orbital involvement in multiple myeloma. Arch. Ophthalmol. *87:*30–35 (1972).

26. Zimmerman, L. E. In: *Lymphoid Tumors in Ocular and Adnexal Tumors.* M. Boniuk (Ed.), C. V. Mosby Co., St. Louis, 1964, pp. 429–457.

27. Hogan, M. J. and Zimmerman, L. E. In: *Ophthalmic Pathology.* 2nd ed. Saunders, Philadelphia, 1962, pp. 456–460.

28. Altrocchi, P. A., Reinhardt, P. H., and Eckman, P. B. Blindness and meningeal carcinomatosis. Arch. Ophthalmol. *88:*508–512 (1972).

29. Susac, J. O., Smith, J. L., and Powell, J. O. Carcinomatous optic neuropathy. Am. J. Ophthalmol. *76:*672–679 (1973).

30. Little, J. R., Dale, A. J. D., and Okazaki, H. Meningeal carcinomatosis. Arch. Neurol. *30:*138–143 (1974).

31. Olson, M. E., Chernik, N. L., and Posner, J. B. Infiltration of the leptomeninges by systemic cancer. Arch. Neurol. *30:*122–137 (1974).

32. Eggers, H., Jacobiec, F. A., and Jones, I. S. Tumors of the optic nerve. Doc. Ophthalmol. *41:*43–128 (1976).

33. Hogan, M. J., Spencer, W. H., and Hoyt, W. F. Primary reticuloendothelial sarcomas of the orbital and cranial meninges (ophthalmologic aspects). Am. J. Ophthalmol. *61:*1146–1158 (1966).

34. Vogel, M. H., Font, R. L., Zimmerman, L. E., *et al.* Reticulum cell sarcoma of the retina and uvea. Am. J. Ophthalmol. *66:*205–215 (1968).

35. Walsh, F. B. and Shewmake, B. J. An unusual case of reticulum cell sarcoma. Am. J. Ophthalmol. *74:*741–743 (1972).

36. Bullock, J. D., Yanes, B., Kelly, M. *et al.* Presented at the Ninth Annual Neuro-ophthalmologic Pathology Symposium. St. Louis, February, 1977.

37. Feinstein, A. R. and Krause, A. C. Ocular involvement in lymphomatous disease. Arch. Ophthalmol. *48:*328–337 (1952).

38. Liebow, A. A., Carrington, C. R. B., and Friedman, P. J. Lymphomatoid granulomatosis. Hum. Pathol. *3:*457–558 (1972).

39. Haynes, B. F., Fishman, M. L., and Fauci, A. S., *et al.* The ocular manifestations of Wegener's granulomatosis. Am. J. Med. *63:*131–140 (1977).

40. Chawla, H. B. and Cullen, J. F. Eosinophilic granuloma of the orbit. J. Pediatr. Ophthalmol. *5:*93–95 (1968).

41. Heuer, H. E. Eosinophilic granuloma of the orbit. Acta Ophthalmol. *50:*160–165 (1972).

42. Walsh, F. B. and Hoyt, W. F. *Clinical Neuro-ophthalmology.* 3rd ed. Williams and Wilkins, Baltimore, 1969, pp. 837–841.

43. Lahav, M. and Albert, D. M. Unusual ocular involvement in acute disseminated histiocytosis X. Arch. Ophthalmol. *91:*455–458 (1974).

44. Mittleman, D., Apple, D. J., and Goldberg, M. F. Ocular involvement in Letterer-Siwe disease. Am. J. Ophthalmol. *75:*261–265 (1973).

45. Enriquez, P., Dahlin, D. C., Hayles, A. B., *et al.* Histiocytosis X. A clinical study. Mayo Clin. Proc. *42:*88–99 (1967).

14 Optic Canal Tomography: Detection and Evaluation of Orbital Apex Meningiomas

Robert M. Quencer, M.D.
John A. Costin, M.D.

INTRODUCTION

In the radiographic evaluation of intraorbital and chiasmatic lesions, computed tomography (CT) has assumed a primary role. However, abnormalities of the orbital apex may escape detection and/or characterization if only computed tomography is used. The object of this chapter is to stress the importance of optic canal tomography for suspected lesions at the orbital apex and to review our experience in the diagnosis of optic canal meningiomas.

RADIOGRAPHIC ANATOMY AND TECHNIQUE

The optic canal is a tubular structure which extends lateral to medial from the orbital apex anteriorly to the middle cranial fossa posteriorly. Its borders are formed by various portions of the sphenoid bone (Table I). The canal runs at an angle of approximately 38° to the midsagittal plane and upwards at a 30° angle relative to an axial plane drawn between the outer canthus of the eye and the external auditory canal. Because of this obliquity, neither skull films nor tomography in frontal and lateral projections will optimally image the optic canal. A special projection, a Rhese view, will demonstrate the canal on end when the head is rotated 38° and extended 30°, but this view gives only a gross idea of canal pathology because the cranial and orbital ends of the canal are superimposed upon each other. In this view the contour

of the orbital end of the canal usually dominates the radiographic image because the bone of the orbital portion of the canal is thicker than the bone of the cranial portion of the canal. Since the canal has an anterior to posterior length (Table II) of approximately 1 cm, a method is necessary for examining various portions of this canal. The radiographic answer to this problem is to employ complex motion tomography.

Tomography, simply stated, utilizes the principal that if the film and x-ray source are moved simultaneously along certain planes, blurring will occur except along a specific plane of interest. The film and x-ray source may move along a linear plane (linear tomography) or the motion used may be of a more complex nature (complex motion tomography) usually either trispiral or hypocycloidal tomography. Evaluation of a small and thin structure, such as the optic canal, requires the use of complex motion tomography since the streaking inherent in linear tomography degrades the image to an unacceptable extent.

Because of the anatomical considerations I have described, tomographic sections of the optic canal should be obtained either at right angles to the long axis of the canal (Rhese tomography—Fig. 1) or the sections are taken parallel to the long axis of the canal (base tomography—Fig. 2). Since the approximate length of the canal is 10 mm, and the height 5 mm, thin sections of 1 mm are necessary for proper visualization of the entire canal. The disadvantage of computed tomography in optic canal evaluation, as routinely employed, is that the axial or coronal sections are never less than 5 mm in thickness. This means that either the optic canal may not be seen, or that it is averaged in with the surrounding structures so that subtle changes in the size and contour of the canal cannot be appreciated. Until the time when CT is capable of resolving structures 1 mm apart, complex motion tomography will remain the paramount method of examining the optic canals.

Figure 1 shows that the shape of the optic canal changes from its orbital to cranial end. The opposite side is tomogrammed for comparison since the optic canals are usually symmetrical in size and shape. A difference of 2 mm in size between the two sides at equal levels of section is abnormal, as is a loss of the normal oval contour at either the cranial or orbital end of the canal. The tomograms are also examined for evidence of erosion of the optic strut, hyperostosis, and intracanalicular calcification.

TABLE I. *Borders of the optic canal*

Roof	—superior root of the lesser sphenoid wing
Floor	—inferior root of the lesser sphenoid wing (the "optic strut")
Medial Wall	—body of the sphenoid bone
Lateral Wall	—medial wall of the anterior clinoid

TABLE II. *Measurements of the optic canal*

Height	—5–6 mm
Roof	—8–10 mm
Floor	—6–8 mm
Lateral and Medial Wall	—6–8 mm

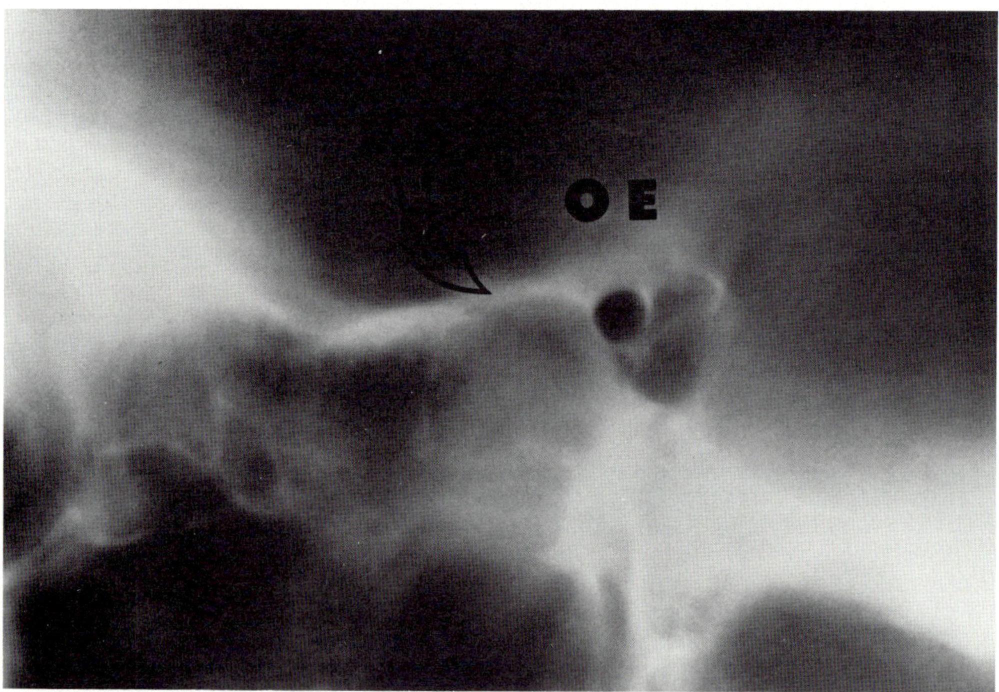

Fig. 1A

Fig. 1 (A, B, and C). *Optic canal tomography—Rhese projection.* With the head positioned as described in the text, 1 mm sections are taken from the orbital end to the cranial end of the optic canal. The orbital end (OE) of the canal (Fig. 1A) has an oval shape the long axis of which is vertical. The arrow points to the planum sphenoidal (PS) which is directly medial to the optic canal. The midportion (MC) of the canal (Fig. 1B) has a more rounded appearance. The optic strut forms the inferior border of the canal and separates it from the superior orbital fissure. The cranial end (CE) of the canal (Fig. 1C) has an oval shape the long axis of which is horizontal. The anterior clinoid (AC) is directly lateral to the optic canal. Properly performed optic canal tomography should clearly show each of these segments of the canal (OE, MC, and CE).

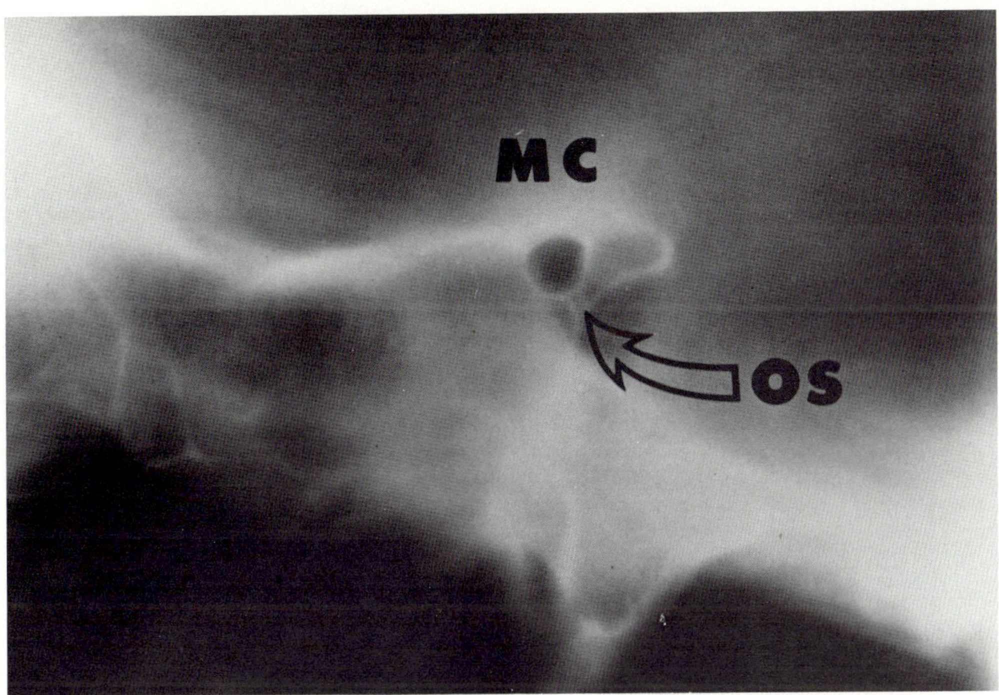

Fig. 1B

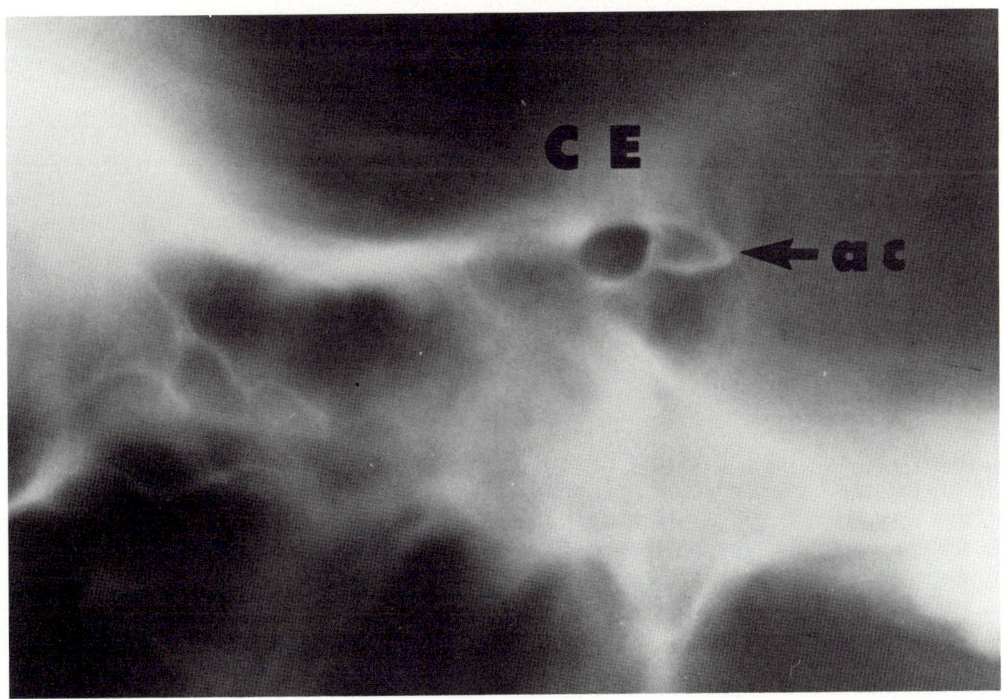

Fig. 1C

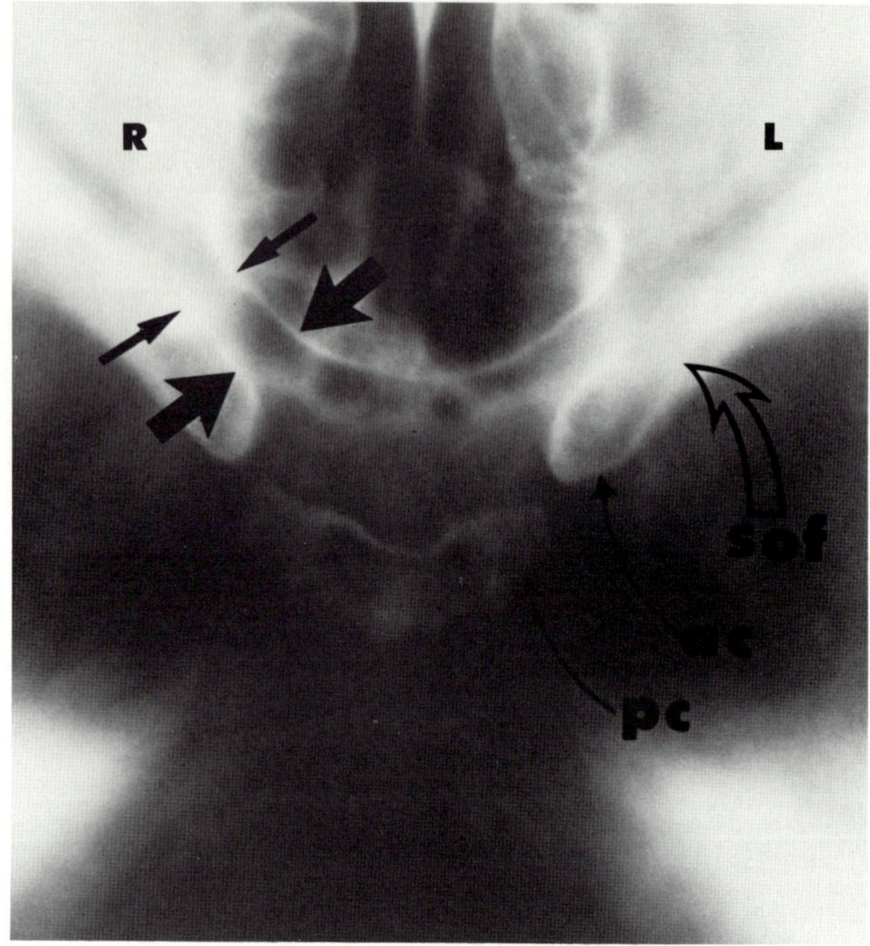

Fig. 2A

Fig. 2 (A and B). *Optic canal tomography—base projection.* Base tomography of a dried skull (Fig. 2A) shows the anatomical details of the optic canal more readily than on a living subject (Fig. 2B). In Figure 2A the thin arrows on the right demarcate the orbital end of the canal while the wide arrows show the cranial end of the canal. On the left side the arrows point the posterior clinoid (PC), anterior clinoid (AC), and the most superior portion of the superior orbital fissure (SOF). In Figure 2B, base tomography in a normal living subject, the arrows point to the medial walls of the optic canals. The cranial opening of the canals (O) are bounded laterally by the anterior clinoids (C). Note how the symmetry of the two canals can be easily compared on this single film.

Although more difficult to interpret, tomography in the base projection (Fig. 2), is the ideal way of visualizing the optic canals. The reason for this is that both canals are on the same film, allowing a direct comparison of the two sides. Measurements of the length of the medial and lateral walls, along with any change in the contour, can be made only with base tomography, thus allowing identification of erosion or amputation of the canal. The only disadvantage of this projection is that it is frequently difficult for elderly or very ill patients to hold the base position for the period of time necessary to take the films.

CLINICAL MATERIAL

On review of our cases of optic canal meningiomas, the following four abnormal patterns were found: (1) erosion or amputation of the canal; (2) canal widening; (3)

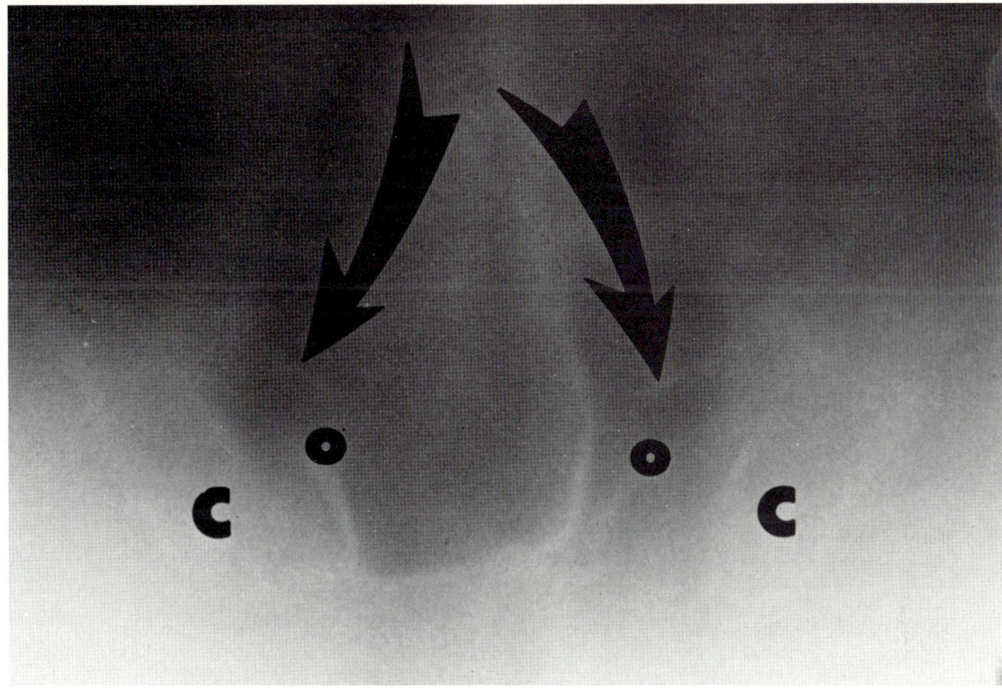

Fig. 2B

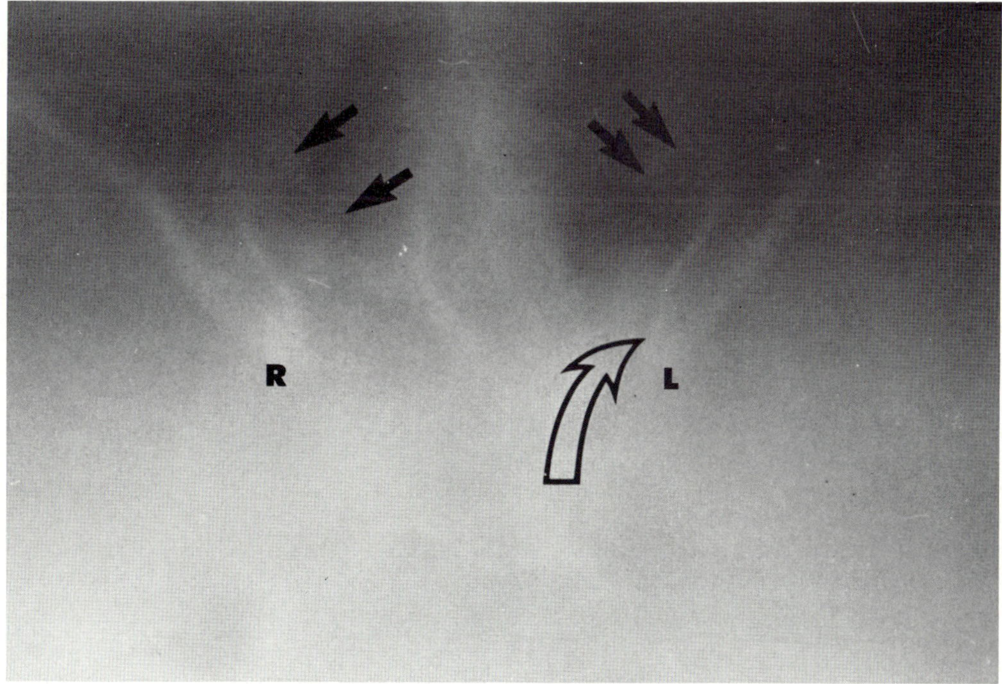

Fig. 3. *Case 1: Base tomography.* Compare the normal right optic canal, the length of whose medial wall is outlined by two straight arrows, to the amputated left optic canal, the length of whose medial walls are also outlined by straight arrows. Note also the associated erosion of the medial border of the left anterior clinoid. Diagnosis: Optic canal meningioma with intracranial extension.

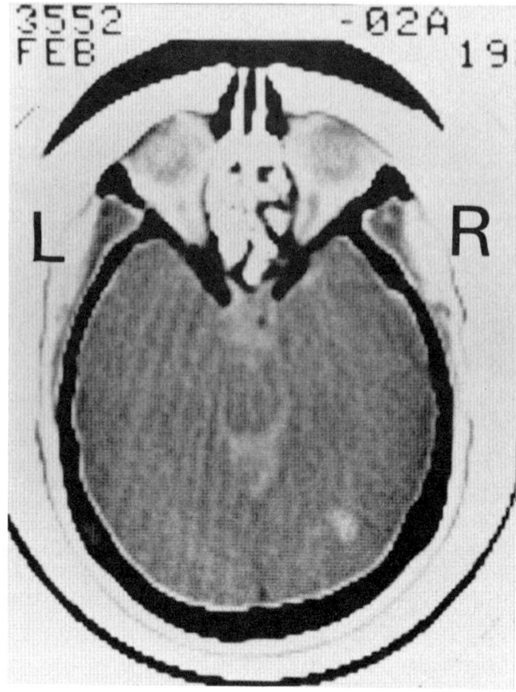

Fig. 4A

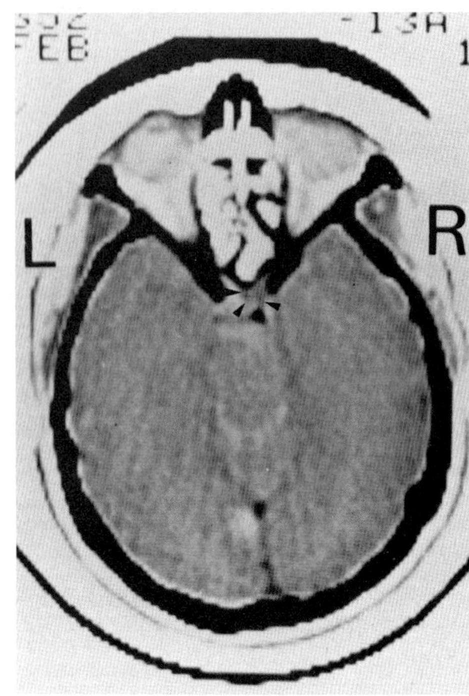

Fig. 4B

Fig. 4 (A and B). *Case 2: CT scan.* The pre-contrast scan (A) through the level of the optic canals is normal. The post-contrast scan (B) shows an area of abnormal enhancement (arrowheads) medial to and posterior to the right anterior clinoid. There was no intra-orbital abnormality, and further information was needed to determine if there was a contiguous intracanalicular mass. This required the use of optic canal tomography (Figs. 5 and 6).

hyperostosis; (4) calcification. In each case CT either failed to identify the lesion or it insufficiently localized the lesion, making further preoperative radiographic investigation necessary. I have found base tomography more sensitive than Rhese tomography in detecting the subtle changes in or directly adjacent to the optic canal.

1. Erosion/Amputation—Case 1

In a patient with vision loss of the left eye and a normal CT scan, base tomography (Fig. 3) showed shortening of the medial wall of the left optic canal and erosion of the medial border of the left anterior clinoid.

Diagnosis: Optic canal meningioma with minimal intracranial extension.

2. Widening—Case 2

This patient had diminished vision in the right eye and a CT scan (Fig. 4) which showed an area of enhancement medial to

the right anterior clinoid. It was not clear if there was extension to the level of the optic canal. On Rhese tomography (Fig. 5) although a normal oval configuration of the canal was present, the cranial end of the canal appeared widened. Base tomography (Fig. 6) showed a widened cranial end of the canal with erosion of the anterior clinoid confirming the presence of a mass in the canal.

Diagnosis: Meningioma with extension into the optic canal.

3. Hyperostosis—Cases 3 and 4

Case 3. There was prior removal of a left intra-orbital meningioma, and the patient was now being evaluated for the possibility of intracranial extension through the optic canal. The skull films (Fig. 7) showed intra-orbital surgical clips and some increased density of the left anterior clinoid. Base tomography (Fig. 8) clearly identified hyperostosis of the anterior clinoid in associ-

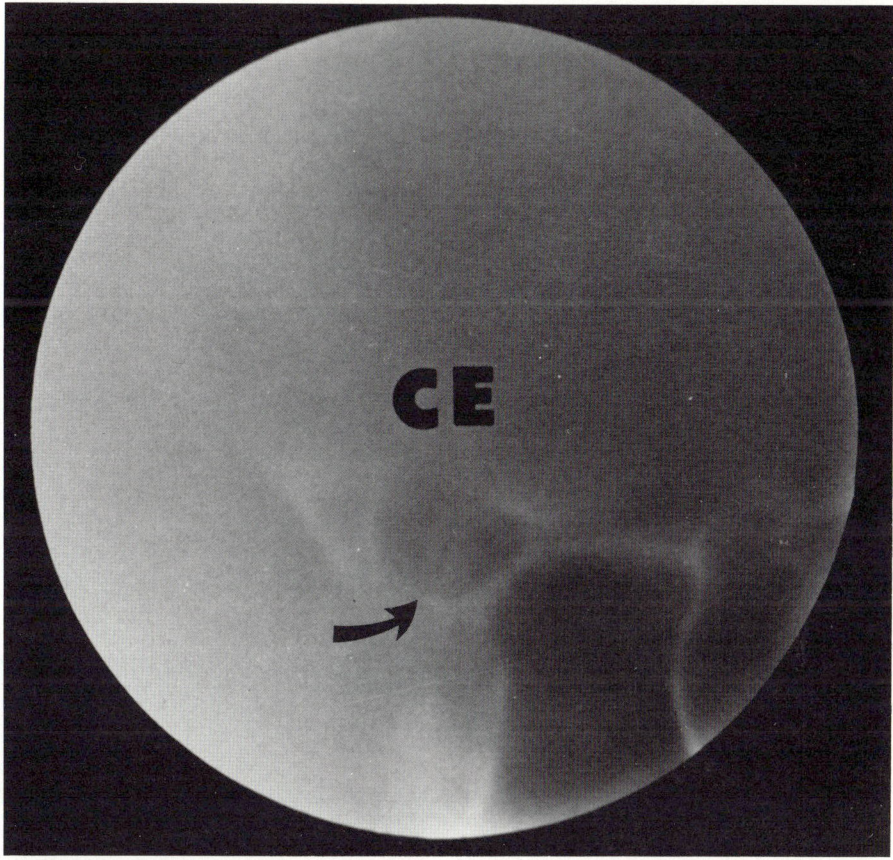

Fig. 5. *Case 2*: The cranial end (CE) of the optic canal is enlarged (compared to Fig. 1C), and there is thinning of the optic strut (curved arrow). This was highly suggestive of optic canal involvement, even though a normal oval configuration of the canal was present.

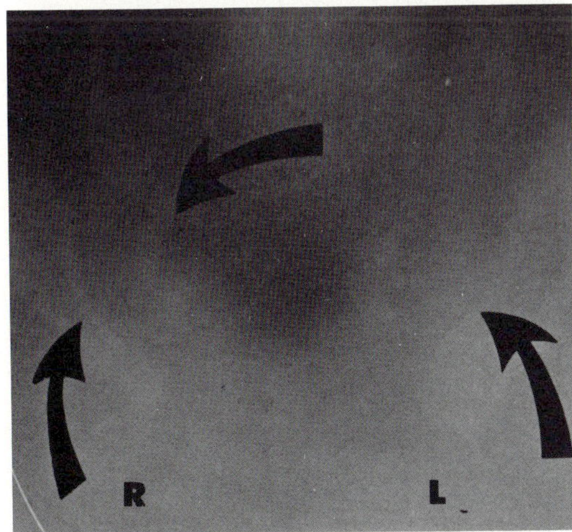

Fig. 6. *Case 2*: Base tomography shows erosion of the medial border of the right anterior clinoid (compare to the normal left anterior clinoid—single arrow). The upper arrow points to the medial border of the right optic canal. Diagnosis: Meningioma with extension into the right optic canal.

ation with partial destruction of the medial wall of the left optic canal.

Diagnosis: Extension intracranially of an orbital meningioma.

Case 4. In a known right sphenoid meningioma, optic canal involvement was demonstrated best on base tomography (Fig. 9). Hyperostosis was seen extending into the optic canal.

Diagnosis: Sphenoid meningioma with intracanalicular extension.

4. Calcification—Case 5

Although a mass was identified in the left orbital apex on CT, the optic canal was not clearly defined and CT evidence of intracranial extension was lacking. Base tomography (Fig. 10) showed a calcified mass at the cranial end of the left optic canal with secondary erosion of the anterior clinoid and amputation of the medial wall of the optic canal.

Diagnosis: Orbital apex meningioma with intracranial extension through the optic canal.

COMMENTS

Our experience has shown that optic canal tomography in the base projection is the most sensitive radiographic examination for detection of meningiomas located in the optic canal or directly adjacent to its orbital or cranial openings. Its advantage over computed tomography is that much thinner sections are obtained which in turn allows the visualization of subtle bony erosion or hyperostosis.

There are two errors which are frequently encountered in the interpretation of the CT scans and base tomography: (1) On CT scanning, because of the proximity of the superior orbital fissure to the optic canal, they may be mistaken for one another. To distinguish them, it should be remembered that the optic canal is oblique to the midsagittal plane, whereas the most medial portion of the superior orbital fissure lies inferior to the optic canal and runs directly posterior into the cavernous sinus. In addition, when the superior orbital fissure is visualized on the same section as the optic canal only the most lateral portion of the superior orbital fissure is seen (see Fig. 11). (2) On base tomography, the anterior clinoid may be mistaken for the optic canal because it runs at approximately the same angle as the canal (see Fig. 2(B)). However, the relatively thick cortex of the clinoid along with its "closed" posterior end will distinguish it from the more medially located and delicately structured optic canal.

In a patient suspected of having an orbital apex or optic canal mass, a negative CT should not dissuade the clinician from further radiographic investigation. As we have shown, complex motion tomography is capable in those cases of detecting the mass, or will, when the CT is positive, clarify the extent of the mass.

CONCLUSIONS

1. Computed tomography, at its present stage of development, is not capable of detecting and characterizing *all* lesions at the orbital apex.

2. If the clinical suspicion of an optic canal meningioma is high, optic canal tomography is necessary even if the CT is normal.

3. Optic canal tomography should be done in the Rhese and/or base projection. The base tomogram, although it is the preferred projection, is frequently difficult to obtain on elderly or ill patients.

4. Only complex motion tomography with sections of 1 mm thickness is acceptable. The abnormalities which we search for are usually too subtle to be detected via linear tomography or with sections of greater than 1 mm thickness.

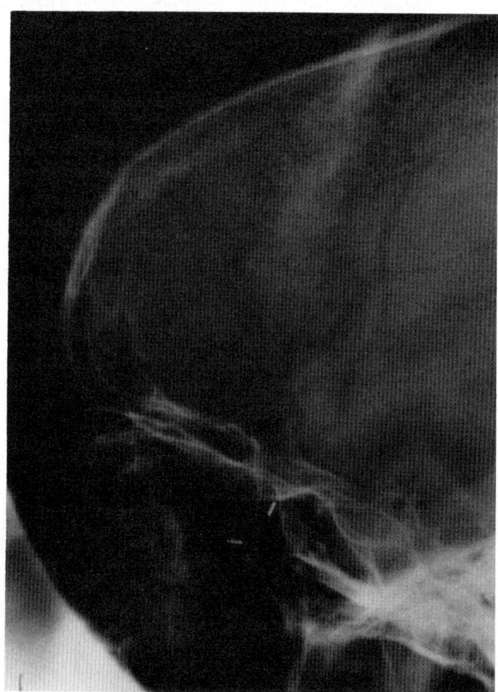

Fig. 7A

Fig. 7 (A and B). *Case 3: Skull series.* Two surgical clips present in the left orbit indicating posterior limits of the intra-orbital meningioma resection. The left anterior clinoid is pneumatized (straight arrow in B) and there is a suggestion of hyperostosis of the left anterior clinoid (arrowheads in B).

Fig. 8. *Case 3: Base tomography.* Partial destruction of the medial wall (X) of the left optic canal is associated with hyperostosis of the left anterior clinoid (straight open arrow). The curved solid arrow points to the air cell in the left clinoid, and the curved open arrow points to a metallic clip adjacent to the orbital end of the left optic canal. Compare the normal medial wall of the right optic canal (Y) and the normal cranial end of the right optic canal (O). Diagnosis: Intra-canalicular and intra-orbital extension of an orbital meningioma.

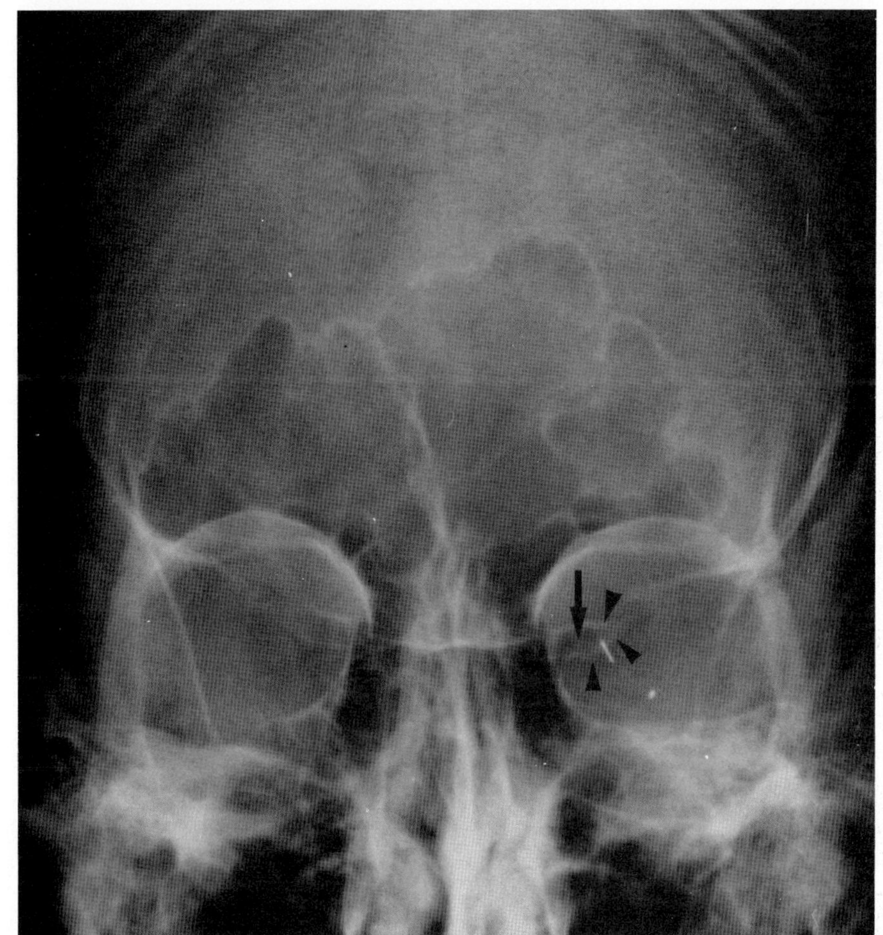

Fig. 7B

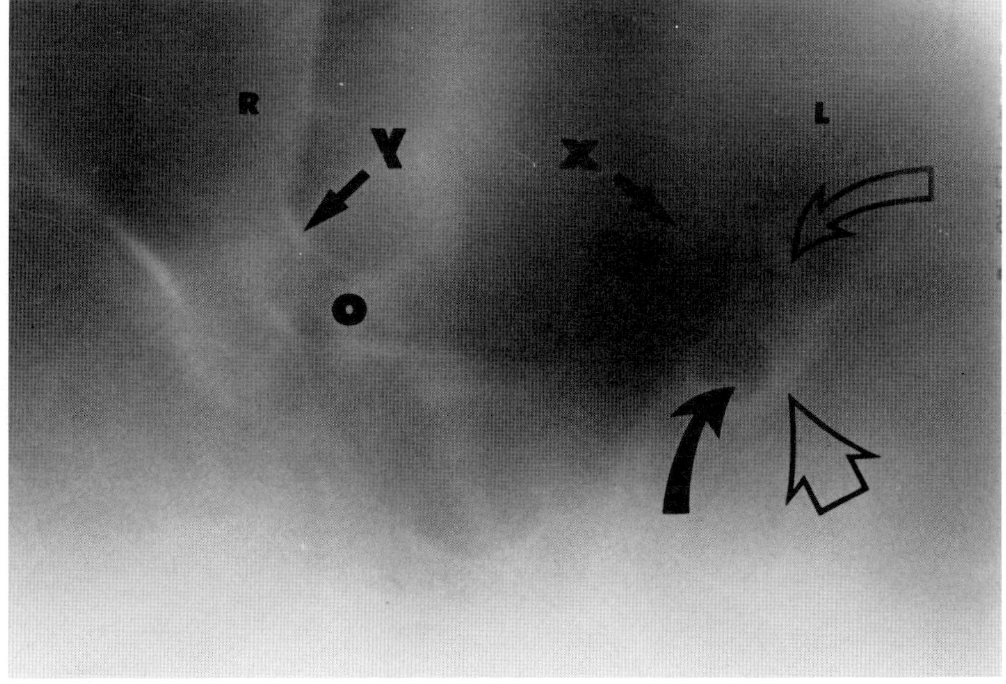

Fig. 8

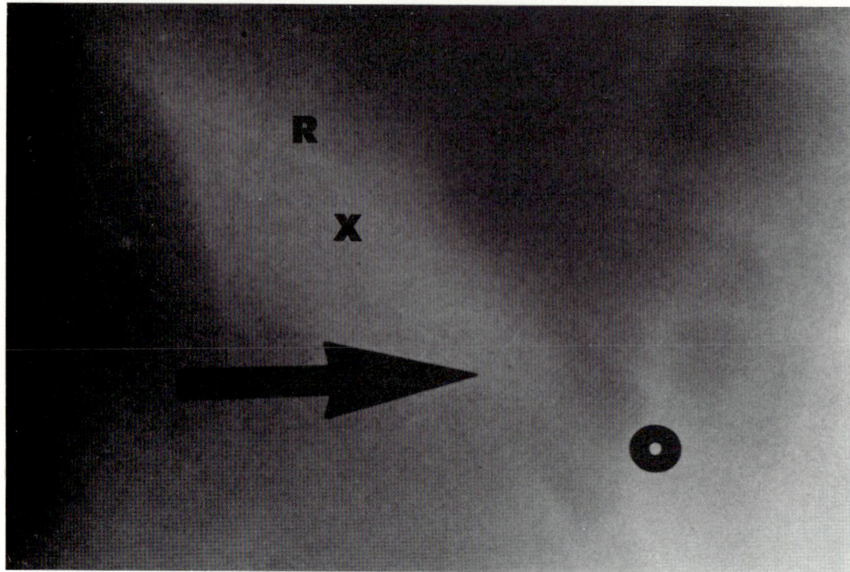

Fig. 9. *Case 4*: On this base tomogram of the right side only, the hyperostosis of the right sphenoid wing (X) is seen extending into the optic midportion of the optic canal. The most cranial end of the canal (O) is normal. Diagnosis: Extension of a sphenoid meningioma into the optic canal.

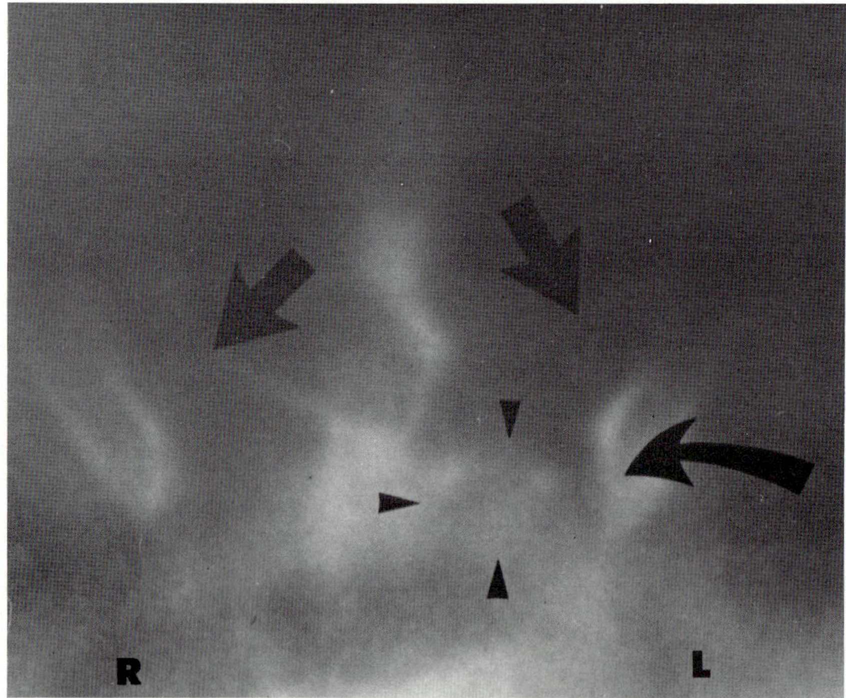

Fig. 10. *Case 5*: A calcified mass (arrowheads) is partially eroding the left anterior clinoid (curved arrow) and amputating the medial wall of the left optic canal (compare the position of the two straight arrows). Diagnosis: Meningioma at the orbital apex with extension intracranial via the optic canal.

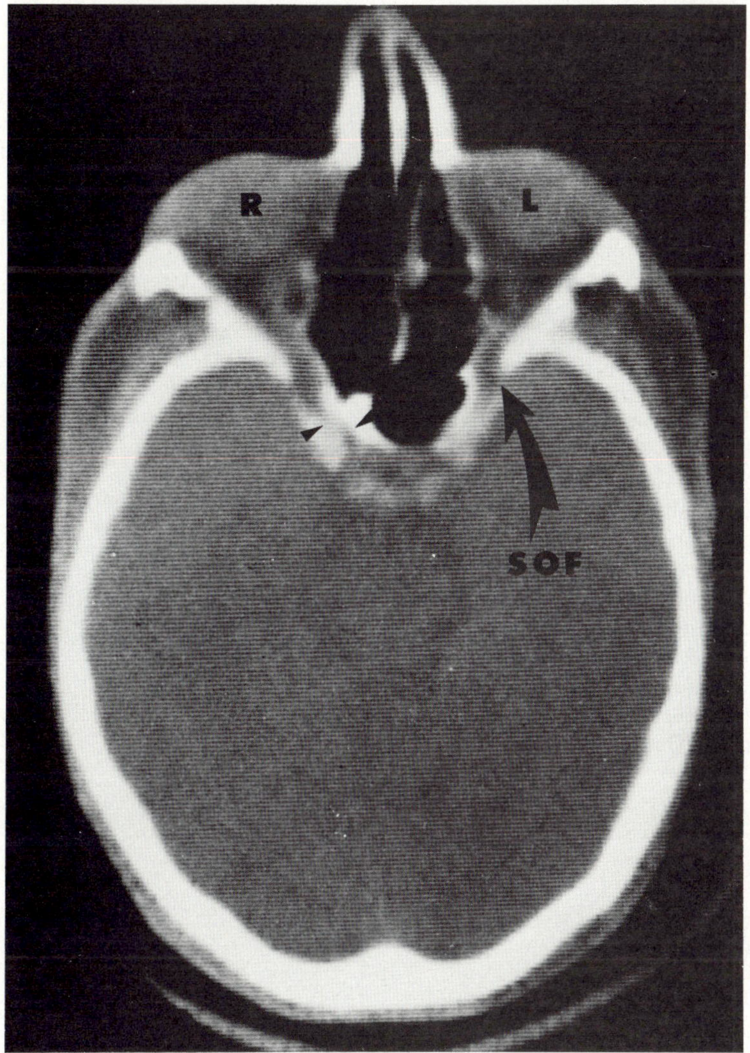

Fig. 11. *CT scan*. To best visualize the optic canal (arrowheads on the right), the plane of the scan should parallel the course of the optic canal. Although the same border forming structures are seen here as on the base tomogram of the optic canal (Fig. 2), the bony detail on computed tomography is much less precise. Only the superolateral portion of the superior orbital fissure (SOF) is seen on the same plane as the optic canal.

EDITOR'S NOTE

This chapter is very, very important! I see case after case of optic nerve sheath tumors missed by NOT having had optic canal tomograms! Also, not only have optic canal tomograms not been ordered, but when they have been obtained, often they are not of good quality. You should order skull films, optic canals (Rhese views), optic canal polytomography, and then a CT scan of orbit and brain, with enhancement—in that order, when you are thinking of an anterior meningioma or optic nerve sheath tumor. Do NOT bypass the plain films and go to the CT scan—you'll be sorry if you do!

One final point that may help. If you look at the nice pictures of the optic canal in Figures 1A, B, and C—you will note that the optic canal has a *vertical* long *oval* in 1A, but has a more *horizontal* long *oval* in 1C. This may help you—you *"punt in the orbit"* but *"pass intracranially!"* That may apply to many ophthalmologists, too! If you see a tough orbital problem, you may punt! Remember, that football has a vertical long oval when it is being held for that attempted field goal. However, when you run into a real intracranial problem, many ophthalmologists at that point may feel that they really need to "pass"! The optic canal shares that feeling, for it is shaped like a short "flat pass" at its intracranial end, where you now see a horizontal long oval shape to the canal. In the midportion of the canal, its more rounded (somewhat like a "home-made" conoid of Sturm with the circle of least confusion midway between a vertical axis anteriorly and a horizontal axis posteriorly). Remember, that the optic canal is about 10 mm long on its upper border but about 6 mm long along its lower border. That leaves the telephone number of the nerve still reasonable—"1,30,6,10" standing for 1 mm intraocular, 30 mm intraorbital, 6 mm intraosseous, and 10 mm intracranial. Do not forget optic canal tomograms—they are important in neuro-ophthalmology!

JLS

REFERENCES

1. Maniscalo, J. E. and Habal, M. D. Microanatomy of the optic canal. J. Neurosurg. *48*:402–406 (1978).
2. Takahasi, M., Lombardi, G., Passerini, A., and Ohno, S. Primary intra-orbital meningiomas: A roentgenologic study. Neuroradiology *5*:95–101 (1973).
3. Susac, J. O., Marins, A. N., and Whaley, R. A. Intracanalicular meningioma with normal tomography. J. Neurosurg. *49*:659–662 (1977).
4. Trobe, J. D., Glaser, J. S., Post, M. J. D., and Page, L. K. Bilateral optic canal meningiomas. A case report. Neurosurg. *3*:68–74 (1978).
5. Potter, G. D. *Sectional Anatomy and Tomography of the Head.* Grune and Stratton, New York, 1971, p. 334.
6. Potter, G. D. and Trokel, S. L. Optic canal. In: *Radiology of the Skull and Brain.* T. H. Newton and D. G. Potts (Eds.), C. V. Mosby Co., St. Louis, 1971, Vol. 1, pp. 487–507.
7. Tadmor, R. and New, P. F. J. Computed tomography of the orbit with special emphasis on coronal sections. Part 1. Normal anatomy. J. Comput. Asst. Tomog. *2*:24–34 (1978).
8. Gyldenstead, C., Lester, J., and Fledus, H. Computed tomography of orbital lesions. Neuroradiology *13*:141–150 (1977).

15 Optic Canal Enlargement

Thomas J. Walsh, M.D.

Asymmetry or enlargement of the optic canals has always been of intense interest to the neuro-ophthalmologist. The major concern has always been optic canal enlargement due to tumors and particularly optic nerve gliomas. In the course of this discussion, other causes of optic canal enlargement including congenital defects, other types of tumors, and nontumor causes will be commented upon. It is true that most of the optic canal enlargements that we see are due to optic nerve gliomas, but occasionally one of the other causes comes along and must be kept in mind. Failure to recognize these other possibilities will cause the wrong diagnostic tests to be ordered in making the diagnosis resulting in an incorrect or delay in proper diagnosis and treatment.

In order to understand the congenital defects which cause optic canal enlargement, a brief review of the embryologic development of the optic canal is in order. This was reviewed so graphically and rhoentgenographically by Kier in his work.[1] The three stages of the optic canal are the formation of the cartilagenous optic foramen, ossification of the cartilagenous foramen, and lastly the transformation of the bony foramen into the bony optic canal.

The first stage, which is the formation of the cartilagenous optic foramen, occurs during the third fetal month. The second stage, which is the ossification of the cartilagenous foramen, develops from only two of the 19 ossification centers of the sphenoid anlage.

These two centers are the lesser and presphenoid centers. From these two centers ossification develops to form the optic strut. The anterior strut is formed by the ossification developing from the lesser sphenoid center to the postsphenoid center. The posterior segment of the strut develops either from the presphenoid center alone or from the lesser and presphenoid centers simultaneously. In the early stages of ossification before the posterior segment of the optic strut is fully formed, the foramen has the appearance of a figure-of-eight or keyhole appearance. When this posterior segment of the optic strut is fully formed, the optic canal has two distinct openings. This opening between the two segments of the optic strut is obliterated during the last two months of fetal life to leave an optic canal as we usually see it on roentgenograms. If there is a cessation of development when the posterior segment of the optic strut is forming, a keyhole or figure-of-eight configuration of the optic canal is seen (Fig. 1A, B). If the posterior segment of the optic strut forms but the foramen between the anterior and posterior segments fails to become obliterated by the ossification process, a double optic canal is produced (Fig. 1C). The final stage of ossification fuses the anterior and posterior segments into one segment, leaving only the true optic canal (Fig. 1D).

The double optic canal configuration does not cause the confusion that a figure-of-eight type of optic canal causes unless the false canal is picked to compare to the true optic canal in the other orbit. This would give the false impression of optic canal asymmetry. In order to avoid this problem when viewing roentgenograms, there is a simple method for properly identifying the true optic canal. The planum sphenoidale is an obvious landmark in any roentgenogram for optic canals. Follow this sloping line on the roentogenogram medially to its end. Just beneath the end of the planum sphenoidale is the optic canal. The figure-of-eight type anomaly produces an

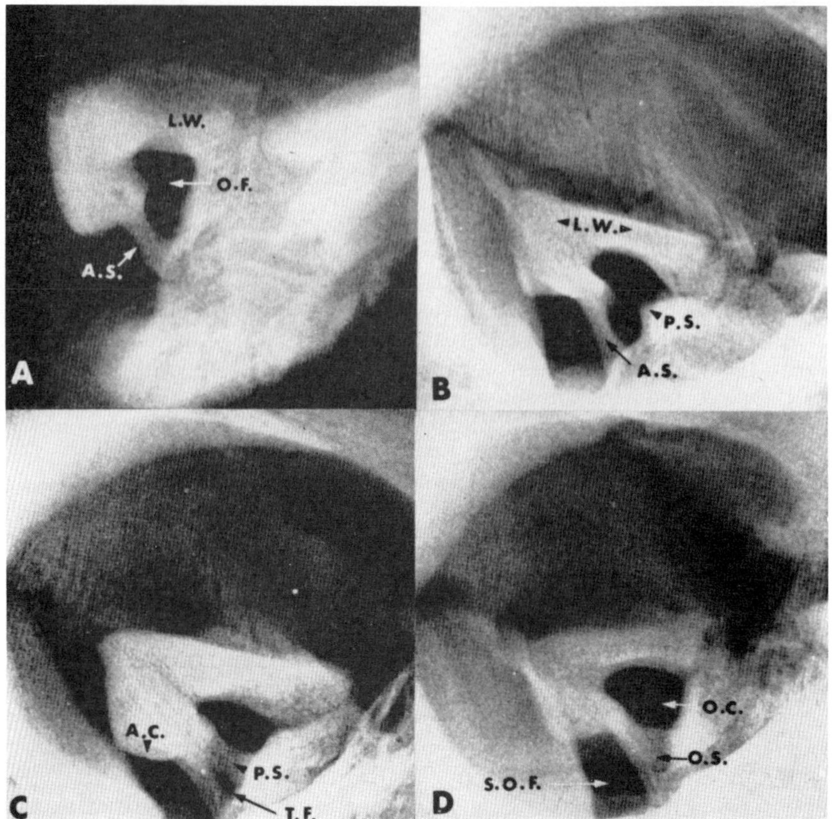

Fig. 1. (A) shows some beginning pinching in the middle portion of the keyhole appearance. (B) is a continuation and more pronounced version of the same process with a figure-of-eight appearance. (C) has both struts formed but the foramen between them is not obliterated causing an appearance of a double canal. (D) is the normal appearance of the strut with the foramen between completely ossified.

elongated diameter to the optic canal rather than two distinct openings. Therefore, in order to avoid falling into the error of erroneously calling an optic canal enlarged when it is only a figure of eight, always measure the canal diameter in the horizontal and not in the vertical diameter.

Besides the congenital anomalies and optic nerve gliomas, there are other causes of optic canal enlargement. Not all of these have roentgenographic changes limited only to the optic canal.

Other Causes of Optic Canal Enlargement:

1. Pituitary adenoma with extrasellar extension
2. Extension of suprasellar cholesteatomas, ectopic pinealomas and craniopharyngiomas (Ref. 2)
3. Infraclinoid aneurysms
4. Orbital reticulosarcoma
5. Meningioma of optic nerve sheath (Ref. 3)
6. Nasopharyngeal malignancy
7. Carcinoma of the sphenoid bone
8. Sphenoid bone mucocele
9. Tuberculosis of sphenoid bone
10. Retinoblastoma infiltrating along the optic nerve sheath

CASE 1

K. D. was first examined at age fourteen months because of "dancing eyes" and esotropia first noted at four months of age. He was the product of a normal pregnancy and delivery but was developing about six months slower than his older siblings.

On examination he had at least ambient vision. However, there was no response to large OKN targets. There was a large and variable right esotropia along with some wandering of both eyes. The right pupil had an amaurotic response and the left pupil was intact to light. The fundus examination revealed optic atrophy with bilateral small discs.

Skull roentgenograms were obtained, and the initial report was an enlarged right optic canal. An optic nerve glioma was suspected. EEG was normal. The ERG was extinguished on the right and severely impaired on the left. The VER was unrecordable from the right eye and normal from the left.

In reviewing the films, it was quite obvious that the enlargement of the optic canal was due to a failure of development of the posterior optic strut resulting in the figure-of-eight or keyhole anomaly (Fig. 2). The reason for the optic atrophy and poor vision was bilateral hypoplasia of the optic nerves and not an optic nerve glioma (Fig. 3).

The lesson learned from this case was that defects in the formation of the optic strut cause abnormalities in the vertical and not the horizontal diameter. When you are in doubt as to the size of an optic canal, check the horizontal diameters.

CASE 2

R. S. is an eight-year-old boy who was seen by his local ophthalmologist for a red left eye. It was diagnosed as conjunctivitis and treated with topical antibiotics, and the patient was told to return in two weeks. At that next visit, the vision in the left eye was no light perception, and the fundus showed unilateral disc edema. The diagnosis of optic neuritis was made, and the patient was treated with systemic steroids with no im-

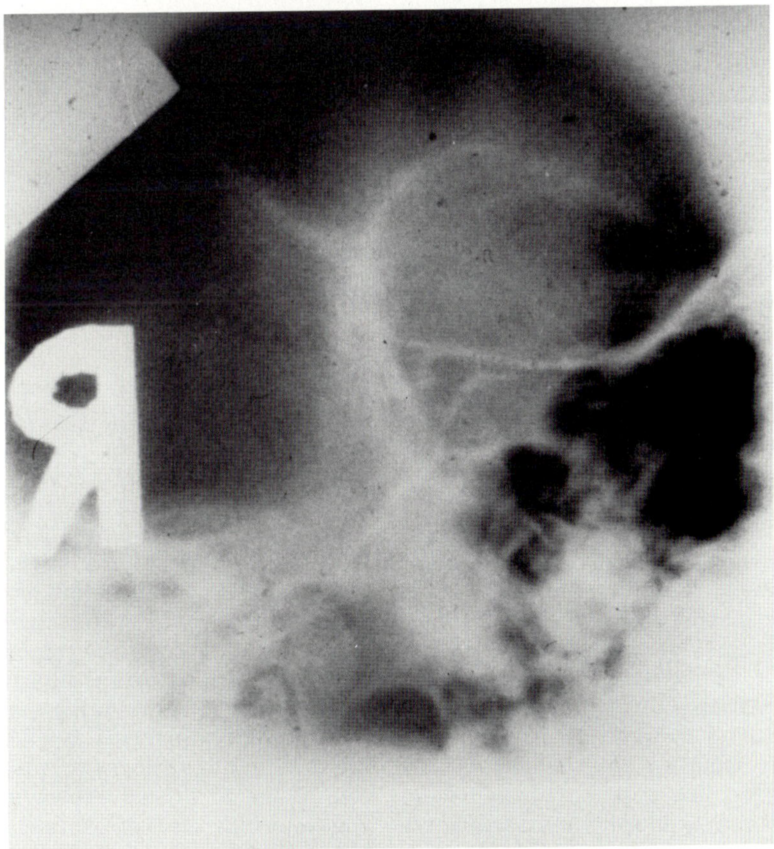

Fig. 2. The optic canal here renals "normal size in the horizontal dimension but elongated keyhole or figure of eight appearance in the vertical dimension."

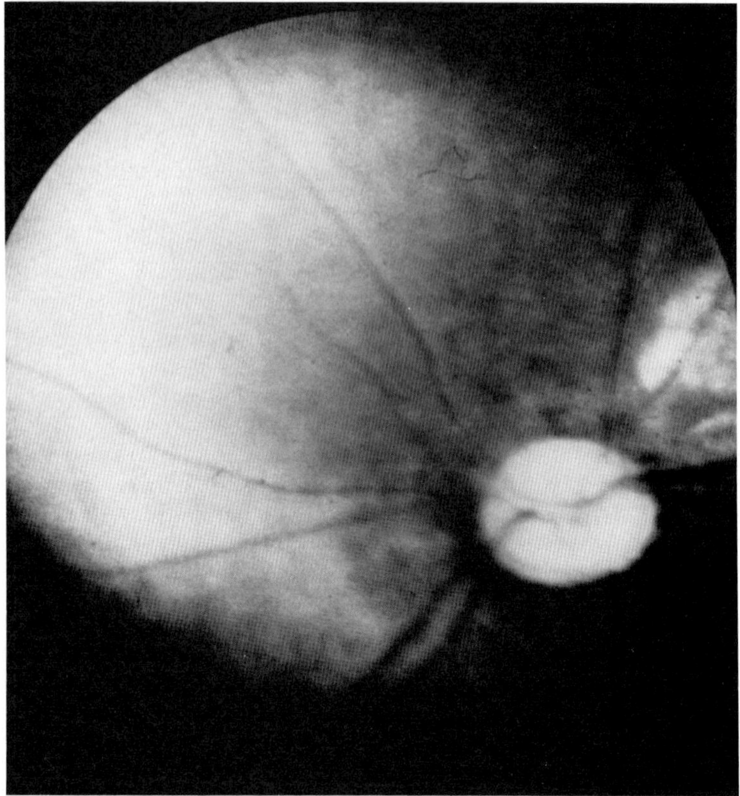

Fig. 3. A fundus photograph of the right optic nerve which shows an atrophic and small nerve. The left nerve was essentially the same.

provement. He was then referred for consultation and was seen one week later. Our examination revealed the same clinical findings and also 3 mm of measurable proptosis which was not grossly obvious on simple inspection. Motility in both eyes and the field examination in the other eye was normal. The right pupil response was normal, and the left pupil had an amaurotic response.

Routine roentgenograms were read as normal. However, tomograms revealed some widening of the apex where there was molding just at the point where the optic nerve enters the optic canal (Fig. 4). An arteriogram revealed widening of the usual bayonet appearance of the ophthalmic artery as it courses around the optic nerve, thereby suggesting an enlargement of the optic nerve (Fig. 5).

A Kronlein procedure was performed, and an enlarged nerve was seen extending from just behind the globe to as far back to the canal as the nerve could be resected. The pathology report was optic nerve glioma with no normal nerve seen at the proximal end. An intracranial procedure was then performed, and the intracranial portion of the optic nerve was resected up to the chiasm. This pathology report also revealed intracranial extension of the glioma but a normal nerve free of tumor before it entered the chiasm. The postoperative field in the other eye was normal with no upper temporal defect.

In this case despite intracranial extension, routine optic canal roentgenograms were normal. It required tomograms to suggest the diagnosis. If we had stopped our work up with routine optic canal roentgenograms, the diagnosis would have been missed. The arteriogram was also suggestive of the diagnosis. However, nowadays, CT scanning or ultrasound would have been more useful and easier to perform than an arteriogram. It was Vignaud's work

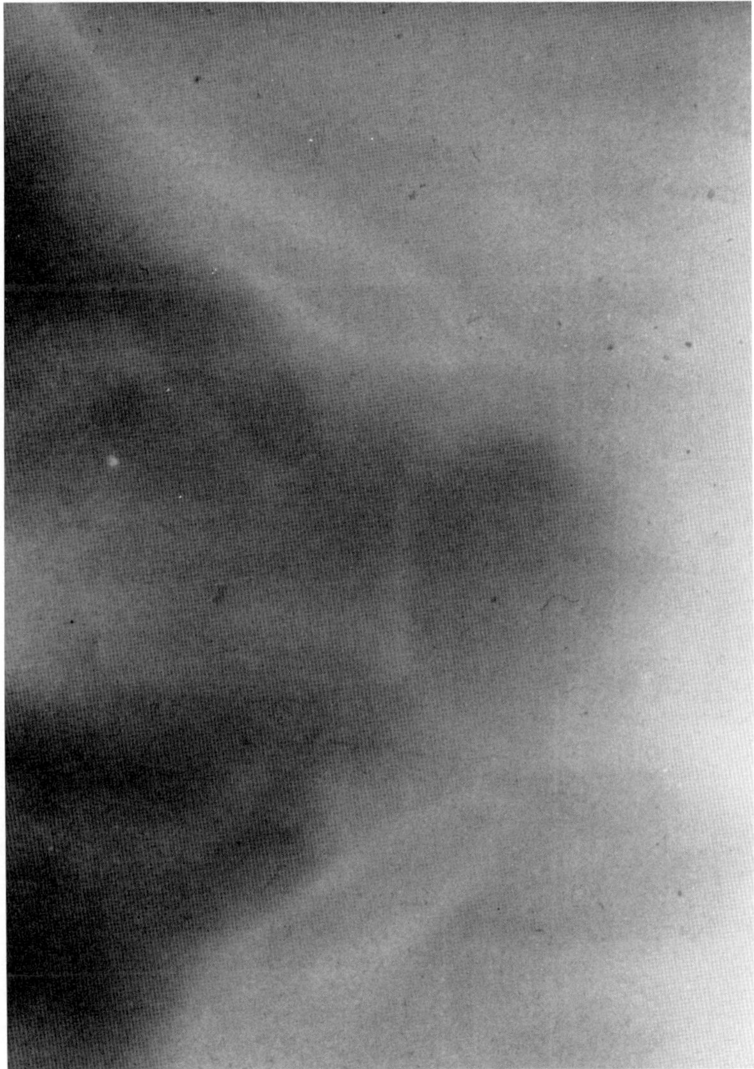

Fig. 4. Routine roentgenograms of the optic canal were normal, but tomograms show some widening of the right canal as the nerve enters into it.

that suggested the orbital arteriography sign for an enlarged optic nerve (Ref. 4). He demonstrated that most of the time the intra-orbital ophthalmic artery has a bayonet appearance as it crosses the optic nerve. The first portion is straight and beneath the nerve. The second portion is the circumneural portion and comes up on the lateral aspect of the nerve and then crosses over to the medial side.

The last portion goes anterior in the medial aspect of the orbit giving off muscular branches and ending in the angular artery (Fig. 6). Vignaud felt that the average distance between the first and third portion of the artery as it crossed the optic nerve was 3–7 mm. More than this amount or a distortion of this bayonet appearance indicated an enlarged nerve. Of course, this sign could not distinguish an intrinsic tumor of the nerve from one on its surface. This is a valid sign and was also seen in Case 3 and was our only clue prior to CT scanning and ultrasound orbital examinations.

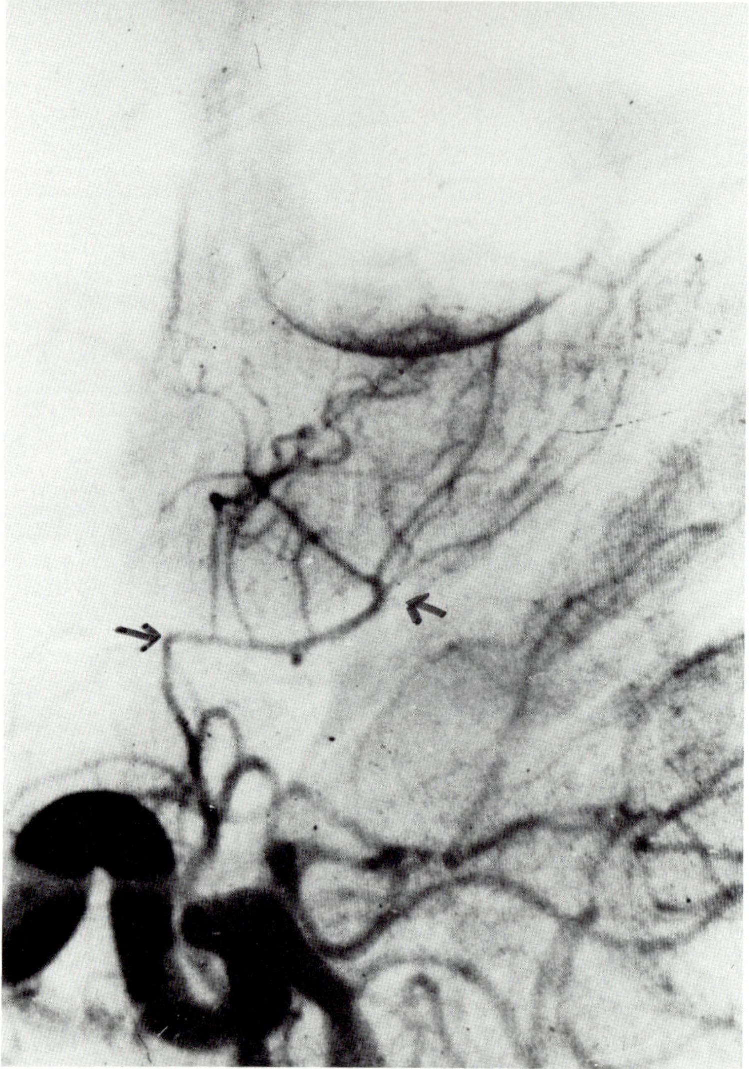

Fig. 5. There is a stretching of the distance between the first and third segments of the ophthalmic artery as it courses around the optic nerve.

CASE 3

B. C. is a 29-year-old lady who noted blurred vision in her left eye in November 1969. The vision in the left eye was recorded by her physician as 20/200 with a large central scotoma in the left eye only. Because she was eight months pregnant, no roentgenographic diagnostic studies or treatment was begun. She had no other symptoms or signs except a Marcus Gunn afferent pupillary defect in the left eye. At the end of December, she delivered a healthy male child.

In January 1970, she was treated with steroids with no change in acuity. At the same time a workup including optic canal roentgenograms, tomograms, orbital venogram, thyroid studies, spinal fluid electrophoresis, and neurological examination was normal. In June 1971, she was again seen by her physician, and the vision in the left eye was no light perception. The same workup was repeated and in addition, a brain scan, all of which were entirely negative once again.

We saw the patient in April of 1972 with a six-month history of mild left eye proptosis. The history and 2 mm of proptosis certainly suggested a retrobulbar mass. The eye examination including a field examination of the other eye was normal except for

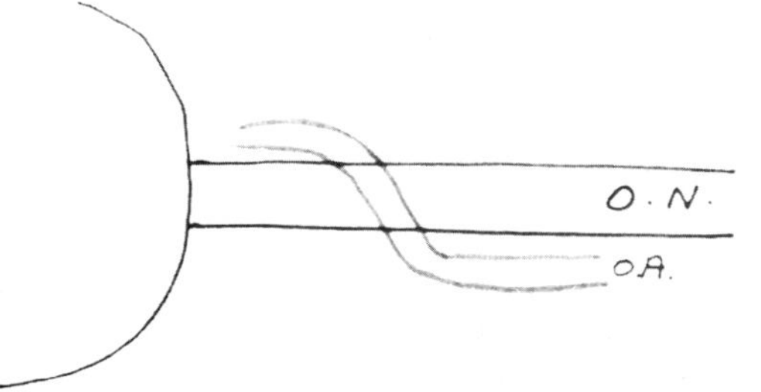

Fig. 6. The normal bayonet appearance of the artery as it winds around the nerve. Figure 5 reveals a marked stretching of this relationship.

a blind left eye, marked left optic nerve atrophy, and a left amaurotic pupil. All studies were again repeated and again were normal. In addition, an arteriogram was performed which revealed a 13-mm widening of the bayonet appearance of the ophthalmic artery (Fig. 7).

A Kronlein procedure was performed, and an enlarged nerve from just behind the globe all the way to the optic canal was observed. As much of the nerve as possible was excised and optic nerve glioma was the pathology report. The tumor extended from one end of the resected specimen to the other with no normal nerve seen. Because of this report, an intracranial procedure was performed, and the nerve was resected up to the chiasm. The pathological reports still

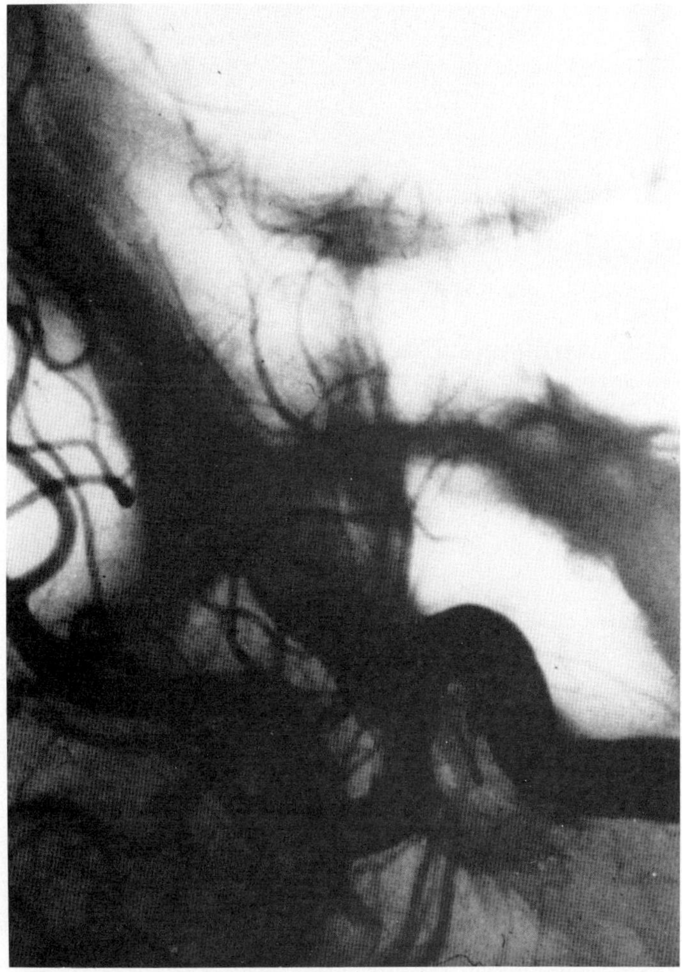

Fig. 7. Another example of stretching of the ophthalmic artery even when routine roentgenograms and in this case tomograms were negative.

revealed no normal nerve, suggesting extension into the chiasm itself. Despite this finding, the fields in the right eye revealed no upper temporal defect before or after surgery.

This case is similar to Case 2 except that regular as well as tomograms were normal despite intracranial extension of the tumor. No enlargement of the canal is not necessarily any guarantee that the tumor is confined to the orbit. In this age of CT scanning and ultrasound examinations, this enlargement of the optic nerve by a tumor would have been picked up much earlier and may have spared this lady an intracranial procedure. It also would have allowed us to treat her before the tumor reached the chiasm. Certainly when there is progressive loss of vision, a tumor must be the first consideration and pursued with every modality available even resorting to surgery for direct observation of the nerve. As is demonstrated by this case, routine roentgenograms and tomograms are not the definitive and final answer to ruling out optic nerve tumors or orbital masses.

CASE 4

M. S. is a two-year-old child who was first seen in the emergency room with a one-day history of right eye proptosis. The eye exam except for the proptosis was within normal limits. He was seen in con-

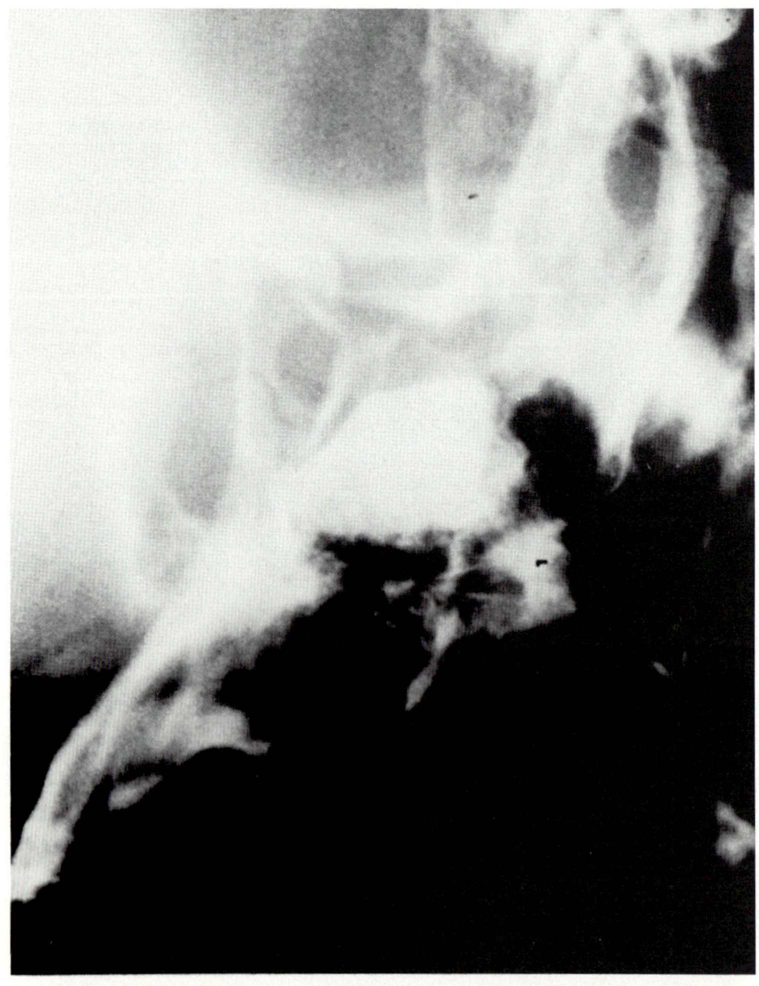

Fig. 8

Figs. 8, 9. The right optic canal in Figure 8 is enlarged as compared to the left canal in Figure 9.

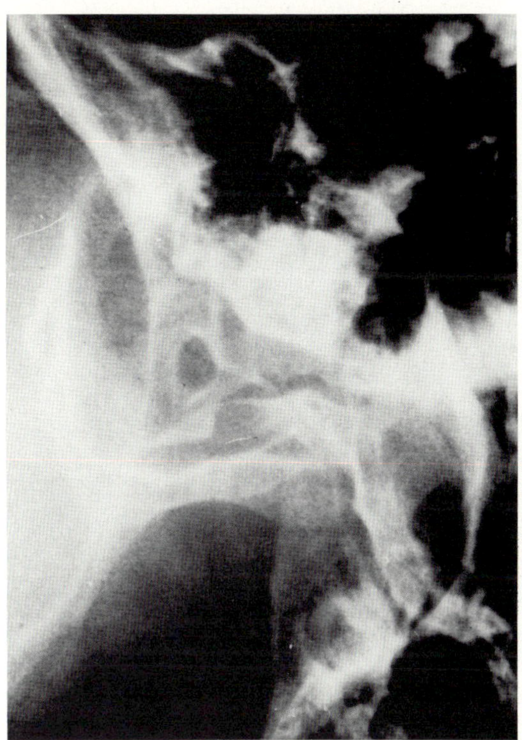

Fig. 9

sultation two days later with increased proptosis of the right eye. However, the right disc now showed obvious papilledema. Due to the rapidity of the proptosis, rhabdomyosarcoma was a consideration. The motility and pupil examinations were within normal limits, and no periorbital mass could be palpated.

The family history was extremely interesting. He was one of twins and his twin was a cerebral palsy child with a right esotropia. Both twins were noted to have *café au lait* spots. The father had multiple skin neurofibromas.

Now expecting an optic nerve glioma, skull roentgenograms were ordered and showed right optic canal enlargement (Figs. 8, 9). A CT scan revealed an enlargement of the right optic nerve which was presumed to be an optic nerve glioma (Figs. 10, 11). What was a bigger surprise was the report that the supposedly normal left optic nerve also was enlarged. This finding was also confirmed by orbital ultrasound.

Here is a child with presumed neurofibromatosis and with bilateral involvement of the optic nerves. In retrospect, this is not unexpected since patients with neurofibromatosis have multiple tumors. For example, there is a limited relationship between cerebella pontine angle tumors and neurofibromatosis. However, if there occurs bilateral cerebella pontine angle tumors, then they are almost always related to neurofibromatosis.

The lesson we learned from this patient was that optic nerve gliomas can be multiple and bilateral even if the symptoms and signs suggest unilateral disease.

CASE 5

A. K. is a five-year-old girl who was seen in the summer of 1977 by her local doctor because of the onset of nystagmus. He felt that it was unilateral and vertical and made the diagnosis of spasmus nutans. During the summer, this previously well-developed, gay, active, pleasant child became thin, apathetic, and housebound rather than playing with her neighborhood friends. She was seen in consultation in October of 1977. The child had vertical nystagmus which was not truly unilateral but bilateral and very asymmetric. The fact that it was bilateral changes the diagnosis considerably. No better than count fingers vision in either eye was noted. Further examinations revealed a normal external examination and motility. The pupils were equal and poorly reactive to light but no unilateral afferent pupillary defect was demonstrated. The fundus examination showed florid bilateral papilledema.

Skull roentgenograms revealed the largest optic canals I have ever seen. They were both 13 mm (Fig. 12). At that point, we felt we had either a chiasmal glioma extending down both optic nerves causing bilateral enlargement of the optic canals or bilateral optic nerve gliomas. Arteriography demonstrated a large vascular lesion in the inferior aspect of the anterior fossa in the midline predominately to the right. There appeared to be a blood supply from the ophthalmic artery as well as from frontal branches of the cerebral artery. There was also a large avascular component present superiorly. The air study showed a large mass projecting into the anterior third and

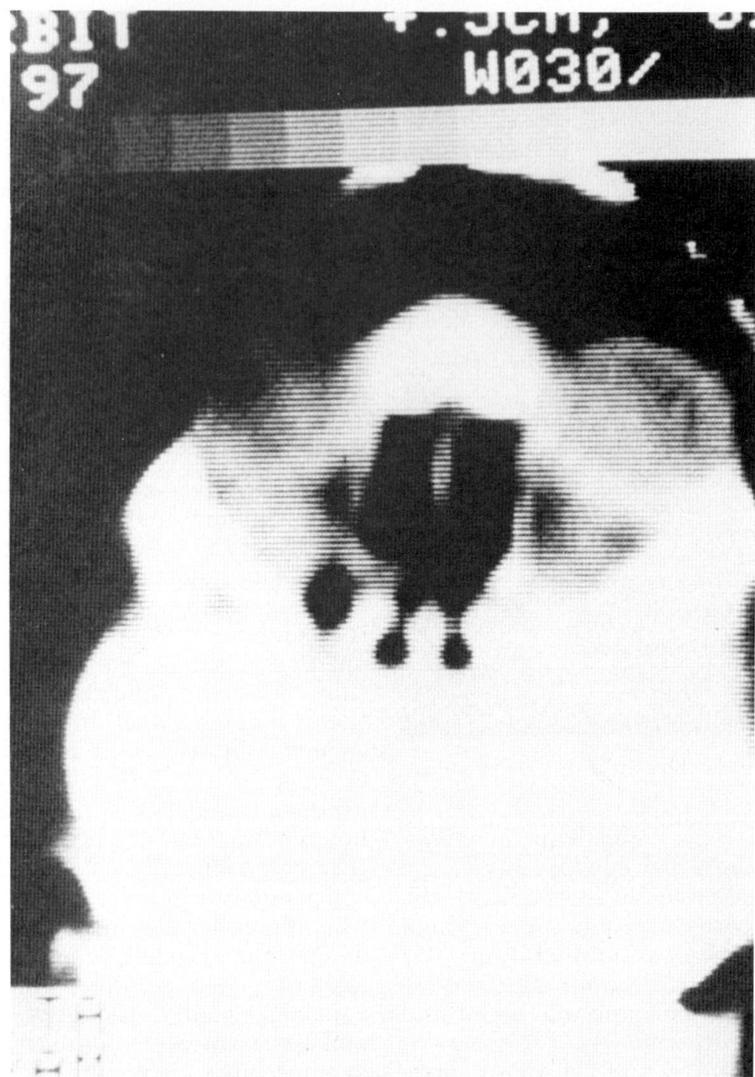

Fig. 10

Figs. 10, 11. The Acta Scan shows enlargement of the right optic nerve and perhaps the left nerve also in Figure 10. Figure 11 leaves no doubt that the left optic nerve also is enlarged.

floor of the right lateral ventricle, displacing the structures across the midline to the left.

At the time of surgery, the neurosurgeon found a large cystic neoplasm from which he drained large amounts of fluid. The pathology report was astrocytoma probably a hypothalamic glioma. Exploration of the optic nerves did not reveal any optic nerve tumors but only severe optic nerve atrophy. The nerves not only did not show a large nerve expanding the optic canals but were indeed so atrophic that they did not fill the canal. It was felt that the enlarged canals were due to prolonged increased intracranial pressure. This cause has been reported previously but is admittedly a rare cause even with all the cases of increased intracranial pressure that do occur.

The lesson to be learned from this case is not to presume that enlarged canals always represent an optic nerve tumor even in a five-year-old child.

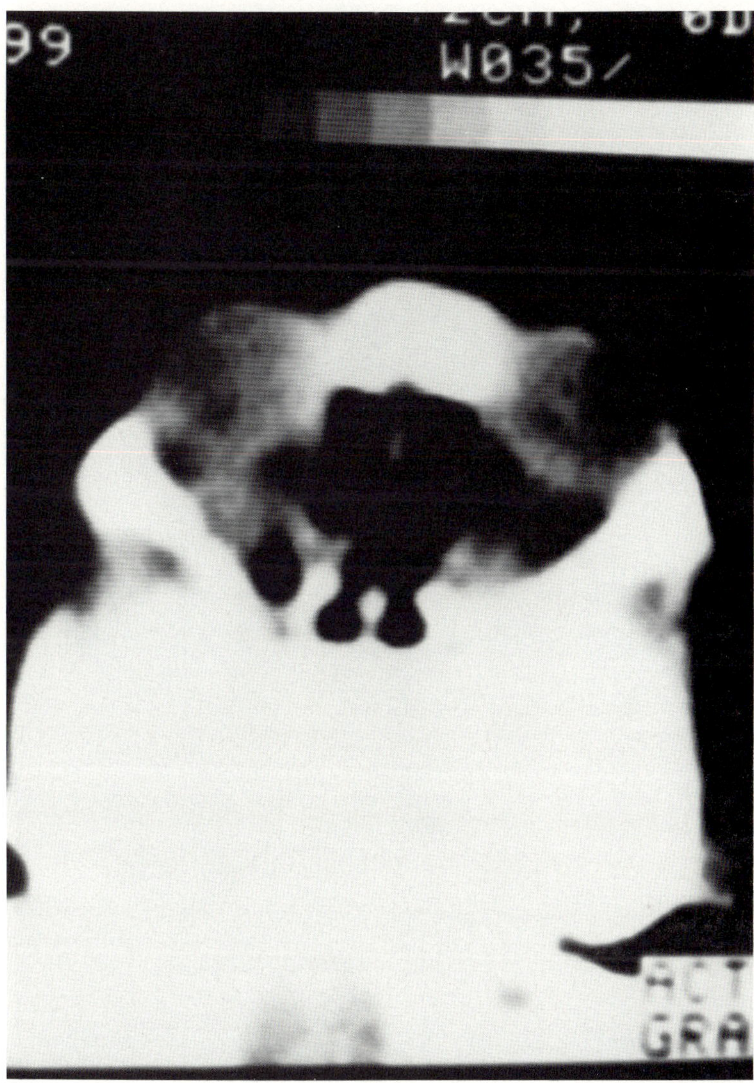

Fig. 11

CASE 6

A. B. is a 47-year-old man with a five-month history of progressive proptosis of the right eye. On examination the vision in the right eye was 20/80 and the left eye was 20/20. There was moderate proptosis and chemosis of the right eye. A firm rubbery mass was easily palpated temporal to the right eye and up into the upper fornix. The motility of the right eye was markedly limited in all directions of gaze.

The view of the fundus in the right eye was partially obscured by a cataract and the media was equal to the visual acuity. The disc in both eyes appeared normal without any atrophy or edema. There was an inferior temporal nonrhegmatogenous retinal detachment of the right eye. The Hertel exophthalmometer measurements were right eye 27 and left eye 17.

Plain roentgenograms showed an increased density in the upper temporal quadrant of the right orbit (Fig. 13). The optic canal on the right side was markedly enlarged (Figs. 14, 15). However, there was

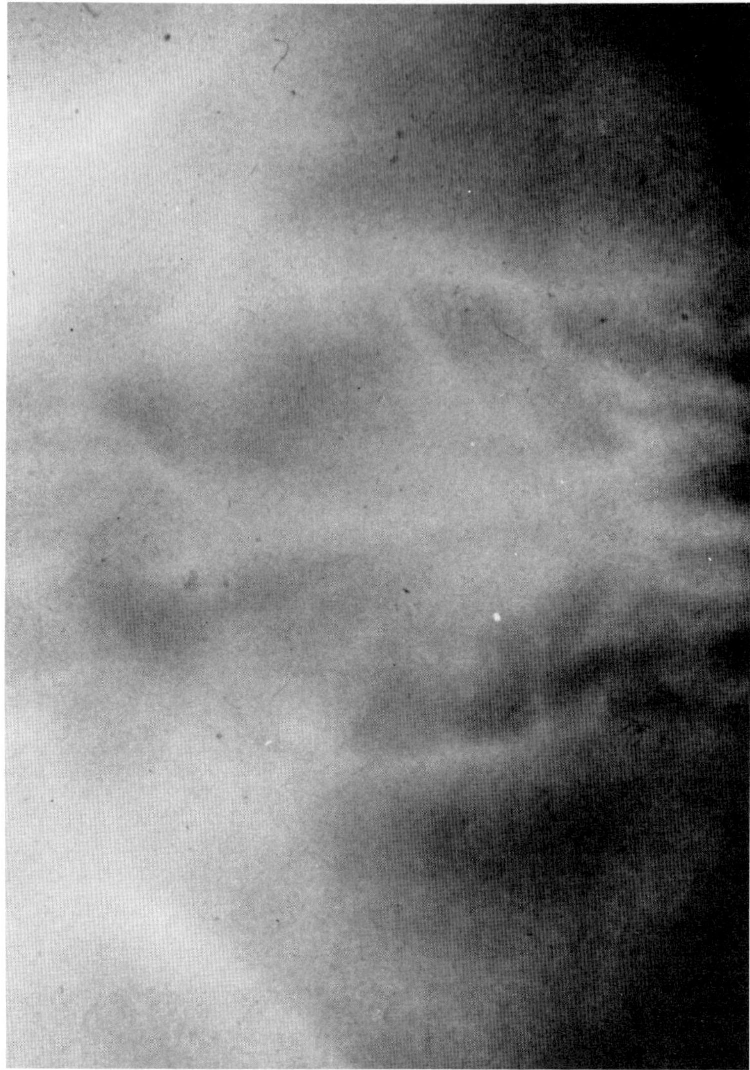

Fig. 12. Tomograms of both optic canals demonstrate bilateral enlargement.

no sclerosis of the surrounding bone. An arteriogram demonstrated increased vascularity in the area of the soft tissue density and a presumptive diagnosis of meningioma was made (Fig. 16).

A biopsy confirmed this diagnosis. A combined orbital and neurosurgical procedure was performed, and the tumor was removed and dissected off the optic nerve. The vision remained at 20/80 post-operatively due to the cataract, and the retinal detachment disappeared. It was felt that the meningioma was primarily orbital in orgin.

The presumed mechanism for the non-rhegmatogenous retinal detachment was compression by the tumor of the inferior vortex vein.

Eighteen months later his cataract in the right eye was successfully operated, and he obtained 20/20 vision with a contact lens and had normal motility.

The lesson learned here is that meningiomas involving the optic canal do not have to have associated sclerosis of the surrounding bone.

The foregoing discussion outlines the

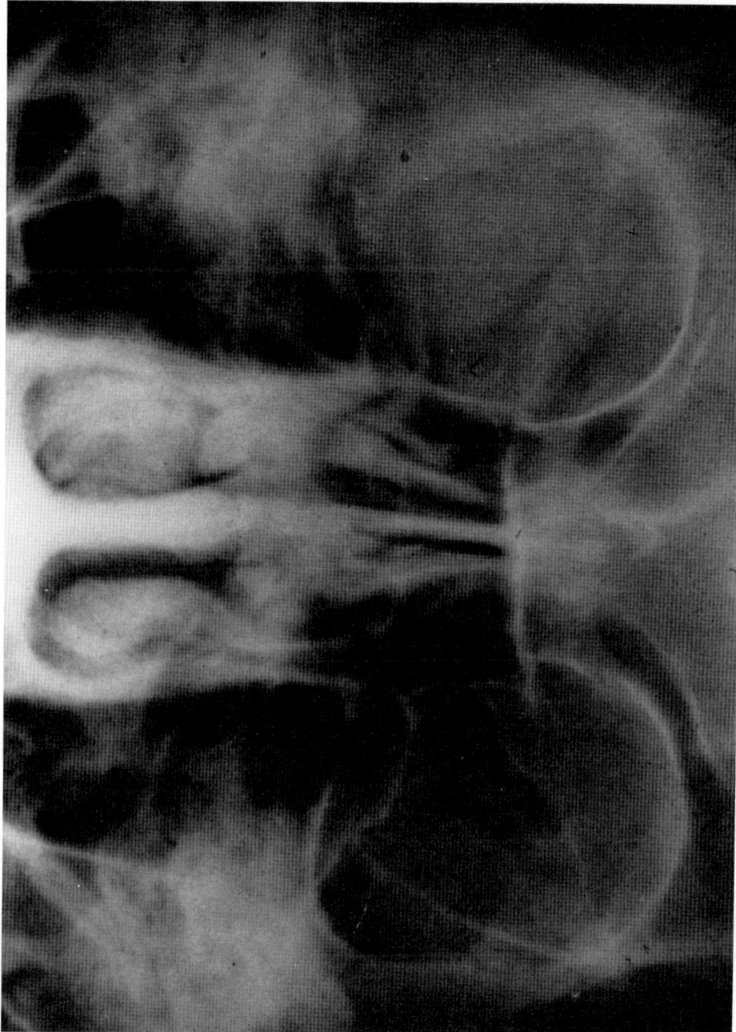

Fig. 13. There is an increased soft tissue density in the upper outer quadrant of the right orbit.

many causes of optic canal asymmetry. It is true that most of the causes outlined are rare as compared to optic canal enlargement secondary to an optic nerve glioma. I hope that I have not distracted the reader from that important fact particularly in the young person less than 20 years of age. However, the other causes of optic canal enlargement do occur and should be kept in mind.

EDITOR'S NOTE

All I can say to Dr. Walsh's chapter is *"Amen!"* This shows again that the CT scan has not done away with the routine radiographs of the optic canals at all, and particularly the need for good optic canal tomograms in cases of unexplained anterior visual loss. One major point, however, is to be sure and get those optic canal tomograms reviewed by a competent neuroradiologist. The commonest error I have made with x-rays is to accept the nice typed-up report by that board radiologist. Many, many times when the same films are shown to another "knock-out" neuroradiologist, he says—"Why, there's the meningioma!"—and points to it with his finger and shows it to you, too! Have those x-rays

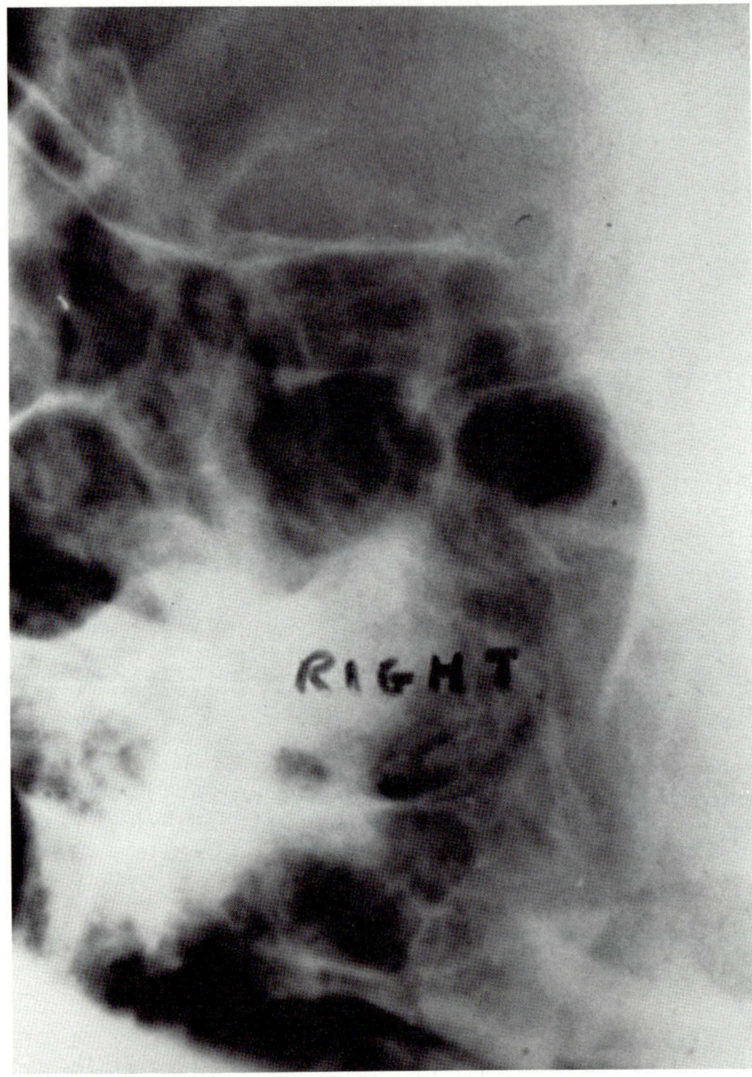

Fig. 14

Figs. 14, 15. The right optic canal in Figure 14 is not only larger than the left optic canal in Figure 15 but is also above the upper limits of normal.

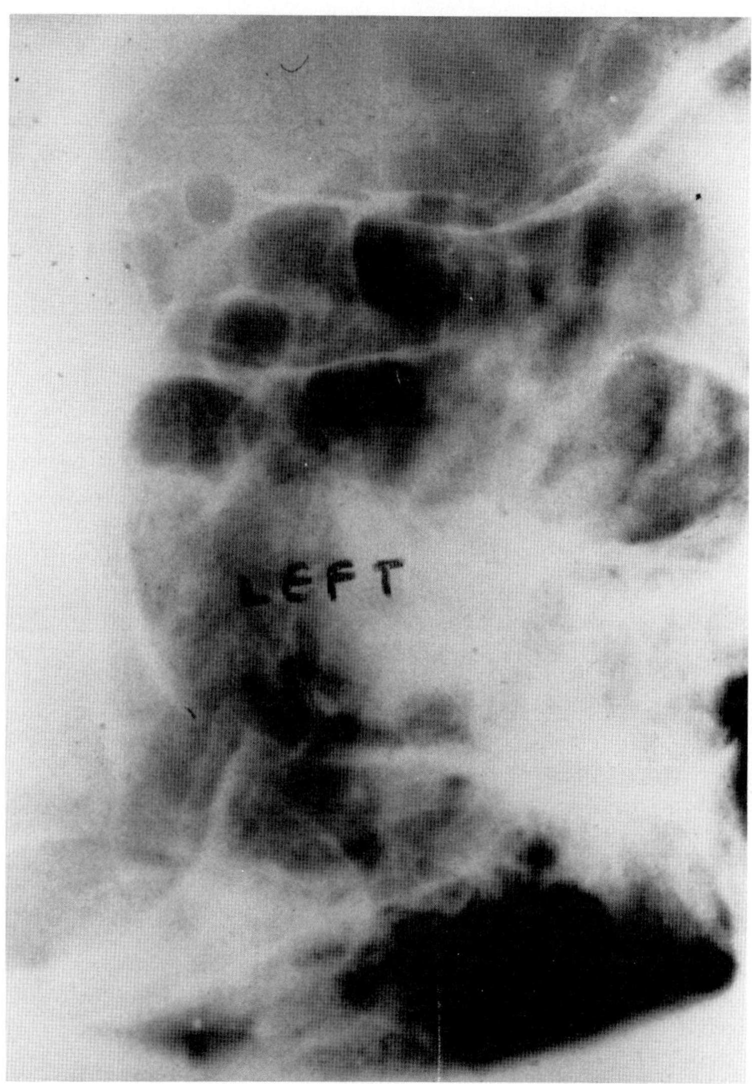

Fig. 15

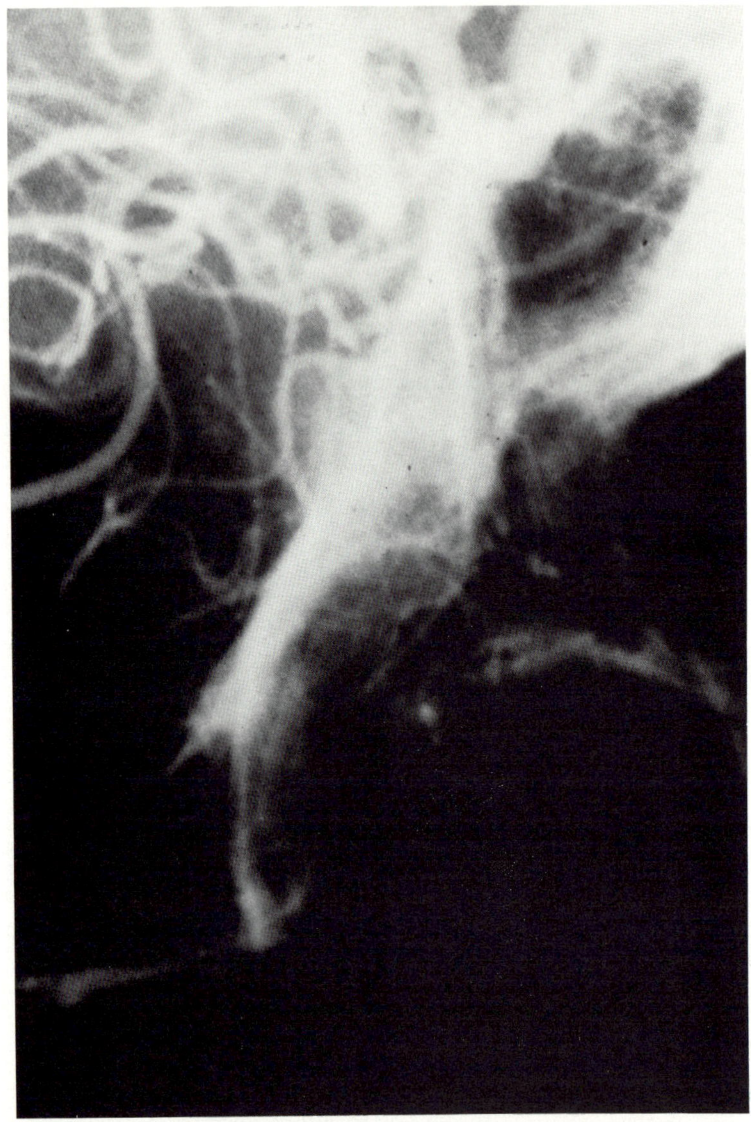

Fig. 16. The arteriogram demonstrated increased vascularity in the area of the soft tissue density, which suggested menigioma as the most likely diagnosis.

and CT scans reviewed, and have the radiologist show the lesion to you. If he cannot show it to you to your own satisfaction, go slow on that lesion!

JLS

ACKNOWLEDGMENT

Figure 1 is reproduced with the kind permission of Leon Kier and J. B. Lippincott Company: Kier, L. E. Embryology of the nomal optic canal and its anomalies. *Invest. Radiol.* **1**:346, 1966

REFERENCES

1. Kier, L. E. Embryology of the nomal optic canal and its anomalies. Invest. Radiol. *1*:346 (1966).
2. Block, M. A., Goree, J. A., and Jimenez, J. D. Craniopharynogioma with optic canal enlargement simulating glioma of the optic canal. J. Neurosurg. *39*:523 (1973).
3. Hollenhorst, R. W., Hollenhorst, R. W., and MacCarty, C. C. Visual prognosis of optic nerve sheath meningiomas producing shunt vessels on the optic disc. Mayo Clin. Proc. *53*:84 (1978).
4. Vignaud, J. and Clay, C. Orbital arteriography. Radiol. Clin. North Am. *10*:30 (1972).

16 Cecocentral Scotomas— Neuro-ophthalmologic Considerations

Harold E. Shaw, Jr., M.D.
J. Lawton Smith, M.D.

Cecocentral scotomas are a widely recognized feature of toxic (nutritional, tobacco-alcohol) amblyopia,[1-6] but other etiologies of cecocentral scotomas and the significance of these field defects are seldom emphasized. In this chapter, we examine from a neuro-ophthalmologic perspective the causes and implications of cecocentral scotomas.

MATERIALS AND METHODS

Sixty-five cases of unilateral and bilateral cecocentral scotomas seen in a referral neuro-ophthalmologic practice during the 15-year period 1963–78 were reviewed. All patients had complete eye examinations, which included central and peripheral visual fields, using a tangent screen and the Aimark projection perimeter. A projector light target corresponding to a 5/1000 white isopter was routinely employed on tangent screen testing. In selected cases, formed white and color targets were used. The 3/330 white and 5/330 red isopters were most commonly used on the Aimark perimeter. We define a cecocentral scotoma as a field defect restricted to the horizontally oval area between and including fixation and the blind spot. Only cases of field defects which strictly conformed to this definition were included in this study. The peripheral visual fields were normal in all cases.

RESULTS

The cecocentral scotomas were bilateral in 52 and unilateral in 13 cases. Thirty-nine males and 26 females were affected. Sixty-two patients were white, and three were black. Their ages ranged from 9 to 70 years and averaged 42. Visual acuities varied from 20/15 to finger counting. The median visual acuity in unilateral cases was 20/40 and in bilateral cases was 20/80. Of the 52 bilateral cases, the difference in visual acuity between the two eyes was one line or less on the distance Snellen chart in 35 (68%) cases. Follow-up data were available on 54 of the 65 cases and ranged from two months to 15 years. The average follow-up time was 36 months. Eight patients were followed for more than eight years, and, excluding those, the average follow-up time was 15 months. Vision improved in 18 cases (28%), remained the same in 29 (44%), and worsened in seven (11%). Follow-up was unavailable in 11 (17%). The visual outcome was comparable in those with unilateral and those with bilateral cecocentral scotomas.

Toxic amblyopia was the most common cause of bilateral cecocentral scotomas, occurring in 22 of 52 cases (42%). In this group, 17 patients had histories of suboptimal nutrition, alcohol abuse, or tobacco usage alone or in combination. In five cases, drugs or other toxins were incriminated as the cause of cecocentral scotomas. Genetic optic nerve disease accounted for 14 cases (27%) of bilateral cecocentral scotomas. In this group were patients with dominant optic atrophy and other forms of congenital or hereditary optic atrophy, including optic nerve hypoplasia. Other causes of bilateral cecocentral scotomas included optic neuritis due to demyelinating disease (8%), optic pits (4%), syphilitic optic neuritis (4%), and pernicious anemia (2%). Seven patients (13%) had intrinsic optic nerve disease, the etiology of which remained obscure. Two of those had histories of thyroid disease, and a metabolic optic neuropathy was postulated, but in none was a definitive diagnosis possible (Table I).

The most common cause of unilateral cecocentral scotomas was inflammatory, idiopathic, or demyelinating optic neuritis. Other causes included retinal vascular occlusions and optic pits. One patient had an atypical form of ischemic optic neuropathy. None of the patients with toxic amblyopia or genetic optic atrophy had unilateral cecocentral scotomas (Table II).

DISCUSSION

A cecocentral scotoma indicates pathologic change in the papillomacular nerve fiber bundle.[5] Excluding obvious macular lesions, the most common cause of a unilateral cecocentral scotoma in our experience is optic neuritis. Chamlin reported a 52% incidence of cecocentral scotomas in patients with optic neuritis.[7] Undoubtedly, with more careful perimetric scrutiny, many of the "central" scotomas associated with optic neuritis would be "cecocentral." More subtle abnormalities, such as optic pits, may produce unilateral cecocentral field defects which characteristically assume a "pistol" configuration (Fig. 1). The denser defect above the horizontal meridian corresponds to the typical inferotemporal location of pits in the optic disc. Cilioretinal artery occlusions can also cause cecocentral scotomas (Fig. 2). The diagnosis of vessel occlusion usually is obvious in the acute phase, but may be less apparent later. How-

TABLE I. *Bilateral cecocentral scotomas*

Etiology	No.	Clinical course			
		Better	Same	Worse	Un-known
Toxic (Nutritional, tobacco-alcohol)	22	11	5	1	5
Genetic optic atrophy	14	—	9	1	4
Optic neuritis (Demyelinating)	4	1	2	1	—
Optic pits	2	—	2	—	—
Syphilis	2	1	—	1	—
Pernicious anemia	1	1	—	—	—
Intrinsic optic nerve disease, ? etiology	7	1	5	1	—
Total	52	15	23	5	9

TABLE II. *Unilateral cecocentral scotomas*

Etiology	No.	Clinical course			
		Better	Same	Worse	Un-known
Optic neuritis	6	1	2	2	1
Retinal vascular occlusion	3	1	2	—	—
Optic pit	3	—	2	—	1
Ischemic optic neuropathy	1	1	—	—	—
Total	13	3	6	2	2

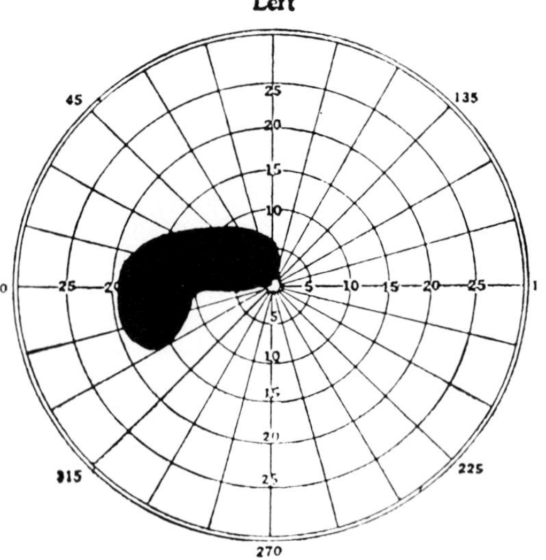

Fig. 1. "Pistol-like" cecocentral scotoma due to optic pit.

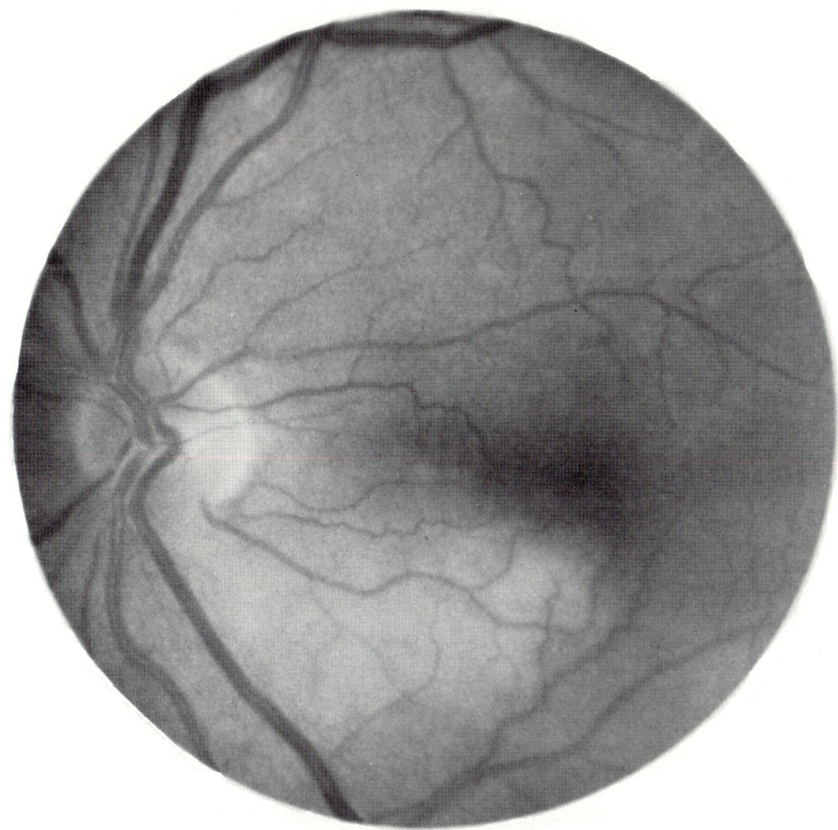

Fig. 2. Left eye. Cilioretinal artery occlusion involving inferior portion of papillomacular bundle.

ever, with a careful history and fundus examination, including use of a Hruby lens, the diagnosis in cases of unilateral cecocentral scotomas generally is evident.

The most common cause of bilateral cecocentral scotomas in our experience is toxic amblyopia. This entity affects patients with a history of excessive alcohol use, smoking, suboptimal nutrition, or any combination thereof.[8] In some instances, ingestion of drugs or other toxins may be a factor. Temporal pallor of the optic discs and bilateral cecocentral scotomas are the diagnostic hallmarks of toxic amblyopia (Fig. 3).

Another important cause of bilateral cecocentral scotomas is genetic optic nerve disease, particularly dominant optic atrophy.[9] This condition, which is said to be the most common heredofamilial optic atrophy,[10] characteristically produces cecocentral scotomas. Other forms of genetic optic nerve disease, such as Leber's disease and optic nerve hypoplasia,[11] may cause ceco-

central field defects. The patient with cecocentral scotomas due to genetic optic nerve disease may be asymptomatic or have a long history of mildly progressive visual dysfunction. A thorough history and examination of the family members are essential requirements for diagnosis in these patients.

Optic neuritis due to demyelinating disease, optic pits, syphilitic optic atrophy, and optic neuropathy associated with pernicious anemia are less frequent causes of bilateral cecocentral scotomas in our experience. In seven of our bilateral cases, we have been unable to establish a precise diagnosis despite extensive clinical investigation.

Cecocentral scotomas due to glaucoma have been reported,[12] but we have not observed pure isolated cecocentral scotomas, with totally normal visual fields otherwise, as a manifestation of glaucoma. Upper and lower Bjerrum scotomas may produce cecocentral-like defects, but they should be differentiated from true cecocentral scotomas.

Our experience indicates that, in the absence of other visual field defects, cecocentral scotomas point strongly to nonsurgical intrinsic optic nerve disease, most commonly toxic amblyopia or genetic optic atrophy. However, when bilateral cecocentral scotomas are found, one must be certain he is not dealing with a compressive lesion of the chiasm which can cause central field defects that simulate cecocentral scotomas.[1,13–15] The "cecocentral dilemma" arises, therefore, when one must distinguish between cecocentral scotomas, central scotomas, and bitemporal hemianopic para-

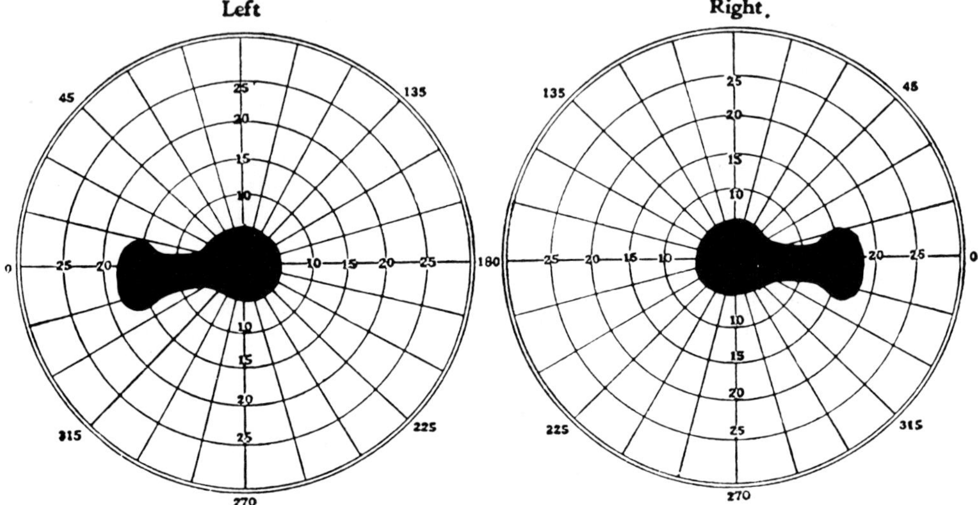

Fig. 3. Toxic amblyopia. (a) Bilateral temporal disc pallor and (b) cecocentral scotomas are diagnostic hallmarks.

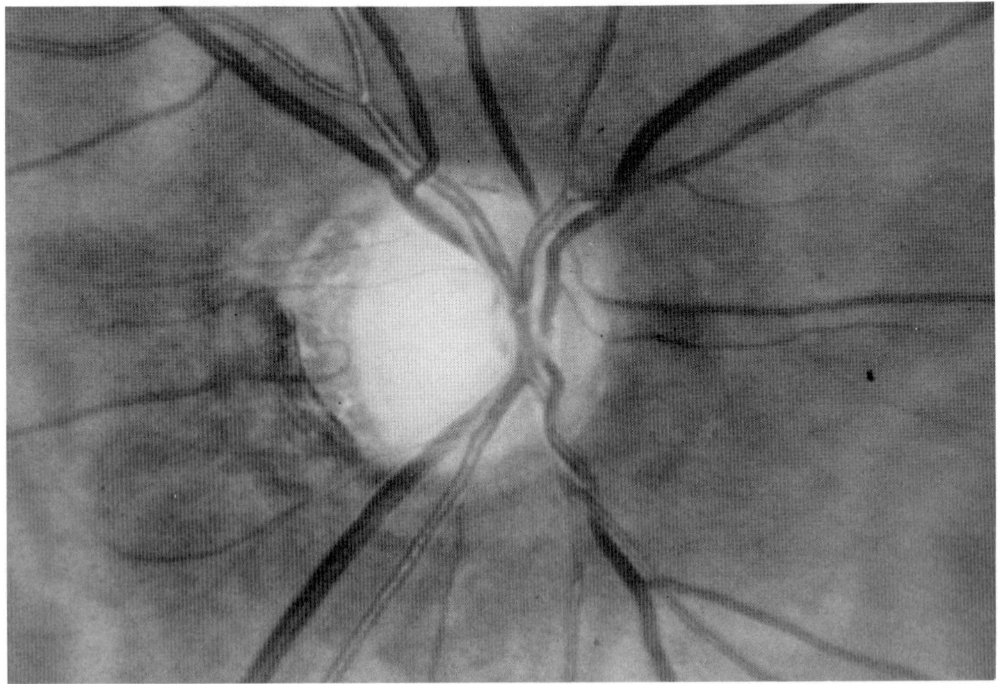

Fig. 3A

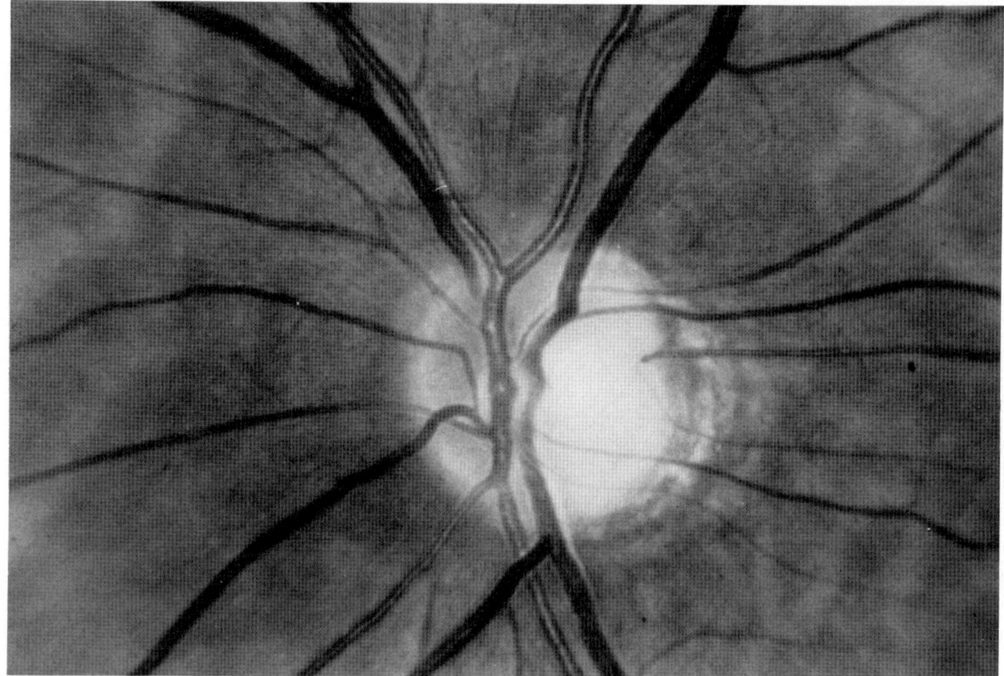

Fig. 3B

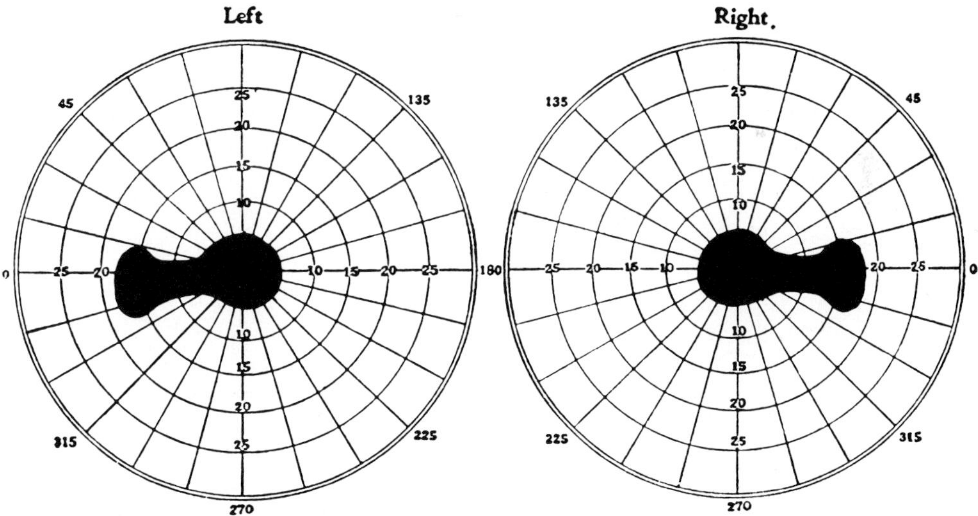

Fig. 4. Bilateral cecocentral scotomas.

central scotomas (Figs. 4–8). From a perimetric standpoint, this differentiation can be difficult but is obviously of critical importance. We have seen patients followed for what were thought to be bilateral cecocentral scotomas who, under more careful scrutiny, were found to have compressive lesions of the chiasm. On the other hand, 14 of the 65 patients with cecocentral scotomas in our series had workups through carotid angiography and pneumoencephalography. Two had negative exploratory craniotomies, and two others were advised to have cranial explorations, but they refused. Thus, a significant number of these patients were subjected to invasive neuro-

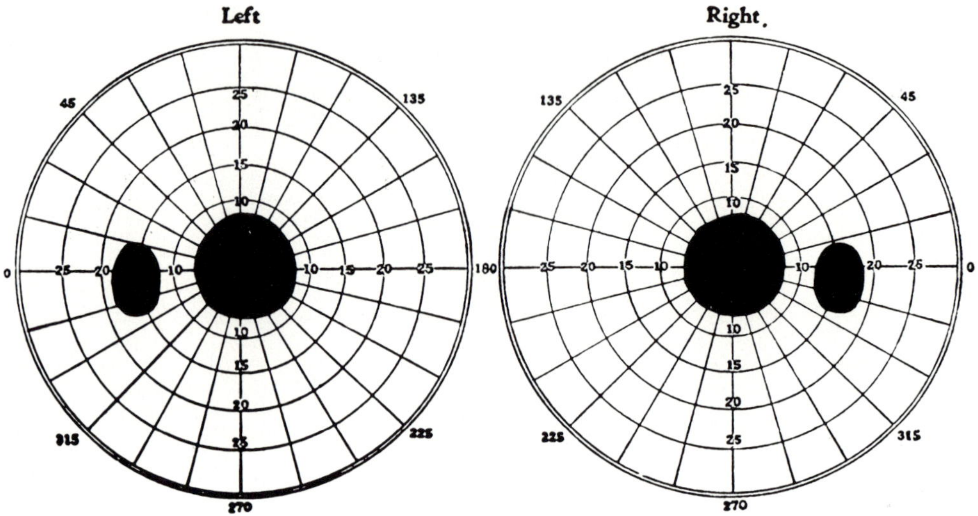

Fig. 5. Bilateral central scotomas.

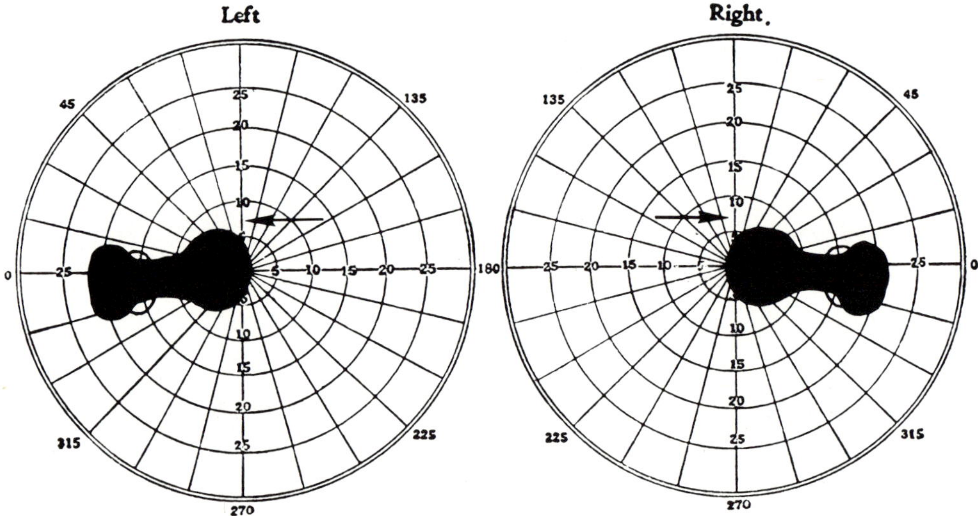

Fig. 6. Bilateral cecocentral scotomas with fixation shift.

logic procedures, which ideally might have been avoided.

We believe that cecocentral scotomas are best delineated on tangent screen testing. These scotomas are frequently ill-defined, and it can be hard to differentiate cecocentral scotomas from other central and hemianopic paracentral defects. As emphasized by Traquair,[1] a characteristic feature of many cecocentral scotomas is the presence of one or two areas of greater density or "nuclei" within the scotoma. A single nucleus may lie between fixation and the blind spot, or there may be two nuclei, one just temporal to fixation and the other at the nasal aspect of the blind spot. A subtle "waist" may connect these two nuclei, or the nuclei may merge to form a dense horizontal core connecting fixation and the blind spot (Fig. 9). Reduced intensity stimuli, such as red or small white formed targets or projector light targets, best define the scotomas.

It is important to assess the patient's fixation in these cases. We utilize one-half inch adhesive strips to make a 4 × 4 inch

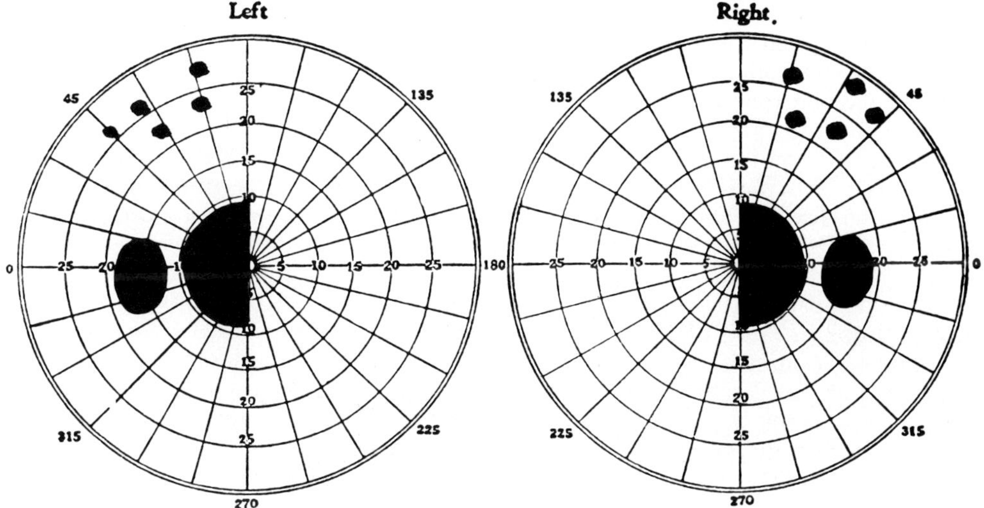

Fig. 7. Bitemporal hemianopic paracentral scotomas.

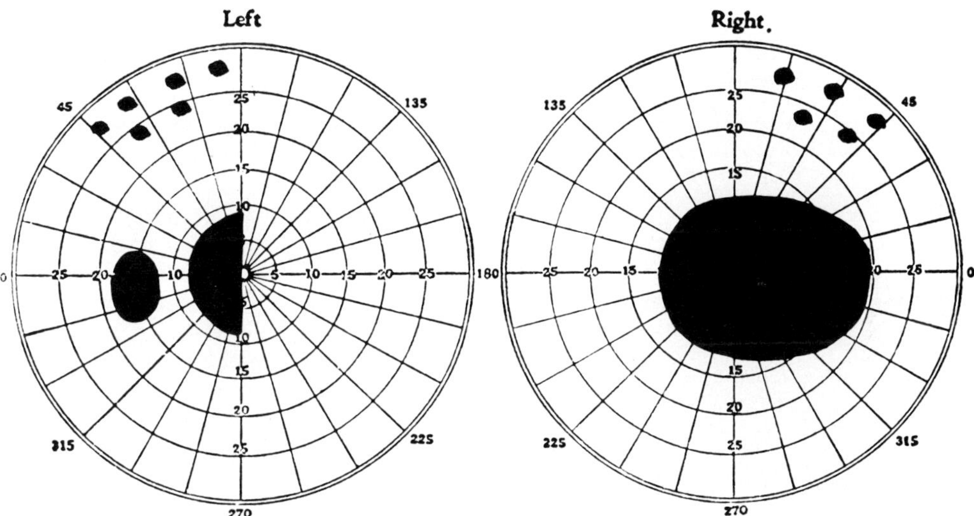

Fig. 8. Junction-like scotoma.

cross at fixation on the tangent screen. By simply having the patient view the center of the cross and report what he sees, valuable information about his fixation and scotoma is ascertained. Patients with a cecocentral scotoma and good fixation will frequently report that the temporal leg of the cross is blurred or absent. On the other hand, patients with significantly reduced vision due to a central field defect may see all four legs equally well, suggesting eccentric fixation. The critical area for testing in patients with suspected cecocentral scoto-mas is the "waist" located equidistant between fixation and the blind spot. With central scotomas, the target will consistently be seen in the waist, whereas with cecocentral defects it will not. In some cases the waist is very subtle and can only be detected with a reduced intensity projector light target. A perimeter is frequently unreliable for defining these defects. On the tangent screen, however, one can magnify the scotoma to establish its cecocentral nature.

Examination of only the central fields is

not sufficient in cecocentral scotoma cases. It is mandatory to also check the peripheral fields to exclude chiasmal lesions. We have found midzonal red targets on the Aimark perimeter helpful in this regard. Large red isopters on the perimeter are intact outside the central defects in patients with cecocentral scotomas. However, a midzonal temporal cut to red targets is suggestive of a chiasmal lesion. Important points for the perimetric diagnosis of cecocentral scotomas are outlined in Table III.

The optic disc changes associated with cecocentral scotomas can be extremely subtle. In our experience the Hruby lens has been indispensable in properly evaluating these cases. This has been particularly true in patients with mild optic atrophy, small vessel occlusions, and optic pits.

The history is paramount in establishing a cause for cecocentral scotomas. One

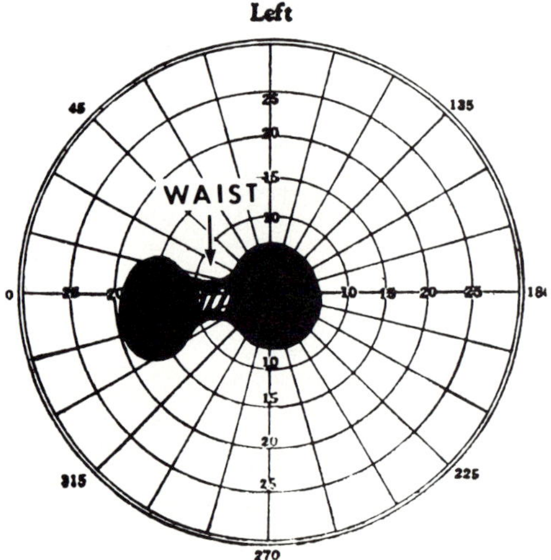

Fig. 9. Cecocentral scotoma. Note "waist" connecting blind spot and fixation area.

TABLE III. *Key points for perimetric diagnosis of cecocentral scotomas*

1. Scotomas are best demonstrated on tangent screen, often at distances >1 m
2. Good fixation by patient is mandatory
3. Peripheral fields, including midzonal red isopter, should be intact
4. Defect in "waist" between fixation and blind spot is essential for diagnosis
5. Scotomas may be extremely subtle and only detected with reduced intensity stimulus, such as projector light target.

should inquire specifically about tobacco and alcohol use and diet. In response to the question, "How is your diet?", many patients will state it is adequate. When asked specifically what they eat for each meal, however, they often describe a clearly suboptimal diet. Other important considerations include exposure to drugs or toxins, malabsorption states, the presence of other neurologic symptoms, and the family history. Attention to these historic details cannot be overemphasized.

How should patients with cecocentral scotomas be managed? Those with genetic optic atrophy and optic pits simply require recognition and periodic follow-up. Patients with optic pits should be monitored for increased intraocular pressure. Those with optic neuritis must be individualized, but sub-Tenon's steroid therapy is a consideration in selected cases. In patients with retinal vascular occlusion, attention should be directed towards potential sources of emboli. We routinely order a complete blood count on all patients with cecocentral scotomas, but any history suggestive of pernicious anemia should prompt a more thorough hematologic evaluation. We also obtain a fluorescent treponemal antibody absorption test on patients with cecocentral scotomas and treat them accordingly if the test is reactive. In cases of toxic amblyopia, we advise discontinuation of all alcohol and tobacco, maintenance of a proper diet, a daily multivitamin, and 1-cc intramuscular injections of hydroxocobalamine (Neo-Betalin 12, by Lilly) once a week for 10–20 weeks.

Finally, some patients have cecocentral scotomas due to intrinsic optic nerve disease, the etiology of which is obscure. We treat these patients empirically with the toxic amblyopia regimen outlined above and follow them. Fortunately, the visual prognosis in these and other cecocentral scotoma cases is generally good.

SUMMARY

Sixty-five cases of cecocentral scotomas seen in neuro-ophthalmologic consultation were reviewed. Optic neuritis was the major cause of unilateral cecocentral scotomas. Toxic (nutritional, tobacco-alcohol) amblyopia and genetic optic atrophy were the most common causes of bilateral cecocentral scotomas. The presence of cecocentral scotomas strongly indicates nonsurgical intrinsic optic nerve disease, and the visual prognosis in these cases is generally good. However, surgical lesions involving the chiasm can produce central field defects which mimic cecocentral scotomas, and such lesions should always be carefully excluded.

EDITOR'S NOTE

It is important to differentiate between a *central scotoma* and a *caecocentral scotoma*. The former may point to a hole in the macula, early macular degeneration, and the like—whereas a caecocentral scotoma means exactly what it says—the defect extends from the blind spot to the center of fixation. The word "caecum" means a "blind pouch" and hence "caeco-" means going from the blind spot of Mariotte to the appropriate suffix "central." You can actually differentiate a *caecocentral* scotoma from a *centrocaecal* scotoma in some cases. You may ask—what does that double talk mean? If you have a focal papillitis involving the papillomacular bundle, the defect will start at the disc and extend out towards fixation. Conversely, if you have a long standing macular lesion (for example, a late instance of toxoplasmic macular retinitis), there will be a dense central scotoma, and you can also plot out retrograde involvement of papillomacular bundle fibers on in to the disc. Obviously, if the central visual defect is *huge*, you can no longer tell whether it is central or caecocentral because it has now "eaten up" the disc, so that if you have a 30–40 degree central scotoma, it will now be difficult to tell how it began.

Dr. Shaw has emphasized the *"waist"* of the caecocentral scotoma in this paper. This merits even more emphasis. It may help you to have the patient fix on the wall entirely across your examining room and look at, for instance, a door knob or a light switch. Give them something large enough for them to find it—obviously! They will have to fix eccentrically if their central vision is down considerably, but you will find something there they can see. Then use a hand-held projector light (as a large Ednalite pointer used for lectures)—cover it a bit with your fingers to reduce intensity if needed— and throw a spot or two halfway between fixation and the large blind spot you'll find 10 feet away. If they miss in this area, you have hit "pay dirt" (perimetrically speaking). This means you have a caecocentral scotoma—not a purely central scotoma—and that is a large vote for medical optic nerve intrinsic disease, and a large vote against an intracranial neurosurgical situation. You may want to use a "history field" on these cases. This is simply extending the Amsler grid test all the way across the room—by confrontation and history. I stand before the patient about 5–6 feet away (with his left eye covered) and simply ask him to tell me what he now sees with the right eye. If he sees my glasses and my chin, but not my nose or mouth—this tells me he has a rather sharp central scotoma. If he sees my left ear but not my right, he may be telling me of a paracentral temporal hemianopic defect. If he sees my head but not my trunk, he has a lower altitudinal defect. If he seems my pants, but not my head, he has an upper altitudinal problem. One can often get the "crux" of the field problem by two to three questions at distance, and this will often be more accurate than what is plotted at ⅓ m. At any rate, caecocentral scotomas are not uncommon, and you must find them on the tangent screen or at greater distances, as you will simply be unable to differentiate central from caecocentral scotomas on any perimeter—for things are "smushed down" too small at ⅓ m! Remember, there are more than a few ways to skin a cat!

JLS

REFERENCES

1. Scott, G. I. *Traquair's Clinical Perimetry.* 7th ed. C. V. Mosby Co., St. Louis, 1957, pp. 153–167.
2. Bloom, S. M., Merz, E. H., and Taylor, W. W. Nutritional amblyopia in American prisoners of war liberated from the Japanese. Am. J. Ophthalmol. *29:*1248 (1946).
3. Victor, M., Mancall, E. L., and Dreyfus, P. M. Deficiency amblyopia in the alcoholic patient. Arch. Ophthalmol. *64:*1 (1960).

4. Harrington, D. O. Amblyopia due to tobacco, alcohol and nutritional deficiency. Am. J. Ophthalmol. *53:*967 (1962).

5. Victor, M. and Dreyfus, P. M. Tobacco-alcohol amblyopia. Arch. Ophthalmol. *74:*649 (1965).

6. Carroll, F. D. Nutritional amblyopia. Arch. Ophthalmol. *76:*406 (1966).

7. Chamlin, M. Visual field changes in optic neuritis. Arch. Ophthalmol. *50:*699 (1953).

8. Potts, A. M. Tobacco amblyopia. Surv. Ophthalmol. *17:*13 (1973).

9. Kjer, P. Infantile optic atrophy with dominant mode of inheritance: A clinical and genetic study of 19 Danish families. Acta Ophthalmol. [Suppl.] (Kbh.) 54, 1959.

10. Glaser, J. S. Heredofamilial disorders of the optic nerve. In: *Genetic and Metabolic Eye Disease.* M. F. Goldberg (Ed.), Little, Brown & Co., Boston, 1974, pp. 463–486.

11. Seeley, R. L. and Smith, J. L. Visual field defects in optic nerve hypoplasia. Am. J. Ophthalmol. *73:*882 (1972).

12. Carroll, F. D. and Forbes, M. Centrocaecal scotomas due to glaucoma. Trans. Am. Acad. Ophthalmol. Otolaryngol. *72:*643 (1968).

13. Adler, F. H., Austin, G., and Grant, F. C. Localizing value of visual fields in patients with early chiasmal lesions. Arch. Ophthalmol. *40:*579, 1948.

14. Rucker, C. W. and Kearns, T. P. Mistaken diagnoses in some cases of meningioma. Am. J. Ophthalmol. *51:*15 (1951).

15. Wendland, J. P. Some instructive manifestations of chiasmal disease. Arch. Ophthalmol. *54:*13 (1955).

17 The Swiss Cheese Visual Field or Time-varying Abnormalities of Vision after "Recovery" from Optic Neuritis

Carl Ellenberger, Jr., M.D.
Timothy Ziegler

Every consulting opthalmologist has, at some point in his career, been asked to interpret a "Swiss cheese" visual field*; he may even have been guilty of plotting one himself. Such a field is characterized by multiple, small, discrete scotomas, usually close to the point of fixation, that elusively change location with repeated examination. These defects almost always appear near the center of a visual field of an eye that has sustained past or recent visual loss. In our experience, the most common cause of the "Swiss cheese" visual field is demyelinating disease.

Zappia *et al.*,[1] identified this effect with the phenomenon described by Riddoch[2] in 10 patients with traumatic occipital lobe lesions. Several of Riddoch's patients could see moving, but not stationary, stimuli in their affected visual fields. Riddoch hypothesized that systems for detecting moving and stationary images were dissociated from one another in the occipital cortex. Zappia *et al.* noted that Riddoch did not confirm his hypothesis by testing patients with lesions elsewhere in the visual pathways, and described the same effect in patients with lesions affecting the optic tract and chiasm.

It is this tendency for a stationary or slowly moving stimulus to disappear that

traps that unwary or inexperienced perimetrist into plotting a Swiss cheese field. The perimetrist, encountering an area of uncertain detection, slows the test stimulus in order to more carefully define a possible scotoma. The stimulus disappears, only to reappear shortly after it begins to move again, thus further suggesting a defect.

The relatively common discovery of this effect in patients who have sustained evidence of demyelinating optic neuropathy suggested to us that this Riddoch-like phenomenon is another aspect of so-called "hidden visual loss" in patients with multiple sclerosis, perhaps related to delayed conduction detected by evoked potential testing, or to the reduced sensitivity to sine-wave gratings. Sunga and Enoch[3] devised tests to investigate this phenomenon. They found both abnormally rapid local adaptation and "short-term saturation or fatigue effect" in abnormal regions of the visual fields of patients with various lesions in the visual pathways. To study this phenomenon further, we selected 10 patients who had recovered normal visual acuity (in 12 eyes) after an acute attack of optic neuritis.

METHODS

Ten patients with multiple sclerosis, ages 18–53 (average 33), and histories of acute monocular visual loss ("optic neuritis")

* The term "Swiss cheese" visual field was coined by Enoch.

were studied after experiencing full recovery of visual acuity (20/25 or better). Among the patients, 12 eyes had sustained temporary visual loss (affected group) and eight had remained asymptomatic (unaffected group). Quantitative kinetic and static perimetry was normal in all patients except for slight reduction of central light sensitivity in three of the previously symptomatic eyes. These patients were compared to 10 normal subjects, ages 19–49 (average 28).

Short-Term Saturation or Fatigue Effect. A circular spot, 10 minutes of arc in diameter, 0.2 sec in duration, was flashed at a rate of two per second at the point of fixation. Background luminance for this and the following test was 10 apostilbs. The subject was instructed to signal when the flashing light disappeared. With each response, the experimenter recorded the luminance of the test target and increased it by 0.1 log units. Recording was continued for five minutes. The test was repeated with the stimulus appearing 5° temporally along the horizontal meridian.

Local Adaptation Test. Subjects and patients viewed constantly illuminated test stimuli (1000 apostilbs in luminance; 0.2° of arc in diameter) at each of seven locations along the horizontal meridian of the visual field from 6° nasally to 6° temporally. They were instructed to open the eye upon command and view a central fixation target. The time between eye opening and the disappearance of the test target was recorded.

RESULTS

Normal results for both tests are indicated in Figures 1 and 2. Note in Figure 1 that sensitivity of the normal group falls slightly during the first minute of the short term saturation test, but eventually stabilizes for both the central and 5° temporal targets. Note in Figure 2 that accuracy of the local adaptation test is diminished by the wide scatter of normal results, most likely resulting from varying stability of visual fixation.* Our values, however, are

---

* A perfectly stabilized retinal image disappears within several seconds.[4]

similar to the normal results of Bay.[5] The test stimulus disappeared at the fixation point before 30 sec (the limit of the test) in only two (of 20 normal eyes).

Short-Term Saturation or Fatigue Effect. Among the patients, three showed progressive reduction of sensitivity of the affected eye to the 5° stimulus. In two instances, patients B. L. and M. Y., sensitivity fell below the limits of testing. One unaffected eye, J. C. (right eye), showed the same decline in sensitivity.

Local Adaptation Test. Among the patients, the constant target disappeared sooner than any of the normals in three affected eyes (of three patients) and four unaffected eyes. The abnormality was present for a directly fixated target in all of these cases, and in addition, for a peripheral target in five of the seven eyes.

All three patients with abnormal short-term saturation had abnormal focal adaptation.

DISCUSSION

We have demonstrated that patients who have recovered normal visual acuity as well as visual fields after acute optic neuritis may nevertheless experience abnormally rapid disappearance of focal visual stimuli and fatiguing sensitivity to repetitively flashing focal stimuli. We detected abnormalities in the apparently normal, scotoma-free, portions of the visual fields. Sunga and Enoch[3] found similar abnormalities in the visual fields, but, in most cases, they projected test stimuli within the field defects.

These abnormalities may possibly be another aspect of so-called "hidden visual loss" in multiple sclerosis. They may underlie the Riddoch effect that may result from disease, particularly demyelinating lesions, seen anywhere along the course of the visual pathways, and may lead to the plotting of a "Swiss cheese" visual field by an inexperienced perimetrist. Swiss cheese field defects can be avoided by maintaining uniform motion of the test spot. Scotomas present only for stationary stimuli should not be plotted on a kinetic field exam; they are better displayed by static perimetry, or perhaps even better by other methods of assessing visual function. We suspect (but

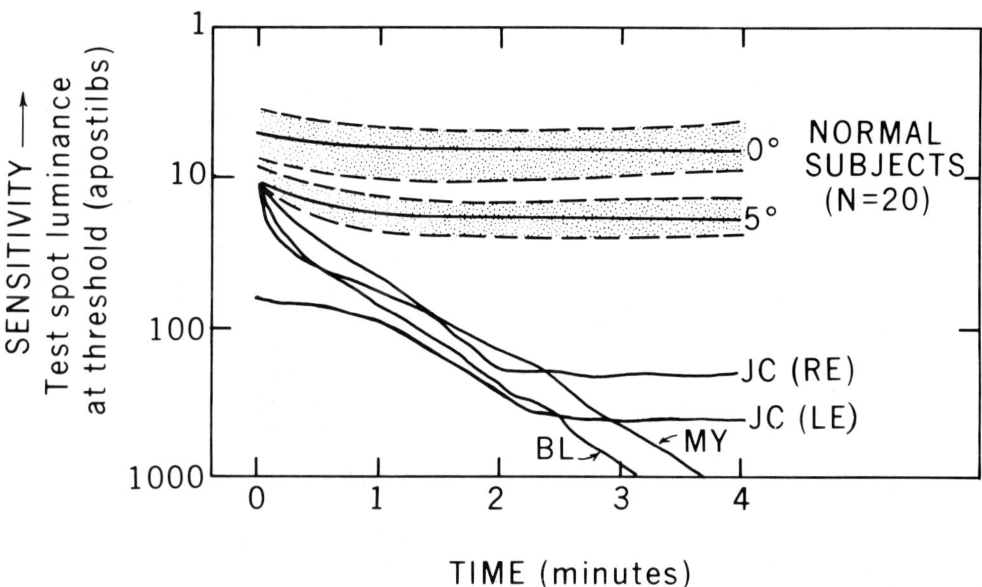

Fig. 1. Short-term saturation or fatigue effect in the group of normal subjects at fixation and 5° and in the four abnormal eyes. Stippled area indicates one standard deviation on either side of the normal mean. Note how sensitivity of the patients' vision to a repetitively flashing stimulus, 5° from the fixation point, progressively falls.

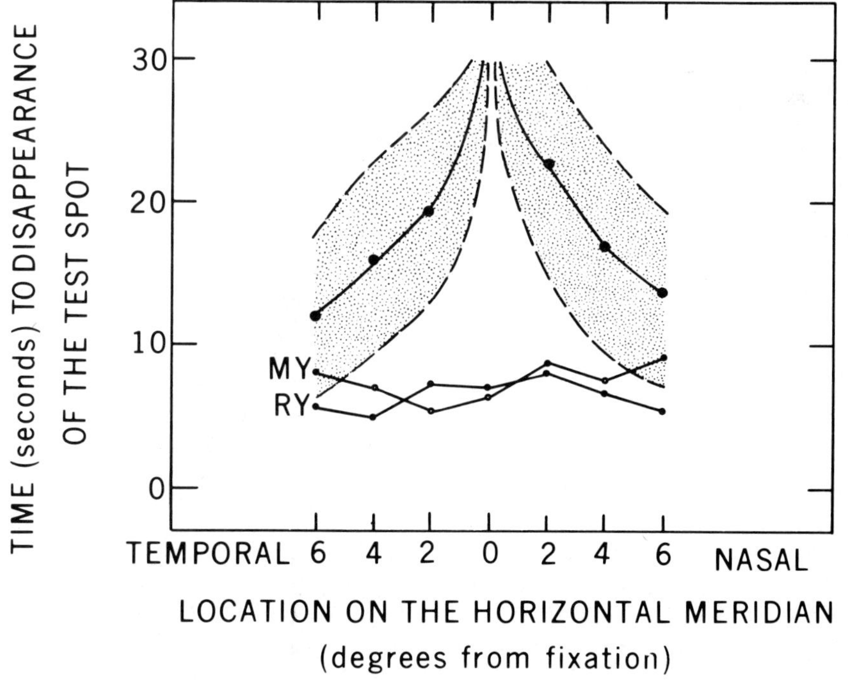

Fig. 2. Local adaptation times of the group of normal subjects and examples of two abnormal responses. Stippling indicates one standard deviation on either side of the mean.

did not systematically test our suspicion) that the presence of one "Swiss cheese" scotoma indicates that in such cases the Riddoch effect can be demonstrated throughout much or all of the central region of the same visual field.

Recently Enoch *et al.* studied the visual acuity of a patient with recovered optic neuritis using a laser interference technique. When fixation was precisely maintained, acuity fell from 20/25 to 20/800 in 2 min.[6] Enoch did not record the visual symptoms in the patient he studied, but observed that other patients with visual fatigue or saturation effect may be able to restore their vision by closing their eyes for 3–5 min and to maintain it by wearing tinted spectacles. We were not able to correlate visual symptoms in our patients with the presence of time-varying abnormalities.

EDITOR'S NOTE

Dr. Ellenberger has "grabbed the bear by the tail" (perimetrically speaking) in this paper. He is drawing attention to multiple, small scotomas—usually close to fixation—that elusively change location with repeated examination. Now that is really opening Pandora's box to many, many possibilities—including not only retinal adaptation time, the Riddoch phenomenon, but even more common things such as small shifts of fixation, which may be very difficult to spot, and functional visual field defects, as well. I'd simply like to comment about two of these briefly here.

Retinal adaptation in visual field testing. Dr. Norton first really drew my attention to this as a problem in tangent screen work about 14 years ago. The way it is usually encountered is as follows—you may do a confrontation or a peripheral field, or even a tangent screen exam, and find this quite normal. You then dilate the patient, look in with indirect, and lo and behold!—there is a pigmented lesion in that upper temporal equatorial region! Now as soon as you see this, you begin to wonder—is that a nevus or is that an early malignant melanoma? I wonder if there is a field defect corresponding to that lesion that I missed? Or even worse, is there a field defect that is larger than the gross appearance of the lesion itself, which might worry me even more? So, you then go back on the tangent screen, and use a 3- or 6-mm white target at 1 m and really "fish" that lower nasal quadrant (since you now know the mischief is in the upper temporal fundus). You look carefully—so, so carefully—that you begin to slow down the target in the area where you really suspect the field defect. *Voila!* The patient reports—"I missed it there!" or "It just dropped out!" What you may be simply doing is stopping the target just long enough for the patient's retina to adapt to it, and, the second you start it moving again, he perceives it. This is not a field defect at all, but simply retinal adaptation. The way to prove this to yourself, and this will "eat into your brain like a rat," is to look at the fixation target on your tangent screen—and hold it very, very tight. Now as you fixate on that target, hold a quarter about 15–20 degrees away very still, and you will find that the quarter will disappear within a very few seconds. No, I'm not talking about putting it in the blind spot of Mariotte— even a large target (as the tip of your finger) will disappear if you put it eccentrically in the field but do not move at all. This is why you must never completely stop the target in perimetry—but must keep it slowly moving a bit. This can be a definite artefact in kinetic perimetry.

The *Riddoch phenomenon* is, in my opinion, the real McCoy. Riddoch emphasized that certain patients with *occipital* field defects could perceive *motion* but not *form*. The first time I really saw this was in a tragic instance of a young house officer on Pathology at Duke Hospital in 1961 or 1962. He awoke one morning—noted a disturbance in his vision—and dropped by my office within two hours after noting it. I found his acuity to be 20/15 in both eyes without glasses, but as I did his peripheral fields on the Aimark perimeter with the largest possible target (10/330 white at brightest intensity), I found that he had a total right homonymous hemianopia—*if* the large target were moved ever so slowly in. However, if a much smaller target were moved a bit more rapidly, he immediately said—"I can see it when it moves!" This was not just moving a smaller target faster, but was a true distinct separation of the form sense and the motion sense. Unfortunately, this young man died within about six weeks of that day when his first symptom presented, and at autopsy had a left occipital metastasis from a highly undifferentiated malignant sarcoma of the bladder. I believe that one must go very slowly in attributing the Riddoch phenomenon to lesions other than occipital lobe problems. One of the reported cases of Riddoch phenomenon with anterior visual involvement had an arteriogram which showed the posterior cerebral filling off the internal carotid on that side (which happens in about 15–20% of persons) so that one could not exclude compromise of the posterior circulation from a large aneurysm anteriorly in that case.

What I am trying to say is simply this—perimetry is so poorly taught in many eye residencies now, that many ophthalmologists have just given up. They figure that if they have a $4,000 perimeter in a room, they're bound to get good fields. In fact, they might even think that if they have a $8,000 perimeter in their office, the fields might be twice as good. Now, they're even talking about $80,000 octopus field machines. The "history field," a good Amsler grid test, good confrontation, and proper knowledge of how to really do simple peripheral and central fields well will end a lot of the problems that now exist. I think

the test should be simple and rapid and that you do NOT need to send your patient for a 30-minute, 45-minute, 1-hour, or longer expensive test in nearly every instance. Dr. Ellenberger is drawing attention to two important "perimetric pearls," however—so I hope he continues looking into retinal adaptation and the Riddoch phenomenon. I'd personally go slow into blaming these central field defects that are elusive as a sign of demyelination, however—as yet.

JLS

REFERENCES

1. Zappia, R. J., Enoch, J. M., Stamper, R., *et al.* The Riddoch phenomenon revealed in non-occipital lobe lesions. Br. J. Ophthalmol. *55*:416–420 (1971).
2. Riddoch, G. Dissociation of visual perceptions due to occipital injuries, with especial reference to appreciation of movement. Brain *40*:15–57 (1917).
3. Sunga, R. N. and Enoch, J. M. Further perimetric analysis of patients with lesions of the visual pathways. Am. J. Ophthalmol. *70*:403–422 (1970).
4. Barlow, H. B. Slippage of contact lenses and other artifacts in relation to fading and regeneration of supposedly stable retinal images. Q. J. Exp. Psychol. *15*:36–51 (1963).
5. Bay, E. Disturbances of visual perception and their examination. Brain *76*:515–550 (1953).
6. Enoch, J. M., Campos, E. C., and Bedell, H. E. Visual resolution in a patient exhibiting a visual fatigue or saturation effect. Arch. Ophthalmol. *97*:76–78 (1979).

18 Carotid-Ophthalmic Artery Aneurysm Presenting as Unilateral Disc Edema With Choroidal Folds

Robert L. Tomsak, M.D., Ph.D.
John A. Costin, M.D.
and Maurice Hanson, M.D.

INTRODUCTION

Carotid-ophthalmic artery aneurysms are rare, representing 1.3–8.0% of all intracranial aneurysms.[1,2] Because of the close proximity to optic nerve, chiasm, and cavernous sinus, visual involvement is present in about one-third of cases and can present a difficult diagnostic dilemma for the ophthalmologist.[1] Unfortunately, when visual involvement occurs, the diagnosis is often missed, leading to irreversible optic atrophy, visual field defects, and even death from subarachnoid hemorrhage.[1-3]

The following case exemplifies a perplexing ophthalmic presentation of this unusual lesion:

Case report. A 60-year-old right-handed housewife presented with the chief complaint of blurred vision in the left eye. One month prior she noted the onset of mild left supraorbital discomfort, blurred vision in the left eye, and pain on movement. She had no history of hypertension, diabetes mellitus, thyroid disease, or trauma, and was on no medication.

Ophthalmic exam revealed a best corrected visual acuity of 20/20 in the right eye and 20/25 in the left eye. A 2+ afferent pupillary defect was noted in the left eye. External and slit lamp examination was unremarkable, and facial sensation was normal. Extraocular movements were full, but the patient experienced mild discomfort in the left eye on extremes of lateral gaze. Examination of the left fundus revealed a choked disc with focal peripapillary exudates and choroidal folds (Figs. 1 and 2). Spontaneous venous pulsations were absent. The right optic disc was flat and pink with prominent spontaneous venous pulsations (Fig. 3). Goldmann visual fields were normal in the right eye. However, an inferotemporal defect and an enlarged blind spot were noted in the left eye.

Initially, a diagnosis of papillitis was entertained. However, the patient's age, the visual field defect, and the presence of choroidal folds left enough doubt to warrant further evaluation. She was admitted to the hospital where a complete neurologic examination was entirely normal. The sedimentation rate, FTA-ABS, glucose tolerance test and antinuclear factor were within normal limits. Plain films of skull, sinuses, and optic canals were unremarkable. Computerized tomography of the orbits was normal, but an abnormality was noted near the left anterior clinoid after Conray injection (Fig. 4). Polytomography disclosed erosion of the inferior aspect of the left anterior clinoid.

A selective left internal carotid angiogram was done by the femoral approach (Fig. 5). This disclosed a 4 × 4 × 4 mm aneurysm at the ophthalmic-carotid artery junction. The patient underwent a left temporal-frontal craniotomy on June 6, 1978.

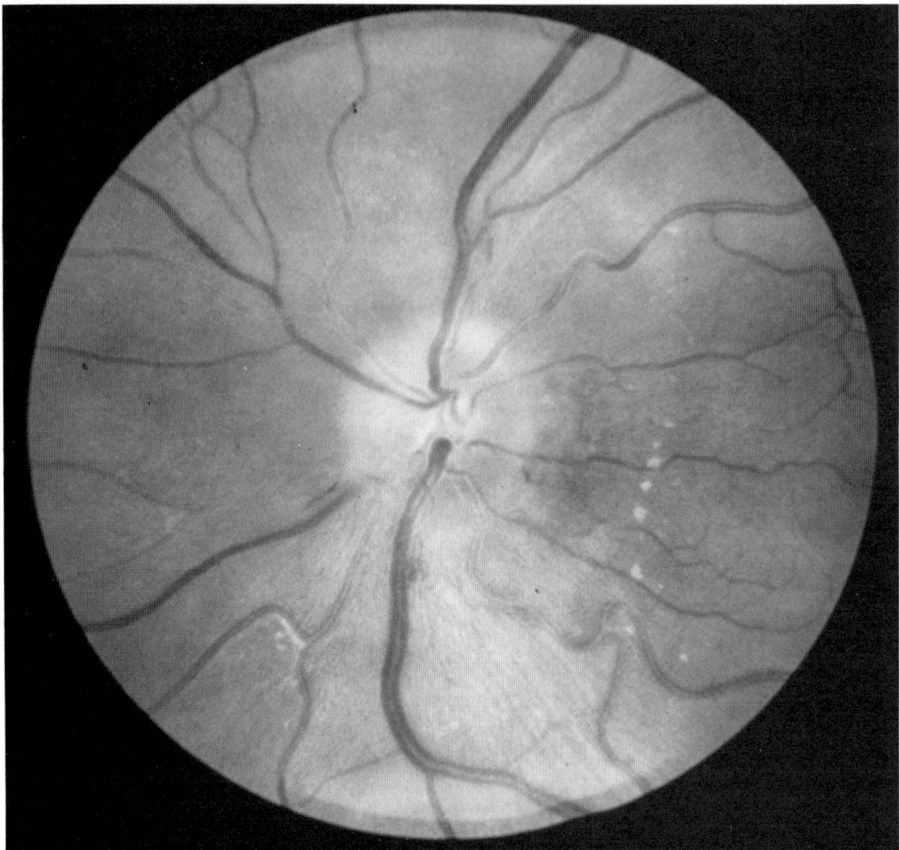

Fig. 1. Choked disc with peripapillary exudates.

The aneurysm was located in the left ophthalmic artery at the junction of the internal carotid. Arising inferotemporal to the left optic nerve, it compressed the nerve superio-medially against the intracranial optic canal (Fig. 6).

Optic disc edema began to resolve by 48 hours after aneurysm clipping. One month later the left disc was flat with good spontaneous venous pulsations and no choroidal folds were seen. A repeat visual field showed improvement and her vision returned to 20/20 in the left eye.

DISCUSSION

Carotid-ophthalmic artery aneurysms are unique in several respects. Females are predominantly affected (50–85%) and the aneurysms are mainly left sided (64–81%) as seen in our patient.[1] Other intracranial aneurysms are found in 21–64% of cases, and symptoms usually present between the ages of 36 and 55 years in 75% of patients.

These aneurysms most often arise from the anteromedian wall of the internal carotid artery just above the junction of the ophthalmic artery, hence the name carotid-ophthalmic artery aneurysms.[4,5] Two general types of this lesion are seen: a laterochiasmal type which bulges forward and up against the lateral margin of the optic nerve as seen in our case, and a subopticochiasmal type which directs itself medially and under the chiasm.[5] Aneurysms of the orbital ophthalmic artery have also been described, but are extremely rare.[6,7]

Several other features of this case warrant specific attention: (1) unilateral disc edema with choroidal folds; (2) afferent pupillary defect with visual loss; and (3) pain on eye movement.

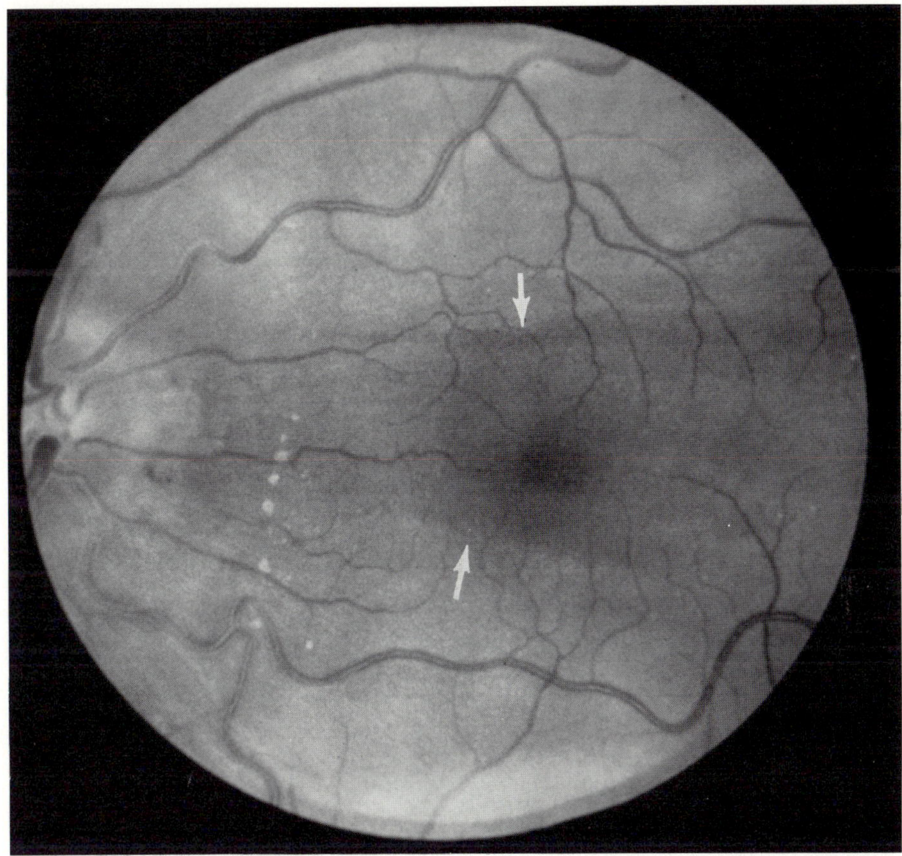

Fig. 2. Choroidal folds (arrows).

Unilateral Disc Edema and Choroidal Folds. The presence of unilateral disc edema resulting from an intracranial lesion is unusual. One other report[8] described unilateral disc swelling and diminished visual acuity in a 44-year-old man who had a saccular aneurysm of the intracranial ophthalmic artery which partially eroded into the posterior optic canal. As in our case, the disc swelling abated, and vision improved after clipping of the aneurysm.

The choroidal folds in our patient was a confusing finding that strongly suggested an orbital mass. In Newell's review of 16 cases choroidal folds were due to orbital tumor in 50%.[9] The remaining cases were due to various causes such as thyroid disease, hypotony, hyperopia, uveitis, and disciform macular disease, with only one case associated with optic disc edema of undetermined etiology.[9]

The exact mechanism for the development of our patient's choked disc and choroidal folds is unclear, but probably resulted from aneurysmal compression of the optic nerve and interference with axoplasmic transport.[10] This suggestion is strengthened by the observation that the disc swelling and choroidal folds began to resolve within 48 hours after aneurysm surgery.

Afferent Pupillary Defect with Decreased Vision. Visual symptoms are present in 7–50% of patients with carotid ophthalmic aneurysms.[1] By far the most common visual presentation is unilateral decreased vision with optic atrophy and peripheral field abnormalities due to chronic compression of the optic nerve.

Subtle visual loss, pain on eye movement, a swollen disc and an afferent pupillary defect were findings which initially suggested the diagnosis of optic neuritis in our

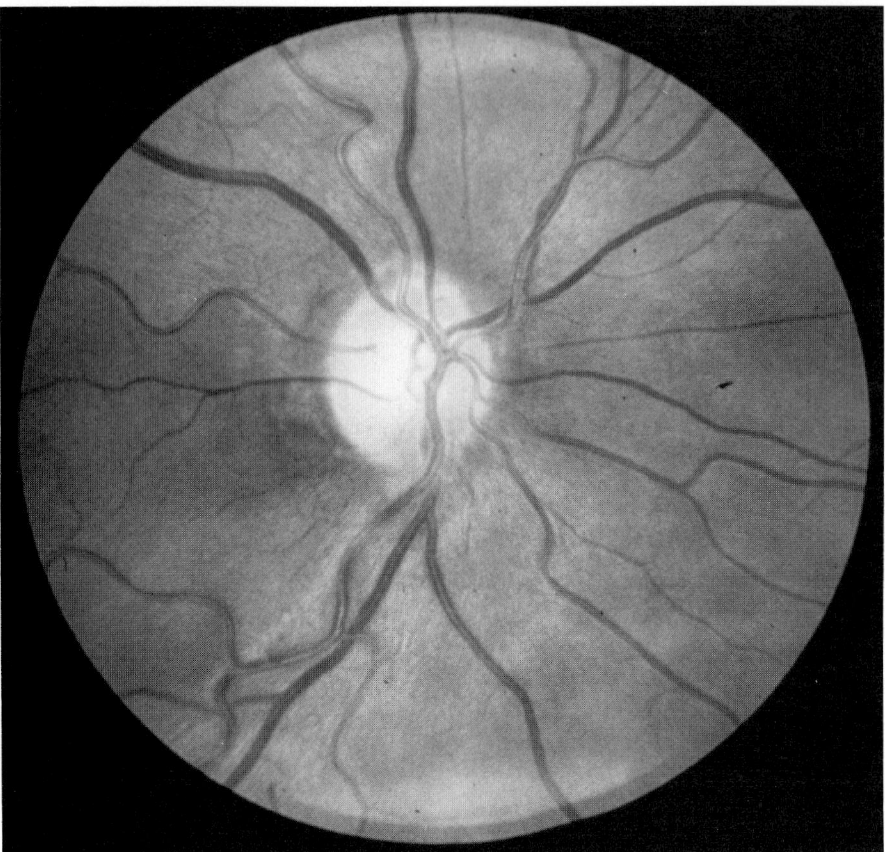

Fig. 3. Normal right disc.

patient, and are an unusual presentation of an intracranial ophthalmic artery aneurysm. Other rare findings are orbital discomfort, sudden visual loss, and bitemporal hemianopia.[2-4]

Pain on Eye Movement. One of the most perplexing findings associated with carotid-ophthalmic artery aneurysms is pain on eye movement. It has been speculated that blood in the optic nerve sheath was responsible in one case[3] with associated subarachnoid hemorrhage. However, the cause for this discomfort in our patient is unknown.

It is important to emphasize that the diagnosis of these lesions is made by selective internal carotid angiography. Oblique views and subtraction techniques are often needed to define the origin and direction of the aneurysm. Because carotid-ophthalmic aneurysms are frequently associated with other intracranial aneurysms,[1] multiple vessel angiography may be warranted as well.

SUMMARY

Carotid-ophthalmic artery aneurysms are comparatively rare but may affect the visual system. The most common visual presentation is progressive unilateral optic atrophy which may erroneously lead to the diagnosis of "chronic optic neuritis" in late cases. Our patient presented a disturbing diagnostic dilemma with unilateral choked disc and choroidal folds, suggesting the presence of an orbital mass. Other findings mimicked optic neuritis. We suggest that unilateral disc edema in association with mild visual loss, pain on eye movement, an afferent pupillary defect or even choroidal folds may be an early presentation of carotid-ophthalmic aneurysm.

The surgical management of these aneu-

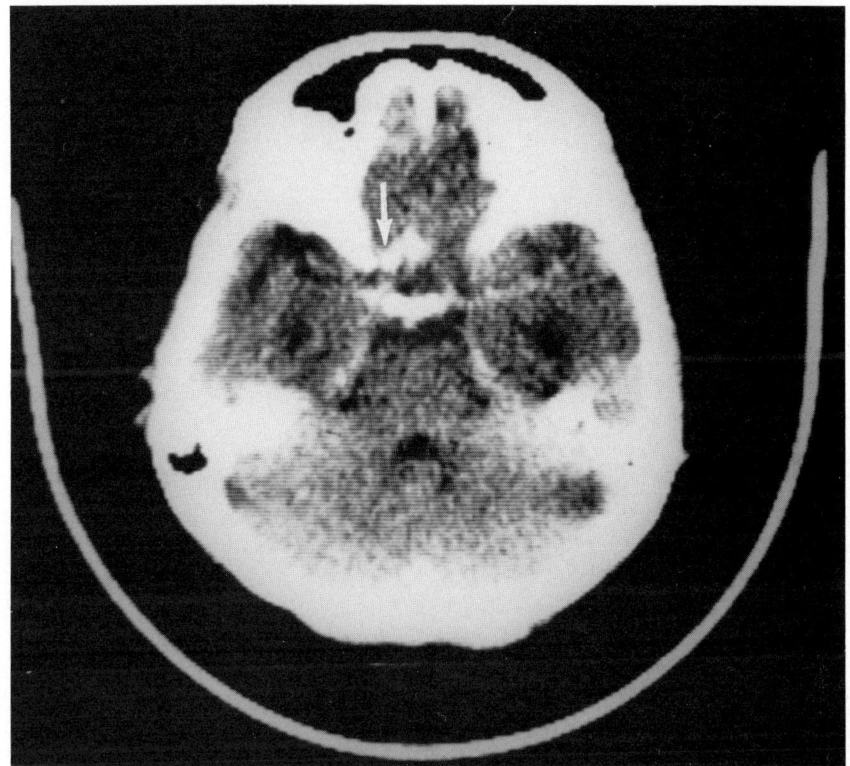

Fig. 4. Computerized tomography showing density near left anterior clinoid after enhancement (arrow).

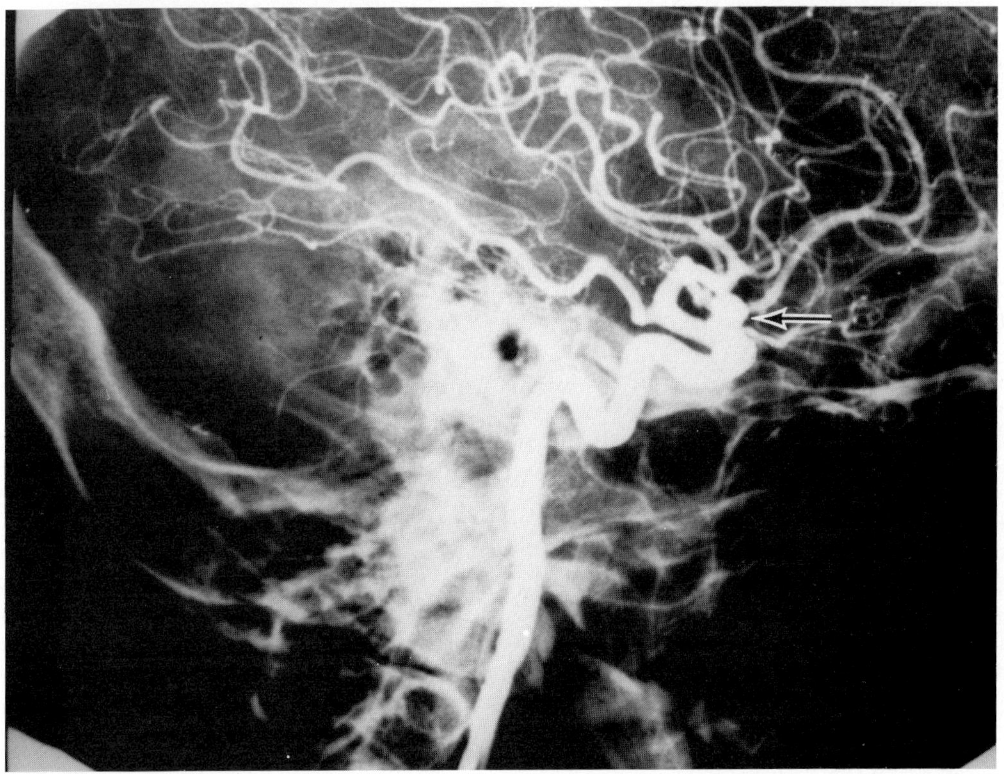

Fig. 5. Left selective internal carotid angiogram showing aneurysm at carotid-ophthalmic artery junction (arrow).

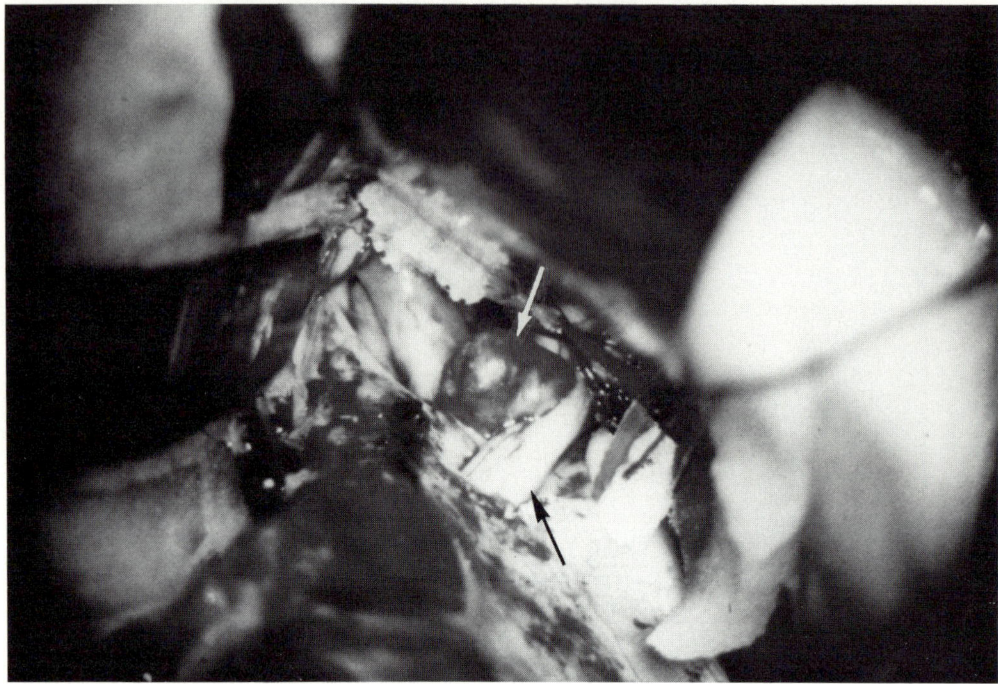

Fig. 6. Carotid-ophthalmic artery aneurysm (white arrow) arising infero-temporal to left optic nerve (black arrow).

rysms has been debated. Some neurosurgeons advocate cervical carotid ligation, whereas others prefer a direct surgical approach as used in our patient.[1, 2, 4, 5, 11] Early diagnosis of these lesions is urged, since either method of surgery may be more beneficial for the patient than no treatment at all.[1, 3, 4]

EDITOR'S NOTE

The patient here reported is one of those cases of optic nerve disease that comes along to keep you honest. We all seem to see some of those "head-scratching" instances which help us to humbly admit that there is still plenty we do not understand. Note that a patient presented with a unilateral choked disc with 20/25 acuity and after clipping an ophthalmic artery aneurysm on that side the disc returned to perfectly normal.

A case with a related optic nerve problem, although due to an entirely different cause, is worth mentioning at this point. A 29-year-old woman was seen through the courtesy of Dr. J. H. Rigsby on June 13, 1978 complaining of blurred vision in the left eye. She had noted the onset of classic transient obscurations of vision in her left eye one year earlier, which has progressed inexorably. The left optic disc was found to be swollen in April 1978. Skull films, optic canal views, and a computed tomographic scan were made, and the left optic nerve was considered to be slightly enlarged.

Examination in Miami revealed a corrected vision of 20/15 in the right eye and 20/20+2 in the left eye. No Marcus Gunn pupil was seen on the left, and this was specifically looked for. The fields revealed only a very large blind spot in the left eye. The right disc was normal and the left disc appeared chronically choked. A lateral orbital exploration was performed June 14, 1978, and this revealed a normal optic nerve sheath. A small portion of the sheath was removed and found to be normal. The patient continued to have transient obscurations after only a short respite. Further study of optic canal tomograms revealed a suspicious change in the intracranial end of the left optic canal. The patient was explored via a left frontal craniotomy on August 10, 1978 by Dr. Yates. A very small tumor was seen at the posterior aspect of the left optic canal. This was removed, and histologically was a meningioma. The patient has subsequently improved and a post-operative acuity was found to have improved from 20/60 to 20/30 in the involved eye. This is an important case for there is good evidence that the unilateral choked disc in this case was due to an intracranial involvement of the optic nerve due to a small meningioma, just as a unilateral choked disc was due in the case of Dr. Tomsak and associates to an ophthalmic artery aneurysm. I started to put all of the pictures of the optic nerve meningioma case in here, but believe that case should probably be the subject of a more complete report, and so will simply cite it here to go along with the ophthalmic artery aneurysm case. The moral of the story is that some of the old-timers described unilateral papilledema due to intracranial causes, and we suspected some orbital process was also going on, but there are a few of those cases around. Whether this is axoplasmic flow restriction or not, I do not know—but I do know that such cases CAN exist, although they are rare.

JLS

REFERENCES

1. Sengupta, R. P., Gryspeerdt, G. L., and Hankinson, J. Carotid-ophthalmic aneurysms. J. Neurol. Neurosurg. Pschychiatry *39:*837 (1976).
2. Yasargil, M. G., Glasser, J. C., Hodosh, R. M., and Rankin, T. V. Carotid-ophthalmic aneurysms: Direct microsurgical approach. Surg. Neurol. *8:*155 (1977).
3. Stern, W. H. and Ernst, J. T. Intracranial ophthalmic artery aneurysm. Am. J. Ophthalmol. *80:*203 (1975).
4. Guidetti, B. and La Torre, E. Management of carotid-ophthalmic aneurysms. J. Neurosurg. *42:* 438 (1975).
5. Benedetti, A. and Curri, D. Direct attack on carotid ophthalmic and large internal carotid aneurysms. Surg. Neurol. *8:*49 (1977).
6. Pfingst, A. O. Anomalous ophthalmic artery with ocular symptoms. Arch. Ophthalmol. *16:*829 (1936).
7. Danziger, J. and Bloch, S. An intra-orbital aneurysm of the ophthalmic artery. South Afr. Med. J. *48:*2569 (1974).
8. Jain, K. K. Saccular aneurysm of the ophthalmic artery. Am. J. Ophthalmol. *69:*997 (1970).
9. Newell, F. W. Choroidal folds. Am. J. Ophthalmol. *75:*930 (1973).
10. Hayreh, S. S. Fluids in the anterior part of the optic nerve in health and disease. Surv. Ophthalmol. *23:*1 (1978).
11. Almeida, G. M., Shibata, M. K., and Bianco, E. Carotid ophthalmic aneurysms. Surg. Neurol. *5:*41 (1976).

19 Current Approaches to the Diagnosis and Management of Ocular Melanomas

C. C. Barr, M.D.

Recent advances in both diagnosis and management of intraocular melanomas have caused some controversy within the ophthalmic community. In this chapter, the more modern aspects of the diagnosis and treatment of uveal melanomas will be discussed. I will not attempt to review all the recent literature on this vast subject, nor will I review the pathology of this disease, but I will try to present some of the newer ideas and modalities that have present and future clinical applications.

Duke-Elder[1] reports the incidence of ocular melanomas to be two to six per 10,000 patients seen in an eye clinic, and a recent study at the Mayo Clinic indicated that incidence of ocular melanomas in the general population is only 1.3 per 100,000 individuals.[2] Nonetheless, the detection of melanomas is not an uncommon event in clinical practice, and the average ophthalmologist should be familiar with the diagnosis and management of these tumors.

There are many intraocular lesions that may simulate melanomas. Hemangiomas, metastatic carcinoma, hemorrhagic and nonhemorrhagic choroidal and retinal detachments, and numerous other diseases have all been confused with malignant melanomas. In the past, intraocular tumors were often diagnosed with the direct ophthalmoscope alone, and errors were frequent. Earlier reports from the Armed Forces Institute of Pathology[3, 4] indicated that the over-all diagnostic error in eyes with clear media, and enucleated with a clinical diagnosis of malignant melanoma of the choroid, was approximately 20%. In analyzing these results, Shields[5] came to the conclusion that many of the eyes removed with an incorrect diagnosis had not been fully evaluated with the more currently available modalities, including indirect ophthalmoscopy. More recent workers, however,[6, 7] have reported a more acceptable rate of 4–6% in patients examined at clinical referral centers.

There are probably several reasons for this increased diagnostic accuracy. Among them are some basic principles that deserve reiteration, although they are by no means "new." A good history, for example, should be obtained on all patients suspected of harboring intraocular malignancies.[5] A history of trauma or recent surgery should suggest a retinal or choroidal detachment. A history of mastectomy or other cancer surgery will raise the possibility of metastatic disease.

Similarly, all patients with fundus lesions that are suspected of being malignant should have a careful medical evaluation, including a complete physical examination. Emphasis should be placed on detecting the presence of metastatic disease, for both extraocular cancers that may have metastasized to the eye, as well as for evidence of metastases from a melanoma itself. Subcutaneous nodules should be sought, as they are often the first sign of extraocular extension. Because a patient with metastatic melanoma has a life expectancy of less than one year, Char[8] has suggested that patients suspected of harboring metastatic melanomas have screening laboratory tests before any therapeutic measures are undertaken. These include a routine chest x-ray and liver function tests (alkaline phosphatase and serum lactic dehydrogenase); if these are abnormal, further examinations such as liver-spleen scan should be performed. If a systemic malignancy is suspected, carcinoembryonic antigen (CEA) assay may be helpful.[8]

It goes without saying that all patients should have a complete eye examination with emphasis on the opposite eye. Choroidal melanomas are almost always unilateral, and the presence of lesions in the opposite eye may greatly aid in the diagnosis. Moreover, the status of the opposite eye has important therapeutic implications.

Of all the most recent diagnostic modalities that have gained attention, perhaps foremost is the indirect ophthalmoscope, which has now come into widespread use. Gass[9] has listed certain ophthalmoscopic features of melanomas that may help the clinician to distinguish these tumors from nevi and other lesions. Melanomas characteristically present as a pigmented choroidal mass lesion that may be covered with a superficial orange pigment and surrounded by subretinal fluid (Fig. 1). A "collar-but-

ton" configuration (produced by the tumor mass breaking Bruch's membrane) is almost pathognomonic (Fig. 2). In contrast to this, metastatic tumors are almost always located in the posterior pole, and are frequently multiple. They are usually amelanotic masses that are covered with a mottled pattern of disrupted retinal pigment epithelial cells (Fig. 3). Choroidal hemangiomas are usually dome-shaped and pinkish to red in color.

It may be especially difficult, if not impossible, to differentiate small malignant melanomas from benign choroidal nevi. There are, however, certain features which may indicate a lesion's proclivity for growth, and, thus, its malignant potential. Although the shape and pattern of pigmentation may not be helpful in distinguishing melanomas from nevi, the presence of drusen scattered over the tumor surface, localized areas of depigmentation of the retinal pigment epithelium adjacent to the tumor, and choroidal neovascularization indicate that the lesion is growing very slowly, if at all (Fig. 4). Serous retinal detachment and

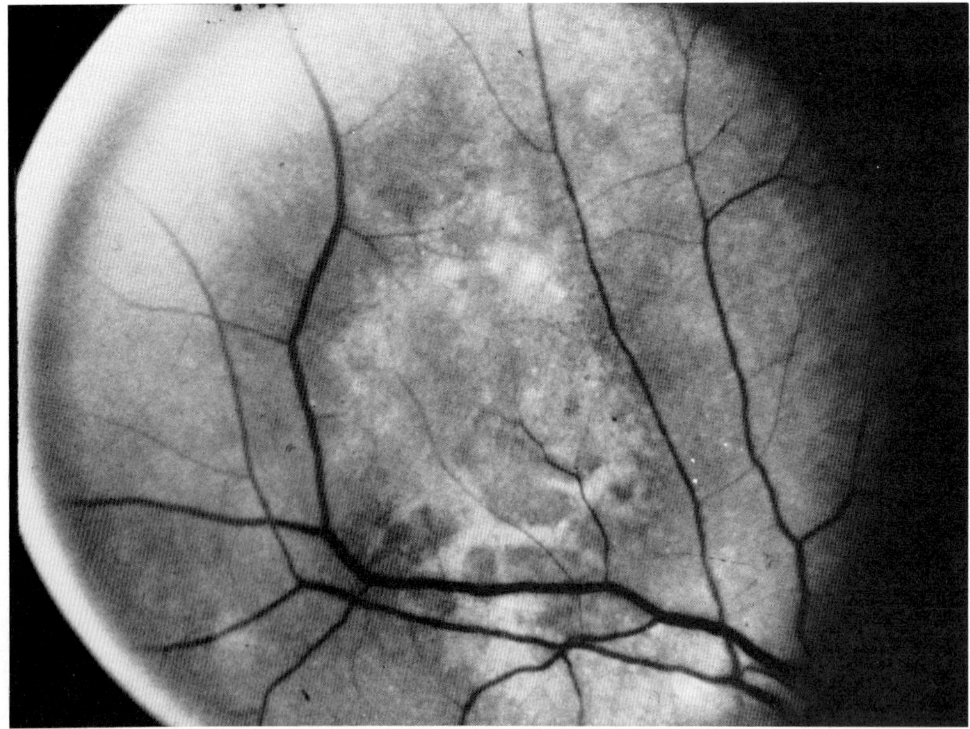

Fig. 1. Typical choroidal melanoma with characteristic orange pigment on tumor surface.

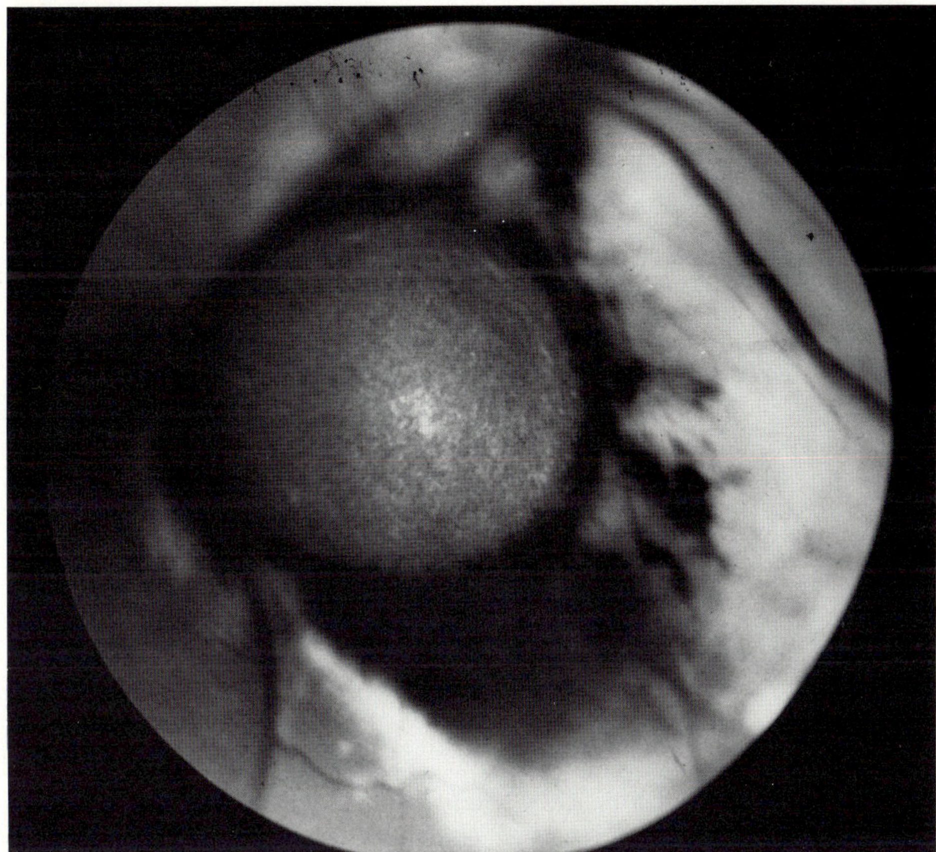

Fig. 2. Choroidal melanoma, "collar-button" configuration. The darker part of the tumor has broken through Bruch's membrane.

the presence of orange pigment over the surface of pigmented lesions, on the other hand, may indicate a more recent decompensation of the overlying retinal pigment epithelium, and should alert the clinician to the possibility of tumor growth. It should be noted, however, that the signs listed above are not always reliable in predicting the future enlargement of a neoplasm, and may be observed in benign lesions.[9, 10] Although the clinician may predict with reasonable accuracy which small tumors will grow, the differentiation between small malignant lesions and small nonmalignant lesions is not always straightforward, and a period of observation to determine growth is often warranted. Slit-lamp biomicroscopy, Hruby lens examination, and three-mirror contact lens examinations may be very helpful in certain cases, and are a useful adjunct to indirect ophthalmoscopy.

Transillumination is a simple technique that helps to differentiate melanomas that are partly pigmented from other nonpigmented lesions, such as serous pigment epithelial and retinal detachments, choroidal and ciliary body detachments, metastatic carcinomas, and disciform scars. There are several ways of performing transillumination both with direct illumination and with the indirect ophthalmoscope. This technique will enable the clinician to differentiate pigmented choroidal melanomas from other partly pigmented tumors or hemorrhages.

Fundus photography may enable the clinician to evaluate some fundus lesions more thoroughly, and serial photographs are helpful in following lesions to determine if growth has occurred. Fluorescein angiography may also be helpful in diagnosis of intraocular tumors. Serous and hemor-

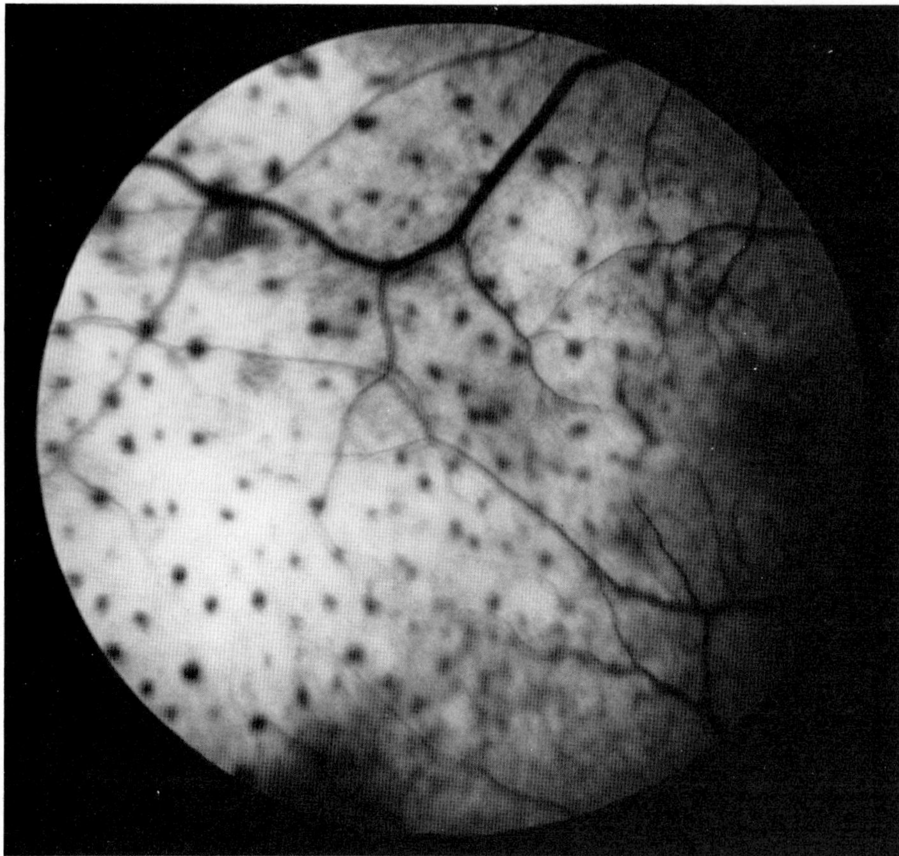

Fig. 3. Breast carcinoma metastatic to the choroid. Disrupted retinal pigment epithelial cells result in mottled pattern over tumor surface.

rhagic detachments of the pigment epithelium may be easily differentiated from other fundus lesions by this method. Choroidal melanomas characteristically show mottled fluorescence in the arteriovenous phase, and increased vascular permeability results in late staining of the tumor. Although often quite helpful in evaluating large fundus lesions, this test is of limited usefulness in distinguishing small choroidal melanomas from benign nevi, for both may have identical angiographic patterns. The angiogram may be more helpful in determining which of these lesions have growth potential. Evidence of widespread destruction of the retinal pigment epithelium favors growth of the tumor; drusen, choroidal neovascularization, and cystic changes in the retina indicate chronicity.

Ultrasonography has now come into widespread use in ophthalmology. It is particularly helpful in evaluating eyes with opaque media, but it may provide invaluable information in other cases as well. There are two basic forms of ultrasound: a linear time amplitude echo, or A-scan, and B-scan, which provides a two-dimensional cross section of the globe. Both A- and B-scan have relatively characteristic patterns for choroidal melanomas. On A-scan, there is a high leading echo that is reflected from the surface of the tumor, with a steep decay of following echoes (Fig. 5A). B-scan may demonstrate not only the contour and location of the tumor, but other characteristics, such as choroidal excavation and acoustic shadowing of retro-ocular structures (Fig. 5B).[11, 12] A- and B-scan patterns result from the relatively dense, homogenous cellular structure of choroidal melanomas. Unfortunately, ultrasonography is of limited usefulness in tumors less than 3

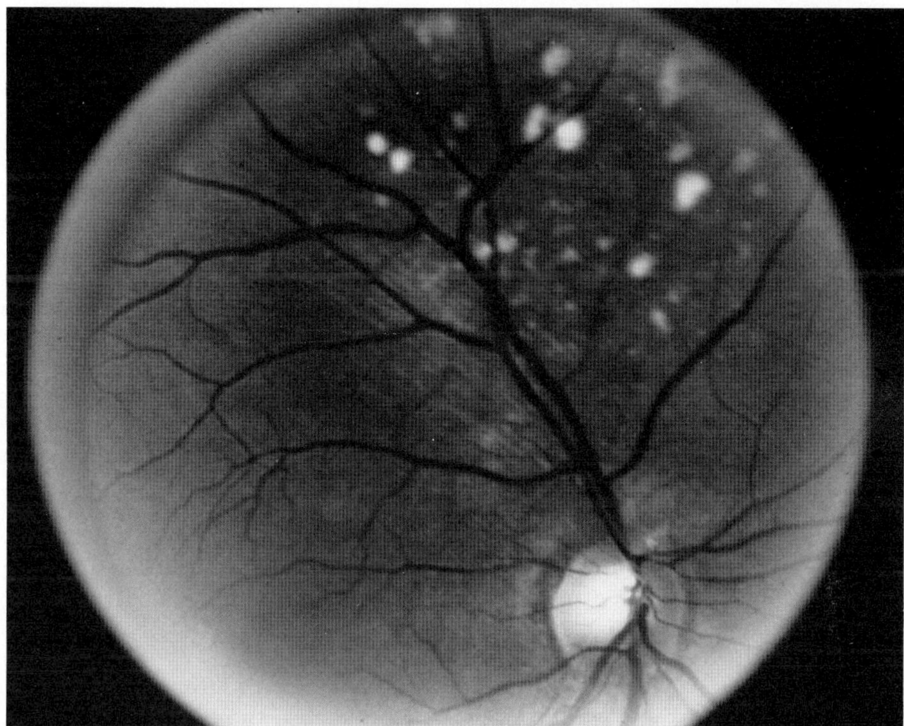

Fig. 4. Choroidal nevus with minimal elevation and multiple drusen.

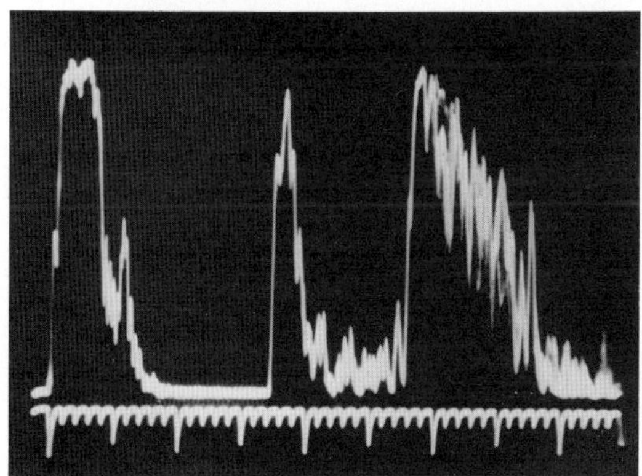

Fig. 5A. A-scan ultrasonogram of choroidal melanoma. Initial high spike indicates retinal surface; the low amplitude echoes that follow are characteristic.

mm in height, and it may be difficult to distinguish melanomas from other tumors with a uniform cellularity, such as metastatic carcinoma. Nonetheless, it is an almost totally benign procedure, and should be utilized whenever necessary.

Perhaps the most controversial of all ancillary diagnostic tests is the ^{32}P test. It is based on the principle that malignant cells, perhaps because of greater metabolic activity, incorporate radioactive phosphorus to a higher degree than normal cells.[13] Radioactive phosphorous is given to patients intravenously and then the activity of the lesion in question is measured with a Geiger counter. The amount of radioactivity is compared to other areas of the globe for

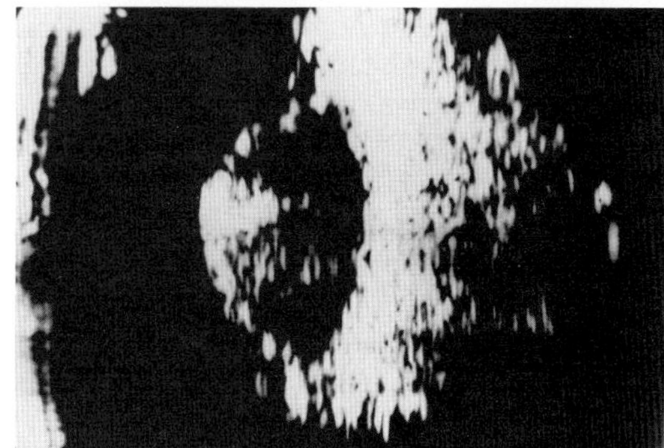

Fig. 5B. B-scan ultrasonogram of choroidal melanoma. The smooth dome-shaped mass of the tumor is accompanied by acoustic hollowness and "choroidal excavation." (Courtesy Dr. Gary Abrams.)

control values. This test requires surgical manipulation of the globe and precise probe localization. Its controversy arises from the fact that certain authors[14–16] have stressed its accuracy and not its limitations, whereas others[17] have emphasized its limitations, perhaps without pointing out its potential values.

What are the indications for, and the limitations of, the ^{32}P test? It may be helpful in the case of a choroidal mass in which a thorough clinical examination, in combination with studies such as fluorescein angiography and ultrasound, has failed to firmly establish the diagnosis. The test is fairly reliable in distinguishing malignant lesions from hemangiomas and atypical disciform lesions. Shields[5] recommends its use in cases of small to medium sized lesions in which treatment is contemplated. Perhaps another indication is in eyes with opaque media in which a lesion has been detected on ultrasound. Finally, the test may be used as a confirmatory test for choroidal and ciliary body melanomas in which both physician and patient wish to have the diagnosis confirmed in every way possible before enucleation. It should be noted, however, that this particular use of the ^{32}P test is still quite controversial.

There are definite limitations of the ^{32}P test. False-positive results have been reported with hemangiomas, melanocytomas, disciform lesions, nevi and intraocular hemorrhage.[18] The test is unable to accurately diagnose iris melanomas, and it fails to distinguish between choroidal nevi and small melanomas. As might be suspected, the test cannot differentiate between metastatic malignancies and primary intraocular melanomas. Operative complications can occur, and because a radioactive substance is injected, the test should not be used in children or young women. The test is not advised for those lesions in the region of the optic nerve or macula. Because of these factors, the ^{32}P test is of only limited usefulness in those cases where the clinician may need it most to aid in differential diagnosis.

Finally, the importance of ophthalmic consultations cannot be overemphasized. The effects of treatment of melanomas can be devastating, and should not be under-taken lightly. If several observers agree that the lesion in question is in fact a melanoma, therapy can be directed accordingly, with psychological reassurance to both physician and patient.

For the future, immunologic techniques may prove helpful in establishing the diagnosis of melanoma. Tumor-associated antibodies have been detected in the serum of melanoma patients by immunofluorescent techniques,[19, 20] and a recent study by Char[21] has demonstrated cutaneous delayed hypersensitivity reactions in patients with ocular melanomas. Although wide clinical applications have not been established, the potential for future use is intriguing.

In the past, once the diagnosis of melanoma had been established, the clinician's primary form of therapy was enucleation. More recently, different forms of management have been proposed, which include photocoagulation, cobalt irradiation, scleral resection, immunotherapy, and simple observation. To discuss these varied forms of management, it is important to divide choroidal melanomas into three categories: large, medium, and small.[22, 23] A small tumor is one that is no greater than 10 × 10 mm in base dimension and no greater than 3 mm in height; a large tumor exceeds either 15 mm in base dimension or 5 mm in height; medium tumors fall in between. All forms of management to be discussed are limited, to a large extent, by the dimensions of the tumor in each individual case. One must also bear in mind that although each of these forms of therapy has its proponents, for the most part, controlled clinical trials are lacking.

I would like to begin our discussion of management of melanomas by reviewing some of the ideas pertinent to small melanomas of the choroid, and how small melanomas differ from larger tumors.

Much of the controversy surrounding the management of small choroidal melanomas has arisen because their mortality rate is much lower than that of larger tumors. In recent series, reporting statistics in patients with enucleated eyes, choroidal melanomas with dimensions greater than 10 × 10 × 3 mm have a six-year mortality rate of 35–50%, depending on age, location, largest tumor dimension, cell type, and other factors.[24] Small melanomas, on the other hand, tend to have a six-year mortality rate of 10–15%.[24–26] The comparatively low mortality rate in patients with an eye enucleated for a small melanoma seems to be related to several factors; among them are tumor size, cell type, location and lack of sceral extension.

Overall tumor size is important in relation to the patient's prognosis. In two of the more recent series,[24, 26] in retrospective analyses of enucleated eyes, there were significant increases in mortality when tumor height exceeded 3 mm.

Numerous studies of choroidal melanomas have demonstrated that one of the most important factors determining prognosis is the tumor cell type, according to the Callender classification. In recent studies,[23, 25] approximately 80% of small tumors were of the spindle cell type and 20% were of the mixed or epithelioid cell types. It may be that all melanomas that eventually metastasize have epithelioid cells somewhere within the tumor, not evident on the few sections that are examined histopathologically.[17] Patients with small tumors, however, less than 3 mm in height, enjoy the benefits of the better prognosis that is associated with melanomas of the spindle cell variety.

Additional factors that account for lowered mortality are posterior location and lack of scleral invasion. If a melanoma is located anteriorly, it tends to be larger when first discovered and carries a worse prognosis.[24, 26] Up to 90% of small melanomas are posterior to the equator when detected.[23, 25] Moreover, only 10% of small melanomas have some degree of scleral invasion; patients with small tumors may have a more favorable prognosis because of their relative lack of this tendency to grow beyond the confines of the eye itself.

The age of the patients at the time the tumor is detected is a very important factor in management of both small and large choroidal melanomas. Melanomas are rare in children, and although they may appear in all adult age groups, they are most common in the sixth and seventh decades of life. Recent work by McLean, Foster, and Zimmerman[26] indicated that there was no real difference in the age of those patients with nonfatal melanomas and those patients who died of metastases, the average being 52 years in each group. Shammas and Blodi,[24] on the other hand, performed a retrospective study of 293 patients with choroidal and ciliary body melanomas, 129 of which had tumors less than 10 mm in largest dimension. They found that, in those patients over 60 years of age who underwent enucleation for small melanomas, survival was essentially the same as that of the general population (Figs. 6A and 6B). The prognosis for patients with larger choroidal melanomas was considerably worse. In addition to the fact that all patients with small choroidal melanomas have a low mortality rate, those patients greater than 60 years of age appear to have almost no increased risk, provided that the tumor remains small. Older patients are more likely to die of causes other than metastases from small melanomas.[27]

Because of the lower mortality of small melanomas, various forms of management have been proposed. Recently, observation of small melanomas, rather than enucleation or other forms of therapy, has been advocated. This approach may be especially helpful when the diagnosis is in question. In spite of the numerous diagnostic modalities currently available, it is often impossible to determine which lesions are in fact melanomas, with a potential to metastasize. This is especially true of small lesions, for although the diagnostic accuracy of fluorescein angiography, ultrasound, and the ^{32}P test is excellent with large tumors, their specificity and sensitivity are poor with smaller ones.[8] It is therefore often advisable to observe small lesions for signs of growth, which may be the only reliable indicator of malignant potential. Gass[17] reported 58 patients with small pigmented choroidal lesions, 12 of whom had their eye removed when tumor growth was detected. None of these patients showed any signs of metastases. Curtin and Cavender[27] reported 17 patients with clinically observed melanomas in varying size, followed for at least five years. There were no tumor deaths in this group, but in a similar group of 12 patients who eventually had the eye enucleated, two died with metastatic disease.

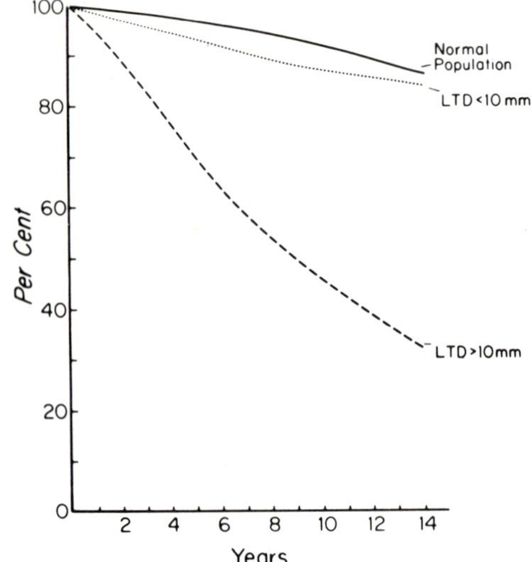

Fig. 6A. Actuarial survival rates according to largest tumor diameter (all deaths) compared to those of normal population of less than 60 years of age.

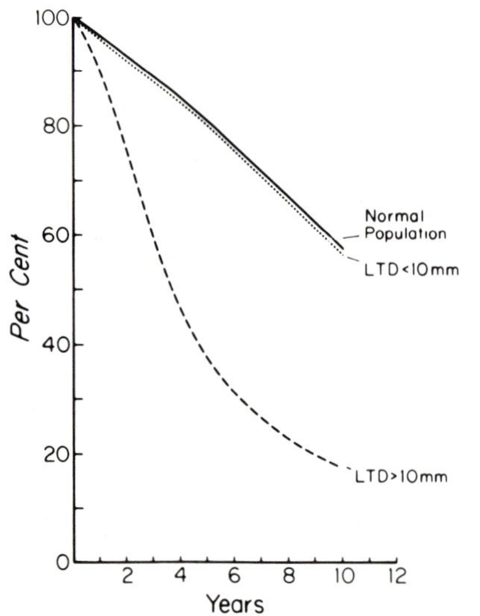

Fig. 6B. Actuarial survival rates according to largest tumor diameter (all deaths) compared to those of normal population of 60 years and older. Largest tumor diameter (LTD) (courtesy Shammas, H. F. and Blodi, F. C. *Arch. Ophthalmol.* **99**:68, 1977).

Char and Hogan[28] reported 20 patients with small melanomas who were followed for two to 20 years after the diagnosis was made (12 had at least five years of follow-up). Nine of these patients underwent enucleation after the tumor was observed to be growing, but none of the 20 patients had developed any sign of metastatic disease at the time of their report. These authors point out the fact that there is little statistical evidence to indicate that a period of observation, rather than immediate enucleation, adversely affects the prognosis in patients with small melanomas.

Meyer-Schwickerath[29] and Vogel[30] described photocoagulation of small melanomas with the xenon arc photocoagulator. Their criteria for treatment were: a melanoma less than 2 mm in height and no greater than 10 mm in diameter, location at least one disc diameter away from the macula or optic nerve, and absence of subretinal fluid that might interfere with treatment. The technique described by the above authors is to surround the tumor with two rows of photocoagulation burns, to retreat this area again after a period of three weeks, and finally to photocoagulate the tumor itself after another three- to four-week period. The authors propose that the encircling photocoagulations cause extensive occlusion of the vascular network surrounding the tumor, and reduce the chance of hemorrhage when it is photocoagulated. Several treatment sessions may be necessary to completely eliminate the tumor. Complications include exudative retinal detachment, vitreous hemorrhage, and iris atrophy. Although Vogel[30] reports that 25 of 54 patients were considered to be free of tumor after photocoagulation treatment, the overall 10-year mortality rate was 37%. We do not know how these patients would have fared if left untreated. Further studies are needed to establish the value of photocoagulation of small melanomas.

Radiotherapy can be used to treat both small and some medium-sized choroidal melanomas. Melanomas are not especially radiosensitive neoplasms, and external beam irradiation is not beneficial. The approach has been to suture the radiation source to the sclera, maximizing the dose to the tumor, while hopefully protecting other ocular structures. Most physicians using this technique have sutured cobalt-60 plaques to the sclera, which is then removed in two to four days after the calculated dose is delivered. Approximately 10,000 rads are delivered to the apex of the tumor, although Ellsworth[31] states that the optimal dose for melanomas has not yet been determined. Initial reports were encouraging, in spite of Stallard's[32] report that only 69 of 100 tumors were successfully treated, and only 31 of the original 100 retained vision of 20/60 or better. More recently, Char, Lonn, and Margolis[33] reported that only one of eight patients they had treated with cobalt-60 plaques retained visual acuity of 20/40 or better. Statistics vary from author to author as to which cases eventually require enucleation, and the frequent complication of radiation retinopathy is probably underestimated in those series with shorter follow-up periods. Often growth of small melanomas is not documented prior to treatment, and we do not know how these patients would have fared if left untreated. Nonetheless, some authors[31, 34] have been encouraged by their initial results, and we may be provided with a better mode of melanoma therapy once the technique is refined. In order for patients to be candidates for this form of therapy, they should have melanomas occurring in their only useful eye or perhaps have refused other forms of therapy, such as enucleation. Controlled prospective clinical trials will be necessary before the ultimate value of cobalt-60 irradiation is determined.

Recently, Boniuk and Cohen[35] reported the combined use of photocoagulation and radiation plaques to treat small choroidal melanomas, and Gragoudas and co-workers[36] have used proton beam irradiation (from a cyclotron) to treat small melanomas. Their initial results are also encouraging, but adequate follow-up is lacking. We can only hope that these methods of treatment will prove to be even more useful when subjected to the scrutiny of controlled prospective clinical trials.

An ideal treatment of uveal melanomas would be to surgically excise the tumor and salvage the eye, if it did not worsen the patient's prognosis. Forrest[37] reported the results of 107 patients with iris and ciliary body melanomas. Although follow-up data is limited, 75% of the globes were saved and 50% retained useful vision. A substantial number of patients with incomplete excision remained in good health, a fact that in part reflects the benign histologic charac-

teristics of these tumors (only 10% were of mixed or epithelioid cell types).

Choroidal melanomas, because of their size and location, are less amenable to surgical resection than more anterior lesions. Peyman[38] and Shields[34] have treated a certain number of patients with small and medium-sized melanomas by sclerochoroidioretinal resection, and their initial results are encouraging. Peyman is to be credited with developing the surgical technique, which involves treating the area around the tumor with photocoagulation and cryotherapy preoperatively, and treating the area around the tumor with diathermy during the surgery. The eye is supported by a "scleral basket." The section of tumor is removed, and a partial vitrectomy is performed. Donor sclera is sutured to the resultant defect. Peyman[38] has reported 16 patients treated by this method. One-third required subsequent enucleation, and in the remaining patients the visual acuities have been variable. None of these cases have had five years of follow-up; the eventual role of this controversial technique will depend on the long-term results of these initial cases.

The answer to the question of what is the best form of management of small and medium-sized choroidal melanomas awaits prospective clinical trials with adequate follow-up. Smaller melanomas have a better prognosis than larger tumors, and some authors argue that early treatment of small lesions would not only prevent the patient from shifting into a high risk group, but also prevent metastases or extrascleral extension of the melanoma in the absence of clinically observable growth.[24] However, there is no evidence to indicate that observation of small pigmented choroidal lesions increases the patient's risk.[17, 28] Moreover, early treatment of all small pigmented choroidal lesions will result in the destruction of many benign tumors and an increased patient morbidity.

We must modify our approach to smaller melanomas in terms of the individual characteristics of each case, but some general rules may be formulated. Since observed growth is the only reliable indicator of malignancy, and the risks of observation are small, the physician probably should document tumor growth prior to giving treatment. This approach is especially indicated in patients over 60 years of age. If the tumor enlarges, enucleation is probably the safest course of action. If tumor growth is observed in a patient who has limited vision in the fellow eye, is elderly, or in poor health, then photocoagulation, irradiation, or surgical resection should be considered.

Even though alternative forms of therapy have been developed, enucleation is still the preferred method of treatment for most small melanomas once growth is observed, and for almost all medium and large melanomas once the diagnosis is established. Recently, however, Zimmerman[39] has questioned the value of enucleation in improving the prognosis of patients with malignant melanomas. He and his co-workers reappraised survival data at the Armed Forces Institute of Pathology on patients treated by enucleation, and found that the mortality rate before enucleation is low, probably less than 1% per year, that after enucleation the mortality rate rises abruptly, and inferred that many cases of metastatic disease may be caused by tumor emboli at the time of enucleation. They concluded that enucleation of choroidal and ciliary body melanomas, no matter what size, may have an adverse rather than a beneficial effect, and called for both improved, less traumatic techniques of enucleation as well as long-term follow-up study of patients observed rather than treated with uveal melanomas.

This report has resulted in some discussion within the ophthalmic community. The argument that the act of enucleation causes a shower of tumor cells, and thus metastases may be based on false assumptions about the growth rate of melanomas (Gass, personal communication, 1978). Although intraocular melanomas are relatively small tumors when compared to other systemic cancers, it may be that by the time some patients are symptomatic from an enlarging melanoma, micrometastases may already be present throughout the body as a result of tumor growth. If left untreated, these patients will probably develop metastatic disease at the same rate as enucleated patients. On the other hand, most patients, in whom micrometastases are not present at the time of diagnosis, are probably unaffected by observation or

enucleation. Nonetheless, all clinicians join Dr. Zimmerman in advocating the least traumatic enucleation possible. Fraunfelder and associates[40] have advocated a "no-touch technique" for the removal of melanomas. While all aspects of this technique may not be feasible for some clinicians, the enucleation of eyes suspected of harboring tumor cells should be done with great care.

Once an eye containing malignant melanoma cells has been removed, there is currently little to offer the patient to ameliorate metastatic disease. The use of adjunct immunotherapy with nonspecific immunostimulants[41] and with adjunct BCG therapy[8] is currently under investigation. A number of chemotherapeutic agents are available to treat systemic melanomas,[42] but the experience with ocular melanomas is limited.

Gass[16] has advocated randomized prospective clinical trials to determine the efficacy of the various forms of therapy that are now available to treat small melanomas. More recently, Gamel, McLean, and Foster[43] and Zimmerman[39] have advocated prospective studies for larger melanomas as well. These studies would establish criterion for treatment of melanomas, organize patients into both clinical and treatment groups, and evaluate their subsequent clinical course. The results of studies such as these will be long in coming, but whatever their flaws, they should provide us with more rational guidelines for the future management of uveal melanomas.

EDITOR'S NOTE

One might wonder why a chapter on uveal tract melanomas is sitting in a book on neuro-ophthalmology. The aim of this book is to try and give the clinician a feeling of the current state of the art as we leave the 70's and move into the 80's. I can think of few things about which concepts have changed more than in the management of choroidal malignant melanomas. This might be exemplified by telling the following story—about 20 years ago, a patient was presented at the Wilmer Institute Grand Rounds who had a large, pigmented mass lesion involving the posterior pole of the eye. Approximately 70 ophthalmologists looked at it and were all in agreement that this was a malignant melanoma of the choroid and the eye should be promptly enucleated. One senior clinician, however, held out a minority report that it was macular degeneration and that the patient should be followed. Dr. Howard Naquin, now deceased, had a great reputation at Wilmer for loving a good argument. He immediately held up his hand and said—"I agree!" (Everyone held their breath at that point!) He continued—"I agree ... I'd follow this case, too .... until tomorrow morning when I could get him on the schedule and enucleate the eye!" The reason I remember that story is that it exemplifies the attitude and approach to such tumors in those days. This might be briefly summarized by one of Dr. Frank Walsh's favorite quotations: "And if thy right eye offend thee, pluck it out..." (Matthew 5:29a).

Over the years, however, the attitude towards these pigmented fundus lesions has steadily grown more and more conservative. One reason for this is that many eyes were taken out for suspected melanomas only to find on careful histologic study that a benign lesion existed as a hematoma under the pigment epithelium and that the diagnosis was simply wrong. However, with good binocular indirect ophthalmoscopy and more experience, the diagnostic batting average has steadily improved, so that Drs. Norton, Gass, and Curtin can nearly pick up melanomas by "braille"—in a manner of speaking. I have watched Dr. Norton get more and more conservative with intraocular melanomas so much so that if a patient comes in to Eye Grand Rounds with a choroidal melanoma hanging down on his cheek, I could imagine Dr. Norton advising a good set of pictures and measurements of this lesion to be made, and then having the patient come back in a season for a follow-up! Now, that is exaggeration without a doubt, but I am trying to make a teaching point. We have simply gone pole to pole from immediate enucleation as an emergency in many pigmented fundus lesions, even with good acuity—to a current approach of being extremely conservative and following many known melanomas if they are of small to moderate size. I personally am opposed to P-32 and believe it should

be relegated to the status of nux vomica, Hadacol, and spats. The point to make to the practicing ophthalmologist is that you ALWAYS have time with an intraocular melanoma to refer the patient to another good ophthalmologist for a second opinion, and if there is any doubt as to management then, get a third opinion. Finally, if you want to keep the patient's eye in, send them to Dr. Norton. If you want the patient's eye to come out, refer them to someone who likes P-32. I personally believe that a carefully done enucleation is the treatment of choice when the lesion is obviously a melanoma, is large, is progressing in size, interferes with the patient's vision, the other eye is good, and the patient's age allows for a reasonable longevity, and there is no evidence of metastatic disease. I do not agree with the general concept that enucleation is the villain in causing the death of patients with malignant melanomas. That is like not calling out the fire department when your house is on fire because water can cause drowning. We all agree, however, that when enucleation is indicated, it should be done meticulously.

JLS

REFERENCES

1. *System of Ophthalmology.* S. Duke-Elder (Ed.), C. V. Mosby Co., St. Louis, 1966, Vol. 9, p. 843.
2. Resseguie, L. J., Marks, S. J., Winkelmann, R. K., *et al.* Malignant melanoma in the resident population of Rochester, Minnesota. Mayo Clin. Proc. *52*:191 (1977).
3. Ferry, A. P. Lesions mistaken for malignant melanoma of the posterior uvea; a clinicopathologic analysis of 100 cases with ophthalmoscopically visible lesions. Arch. Ophthalmol. *72*:463 (1964).
4. Shields, J. A. and Zimmerman, L. E. Lesions simulating malignant melanoma of the posterior uvea. Arch. Ophthalmol. *89*:466 (1973).
5. Shields, J. A. Current approaches to the diagnosis and management of choroidal melanomas. Surv. Ophthalmol. *21*:443 (1977).
6. Blodi, F. C. and Roy, P. E. The misdiagnosed choroidal melanoma. Can. J. Ophthalmol. *2*:209 (1967).
7. Shields, J. A. and McDonald, P. R.: Improvements in the diagnosis of posterior uveal melanomas. Arch. Ophthalmol. *91*:259 (1974).
8. Char, D. H. The management of small choroidal melanomas. Surv. Ophthalmol. *22*:377 (1978).
9. Gass, J. D. M. *Differential Diagnosis of Intraocular Tumors; a Stereoscopic Presentation.* C. V. Mosby Co., St. Louis, 1974, p. 14.
10. Shields, J. A., Rodrigues, M. M., Sarin, L. K., *et al.* Lipofuscin pigment over benign and malignant

choroidal tumors. Trans. Am. Acad. Ophthalmol. Otolaryngol. *81*:op-871 (1976).

11. Ossoinig, K. C. and Blodi, F. C. III. Diagnosis of intraocular tumors. In: *Current Concepts in Ophthalmology.* F. C. Blodi (Ed.), C. V. Mosby Co., St. Louis, 1974, Vol. IV, p. 296.
12. Coleman, D. J., Abramson, D. H., Jack, R. L. *et al.* Ultrasonic diagnosis of tumors of the choroid. Arch. Ophthalmol. *91*:344 (1974).
13. Thomas, C. I., Krohmer, J. S., and Storaasli, J. P. Detection of intraocular tumors with radioactive phosphorus: A preliminary report with special reference to differentiation of the cause of retinal separation. Arch. Ophthalmol. *47*:276 (1952).
14. Hagler, W. S., Jarrett, W. H., and Humphrey, W. T. The radioactive phosphorus uptake test in diagnosis of uveal melanoma. Arch. Ophthalmol. *83*:548 (1970).
15. Ruiz, R. S. and Howerton, E. E., Jr. [32]P testing for posterior segment lesions. Trans. Am. Acad. Ophthalmol. Otolaryngol. *79*:op-287 (1975).
16. Shields, J. A., Hagler, W. S., Federman, J. L., *et al.* The significance of the ^{32}P test in the diagnosis of posterior uveal melanomas. Trans. Am. Acad. Ophthalmol. Otolaryngol. *79*:op-297 (1975).
17. Gass, J. D. M. G. Problems in the differential diagnosis of choroidal nevi and malignant melanoma. Am. J. Ophthalmol. *83*:299 (1977).
18. Minckler, D., Font, R. L., and Shields, J. A. Non melanoma ocular lesions with positive ^{32}P tests. In: *Ocular and Adnexal Tumors.* F. A. Jakobiec (Ed.), Aesculapius, Birmingham, 1978, pp. 245–256.
19. Federman, J. L., Lewis, M. G., Clark, W. H., Jr., *et al.* Tumor-associated antibodies in the serum of ocular melanoma patients. Trans. Am. Acad. Ophthalmol. Otolaryngol. *78*:op-784 (1974).
20. Wong, I. G. and Oskvig, R. M. Immunofluorescent detection of antibodies to ocular melanomas. Arch. Ophthalmol. *92*:98 (1974).
21. Char, D. H., Hollinshead, A., and Cogan, D. G., *et al.* Cutaneous delayed hypersensitivity reactions to soluble melanoma antigen in patients with ocular malignant melanoma. New Engl. J. Med. *291*:274 (1974).
22. Warren, R. M. Prognosis of malignant melanomas of the choroid and ciliary body. In: *Current Concepts in Ophthalmology.* F. C. Blodi (Ed.), C. V. Mosby Co., St. Louis, 1974, Vol. IV, p. 158.
23. Davidorf, F. H., and Lang, J. R. The natural history of malignant melanoma of the choroid: small vs. large tumors. Trans. Am. Acad. Ophthalmol. Otolaryngol. *79*:op-310 (1975).
24. Shammas, H. F. and Blodi, F. C. Prognostic factors in choroidal and ciliary body melanomas. Arch. Ophthalmol. *95*:63 (1977).
25. Barr, C. C., Sipperley, J. O., and Nicholson, D. H. Small melanomas of the choroid. Arch. Ophthalmol. *96*:1580 (1978).
26. McLean, I. W., Foster, W. D., and Zimmerman, L. E. Prognostic factors in small malignant melanomas of choroid and ciliary body. Arch. Ophthalmol. *95*:48 (1977).
27. Curtin, V. T. and Cavender, J. C. Natural course of selected malignant melanomas of the choroid and ciliary body. Mod. Probl. Ophthalmol. *12*:523 (1974).
28. Char, D. H. and Hogan, M. J. Management of small elevated pigmented choroidal lesions. Br. J. Ophthalmol. *61*:54 (1977).
29. Meyer-Schwickerath, G. The preservation of vision by treatment of intraocular tumors with light coagulation. Arch. Ophthalmol. *66*:458 (1961).
30. Vogel, M. H. Treatment of malignant choroidal melanomas with photocoagulation; evaluation of 10-year followup data. Am. J. Ophthalmol. *74*:1 (1972).
31. Ellsworth, R. M. Cobalt plaques for melanoma of the choroid. In: *Ocular and Adnexal Tumors.* F. A. Jakobiec (Ed.), Aesculapius, Birmingham, 1978, pp. 119–126.
32. Stallard, H. B. Radiotherapy for malignant melanoma of the choroid. Br. J. Ophthalmol. *50*:147 (1966).
33. Char, D. H., Lonn, L. I., and Margolis, L. W. Complications of cobalt plaque therapy of choroidal melanomas. Am. J. Ophthalmol. *84*:536 (1977).
34. Shields, J. A. Approaches to the management of choroidal melanoma. In: *Ocular and Adnexal Tumors.* F. A. Jakobiec (Ed.), Aesculapius, Birmingham, 1978, pp. 4–11.
35. Boniuk, M. and Cohen, J. S. Combined use of radiation plaques and photocoagulation in the treatment of choroidal melanomas. In: *Ocular and Adnexal Tumors.* F. A. Jakobiec (Ed.), Aesculapius, Birmingham, 1978, pp. 80–87.
36. Gragoudas, E. S., Goitein, M., Koehler, A. M., *et al.* Proton irradiation of small choroidal malignant melanomas. Am. J. Ophthalmol. *83*:665 (1977).
37. Forrest, A. W. Iridocyclectomy for ciliary body tumors: pathologic criterion for success. In: *Ocular and Adnexal Tumors.* F. A. Jakobiec (Ed.), Aesculapius, Birmingham, 1978, pp. 46–60.
38. Peyman, G. A., Sanders, D. R., and May, D. R. Local excision of malignant melanoma of the choroid. In: *Intraocular Tumors.* G. A. Peyman, D. J. Apple, and D. R. Sanders (Eds.), Appleton-Century-Croft, New York, 1977, p. 167.
39. Zimmerman, L. E., McLean, I. W., and Foster, W. D. Does enucleation of the eye containing a malignant melanoma prevent or accelerate the dissemination of tumour cells? Br. J. Ophthalmol. *62*:420 (1978).
40. Fraunfelder, F. T., Boozman, F. W., Wilson, R. S., *et al.* No-touch technique for intraocular malignant melanomas. Arch. Ophthalmol. *95*:1616 (1977).
41. Davidorf, F. H. Management of high risk uveal melanoma patients: role of immunotherapy. In: *Ocular and Adnexal Tumors.* F. A. Jakobiec (Ed.), Aesculapius, Birmingham, 1978 pp. 119–126.
42. Johnson, F. D. and Jacobs, E. M. Chemotherapy of metastatic malignant melanoma. Experience with 73 patients. Cancer *27*:1306 (1971).
43. Gamel, J. W., McLean, I. W., Foster, W. D., *et al.* Melanocytic lesions of the posterior uvea: the impact of new pathologic concepts on prognosis and management. In: *Ocular and Adnexal Tumors.* F. A. Jakobiec (Ed.), Aesculapius, Birmingham, 1978, pp. 19–30.

20 Elevated Carcinoembryonic Antigen and Visual Loss in Ocular Metastases

Michael E. Barricks, M.D.
William A. Meriwether, M.D.
and David Bouda, M.D.

INTRODUCTION

Visual loss may be the presenting symptom of metastatic carcinoma and precede discovery of the primary malignancy.[1,2] This paper will describe the clinical and histopathological features of an unusual case of carcinoma metastatic to the optic nerve and choroid. Though no history of primary malignancy could be obtained, the unusual fundus picture suggested metastatic carcinoma. Extensive oncologic evaluation revealed no definite signs of metastatic disease except a consistently elevated carcinoembryonic antigen. Because of progressive visual loss, a deteriorating fundus appearance, and the elevated carcinoembryonic antigen, enucleation was performed; a poorly differentiated metastatic adenocarcinoma was found. The presence of an elevated carcinoembryonic antigen in a patient with an unusual fundus picture may be a very important clue to the diagnosis of metastatic carcinoma. Numerous reports have recently emphasized the diagnostic value of this antigen in ocular metastases.[3-7]

CASE REPORT

A 61-year-old white man came to the admitting ward of the Audie L. Murphy Veterans Administration Hospital in San Antonio, Texas on July 9, 1977. He complained of decreased vision in the left eye of one month duration. He was otherwise asymptomatic. Past medical history indicated that he had a squamous cell carcinoma removed from his left temple two years previously. Twenty-four years previously he had been in an auto accident and injured his thoracic spine. He had arteriosclerotic cardiovascular disease and a history of myocardial infarction.

Ocular examination revealed a best corrected visual acuity of 20/20 in the right eye and 20/100 in the left eye. A left afferent pupillary defect was present. Fundus examination was normal in the right eye. The left fundus was abnormal with a hyperemic optic nerve head. There was a serous detachment of the retina in the posterior pole with retinal striae in the macular region (Fig. 1). The serous detachment extended superonasal to the optic disc where there was a four disc diameter nonelevated disturbance of the retinal pigment epithelium (RPE). The RPE disturbance had a "leopard spot" appearance with clumps of pigment against a creamy colored background (Fig. 2). The remainder of the ocular exam was normal. A fluorescein angiogram several days later revealed foci of abnormal fluorescence in the early photos of the left optic nerve (Fig. 3). The later photos revealed diffuse hyperfluorescence (Fig. 4).

A diagnosis of carcinoma metastatic to the optic nerve and choroid was considered, and the patient was admitted to the San Antonio Veterans' Administration Hospital for oncologic evaluation. He was seen again in the eye clinic on August 24, 1977. Vision remained 20/20 in the right eye but had fallen to 20/200 in the left eye. The left

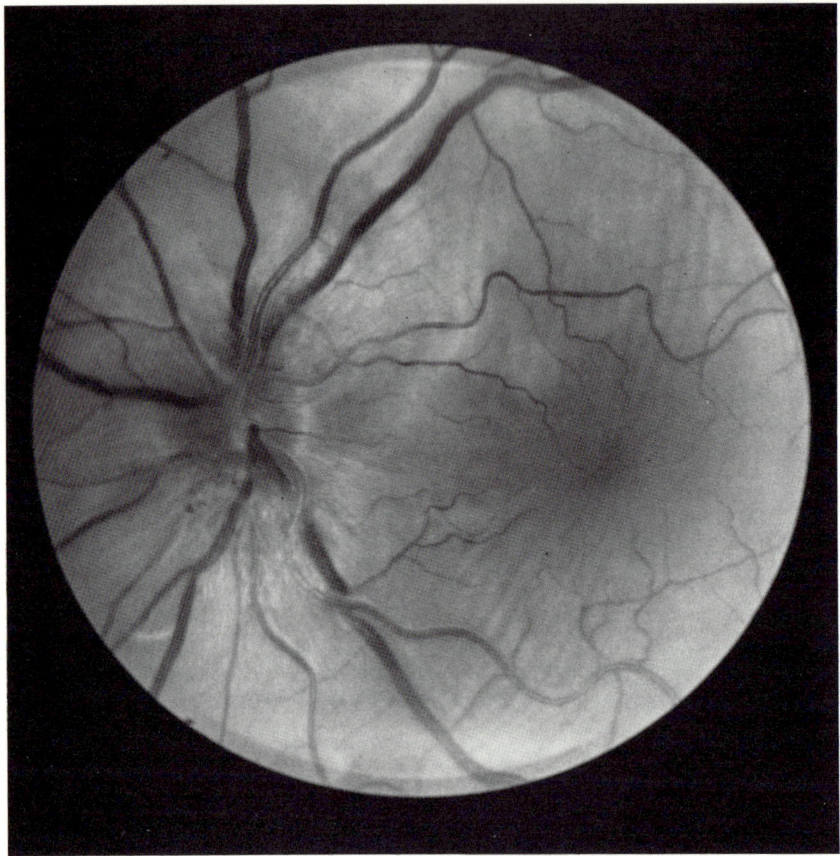

Fig. 1. Left fundus on July 14, 1977. The optic disc is hyperemic, and the margins are not discrete. Note the retinal striae associated with a serous retinal detachment involving the posterior pole.

optic nerve had become increasingly hyperemic and edematous; hemorrhages and whitish material were present on the surface, and the margins were very blurred (Fig. 5). Fluorescein angiography demonstrated extensive leakage from the nerve head and area of RPE disturbance. The area of RPE disturbance was unchanged, but the serous detachment of the retina had become more extensive and involved much of the inferior retina.

On September 5, 1977 he began to develop "shooting" pains involving the left side of his head. A very complete medical evaluation looking for primary or metastatic carcinoma was ongoing. Hemogram and SMA-12 blood chemistries were normal. Chest x-ray, barium enema, intravenous pyelograms, upper GI series, cholangiograms, and a sonogram of the pancreas were all normal as were a brain scan and tomograms of the optic canals and petrous

bones. Proctoscopy and gastroscopy were normal. A liver scan showed diffuse hepatomegaly, but enzymes and a liver biopsy were normal. An EMI scan was read as normal, but there was a suggestion of thickening of the left optic nerve. A lumbar puncture was normal, and the centrifuged specimen showed no cells. A bone scan was positive at T_9, where x-rays demonstrated a possible osteolytic lesion; however, there had been old trauma to the area in a motor vehicle accident 24 years previously. The carcinoembryonic antigen (CEA) assay was markedly elevated to about 50 mg/ml on three separate occasions.

By October 9, 1977 vision in the left eye had fallen to light perception only, and the left-sided head pain continued. Fundus examination demonstrated that the optic nerve head was elevated and its margins were obscured by hemorrhage and cream-colored material on its surface (Fig. 6). The

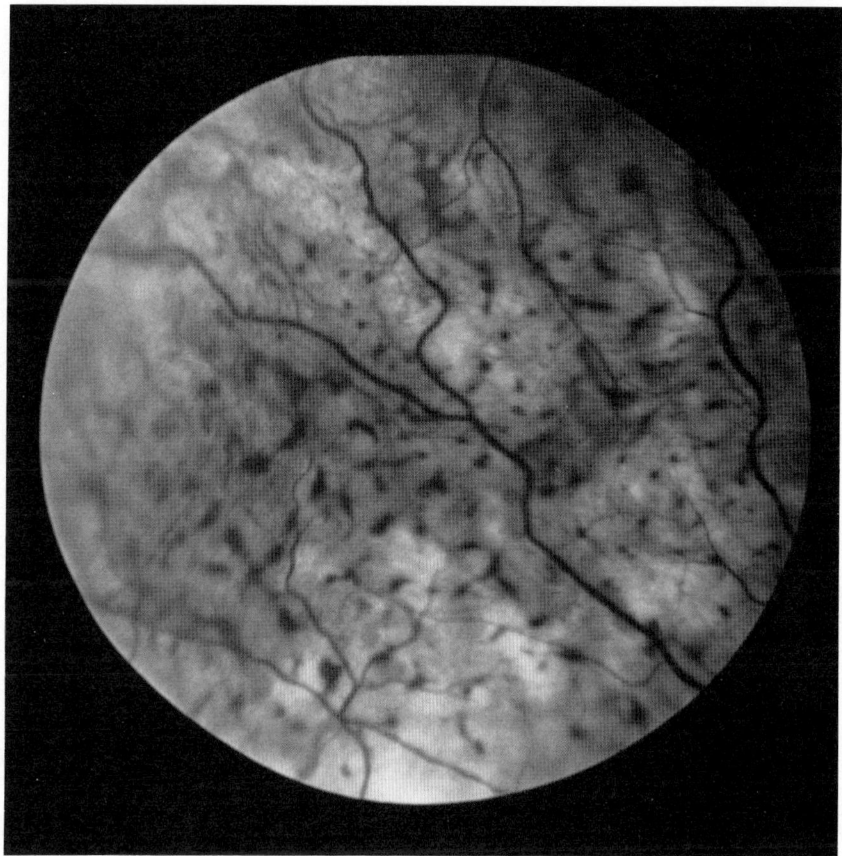

Fig. 2. Left fundus on July 14, 1977. Retinal pigment epithelial (RPE) disturbance involving the superonasal quadrant near the optic disc. There was a low serous detachment of the overlying retina.

entire posterior pole and inferior retina were detached. The area of RPE disturbance was unchanged. Because of the elevated CEA and what had now become a blind and possibly painful eye, enucleation was advised. The patient was taken to the operating room whereupon he developed a cardiac arrhythmia and surgery was cancelled.

On November 2, 1977, he was again taken to the operating room, and the left eye was enucleated without complication. A firm elevated nodule could be palpated on the posterior surface of the globe superonasal to the optic nerve in the region corresponding to the RPE disturbance (Fig. 7). Histopathological examination, which will be discussed in detail below, revealed metastatic adenocarcinoma infiltrating the choroid, sclera, and the optic nerve.

After enucleation the patient's left-sided head pain disappeared. He received radiation to the left orbit since the tumor filled the optic nerve that had been transected. He was placed on various chemotherapeutic regimens but developed evidence of widespread metastatic disease and died on July 31, 1978. An autopsy was obtained.

PATHOLOGY

Gross Description of Eye. The specimen was a left eye with a 1.5-mm segment of optic nerve attached. Externally a nodular thickening of the sclera was present adjacent to the optic nerve extending anteriorly in the 1:00 meridian for 4 mm. The thickening was 2 mm in width and 1 mm in depth (Fig. 7). On sectioning the globe, the retina was completely detached. The posterior choroid was diffusely thickened by an infiltrative lesion which was especially prominent under the previously mentioned scleral thickening. The eye was sectioned

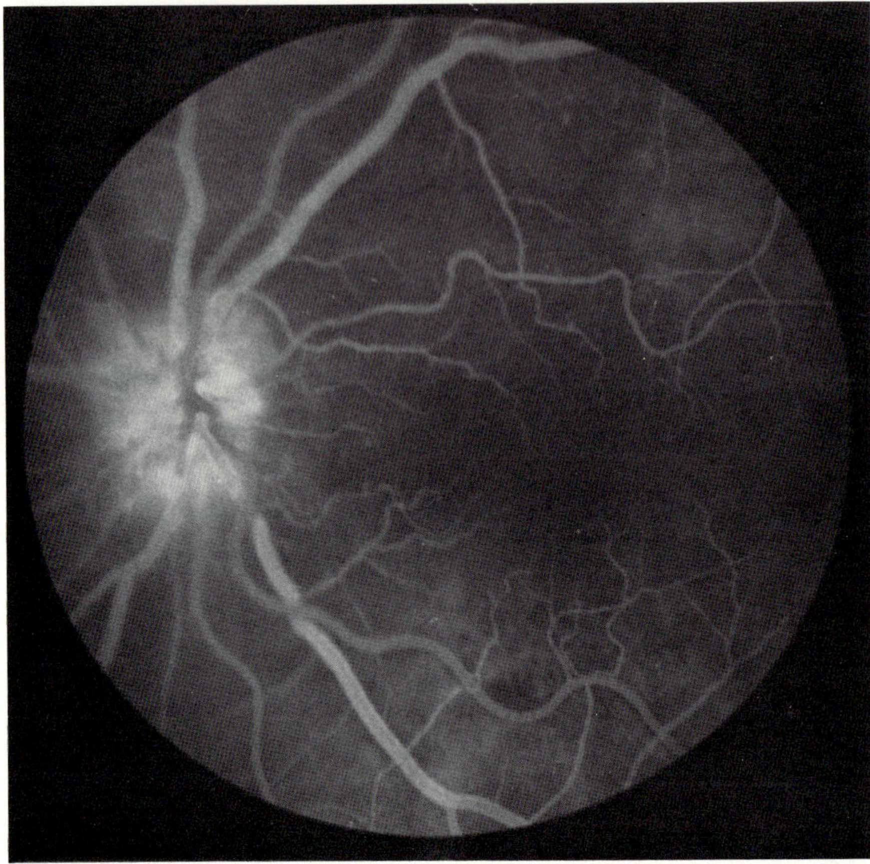

Fig. 3.   Fluorescein angiogram (venous phase) of left fundus on July 14, 1977. The disc is hyperfluorescent, and the choroidal pattern is slightly irregular.

to include the plane of the scleral nodule (Fig. 8).

Microscopic Description of Eye. The anterior segment was normal. The retina was totally detached and invaded by tumor adjacent to the optic nerve head. The entire posterior half of the choroid was involved by a tumor (Fig. 8) composed of large poorly differentiated malignant cells with round to irregularly oval nuclei, few nucleolated cells, no specific arrangement of the cells, abundant cytoplasm, and no evidence of intra-cytoplasmic melanin (Fig. 9). "Signet ring" cells were prominent (Fig. 9). Mucus production was seen on mucicarmine and PAS stains. The tumor extended through the sclera in the area of the nodule adjacent to the optic nerve (Fig. 8). The nerve head was invaded by the tumor and the segment of optic nerve was diffusely replaced by tumor cells (Fig. 10). A tumor

embolus lay in the central retinal vein. The subarachnoid space around the optic nerve also contained tumor cells (Fig. 10).

General Autopsy Report. At autopsy, generalized carcinomatosis was found with tumor involvement of most organs. In the gastric wall, a neoplastic process replaced the mucosa with mucin-containing signet ring cells similar in pattern to the choroidal metastasis. This gastric carcinoma was considered the primary neoplasm. The left optic nerve stump attached to the brain was free of tumor posterior to the optic canal. The left orbit was not entered at autopsy.

DISCUSSION

Ferry[1] and Ferry and Font[2] have recently reviewed the pathological material on file at the Armed Forces Institute of Pathology (AFIP). Their study of 227 cases of carci-

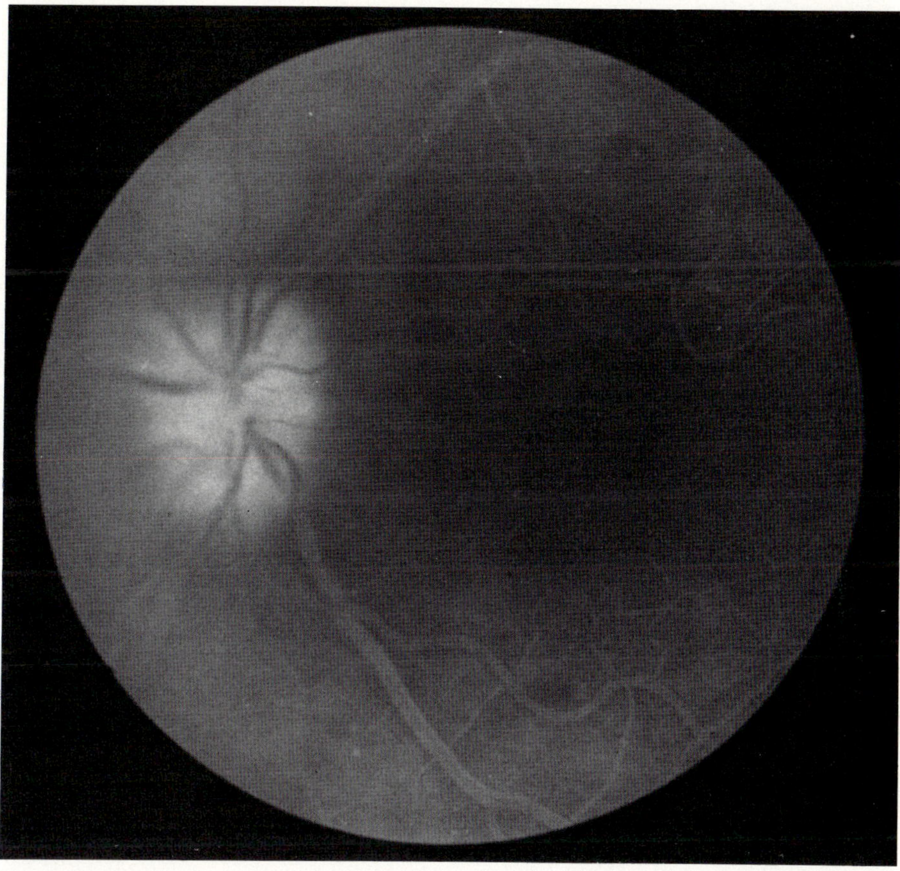

Fig. 4. Fluorescein angiogram (late photo) of left fundus on July 14, 1977. There is late staining of the optic disc.

noma metastatic to the eye and orbit serves as a useful background against which our case can be evaluated. In 46% (105/227) of the cases reported from the AFIP, ocular symptoms preceded recognition of a primary tumor; thus, it is not uncommon for a patient to present, as ours did, with ocular symptoms as the first evidence of malignant disease. Decreased vision is the most common presenting ocular manifestation of metastatic carcinoma[1,2]; pain and secondary retinal detachment are also frequently seen.[1,2] Our patient was typical in his symptoms. Carcinomatous optic neuropathy is not mentioned as a presenting sign in Ferry and Font's series[2] though 11.4% of their cases had tumor involving the optic nerve (1.3% involved only the nerve and/or sheaths). Involvement of the optic nerve and posterior segment as seen in the present case was found in 3.5% of their cases. Of the 105 cases in which ocular symptoms

preceded recognition that a primary tumor was present, the primary site was never determined in 41.[2] Thus a case like the one reported herein (in which the patient presents with an unusual fundus appearance and extensive medical evaluation fails to reveal direct evidence of primary or other metastatic disease) is not particularly rare. In this setting the carcinoembryonic antigen assay is of great value for it may lead to the proper diagnostic and therapeutic manuevers.[3-7]

The carcinoembryonic antigen was described by Gold and Freedman in 1965.[8,9] This antigen was first discovered in extracts of adenocarcinoma of the colon and subsequently found in fetal gut, liver, and pancreas. Later studies demonstrated elevated plasma CEA levels in a variety of tumors and in some nonmalignant conditions.[10] The level of plasma CEA elevation is of great diagnostic significance.[10,11] A value of

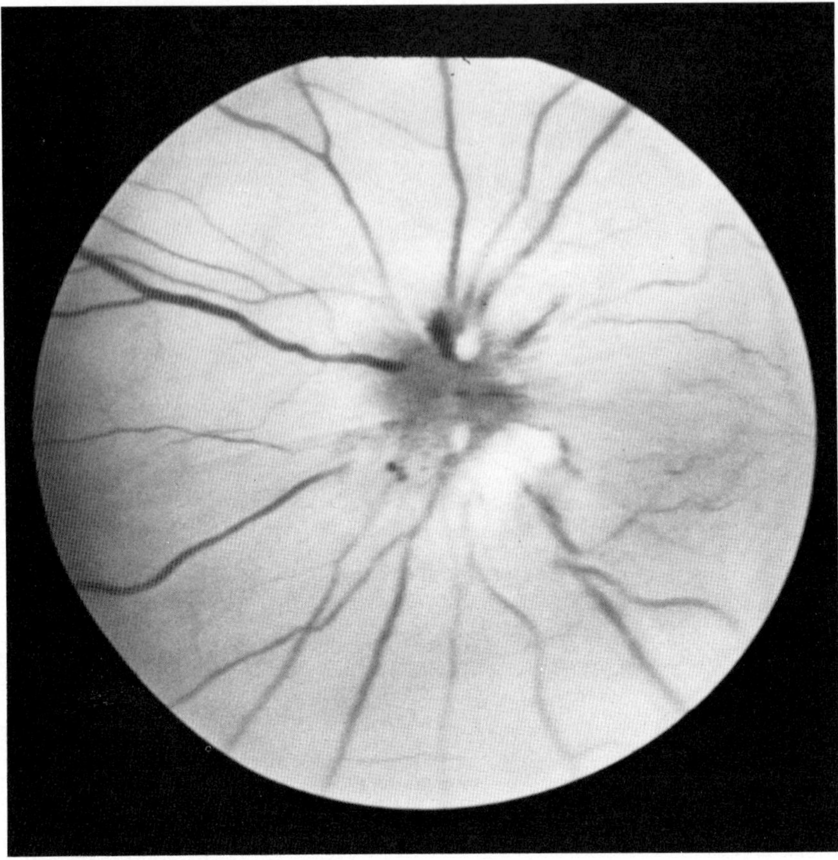

Fig. 5. Left optic disc on August 24, 1977. The margins are very blurred. Hemorrhages and creamy whitish exudates are present on the surface of the disc.

0–5 ng/ml is regarded as normal. Smokers and former smokers tend to have higher values than nonsmokers. Values of 10–20 ng/ml are found in patients with inflammatory bowel disease and entodermal carcinomas. Elevated values are also seen in patients with nonmalignant diseases of the liver and pancreas. Values greater than 20 ng/ml are found almost exclusively in patients with metastatic disease and pancreatic or colorectal carcinoma. Repeated CEA values of about 50 ng/ml in the patient described in this report made it a virtual certainty that he had metastatic carcinoma and helped with the decision for enucleation.

Several recent reports have emphasized the diagnostic value of the CEA assay in carcinoma metastatic to the eye and orbit. Michelson and co-workers[3] have described a case remarkably similar to this one. Using an immunohistologic assay, they were able to demonstrate the presence of the carcinoembryonic antigen within the choroidal metastases. Denslow and Kielar[6] recently reported a case presenting as chronic unilateral iridocyclitis with secondary glaucoma. An increased plasma carcinoembryonic antigen level led them to the correct diagnosis of carcinoma metastatic to the anterior segment. Bullock[7] has also emphasized the value of the CEA assay in diagnosing tumors metastatic to the eye. Michelson, Felberg, and Shields[5] have studied CEA values in 24 patients with metastatic carcinoma to the uvea and compared these values with those seen in 135 patients with uveal malignant melanoma; 58.3% of the patients with metastatic cancers had CEA values above 10 ng/ml, but none of the primary uveal melanoma patients had values this high. Thus the CEA assay is of

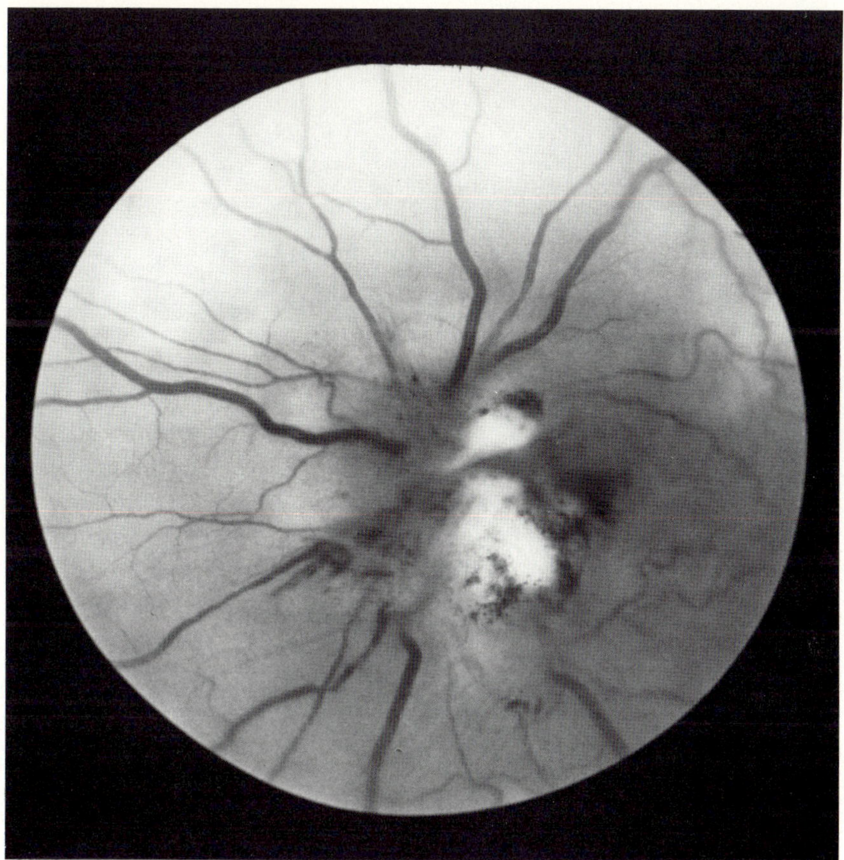

Fig. 6. Left optic disc on October 9, 1977. The disc surface is covered by hemorrhage and creamy exudates.

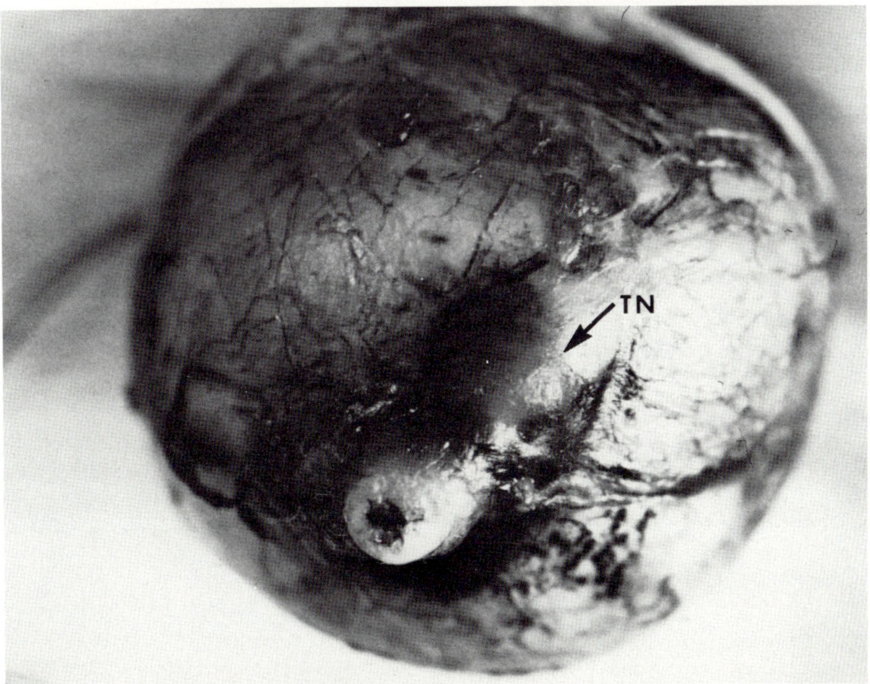

Fig. 7. Enucleated left eye viewed from behind. Extrascleral extension of a tumor nodule (TN) is seen in the superonasal quadrant near the optic nerve. This area of tumor extension corresponds to the RPE disturbance seen in Figure 2.

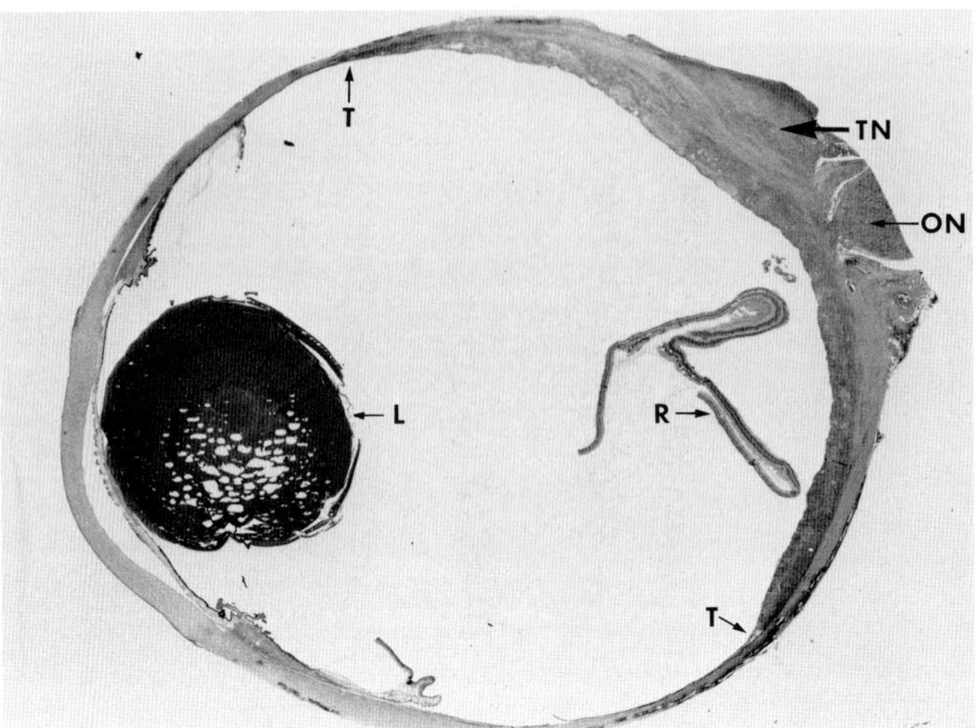

Fig. 8. Low power photomicrograph of cut globe. Tumor has infiltrated the posterior choroid from T to T. The extrascleral tumor nodule (TN) is seen adjacent to the optic nerve (ON). The retina (R) is detached. The lens (L) is artifactitiously rotated.

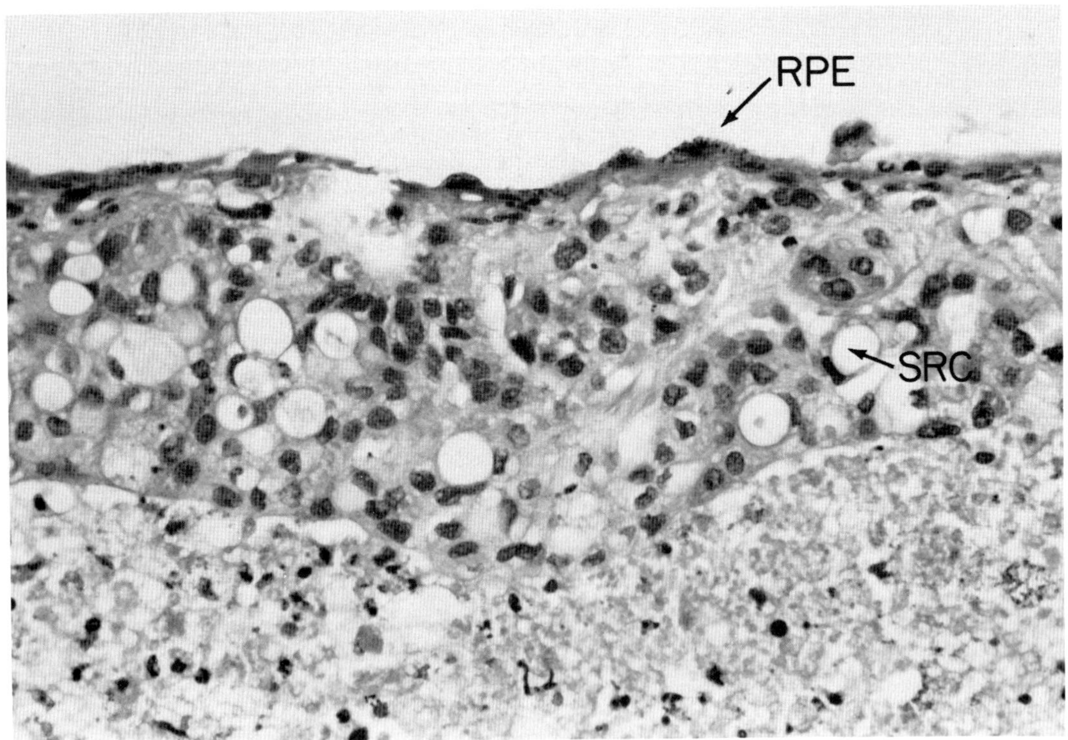

Fig. 9. Photomicrograph of choroid replaced by tumor. Some retinal pigment epithelial cells (RPE) are seen. The tumor was composed of large poorly differentiated malignant cells with no particular arrangement. "Signet ring" cells (SRC) were prominent.

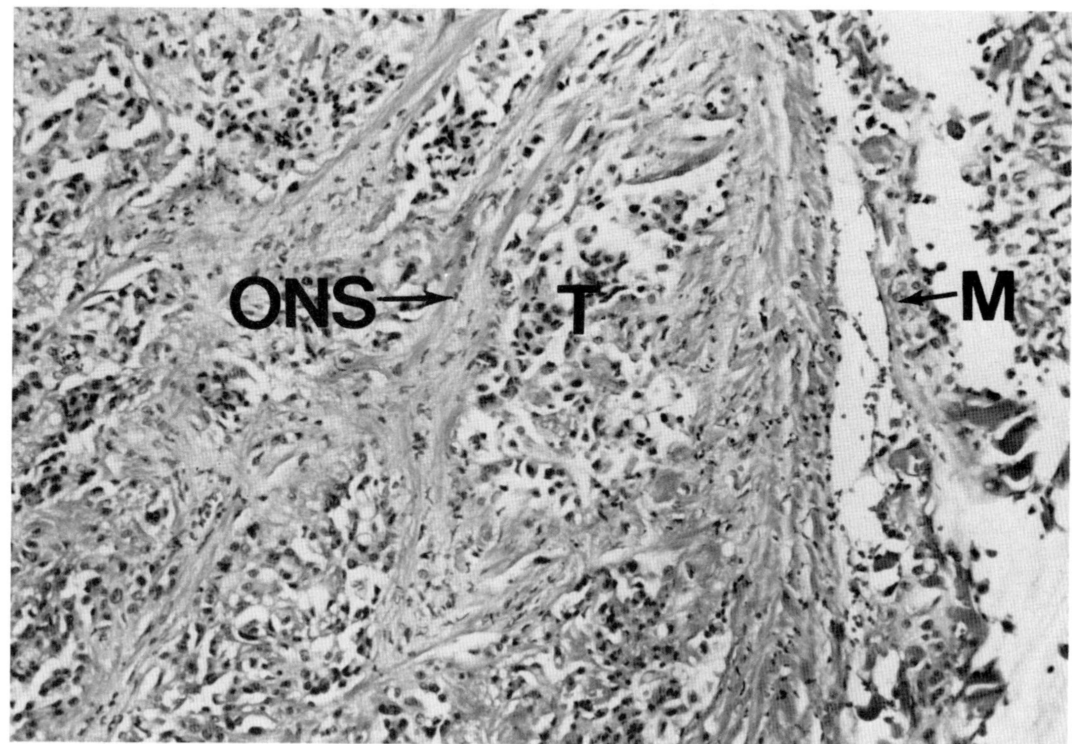

Fig. 10. Photomicrograph of cross section of optic nerve. The optic nerve septae (ONS) are preserved, but tumor (T) has replaced the substance of the nerve. The tumor has spread to the meninges (M).

great value in patients with an unusual fundus appearance in whom metastic carcinoma is suspected. Similarly in patients with a choroidal tumor, the CEA level is useful in differentiating choroidal melanomas from metastatic lesions.

SUMMARY

A case is described in which a patient complained of visual loss; examination revealed an unusual fundus appearance. Though metastatic carcinoma was suspected, there was no history of primary disease, and the only abnormality on extensive oncologic evaluation was an elevated carcinoembryonic antigen (CEA) level. On this basis a diagnostic enucleation was performed demonstrating the presence of metastatic carcinoma to the eye and optic nerve. A discussion of this case emphasizing the value of the carcinoembryonic antigen in diagnosing ocular metastases is given.

EDITOR'S NOTE

The authors have given you a practical clinical "pearl" in this paper. When you encounter a patient who shows evidence of a tumor—whether in the orbit or in the eye—and you are wondering whether the neoplasm is *primary* or *metastatic*, the first thing you want to do is to *order this new blood test!* You want a *plasma CEA* (carcinoembryonic antigen) level. *Normal is 0–5*, and *above 10* points a strong vote for a *metastatic* problem. Hopefully, use of this test could lead to earlier enucleation than was performed in this case. This test merits further use by ophthalmologists, in my opinion.

JLS

P.S. I just called the lab here at Bascom Palmer and asked them about getting the *CEA test.* They told me that they draw two lavender tubes (7 cc each) of blood, and then draw off *6 cc of pure plasma.* They mail that to: CEA Lab, Division of Scientific Laboratories, Inc., PO Box 9208, Wichita, Kansas 67277. The charge for this test here is $27 to the patient. It takes about a week to get the report back. This should help you to get this test out there in your office!

JLS

REFERENCES

1. Ferry, A. P. The biological behavior and pathological features of carcinoma metastatic to the eye and orbit. Trans. Am. Ophthalmol. Soc. *71:*373 (1973).
2. Ferry, A. P. and Font, R. L. Carcinoma metastatic to the eye and orbit. Arch. Ophthalmol. *92:*276 (1974).
3. Michelson, J. B., Felberg, N. T., Shields, J. A., *et al.* Carcinoembryonic antigen-positive metastatic adenocarcinoma of the choroid. Arch. Ophthalmol. *93:*794 (1975).
4. Michelson, J. B., Felberg, N. T., and Shields, J. A. Carcinoembryonic antigen: its role in the evaluation of intraocular malignant tumors. *Arch. Ophthalmol. 94:*414 (1976).
5. Michelson, J. B., Felberg, N. T., and Shields, J. A. Evaluation of metastatic cancer to the eye. Arch. Ophthalmol. *95:*692 (1977).
6. Denslow, G. T. and Kielar, R. A. Metastatic adenocarcinoma to the anterior uvea and increased carcinoembryonic antigen levels. Am. J. Ophthalmol. *85:*363 (1978).
7. Bullock, J. D. Carcinoembryonic antigen in neuro-ophthalmic diagnosis. Audio-digest Ophthalmol. *16:* (May 25, 1978).
8. Gold, P. and Freedman, S. O. Demonstration of tumor-specific antigens in human colonic carcinomata by immunological tolerance and absorption techniques. J. Exp. Med. *121:*439 (1965).
9. Gold, P. and Freedman, S. O. Specific carcinoembryonic antigens of the human digestive system. J. Exp. Med. *122:*467 (1965).
10. Hansen, H. J., Snyder, J. J., Miller, E., *et al.* Carcinoembryonic antigen (CEA) assay. Hum. Pathol. *5:*139 (1974).
11. Ashman, L. K., Ludbrook, J., and Marshall, V. R. Probabilistic application of plasma carcinoembryonic antigen assay in cancer patients. Br. Med. J. *2:*721 (1975).

21 Ultrasonography in the Diagnosis of Endocrine Orbitopathy

Harold W. Skalka, M.D.

The hyperthyroid patient or the patient with a clear history of thyroid dysfunction who shows the characteristic physical findings and laboratory correlates of endocrine orbitopathy ("Graves' disease," "dysthyroid ophthalmopathy," "endocrine exophthalmos," etc.) may pose a problem in nomenclature, but does not present a problem in diagnosis. Lid lag and retraction, puffy lid edema, orbicularis fasciculations, stare, proptosis, conjunctival injection most marked over the medial and lateral rectus insertions, subconjunctival edema, motility restrictions with diplopia, elevation of intraocular pressure on attempted gaze into the field of restricted motility, positive forced ductions, evidence of bilateral involvement, etc. produce a classical clinical picture. Elevation of serum triiodothyronine (T_3), thyroxine (T_4), and T_7 levels, together with an abnormal Werner suppression test, limn the biochemical abnormalities present.

In point of fact, the textbook patient with endocrine orbitopathy is in the minority, and the findings in nearly all patients with this disorder deviate to a greater or lesser extent from this idealized picture. Often, the diagnosis is quite difficult to make, is presumed rather than established, and is made after long, costly, and often inconvenient laboratory and neuroradiologic evaluation.

Most patients with endocrine orbitopathy are euthyroid, judged both by clinical and serum (T_3 and T_4) parameters. In our experience, nearly half the patients with this disorder have no known history of thyroid disease. While some[1] have found the Werner suppression test to be positive in as many as 86% of "euthyroid" patients with ophthalmopathy, others[2] (ourselves included) have obtained positive tests in only half such patients. In any event, the incidence of false negatives is too high to allow reliance on a negative (normal) Werner suppression test.

The plethora of tests which continue to be developed to aid in the diagnosis of euthyroid Graves' disease are testimony to the inadequacy of all. Serum LATS determinations,[3] immunologic and genetic studies,[4-6] and the thyrotropic releasing hormone (TRH) test[7] represent some of the more recent attempts to provide reliable procedures for the diagnosis of endocrine orbitopathy.

Computerized tomography (CT) has made tremendous advances over the past few years, and modern fine-matrix, thin-section scans can demonstrate significant extraocular muscle and "optic nerve" thickenings. By using the newer coronal section techniques, the thickened muscles can be demonstrated in cross section. However, the factors of cost, availability, radiation, reproducibility, and residual diagnostic confusion (e.g., with mass lesions of the orbital apex) continue to limit the diagnostic and prognostic (e.g., is therapy having the desired tissue effects?) contributions of CT in this disorder.

In all affected patients, but especially in the euthyroid patient who presents with unilateral lid retraction or proptosis, or has diplopia, ultrasonic evaluation of the rectus muscles, retrobulbar optic nerves, and other orbital tissues[8-14] is the simplest, safest, and most accurate and reproducible method of diagnosing (or disproving) the existence of endocrine orbitopathy. B-scan examination, whether performed by the contact or water-bath method, can qualitatively show muscle and optic nerve alterations (somewhat analogous to good CT studies) (Figs. 1 and 2), as well as alterations in the reflectivity of the orbital fat. However, A-scan ultrasonic biometry allows quantitative measurements to be made of both extraocular muscle thicknesses and perineural optic nerve alterations (Figs. 3 and 4). By using these atraumatic A-scan techniques, serial determinations may be made over time, allowing observation of evolution and devolution of specific sites of involvement.

McNutt[9] has developed data for rectus muscle sizes and variations in the normal population. We have previously determined[10] that the normal retrobulbar optic nerve dural diameter exceeds the neural diameter by 1.50 mm or less, and that this diameter difference is greater in endocrine orbitopathy.[14] The increasing popularity and availability of A-scan instrumentation for the axial length determinations used in computing intraocular lens powers insures wide availability of this modality for these other facets of orbital biometry.

Endocrine orbitopathy is the commonest cause of unilateral proptosis,[15] and of spontaneous diplopia in middle age and early

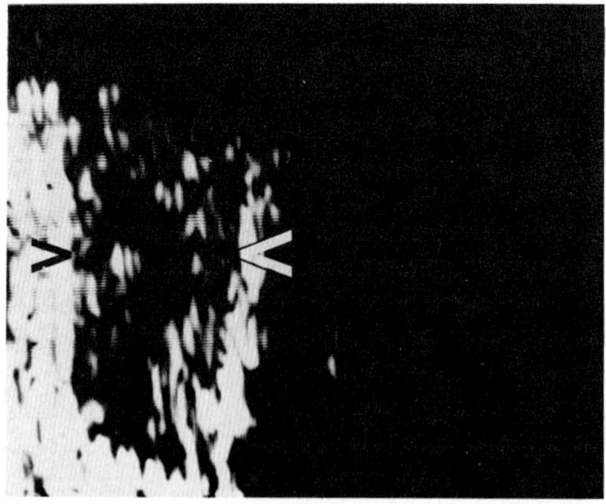

Fig. 1. Contact B-scan photo of left medial rectus muscle (between arrowheads) of patient with endocrine orbitopathy. Interior of globe is off picture to the left, and white arrowhead straddles medial orbital wall.

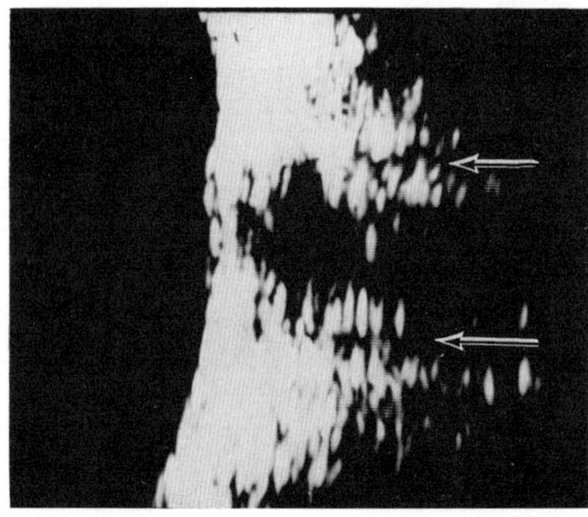

Fig. 2. Contact B-scan photo showing retrobulbar optic nerve in a patient with endocrine orbitopathy. Vitreous cavity is on left side of photo. Arrows lie in perineural space, between neural and dural surfaces.

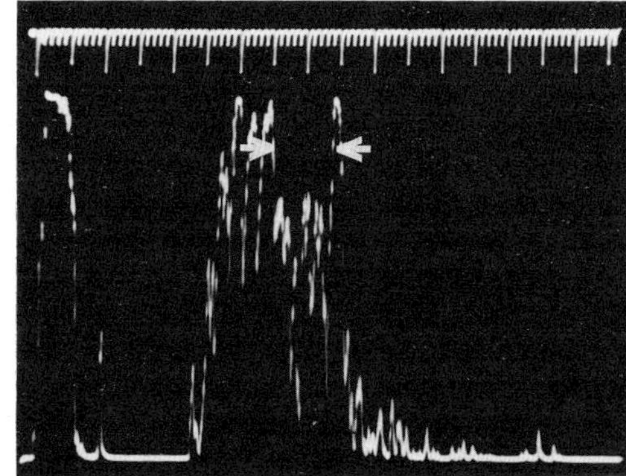

Fig. 3. A-scan photo of medial rectus muscle seen in Figure 1. Probe placed on temporal sclera and aimed medially, with sound beam passing perpendicularly through the medial rectus muscle. Interior of globe is on left side of tracing. Thickness of the medial rectus muscle may be measured between the steeply rising muscle surface echo spikes (arrows).

senescence.[16] The clinical presentation is often unilateral, and we have seen a number of patients with this disease who had undergone, or were scheduled for, neurosurgical or orbital exploration for their presumed tumors (many having had unrevealing or misleading CT studies). Patients with a history of a previous malignancy seem especially prone to be diagnosed as having metastatic disease when orbital abnormalities are found. It is important to realize that endocrine orbitopathy is a bilateral disease, even if clinical involvement is only

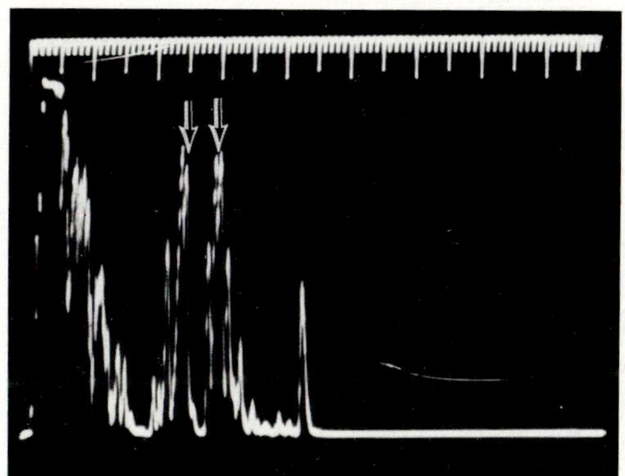

Fig. 4. A-scan photo of retrobulbar optic nerve of patient with endocrine orbitopathy. Probe is placed at lateral canthus and angled back, with sound beam passing perpendicularly through retrobulbar optic nerve. Arrows point to double spiked echoes from proximal and distal nerve surfaces. The outer spikes are echoes from the dural surface, and the inner spikes are neural surface echoes. The perineural space is the gap between the spikes at each arrow, and is only slightly enlarged in this patient.

unilaterally apparent. A-scan biometry will almost invariably show bilateral abnormalities in such cases, and thus help rule out spurious diagnoses which the patient's clinical appearance might otherwise suggest.

Thickening of extraocular muscles (and perineural enlargement) may occur with orbital inflammations such as inflammatory pseudotumors, or diseases of striated muscle such as myotonia congenita, but the clinical picture in such entities is usually sufficient for diagnosis. In the vast majority of cases, there is little with which to confuse the ultrasonic diagnosis of endocrine orbitopathy.

While specific rectus size parameters and techniques of muscle and nerve measurements may be obtained from the references herein cited, a few specific examples are briefly presented to illustrate the often frustrating clinical dilemmas and the straightforward ultrasound resolutions which may be expected:

Case I. A 48-year-old white male developed proptosis OD six years previously, and underwent a neurosurgical exploration of the right orbit via a frontal flap. No tumor was found. He had recently developed $3\frac{1}{2}$ mm of proptosis OS. Thyroid function studies were normal, and a CT scan showed left maxillary sinusitis and a "mass" of the pos-

terior left orbit. He was referred for orbital ultrasonography, which revealed enlarged perineural spaces around both retrobulbar optic nerves (2.06 mm OD, 2.25 mm OS) and enlargement of rectus muscles OU (right superior rectus, left medial, inferior and lateral recti). The left inferior and lateral recti were thickened well beyond the 100th percentile of the normal population. The orbital fat echo pattern was prolonged OU, more so OS, and no masses (other than the thickened extraocular muscles) were present. A diagnosis of endocrine orbitopathy was made.

Case II. A 62-year-old white female had undergone radical surgery for carcinoma of the cervix seven years previously. She had noted proptosis OS for the past year. There was no diplopia and no history of thyroid disease. Medical, ophthalmologic and radiologic evaluation elsewhere had been unrevealing. A metastasis was suspected. Ultrasonographic biometry revealed enlarged perineural spaces OU (2.06 mm OD, 2.50 mm OS), as well as enlargement of all rectus muscles OU except the right lateral rectus (with marked thickening of the left superior and inferior recti). There were no other masses present in either orbit. A diagnosis of endocrine orbitopathy was made.

Case III. A 52-year-old white male was referred for surgical treatment of an "orbital tumor" OS. He had developed 8 mm of proptosis OS over the past year (Fig. 5). Visual acuity was good OU, but there was diplopia on upgaze. Orbital x-rays were unremarkable, and thyroid function studies (T_3, T_4, T_7) were within normal limits. There was no history of thyroid disease.

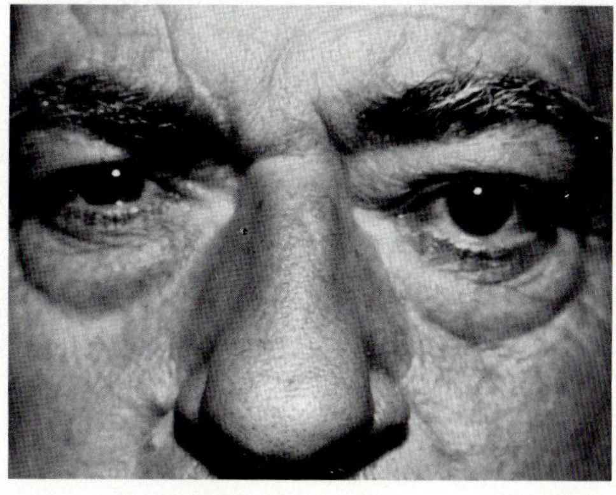

Fig. 5. Case III. Patient with 8 mm of proptosis OS.

Ultrasonography revealed enlargement of all four rectus muscles OS (with marked enlargement of the medial and superior recti), as well as of three rectus muscles OD (Fig. 6). No other orbital masses were noted. A diagnosis of endocrine orbitopathy was made.

The commonest abnormal physical findings in the last 80 patients with endocrine orbitopathy that we have seen have been lid retraction and proptosis (usually unilateral). Only 40% had any current or past history of diplopia. While our patients represent a referral population and may be expected to show less florid or "classical" presentations of this disorder, endocrine orbitopathy is a relatively common orbital disease which may be clinically subtle. The absence of apparent bilaterality or positive forced ductions should not point the examiner away from this diagnosis any more than should normal thyroid function studies.

The diagnosis of endocrine orbitopathy

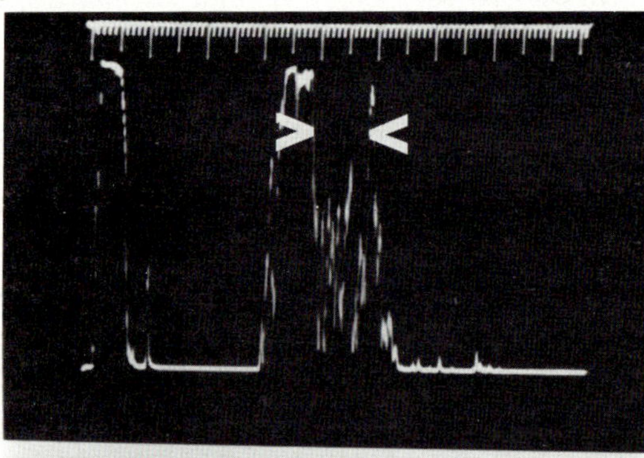

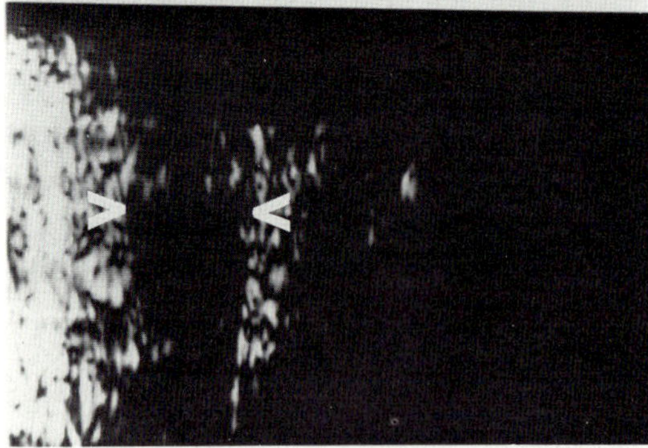

Fig. 6. Left medial rectus muscle of Case III. A-scan above, contact B-scan below. Orientation as in previous figures. Left medial rectus muscle is between arrowheads.

is best made by careful history, thorough physical examination, and A-scan ultrasonographic biometry. The ability of ultrasonography to diagnosis endocrine orbitopathy and differentiate this entity from other etiologies of orbital disease is highly reliable and reproducible. This technique is quantitative, atraumatic, and has no known morbid potential. The thyroid status of the patient in question may be investigated if such information is desired or if an abnormal metabolic state is felt to exist for which specific therapy is indicated. Patients with endocrine orbitopathy do not require angiography, computerized tomography, isotope studies, or other expensive or invasive procedures for diagnosis.

EDITOR'S NOTE

I have to be very careful as to what I say here for several reasons. First of all is that I have a good respect for Dr. Skalka's work and for his ability to express himself. In fact, when I read the last sentence of his first paragraph of this paper where he described several tests that "limn" the biochemical abnormalities present, I thought this was a misprint—and that it should have been "lead." To be sure, however, I looked in Webster's Unabridged and found that *LIMN* is a transitive verb (from Latin, illuminare, to make light) with the following three meanings:

1. To draw or paint, portray, delineate.
2. To illuminate, as manuscripts (obsolete).
3. To portray in words; to describe.

Therefore, Dr. Skalka was quite correct in using this "spiffy" verb to tell us that the T_3, T_4, T_7 and Werner tests do *describe*, *delineate*, or *portray* the biochemical abnormalities present. I was really impressed with his using that word, for today's journals are written, it seems to me, to often actually make things hard to understand. Maybe that's why Webster's Dictionary pointed out that *"to illuminate, as manuscripts"* is an *obsolete* way to use the verb "limn"!

Now, I agree completely with his comments about the diagnosis of endocrine orbitopathy being a *clinical* diagnosis. The majority of patients I see are totally euthyroid—both chemically and clinically. Yet, they show lid retraction, puffy orbits, tight inferior and medial recti, and all of the signs we can recognize by looking at the patient out in the waiting room. We have used the "Thypinone" test (TRH suppression test) and found it also is positive in about half the cases of euthyroid Graves' disease. Unfortunately, the Werner test is also positive in only about half these cases—but there is no good overlap between the "Thypinone" and the Werner tests. The "Thypinone" (I put this in quotation marks as this is the name for Abbott's protirelin, as that is what you really write on the prescription) test has the advantage that you can do it all in one day, however. You simply draw a serum TSH, give the patient an injection of "Thypinone," and draw another serum TSH 30 minutes later. The patient should be lying down during that 30 minutes, they say.

I personally feel that ultrasound and CT scans are really seldom needed to diagnose thyroid eye disease. Of the two, I'd prefer the CT in this area, however, for I believe that ultrasonography really requires somebody expert in its use. The reason I don't like "A"-scans as well as "B"-scans is that I am just an eyeball doctor, and can draw no conclusions whatever from the lines they show me on A-scan. In other words, they could be showing me the documentary record of a seismograph in California, and I wouldn't know that from a metastasis in orbit. The "B"-scan at least shows a picture that will allow me to recognize if it looks like an eye, and whether or not it technically looks good. "A"-scan is very much in vogue, however, for linear measurements of the eye to determine the power of an intraocular lens, however, and I suspect that has really given it its "shot in the arm." I'm not trying to discourage ultrasound in neuroophthalmology, but for orbit, optic nerve, and muscle work, I have found the CT scan preferable. If Dr. Skalka were in Miami, however, I'd probably learn more from him than that! Finally, you might try a drop of 0.5% TIMOLOL (timoptic) for lid retraction cases and see how it works. Dr. Costin suggested this in one lady, and she wrote

back that it helped. We are going to try and look into that a bit more!

JLS

REFERENCES

1. Ivy, H. K. Medical approach to ophthalmopathy of Graves' disease. Mayo Clin. Proc. *47*:980 (1972).
2. Fells, T., Doniach, D., and El Kabir, D. J. Diagnosis of dysthyroid exophthalmos, Trans. Opthalmol. Soc. UK *90*:251–260 (1970).
3. McKenzie, J. M. Hormonal factors in the pathogenesis of Graves' disease. Phys. Rev. *48*:252 (1968).
4. Werner, S. C., Wegelius, O., Fierer, J. A., and Hsu, K. C. Immunoglobulins (E, M, G) and complement in the connective tissues of the thyroid in Graves' disease, New Engl. J. Med. *287*:421–425 (1972).
5. Lamki, L., Row, V. V., and Volpé, R. Cell-mediated immunity in Graves' disease and in Hashimoto's thyroiditis as shown by the demonstration of migration inhibition factor (MIF). J. Clin. Endocrinol. Metab. *36*:358–364 (1973).
6. Grumet, F. C., Payne, R. O., Konishi, J., and Kriss, J. P. HL-A antigens as markers for disease susceptibility and autoimmunity in Graves' disease. J. Clin. Endocrinol. Metab. *39*:1115–1119 (1974).
7. Hyman, B. N. and Johnson, P. C. Thyrotropic releasing hormone: A test to diagnose Graves' ophthalmopathy, In: *XXIII International Congress of Ophthalmology, 1978*, Excerpta Medica, Amsterdam, In Press.
8. Ossoinig, K. C. Echography of the eye, orbit and periorbital region. In: *Radiology of the Orbit*, P. H. Arger (Ed.), Wiley, New York, 1977.
9. McNutt, L. Ultrasound of Graves' Orbitopathy. Seminar, Dept. of Ophthalmology, University of Iowa, April 16, 1975.
10. Skalka, H. W. Quantitative ultrasonographic determination of perineural optic nerve cerebrospinal fluid. In: *Ultrasound in Medicine, Vol. 3A. Clinical Aspects.* Plenum, New York, 1977, pp. 1029–1042.
11. Skalka, H. W. The optic nerve in endocrine orbitopathy. In: *Proceedings of the 16th ISCERG Symposium, Ghent, Belgium, June 1977*, In press.
12. Coleman, D. J., Jack, R. L., Franzen, L. A., *et al.* High resolution B-scan ultrasonography of the orbit: V. Eye changes of Graves' disease. Arch. Ophthalmol. *88*:405–471 (1972).
13. Werner, S. C., Coleman, D. J., and Franzen, L. A.: Ultrasonographic evidence of a consistent orbital involvement in Graves' disease. New Engl. J. Med. *290*:1447–1450 (1974).
14. Skalka, H. W. Perineural optic nerve changes in endocrine orbitopathy. Arch. Ophthalmol. *96*:468–473 (1978).
15. Reese, A. B. *Tumors of the Eye.* 3rd ed. Harper and Row, Hagerstown, Md., 1976, p. 440.
16. Glaser, J. S., In: *Clinical Ophthalmology.* T. D. Duane (Ed.), Harper and Row, Hagerstown, Md., 1976, Vol. 2, Chap. 12.

22 Simple Pediatric Ocular Electrodiagnosis

Alistair R. Fielder, F.R.C.S.

Clinicians are periodically confronted with children in whom a visual problem is either an isolated entity or part of a more generalized illness; investigation into the possible site of visual pathway involvement may be aided by the use of certain electrodiagnostic tests, and in certain instances these may be the only method of establishing a definitive diagnosis.

The semiquantitative nature of the electroretinogram (ERG) was stressed by Charles[1] as it is known that it may vary unpredictably from hour to hour[2] and day to day.[3] It may also be affected by sedation or anesthesia.[4, 5] Marmor[6] reported in 1976 on the instability of the corneal ERG in unsedated children. The effect of anesthesia on the visual evoked response (VER) is said to be considerable.[7]

I have therefore decided to utilize the method described initially by Harden and Pampiglione[8] concerning the noncorneal ERG and VER. As the amplitude of the ERG recorded in this way is small, averaging techniques are required; but neither sedation nor anesthesia are necessary, and both responses may be recorded either simultaneously (Harden and Pampiglione) or at the same sitting, as in this laboratory. Tests can thus be repeated as often as required either to study the kinetics of visual pathway pathology, or to study the evolution of the normal VER in the very young infant.

It should be remembered that the configuration of the VER changes rapidly during development, and for a review of this subject I refer the reader to articles by Maurer, Karmel, and Harter.[9-11] It is imperative for each laboratory to establish its own normal values.

Both ERG and VER are measured on a Medelec MS6 modular electrophysiological system fitted with a DAV6 digital averager, and the investigations are performed in a darkened room. Either 64 or 128 sweeps are averaged, photographed onto Kodak Linagraph Direct Print Paper, and traced onto graph paper for ease of calculation. An SLE stroboscope is used, which at intensity I delivers 0.09 and at intensity IV 0.23 joules per flash, with a stimulus duration of 0.1 msec. For routine testing a flash rate of two per second is used; however, the rate may be increased for flicker. The strobe is hand-held 15 cm from the eyes, and while fixation usually presents little difficulty in the baby, the more discriminating older infant requires interest to maintain fixation (Figs. 1–3). One of our technicians found that by sticking white translucent tape onto the strobe cover, the infant remained fascinated and fixated on the light until he managed to peel the tape off. Although flash VER is described in this article, the use of pattern flash[11] has provided most satisfactory results and is now being used routinely in addition to the former.

Silver, silver chloride electrodes are used with Beckman Electrode paste and are positioned for the VER at 2 cm above the inion, at the vertex, and the earth electrode behind the ear. ERG electrodes are placed at the nasion, vertex, and behind the ear, although other positions have been suggested by Noonan *et al.*[12] and used by Jones and France.[13] It is obviously imperative to test each eye individually in neuro-ophthalmic patients.

There is certainly more inter-eye variation (in amplitude not latency) than reported in adult corneal ERG estimations. The following values for latency and amplitude are included only to indicate approxi-

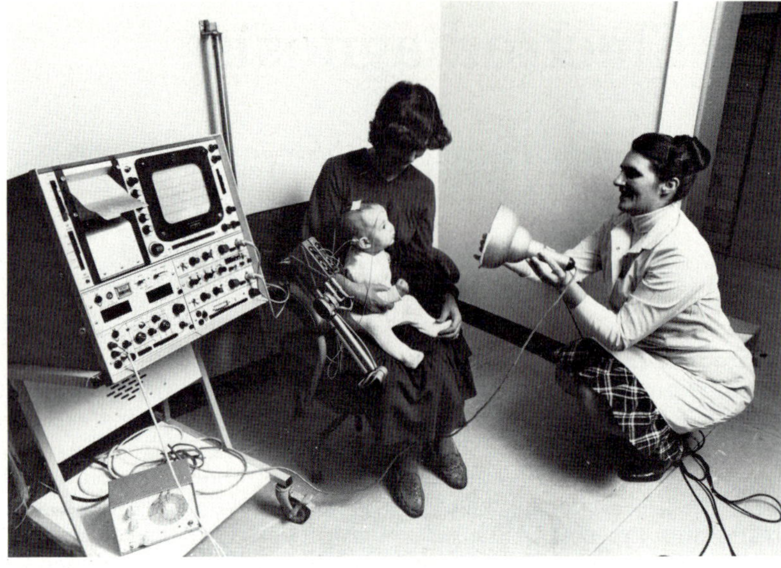

Figs. 1–3. Tests may be performed either on a couch or in mother's arms. The placement of the electrodes can be seen, and as can be clearly seen from the expression on this four-month-old's face, no serious discomfort is experienced. The trolley-mounted Medelec system is shown.

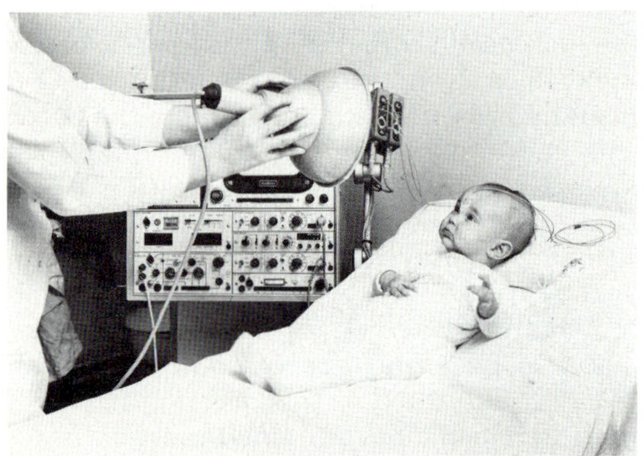

Fig. 2

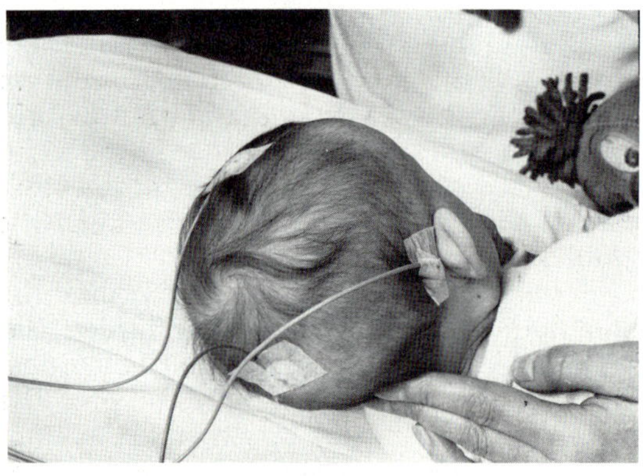

Fig. 3

mately the noncorneal ERG amplitudes obtained in our own laboratory. Implicit times for the "a" wave vary between 10 and 25 msec and "b" wave between 35 and 50 msec. "a" wave amplitude cannot be calculated reliably, but "b" wave (peak to peak) varies from 4.0 to 25.0 μV as compared to 75–600 μV for the corneal ERG. These figures correlate approximately with those given by Harden,[14] although her results refer only to binocular responses.

The indications for electrodiagnostic tests in children with absent or minimal ophthalmoscopic findings have been well described elsewhere,[4, 15] and therefore a few conditions only will be considered.

ACHROMATOPSIA

Achromatopsia (rod monochromatism) requires an ERG for definitive diagnosis as indicated in the following case. Infant N.T. was noted to have nystagmus at six weeks of age, but light aversion and reduction of vision in sunny conditions were not noted until she began to walk. Neurological examination was normal, and with the exception of fine rapid nystagmus, which did not diminish on fixation, no ocular abnormality was detected, and in particular foveal reflexes and maculae were normal. The ERG (binocular) Figure 4 shows both "a" and "b" waves at two flashes per second, but

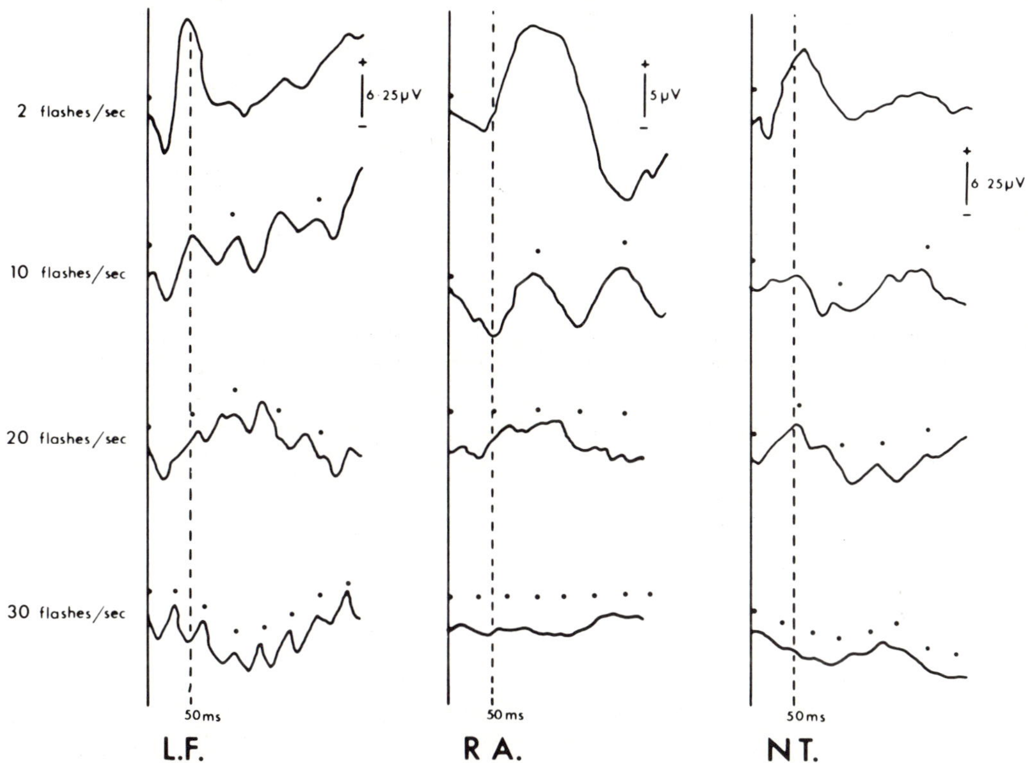

Fig. 4. Binocular ERG's of a normal child (L.F.), adult with achromatopsia (R.A.), and infant (N.T.) with nystagmus and light aversion. Dots above the tracings indicate stimuli.

diminishing "b" wave amplitude with increasing rates until at 30 flashes per second no response can be identified, indicating defective cone function. The tracings of N.T. should be compared with the normal responses in a four-year-old girl (L.F.), and in a 30-year-old woman (N.A.) with achromatopsia.

DELAYED VISUAL DEVELOPMENT

Delayed visual development is an interesting condition, by no means rare, in which babies are noted, characteristically at six weeks of age, to exhibit little or no visual interest. There is no relevant family, pregnancy, or obstetric history. Post-natally, with the exception of the visual deficit, development is normal. On examination at this time vision may range from no reaction to a blink reflex to bright light. No optically elicited movements, including opticokinetic nystagmus, can be demonstrated, and pupillary reactions are normal. Optic discs may appear slightly grey as previously reported.[16] Neurological assessment is normal. Vision improves, often rapidly, within a few months, and following this improvement no visual disability can be detected clinically. Electrodiagnosis at an early stage is of importance as demonstrated in Figure 5 concerning case D. F., which shows at two months of age, when there was minimal reaction to light, a normal ERG, and while N1, P2, and N2 waves can just be identified in the VER, the trace is abnormal and of very low amplitude. As visual responsiveness improves, the VER assumes a more normal configuration as can be seen on comparing the two traces of this infant. The VER tracing of a normal infant seven weeks of age is presented for comparison (Fig. 6). The presence of an ERG distinguishes this condition from Leber's amaurosis, and the VER, although abnormal, is not typical of cortical blindness, enabling the clinician to cautiously reassure the parents. The etiology of this condition is unknown, and discussion of the various proposed theories beyond the scope of this article.

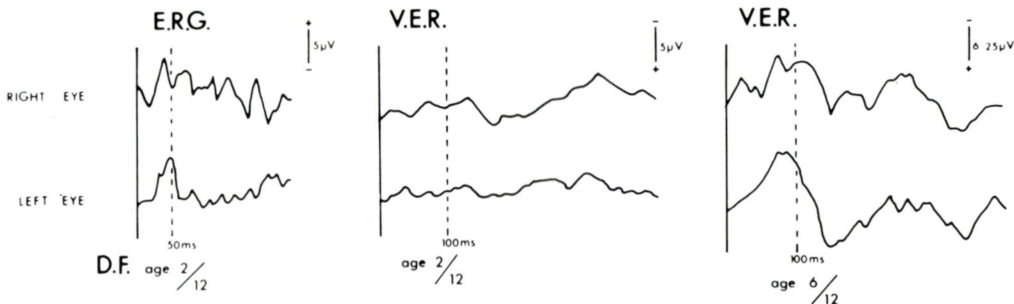

Fig. 5. Delayed visual development (D.F.). Normal ERG but reduced flash VER at two months of age, the latter showing considerable improvement at six months. The point of stimulation is the beginning of the trace in this and all the other figures.

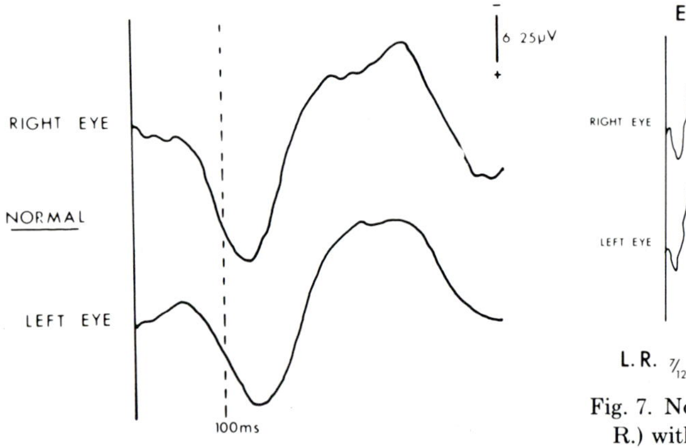

Fig. 6. Normal flash VER at seven weeks.

NEUROLOGICAL ILLNESS

Visual problems can occur during the course of a systemic illness, and electrodiagnostic tests may aid localization of the defect, either to indicate or prevent further neurological investigation. Electrodiagnosis in neurometabolic storage diseases of childhood has been reviewed by Harden and Pampiglione[17] and will not be considered further. In this situation, in contrast to many pediatric ophthalmic problems there are two new complicating factors:

1. Further assessment may be necessary due to a rapidly changing clinical condition.
2. Sedation or anesthesia for electrodiagnosis may not be justified due to the severity of the illness.

Therefore, if these tests are indicated,

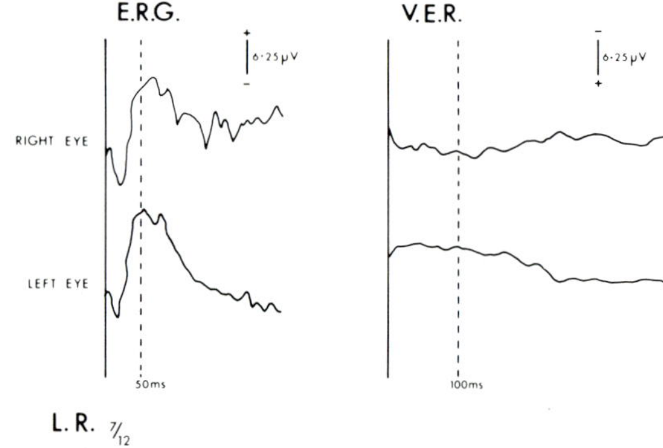

Fig. 7. Normal ERG but absent VER in an infant (L. R.) with severe bilateral optic nerve hypoplasia.

they must be simple, and not inconvenience the patient; therefore, the noncorneal ERG and VER as described in this article are ideal. Due to the simplicity of the apparatus (mounted on a wheeled trolley) tests may even be performed at the bedside.

Optic Nerve Dysfunction. Severe bilateral optic nerve hypoplasia produces a normal ERG but almost flat VER, as shown by infant L.R. (Fig. 7), a severely retarded eight-month-old infant with aqueduct stenosis and hydrocephalus. EMI scan indicated the presence of an intact septum pellucidum.

Cortical Blindness. In the absence of a pediatric case in which one cannot be certain that cortical blindness is not associated with further visual pathway pathology, the case cited concerns an adult, D. T., a 61-year-old man, with a previous history of hypertension, ischemic heart, and cerebrovascular disease, who suddenly, while eating a meal, became completely blind. There was no perception of light in either eye, but

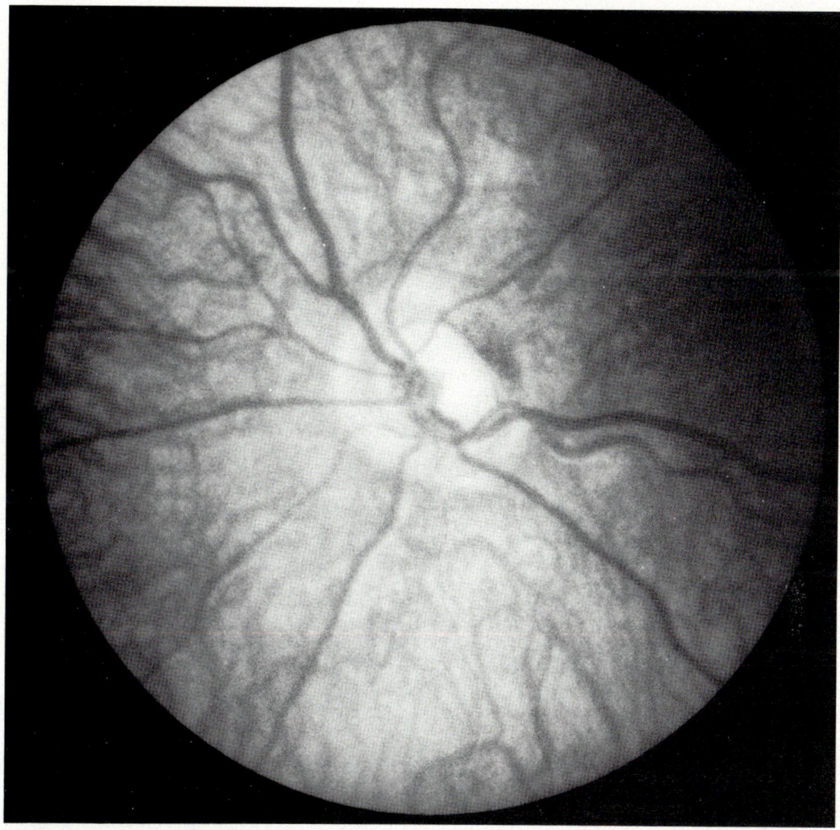

Fig. 8. Optic nerve hypoplasia: the disc appearance of L.R.

ocular findings including pupillary reflexes were entirely normal. As expected, in a defect of such severity, the ERG is normal but the VER absent (Fig. 10).

Acute Neurological Illness. In acute neurological illness, visual pathway involvement may arise as an integral part of the main pathological process, resulting from secondary or tertiary effects of this process, or a combination of these; and it may be extremely difficult to differentiate these clinically. It would be naive to expect electrodiagnostic tests to offer accurate localization; however, they may be affected well before definite physical signs develop, and this is of particular importance in children who may become mute and difficult to evaluate.

Case D. A., a four-year-old boy, developed an intermittent right sixth nerve paresis a week before suddenly becoming unconscious and convulsing. He was transferred to the Neurosurgical Unit of this hospital, unrousable with fixed dilated pu-

pils but no focal signs. On inserting an intraventricular pressure line, intracranial pressure was found to be very high and slow decompression was performed. The next day he was responding to painful stimuli but was thought to be blind. No visual response could be elicited, pupils were 3 mm and fixed, and there was a partial right sixth paresis and papilloedema. As indicated in Figure 11, the VER was essentially absent. Positive contrast ventriculography revealed a large tumor in the region of the posterior third ventricle; a ventriculo-peritoneal shunt were therefore inserted and radiotherapy arranged.

Among the possible causes of the visual loss in this case considered were: cortical blindness following tentorial herniation, tumor compression (most unlikely), or involvement of the anterior visual pathway from either raised intracranial pressure or its decompression. Over the ensuing month this boy remained mute and blind, but the absence of signs of occipital infarction on

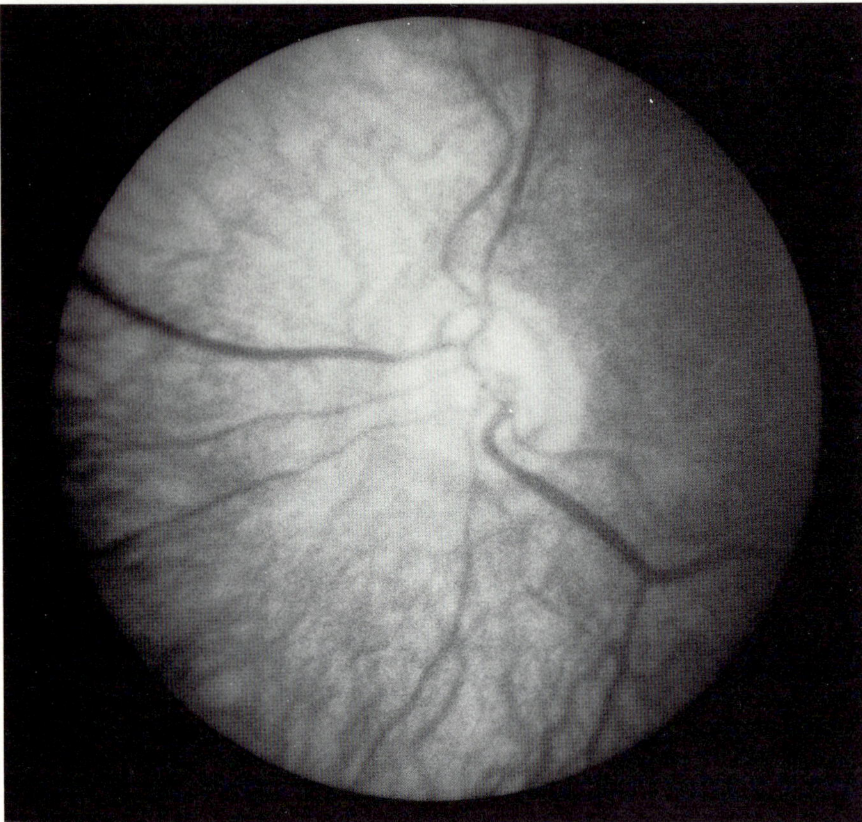

Fig. 9. Optic nerve hypoplasia: the disc appearance of L.R.

the EMI scan and the subsequent development of gross optic atrophy indicated involvement of the anterior visual pathway. In the early stages of this illness when the child was mute and difficult to evaluate, the absent VER preceded the development of optic atrophy by approximately three weeks.

Recently a five-year-old girl became akinetic and mute following a road traffic accident, but, in contrast to the preceding case, there were good opticokinetic responses and normal VER's, enabling cautious optimism to be expressed regarding the presence of vision.

Case P. O. is a boy aged eight years who was admitted to the Neurosurgical Unit under the care of Mr. John Firth, as was case D. A., with encephalitis, raised intracranial pressure, and bilateral optic neuritis. Initially he was very ill, had no perception of light, and both discs were swollen and contained hemorrhages. By the time the first VER was measured (at the bedside due to intracranial pressure monitoring), vision was improving, being approximately right 6/18, left counting fingers, and he was able to identify the color of a large red target on the right but not on the left. The delay of P2 of the VER in optic neuritis is well known, and has recently received considerable attention in the literature[18]; as can be seen from the first trace from the left eye (technical difficulties prevented obtaining a trace from the right eye), the waveform is grossly reduced and P2 at 250 msec is delayed (normal in this laboratory 95–120 msec). The improvement in amplitudes and reduction in P2 latency in each eye over the ensuing weeks can be seen concomitant with the visual recovery to 6/9 part in each eye, indicating how this test may be used to follow clinical progress (Fig. 12).

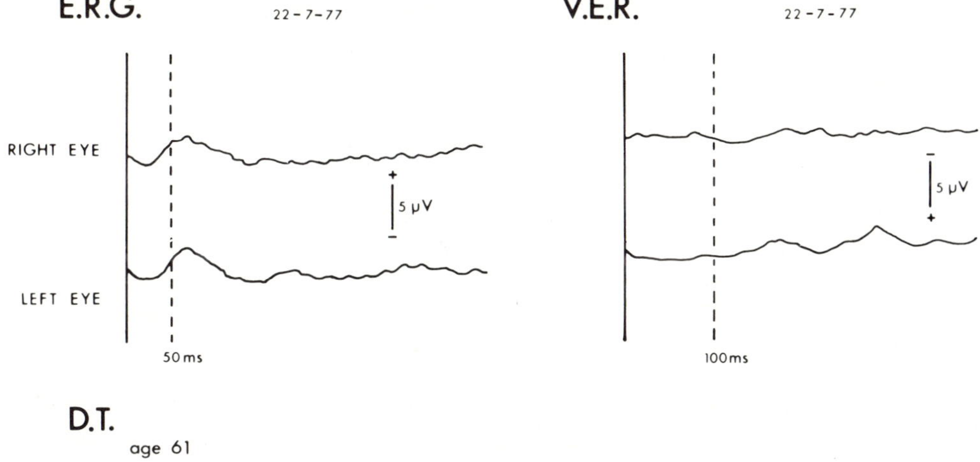

Fig. 10. Cortical blindness (D. T.), showing normal ERG but absent VER.

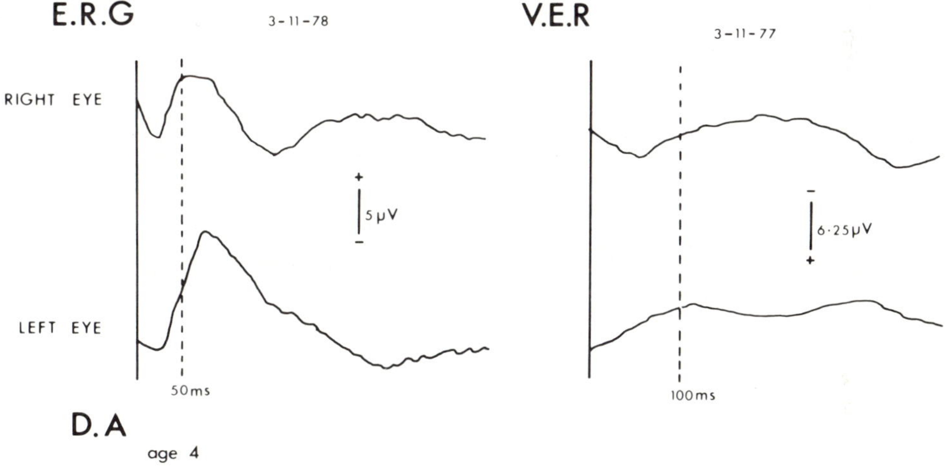

Fig. 11. Absent VER but good ERG in case (D. A.).

These tests are no substitute for clinical examination, but conversely serve to heighten the degree of clinical suspicion in the early stages of neurological illness rather than simply waiting for the development of obvious physical signs.

Combined Retinal and Neurological Pathology. This may occur in trauma, and in the case illustrated this was nonaccidental. Baby P. H. was admitted aged seven weeks with blood in the CSF, bilateral subdural hematomata, and extensive bilateral retinal hemorrhages (Fig. 13). Initially there was no reaction to light, but as the hemorrhages cleared, he appeared to be developing normally visually, although neurologically he was found to be slightly retarded. Clearly the physical signs were so gross that electrodiagnostic tests had no localizing value in the acute phase, as the ERG and consequently the VER would both be affected (Fig. 14). However, as the baby improved, the ERG's of both eyes improved, but the left VER remained abnormal both in waveform, affecting predominantly the early components, and amplitude (Fig. 14). This eye is now developing a convergent squint, there is no ophthalmoscopically visible retinal pathology (Fig. 15), significant ametropia, and therefore it

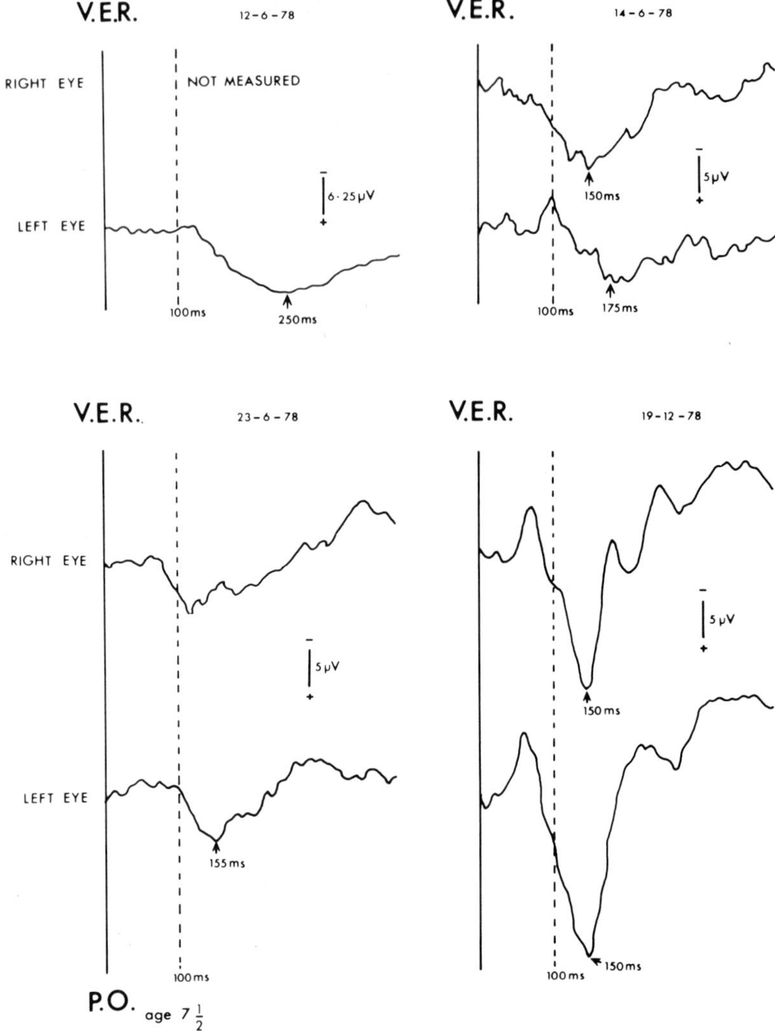

Fig. 12. Bilateral acute optic neuritis (P.O.). Note increase in VER amplitude and decrease in P2 latencies over the ensuing weeks.

is likely that this defect is central to the retina. This case is cited purely to remind the clinician that dual pathology may exist, and that failure of normalization of either of these responses in a clinically improving situation should ensure continued observation.

MULTIPLE HANDICAP

Finally clinical visual assessment in re-tarded mentally handicapped children is often difficult, and these investigations may be performed even in the presence of nystagmus and poor patient cooperation. That normal clinical electrophysiology cannot necessarily be equated with normal vision is well known. However, a defect, if detected, at any level in the visual pathway may lead to more sympathetic or appropriate care of the child.

In this article the electrodiagnostic pro-

Fig. 13. Fundus appearance of nonaccidental injury, baby (P. H.), in October 1977.

Fig. 14. Combined retinal and neurological pathology, infant (P. H.). The top two tracings are ERG's the second, on the right, showing considerable improvement over the first. Although the second VER shows improvement compared to the first, it is still abnormal on the left.

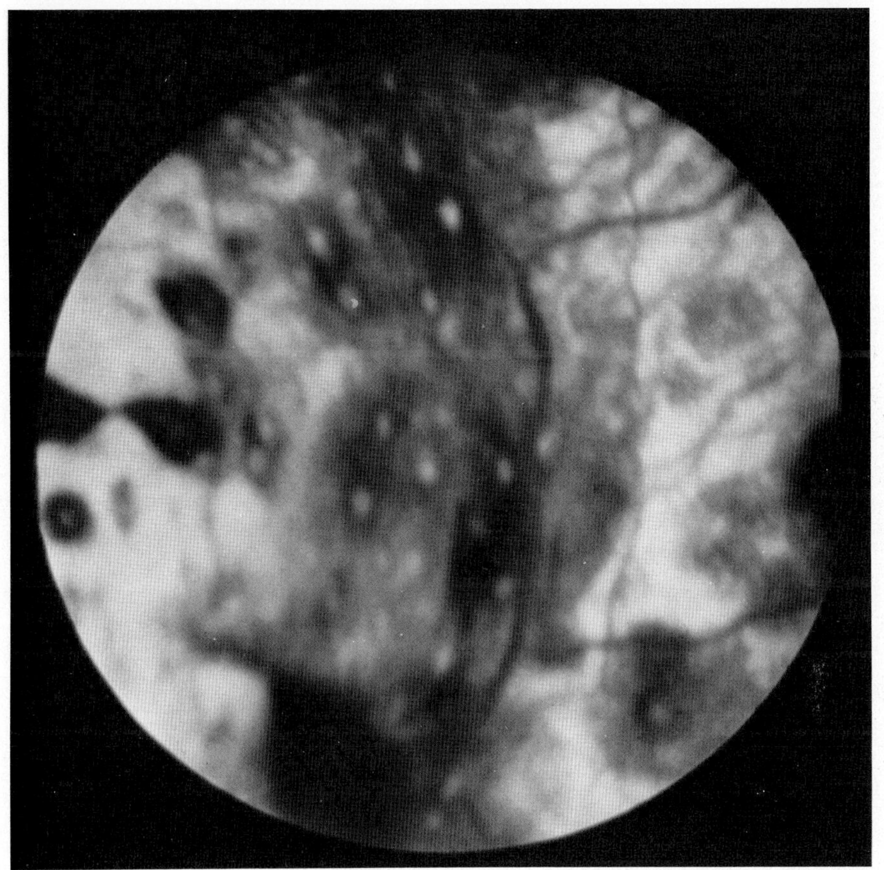
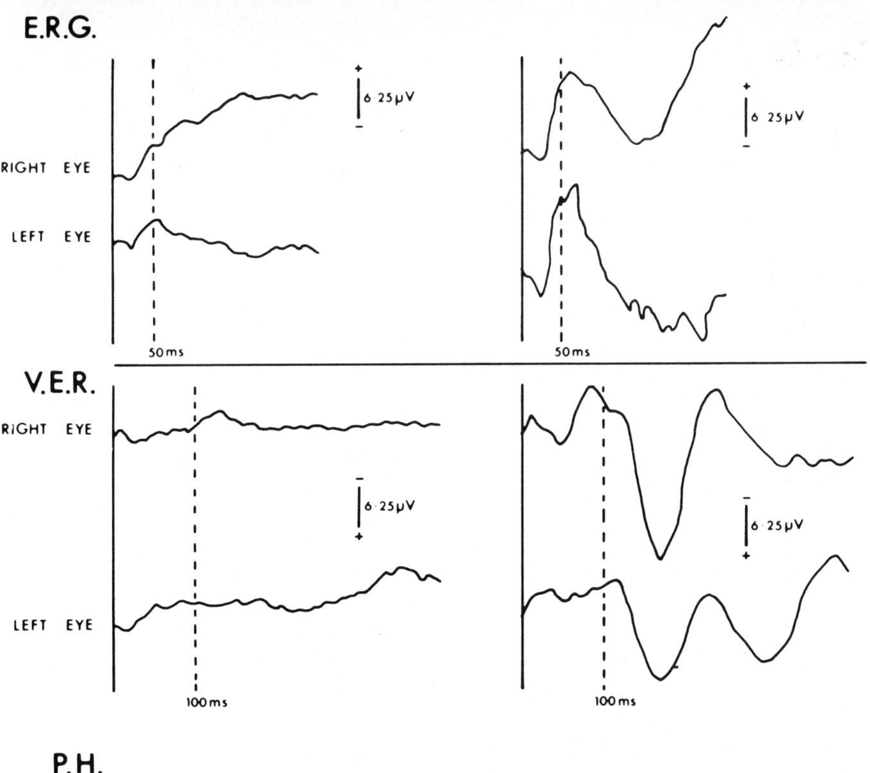

E.R.G.
6·25μV
RIGHT EYE
LEFT EYE
50ms
6·25μV
50ms
V.E.R.
RIGHT EYE
6·25μV
LEFT EYE
100ms
6·25μV
100ms
P.H.
age 7/52
age 13/12

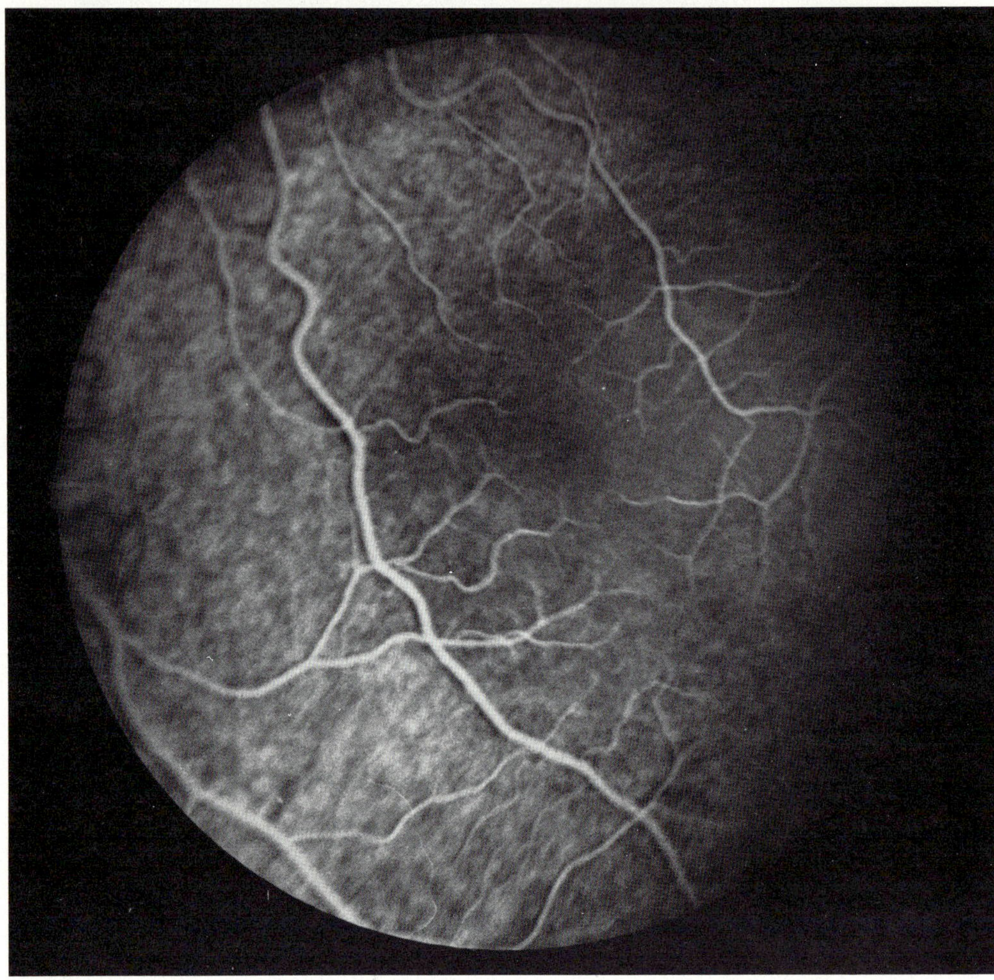

Fig. 15. Fluorescein angiogram of baby (P. H.), one year later than the previous figure, showing, this time, a normal left macula and vascular architecture.

cedures described by Harden and Pampiglione are related to a variety of clinical situations. It is felt by this writer that the loss of quantitative electroretinographic data is more than compensated for by procedural simplicity and, in the absence of the necessity for sedation, safety and ease of repetition. It is hoped that the increased use of these investigations in acute pediatric situations may lead to clearer understanding of visual pathway pathology.

EDITOR'S NOTE

Mr. Fielder has provided us with an excellent paper illustrating the very great usefulness of the electroretinogram and visual evoked response in small infants. Whenever a child is brought to me because the parents suspect poor vision, the initial workup is to do a careful office visit—with emphasis on head circumference, meticulous examination of the pupils, and a careful cycloplegic retinoscopy and indirect ophthalmoscopy, as well as testing the optokinetic responses with various tapes and drums—and then I always get an *ERG* and *VER* if there is any doubt. The next step is to get a good *computed tomographic scan* with emphasis on the occipital lobes. One *must* have an *ERG*, however, to diagnose Leber's congenital amaurosis—for the fundus can be virtually normal *early* in the course of this disease, although the ERG will be extinguished, for practical purposes.

JLS

ACKNOWLEDGMENTS

I would like to thank Dr. M. Espir for the generous use of his EEG Department and Jacqueline Higgins, Christine Clarke, and Sheila Richardson for their skill and enthusiasm in performing these investigations. Also Dr. L. Arthur, Dr. T. Chambers, Dr. K. Dodd, and Mr. J. Firth for permission to report on their patients, the Medical Illustration Department for preparing the figures, and Mrs. Isobel Pritchard for secretarial assistance.

REFERENCES

1. Charles, S. Common Sense in Retinal Function Tests *Neuro-ophthalmology Update.* J. L. Smith, (Ed.), Masson, New York, 1977, pp. 383–385.
2. Ronchi, L. and Ercoles, A. M. Circadian electroretinographic rhythms. Atti Fondazione Contributi Ist. Nazionale Ottica 23:92–104 (1968).
3. Peterson, H. The normal B-potential in the single flash clinical electroretinogram. Acta Ophthalmol. (Kbh) 99:7–57 (1968).
4. Krill, A. E. *Hereditary Retinal and Choroidal Diseases.* Harper and Row, New York, 1972, Vol. I, pp. 227–277.
5. Kelsey, J. H. Electrophysiological tests in clinical ophthalmology. In: *Scientific Foundations of Ophthalmology.* E. S. Perkins and D. W. Hill (Eds.), Heinemann, London 1977, pp. 263–270.
6. Marmor, M. F. Corneal electroretinograms in children without sedation. J. Ped. Ophthalmol. 13:112–116 (1976).
7. Henkes, H. E. and Legein, C. P. Electrodiagnostic procedures in the blind and partially sighted young child. Int. Ophthalmol. Clin. 9:921–933 (1969).
8. Harden, A. and Pampiglione, G. Neurophysiological approach to disorders of vision. Lancet 1:805–809 (1970).
9. Maurer, B. Infant perception: methods of study. In: *Infant Perception: From Sensation to Cognition* L. B. Cohen and P. Salapatek (Eds.), Academic, New York, 1975, Vol. I, pp. 1–75.
10. Karmel, B. Z. and Maisel, E. B. A neuronal activity model for infant visual attention. In: Infant Perception: From Sensation to Cognition. L. B. Cohen and P. Salapatek (Eds.), Academic, New York, 1975, Vol. I, pp. 77–133.
11. Harter, M. R. *et al.* Maturation of evoked potentials and visual preference in 6–45-day-old infants. Electroencephalogr. Clin. Neurophysiol. 42:595–607 (1977).
12. Noonan, B. D. *et al.* The influence of direction of gaze on the human electroretinogram recorded from periorbital electrodes. Electroencephalogr. Clin. Neurophysiol. 35:495–502 (1973).
13. Jones, R. M. and France, T. D. Recording ERG's and VER's from unsedated children. J. Pediatr. Ophthalmol. 14:316–319 (1977).
14. Harden, A. Non-corneal electroretinogram, parameters in normal children. Br. J. Ophthalmol. 58:811–816 (1974).
15. Popkin, A. B. Uses of electroretinography in paediatric ophthalmology. In: *Pediatric Ophthalmology.* R. D. Harley (Ed.), Saunders, Philadelphia, 1975, pp. 824–829.
16. Francois, J. and de Roueck, A. Electroretinography in the diagnosis of congenital blindness. ISC ERG Symp. Ghent. 451–472 (1966).
17. Harden, A. and Pampiglione, G. Visual evoked potential, electroretinogram, and electroencephalogram studies in progressive neurometabolic storage diseases of childhood. In: *Visual Evoked Potentials in Man: New Developments.* J. E. Desmedt (Ed.), Clarendon, Oxford, 1977, pp. 470–480.
18. Halliday, A. M., McDonald, W. I., and Mushin, J. Visual evoked potentials in patients with demyelinating disease. In: *Visual Evoked Potentials in Man: New Developments.* J. E. Desmedt (Ed.), Clarendon, Oxford, 1977, pp. 438–449.

23 Pattern-Reversal Visual Evoked Potentials in Patients with Multiple Sclerosis

Shahram Khoshbin, M.D.
Mark Hallett, M.D.

INTRODUCTION

The cortical evoked response to visual stimulation is becoming a common clinical test for evaluation of the visual pathways in patients with a variety of diseases. At present the test seems to be most helpful in the evaluation of suspected demyelination of the visual pathways. Clinically the most useful circumstance is the demonstration of subclinical disease in the visual pathways in a patient with suspected multiple sclerosis but without apparent lesions disseminated in the central nervous system.

Different visual stimuli have been used in the study of visual evoked potentials in man. The first studies were made with flash stimuli. Flash-evoked responses are complex waves with multiple peaks between 50 and 150 msec following onset of diffuse light flash stimuli. Different factors affect these potentials such as stimulus luminance,[1] electrode location, and the level of arousal of the patient.[2,3] The peaks of the evoked response do not have consistent latencies or amplitudes. Attempts were made to define abnormalities in amplitude and latency of the components of the evoked potentials, but the differences between normal and abnormal responses were not clear.[4-6]

Visual evoked potentials can also be produced by patterned visual stimuli, and Halliday *et al.* found that an extremely consistent waveform could be produced by periodic reversal of a checkerboard.[7,8] This waveform has a characteristic major positive wave which is easy to recognize and has a consistent latency in a normal population. The prolongation of this major positive component in patients with optic neuritis was also first shown by Halliday *et al.*[7]

TECHNIQUE OF RECORDING

Visual evoked potentials are changes in the electroencephalogram (EEG) produced by a visual stimulus. As the amplitude of the evoked potential is usually smaller than the ongoing EEG activity, special techniques such as signal averaging need to be employed in order to see these potentials. Figure 1 outlines the different steps involved in obtaining a visual evoked response.[9] The stimulus in pattern-reversal visual evoked potentials is usually a checkerboard pattern in which the black and white squares reverse positions usually at a rate of about 2/sec. The stimulus can be produced by either a slide projector alternately projecting a checkerboard slide and its negative[10] or by turning a rotatable mirror through a small angle and thus shifting the pattern on the screen, or by use of tachistoscopic display methods.[11] However, commercially available television sets produce alternating patterns which are brighter, and the size of the squares and reversal rate can be manipulated. Differences in distance, location of stimulus and intensity, size of squares, and quality of

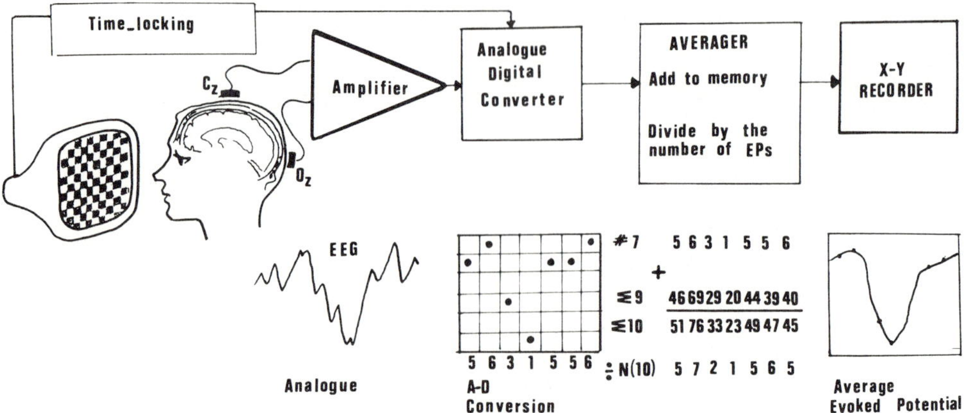

Fig. 1. Schematic diagram of different steps involved in recording a visual evoked potential. See text for details. (Modified from Picton[9].)

stimulus can alter the size and morphology of the evoked potential.[12, 13] Therefore, it is imperative that each laboratory determine its own range of normal values. The checkerboard is the most popular stimulus, but other stimuli seem to be equally as good, for example, a single bright square[14] or a sine wave grating.[15] Factors such as the focusing of the pattern on the retina, drowsiness and inattention have been shown to affect the amplitude but not the latency of the evoked potential.[12, 16] Artifacts such as muscle potentials from the temporalis muscle or palate and eyeblink or eye movement may appear at latencies similar to the evoked cerebral potential, and this should be considered when interpreting the data.

The "active" electrode is placed approximately 3 cm above the inion in the midline, and the reference electrode is placed at the vertex. The position of the active electrode corresponds roughly to the midportion of calcarine fissure.[17] Recording in this fashion produces a high amplitude response since the activity from the vertex is usually reversed in polarity from the activity in the occipital electrode. This EEG activity is recorded on one channel usually with low frequency filter at about 0.3 Hz and high frequency filter at about 70 Hz. The recorded segment of EEG, usually a segment of 200–500 msec after the onset of the stimulus (analysis period), is then converted from analogue to digital form by the analogue-to-digital converter. The purpose of this step is to get the information in a form which can be handled by a digital computer. The computer then extracts the potential (the "signal") from the background EEG ("the noise") by the process of averaging. The background EEG is a random event with respect to the stimulus, while the visual evoked potential is "time-locked" to it. Thus, the averager will gradually reduce the EEG toward zero, while the visual evoked potential signal will constantly grow in size. With further averaging the signal-to-noise ratio increases. The averaged evoked response can then be displayed and produced in hard-copy form. Usually approximately 128 stimuli are averaged, and the resultant waveform shows a major positive peak at approximately 100 msec latency. Two or three trials are done for each eye separately. Figure 2A shows typical visual evoked potentials to pattern reversal in a normal subject.

NORMAL FINDINGS

The mean latency in 25 normal subjects and 10 neurological controls in our pilot studies showed a prominent major positive wave with a mean latency of 98 msec with a standard deviation of ±4.0 msec. There are changes in latency associated with maturation and senility, and in older patients the latency of the major positive peak may increase.[18, 19] A visual evoked potential may be considered abnormal if the latency of the major positive peak is a value greater than any observed in the control group, or

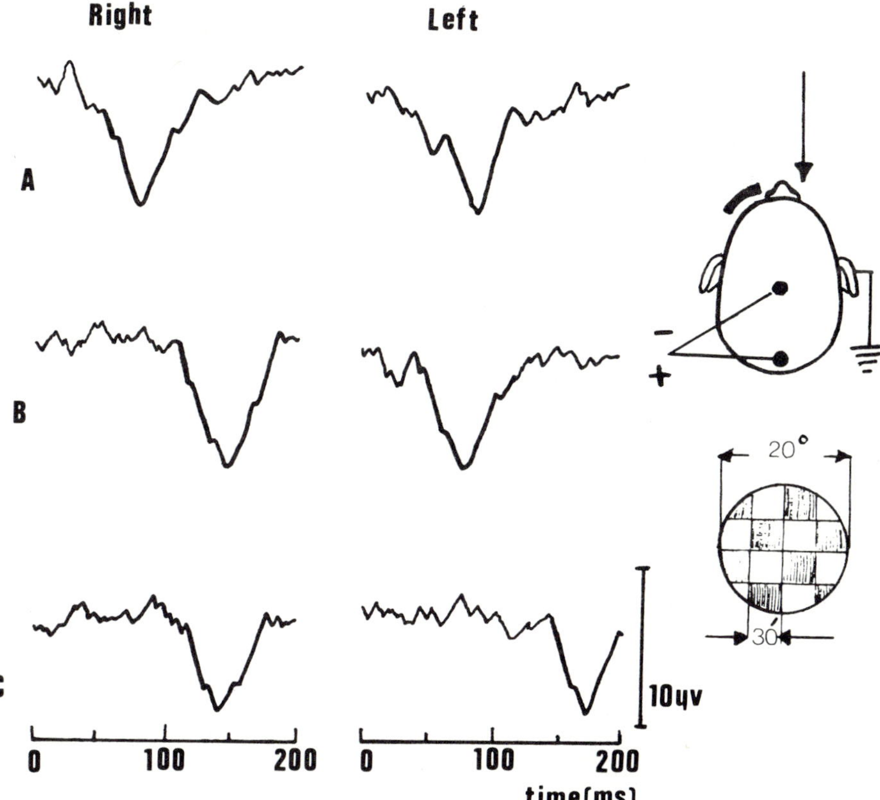

Fig. 2. Examples of visual evoked potentials to pattern reversal stimulation to the right and the left eye separately. A is from a normal subject. B is from a patient with right optic neuritis. C is from a patient with definite multiple sclerosis. On the top right side of the figure is indicated the electrode placement and the technique of stimulation of the right eye with left eye patched. On the bottom right of the figure the stimulus is shown schematically; each check subtends 30 sec at the eye while the whole field is approximately 20°.

if a value is greater than 3 SD above the mean latency or if the latency difference between the two eyes is greater than 8 msec[18, 20] or if there is no response. The amplitude of the evoked potentials is variable, and factors such as refractive errors, drowsiness, and inattention affect this variability. Amplitude asymmetry between the two eyes, however, has been considered by some authors to be abnormal.[17, 21] The morphology of the waveform has been studied,[17, 22] but significant differences can be found only rarely and then only with complex computer techniques. The segment of the averaged EEG where the evoked potential appears seems to be smoother than the segment prior to the evoked potential, and suggests that the stimulus alters the EEG rhythms rather than adding a small superimposed potential.

OPTIC NEURITIS

Multiple sclerosis and optic neuritis commonly produce delayed visual evoked potentials. The first studies by Halliday *et al.*[7] were done on patients with acute optic neuritis. Figure 2B shows the visual evoked potentials in a patient with right optic neuritis. The frequency of abnormalities in optic neuritis is quite high, however, even in those patients who showed latencies comparable to normal subjects, the latency in the affected eye was often prolonged as compared to the unaffected eye. Halliday *et al.* found the pattern reversal visual evoked potential to be abnormal in over 90% of cases of optic neuritis.[23] Mathews *et al.* showed 82% and Sharokhi *et al.* 96% abnormality in isolated optic neuritis.[17, 20] Halliday also showed that in the initial stage, when vision was markedly reduced, the visual evoked potential is often completely absent. In follow-up studies, even after vision partially or nearly completely recovered, the visual evoked potential still showed delayed latency. As recovery occurs, the amplitude of the visual evoked potential gradually returns to normal, while latency remains prolonged.[7] These workers have shown that as long as 15 years after an acute episode of optic neuritis, with a fully normal examination, the visual evoked potential still showed abnormal latency.[23] Thus, the visual evoked potential is more sensitive than the clinical examination and can reveal an optic neuritis long forgotten by the patient. Indeed, it seems clear that the test can even reveal optic neuritis that was never clinically manifest.

MULTIPLE SCLEROSIS

In clinical neurology the most useful application of visual evoked potentials is in the diagnosis of multiple sclerosis. Clinically as well as pathologically, it is well known that incidence of plaques in the optic nerves of patients with multiple sclerosis is quite high and the plaques can be present even without a history of visual difficulties. Plaques are characterized by demyelination of nerve; demyelination causes slow nerve conduction. Thus, the high incidence of plaques in the visual system leads to a high probability of delayed visual evoked potentials (Figure 2C).

Most of the studies of visual evoked potentials in multiple sclerosis have used the diagnostic criteria of McAlpine *et al.*,[24] which divide patients into possible, probable or definite multiple sclerosis. In our own study we combined the criteria for possible and probable and divided our patients into definite multiple sclerosis and suspect multiple sclerosis. Figure 3 shows the results of our first 75 cases, 25 with definite multiple sclerosis, 25 suspect multiple sclerosis, and 25 normal subjects. We found 80% abnormal visual evoked potentials in our definite multiple sclerosis group and 48% in our suspect cases.[25] Continued evaluation of the next 100 additional patients shows roughly the same percentages. Other studies report abnormalities varying between 50% and

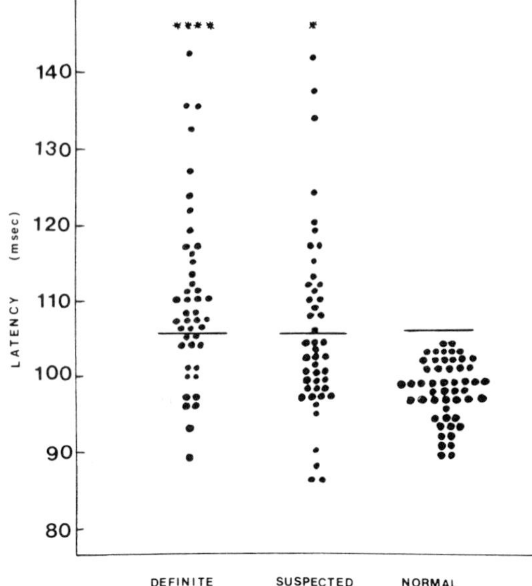

Fig. 3. Latencies of the major positive peak of visual evoked potentials from each eye in 25 normal subjects, 25 with definite multiple sclerosis, and 25 with suspected multiple sclerosis. The * indicates no potential seen. The horizontal lines indicate two standard deviations above the mean of the normal values and represent an upper bound of the normal population.

97% in the patient groups (Table I). Halliday *et al.* studied 51 patients[26] and showed 97% abnormality in patients with definite multiple sclerosis, 100% with probable multiple sclerosis, and 92% with possible multiple sclerosis. Asselman *et al.*, studying the same number of patients, showed 84% abnormal in definite multiple sclerosis, 83% in probable multiple sclerosis, and 21% in possible multiple sclerosis.[18] Most subsequent studies show similar percentages to those in the study by Asselman *et al.*

All studies confirm the remarkable finding that many patients who have abnormal visual evoked potentials have no history of optic neuritis or evidence of optic atrophy. As shown by several recent studies, including our own, somatosensory evoked potentials are probably as sensitive as visual evoked potentials in finding lesions in patients with multiple sclerosis. In our studies we have been able to show that when a combination of visual evoked potentials, somatosensory evoked potentials, brain stem auditory evoked potentials, and blink

TABLE I. *Abnormal visual evoked potentials in multiple sclerosis*

Reference	Total number of patients	Definite multiple sclerosis	Suspect[a] multiple sclerosis
Halliday *et al.* (1973)[26]	51	33/34[b] (97%)	16/17[b] (94%)
Asselman *et al.* (1975)[18]	51	26/31 (84%)	8/20 (40%)
Lowitzch *et al.* (1976)[27]	135	60/73 (82%)	38/62 (61%)
Mastaglia *et al.* (1976)[22]	68	19/23 (83%)	15/45 (33%)
Mathews *et al.* (1977)[20]	110	46/61 (75%)	24/52 (46%)
Hennerici *et al.* (1977)[14]	57	13/16 (81%)	22/41 (54%)
Shahrokhi *et al.* (1978)[17]	149	49/60 (82%)	36/89 (40%)
Nilsson (1978)[28]	38	15/19 (79%)	11/19 (58%)
Khoshbin and Hallett (1978)[25]	50	20/25 (80%)	12/25 (48%)

[a] The suspect category combines the probable and possible categories of McAlpine.[24]

[b] The ratio is the number of abnormal patients to the total number of patients in that group.

reflexes are used (as a battery of tests), the sensitivity markedly increases over the individual tests used alone.[25]

OTHER CLINICAL APPLICATIONS AND CAUSES OF ABNORMAL VISUAL EVOKED POTENTIALS

Multiple sclerosis is not the only cause of delayed visual evoked potentials, and this test can be used in a variety of other clinical settings.

As the amplitude seems to correlate with the clarity of focus of the image on the retina, visual evoked potentials may become another tool in assessment of visual acuity and in detection of astigmatism,[29] particularly in children. Color checkboards have been used in studies of color blindness.[30] Diseases of the retina may cause decrease in amplitude or latency.

In glaucoma delays are noted when stimulating affected areas of retina.[31] Tumors, such as orbital tumors, pituitary tumors, meningiomas, and craniopharyngiomas compressing the optic nerves, can cause delay in visual evoked potentials.[18, 32] Although pattern reversal visual evoked potentials are abnormal in conditions causing visual field abnormalities secondary to lesions behind the chiasm, it has not been possible as yet to localize the lesion or even identify the side of the lesion. Halliday *et al.*, using half field stimulation, found abnormalities ipsilateral to the visual field loss.[33, 34] Holder *et al.* found abnormalities contralateral to the visual field loss.[35, 36] These discrepancies are still unexplained. Visual evoked potential abnormalities have

also been reported in ischemic optic neuropathy[23] and also in Leber's hereditary optic neuropathy.[37]

It is clear that in order to ascribe delay or abnormality of the visual evoked potentials to multiple sclerosis, one must exclude these other conditions, most of which significantly impair vision.

EDITOR'S NOTE

There has been a great rush to get on the band wagon of doing visual evoked responses in order to help make the diagnosis of multiple sclerosis. However, one must remember two very important basic points in doing this, and both of these are pointed out in this chapter by Dr. Khoshbin. He states—"Clinically the most useful circumstance is the demonstration of *subclinical* disease in the visual pathways in a patient with suspected multiple sclerosis but without *apparent* lesions disseminated in the central nervous system." I have italicized the words "subclinical" and "apparent" in this sentence. Finally, his last sentence merits great emphasis—"It is clear that in order to ascribe delay or abnormality of the visual evoked potentials to multiple sclerosis, one must exclude these other conditions, most of which significantly impair vision." The point I am simply making is this—if you find that an elephant's trunk is stopped up, you cannot always blame this on a peanut!

A common mistake is for a neurologist to order visual evoked responses on a patient who might possibly have a demyelination problem and yet the patient has not had a good set of peripheral and central fields—

no Amsler grid test—no meticulous look for a Marcus Gunn pupil—and often indeed the visual acuity has not been accurately measured! It is very, very important that the patient have a good "OV" (office visit) with a complete neuro-ophthalmologic examination before concluding that if you flash a light before the patient or have him look at a patterned target and then you quantitatively measure the evoked occipital potentials, there is some mischief afoot. All I am saying is that those patients who are reported to have an abnormal visual evoked response in an asymptomatic eye due to demyelinating disease will nearly always show a visual field defect in my hands. This note is simply a plea to the neurologist to refer his patients for a careful and complete ophthalmological examination BEFORE getting a visual evoked response. You would hate to find that the delay is due to glaucoma, for example, which could be treated! With this admonition—then we can proceed to evaluate the research data more carefully!

One late point that should be added is an excellent paper by Cohen, M. M., Lessell, S., and Wolf, P. A., "A prospective study of the risk of developing multiple sclerosis in uncomplicated optic neuritis," which appeared in *Neurol.* **29**(2):208–213, Feb. 1979. Dr. Simmons Lessell has made another notable contribution to this subject! Sixty patients with uncomplicated optic neuritis were followed for at least five years in a prospective study. Seventeen of them (28%) developed definite multiple sclerosis and four (7%) developed probable or possible multiple sclerosis during that time.

Six of the 17 patients who developed definite evidence of multiple sclerosis did so within the first year after the optic neuritis. Interestingly enough, 45% of the women but only 11% of the men developed multiple sclerosis. As expected, both sexes were at highest risk if the optic neuritis occurred between ages 21 and 40. Of that age group, 51% of the patients progressed to multiple sclerosis, whereas the risk for other age groups was only 12%. There was an over-all increased risk of developing multiple sclerosis in patients with recurrent optic neuritis. Finally, these authors noted that the course of the multiple sclerosis

appeared to be benign at least during their period of observation, which was a mean of 7.1 years. Therefore, this prospective study probably will be remembered as showing a 28% incidence of developing definite multiple sclerosis after an attack of optic neuritis. Retrospective studies before have ranged from 11.5% to as high as 85%, so I believe the 28% figure is a reasonable one.

JLS

REFERENCES

1. DeVoe, R. C., Ripps, H., and Vaughan, H. G. Cortical responses to stimulation of human fovea. Vision Res. *8*:135–147 (1968).
2. Oosterhuis, H., Ponsun, L., Jonkman, E., *et al.* The average visual response in patients with cerebrovascular disease. Electroencephalogr. Clin. Neurophysiol. *27*:23–24 (1969).
3. Starr, A. Sensory evoked potentials in clinical disorders of the nervous system. Ann. Rev. Neurosci. *1*:103–137 (1978).
4. Richey, E. T., Kooi, K. A., and Tourtellote, W. W. Visually evoked responses in multiple sclerosis. J. Neurol. Neurosurg. Psychiatr. *34*:275–280 (1971).
5. Namerow, N. S. and Enns, N. Visual evoked responses in patients with multiple sclerosis. J. Neurol. Neurosurg. Psychiatr. *35*:269–275 (1972).
6. Feinsod, M., Abramsky, O., and Auerbach, E. Electrophysiological examination of the visual system in multiple sclerosis. J. Neurol. Sci. *20*:161–175 (1973).
7. Halliday, A. M., McDonald, W. I., and Mushin, J. Delayed visual evoked response in optic neuritis. Lancet *1*:982–985 (1972).
8. Behrman, J., Halliday, A. M., and McDonald, W. I. Visual evoked responses to flash and pattern in patients with retrobulbar neuritis. Electroencephalogr. Clin. Neurophysiol. *33*:445 (1972).
9. Picton, T. W. and Hink, R. F. Evoked potentials. How? what? and why? Am. J. EEG Technol. *14*:9–44 (1974).
10. Halliday, A. M. and Michael, W. F. Changes in pattern-evoked responses in man associated with the vertical and horizontal meridians of the visual field. J. Physiol. (Lond.) *208*:499–513 (1970).
11. Jeffreys, D. A. Separable components of human evoked responses to spatially patterned visual fields. Electroencephalogr. Clin. Neurophysiol. *24*:596 (1968).
12. Halliday, A. M., McDonald, W. I., and Mushin, J. Delayed pattern-evoked responses in optic neuritis in relation to visual acuity. Trans. Ophthalmol. Soc. UK *93*:315–324 (1973).
13. Cant, B. R., Hume, A. L., and Shaw, N. A. Effects of luminance on the pattern visual evoked potential in multiple sclerosis. Electroencephalogr. Clin. Neurophysiol. *45*:496–504 (1978).
14. Hennerici, M., Wenzel, D., and Freund, H. S. The comparison of small size rectangle and checkerboard stimulation for the evaluation of delayed

visual evoked responses in patients suspected of multiple sclerosis. Brain *100*:119–136 (1977).

15. Bodis-Wollner, I., Hendley, C. D., Mylin, L. H., *et al.* Visual evoked potential and the visuogram in multiple sclerosis. Ann. Neurol. *5*:40–47 (1979).

16. Harter, M. R. and White, C. T. Effect of contour sharpness and check size on visually evoked cortical potentials. Vision Res. *8:* 701–711 (1968).

17. Shahrokhi, F., Chiappa, K., and Young, R. Pattern shift visual evoked responses. Arch. Neurol. *35:* 65–71 (1978).

18. Asselman, P., Chadwick, D. W., and Marsden, C. D. Visual evoked responses in the diagnosis and management of patients suspected of multiple sclerosis. Brain *98*:261–282 (1975).

19. Celesia, C. G. and Daly, R. F. Effects of aging on visual responses. Arch. Neurol. *34*:403–407 (1977).

20. Mathews, W. B., Small, D. G., Small, M. *et al.* Pattern reversal evoked visual potential in the diagnosis of multiple sclerosis. J. Neurol. Neurosurg. Psychiatr. *40*:1009–1114 (1977).

21. Zeost, J. A. Pattern visual evoked responses in multiple sclerosis. Arch. Neurol. *34*:314–316 (1977).

22. Mastaglia, F. L., Black, J. L., and Collins, D. W. K. Visual and spinal evoked potentials in diagnosis of multiple sclerosis. Br. Med. J. *3:*732 (1976).

23. Halliday, A. M., McDonald, W. I., and Mushin, J. Visual evoked potentials in patients with demyelinating disease. In: *Visual Evoked Potentials in Man.* J. E. Desmedt (Ed.), Clarendon Press, Oxford, 1977, pp. 438–449.

24. McAlpine, D., Lumsden, C. E., and Acheson, E. D. *Multiple Sclerosis: An Appraisal.* Churchill Livingston Ltd., Edinburgh, 1972.

25. Khoshbin, S. and Hallett, M. Somatosensory evoked potentials in the diagnosis of multiple sclerosis: comparison with other evoked potentials and blink reflex. Neurology *28*:388 (1978).

26. Halliday, A. M., McDonald, W. I., and Mushin, J. Visual evoked response in the diagnosis of multiple sclerosis. Br. Med. J. *4:*661–664 (1973).

27. Lowitzsch, K., Kuhnt, U., Sakmann, C. H., *et al.* Visual pattern evoked responses and blink reflexes in assessment of multiple sclerosis diagnosis. A clinical study of 135 multiple sclerosis patients. J. Neurol. *213*:17–32 (1976).

28. Nilsson, B. Y. Visual evoked responses in multiple sclerosis: comparison of two methods of pattern reversal. J. Neurol. Neurosurg. Psychiatr. *41*:499–504 (1978).

29. Reagan, D. Clinical applications of steady state evoked potentials. Speedy methods of refracting the eye and assessing visual acuity in amblyopia. In: *Cerebral Evoked Potentials in Man.* J. E. Desmedt (Ed.), Oxford Univ. Press, London, 1976.

30. Reagan, D. and Spekreijse, H. Evoked potential indications of colour blindness. Vision Res. *14*:89–95 (1974).

31. Cappin, J. and Nissims, S. Visual evoked responses in the detection of field defects in glaucoma. Arch. Ophthalmol. NY *93*:9–18 (1975).

32. Vaughan, H. G., Jr. and Katzman, R. Evoked responses in visual disorders. Ann. NY Acad. Sci. *112*:305–319 (1964).

33. Halliday, A. M., Halliday, E., Kriss, A. *et al.* The pattern evoked potential in compression of the anterior visual pathways. Brain *99*:357–374 (1976).

34. Halliday, A. M. Visually evoked responses in optic nerve disease. Trans. Ophthalmol. Soc. UK *96:* 372–376 (1976).

35. Holder, G. E. The effects of chiasmal compression on the pattern visual evoked potential. Electroencephalogr. Clin. Neurophysiol. *45*:278–280 (1978).

36. Blumhardt, L. D., Barnet, G., and Halliday, A. M. The asymmetrical visual evoked potential to pattern reversal in one-half field and its significance for the analysis of visual field defects. Br. J. Ophthalmol. *61*:454–461 (1977).

37. Dorfman, L. J., Nikoskelainen, E., Rosenthal, A. R., *et al.* Visual evoked potentials in Leber's hereditary optic neuropathy. Ann. Neurol. *1*:565–568 (1977).

24 Visual Evoked Response (VER) in Neuro-ophthalmology

Thomas J. Carlow, M.D.

The visual evoked response (VER) or visual evoked potential (VEP) visual evoked cortical potential and evoked potential is an electrical signal generated by the central nervous system in response to a visual stimulus. This phenomenon has been known for at least 40 years; however, the small size (1–20 μV) necessitated the development of modern computer averaging techniques in the early 1960's to distinguish and separate the VER from noise and normal electroencephalographic (EEG) activity (20–100 μV). The VER has subsequently proven to be a valuable asset in evaluating the functional integrity of the visual system. A survey of the practical clinical usefulness of the VER will follow a brief introduction into methodology.

VER METHODOLOGY

A stimulus mechanism, EEG electrodes, differential amplifiers, a data processor, and an XY plotter or camera are required to record a VER.[1]

Two types of visual stimuli are commonly utilized: flashing light and checkerboard pattern reversal. Both can be used in either a transient or steady state mode, depending upon the frequency of stimulation.[2] The transient response is slow, once or twice a second. Since each clinically useful visually evoked response normally lasts 250 msec, each cortical response will not interfere with the next or following cortical response. At a frequency of 4 cps a steady state VER will begin to develop. The waveshape appears sinusoidal since the cortical responses now interfere with and overlap each other.

EEG electrode locations, either referential or bipolar, utilize the International 10–20 system. Referential recording is commonly preferred; an electrode over a cortical region is compared or referenced to an electrode over a noncortical region. An electrode over the occipital tip, O_Z, the right occipital hemisphere, O_2, or the left occipital hemisphere, O_1, will be referenced to a noncortical region, e.g. linked ears. In bipolar recording one active cortical area is referenced to another active cortical region, e.g., O_2 to O_1.

Two major bioengineering signal processing techniques have been used to enhance and uncover the VER: ensemble averaging of repetitive evoked responses and narrowband filtering of the steady state evoked response coupled with Fourier analysis. In the ensemble averaged technique the VER is recorded relative to a time-locked stimulus. Normal EEG and electromyographic (EMG) activity is assumed to be random while the visually evoked response is time-locked to the stimulus and therefore follows each flash or pattern shift at a designated period. After 50–100 stimulus presentations the EEG and EMG activity (noise) will average to zero while the resultant VER waveforms will add together and emerge from the background. The second most common signal processing technique utilizes a narrowband steady state filtering technique and Fourier analysis. The background activity or noise is suppressed relative to the desired visual evoked response by selecting filters that remove all activity except that which is exactly at the frequency of the visual stimulation. Although this method can produce clinical data in seconds, it requires rather elaborate and expensive equipment. Once processed, the resultant waveshape can be displayed on an oscilloscope and recorded with either an XY plotter or photographed.

Standardization of latency and amplitude waveshape components for flash and pattern VER has not been entirely satisfactory. Some laboratories label each wave with a "P" for positive and an "N" for negative. Others have arbitrarily elected to designate the more prominent waves with Roman numerals (I–VI). The positive deflection may be depicted up or down. This lack of uniform VER standards has made it difficult but not impossible to compare the work of different authors. Representative examples of a transient flash and pattern and a steady state VER can be seen in Figures 1, 2, and 3.

Theoretically, different neuroanatomic subsystems of neural organization are present in the human visual system and operate as a function of the visual stimulus presented. Information processed secondary to an unstructured flash of light is presumed to travel in a neuroanatomic substrate separate from the response to a pattern stimulus. It is probable that the cortical contribution of the VER can arise from more than one source.[3, 4]

The flash transient VER is postulated to originate from at least two sources: a primary response generated by the retino-geniculo-occipital substrate and a secondary or late response that first passes to the brainstem reticular formation, superior colliculi, or perhaps pulvinar of the thalamus prior to being transmitted to the cerebral cortex. A definite neuroanatomic substrate has been suggested but not fully delineated for the pattern VER.[5, 6]

The VER is dependent upon a multitude of variables: luminance of target and background, frequency of the stimulus, electrode placement, and the subject's attention and visual acuity. Large checkerboard targets, greater than 30 minutes of arc, are predominantly luminance specific and may give information that travels on the same neu-

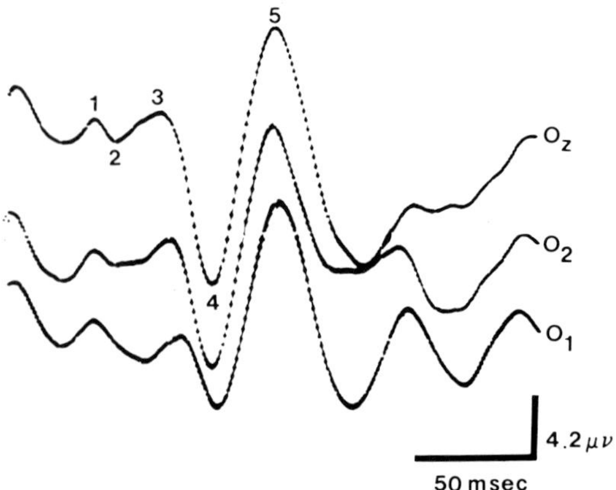

Fig. 1. *Normal transient flash VER.* The first five major waves are labeled for the flash VER recorded from Oz (occipital tip), O₂ (right occipital hemisphere), and O₁ (left occipital hemisphere). The early components, waves 1, 2, 3, are the most consistent and clinically useful.

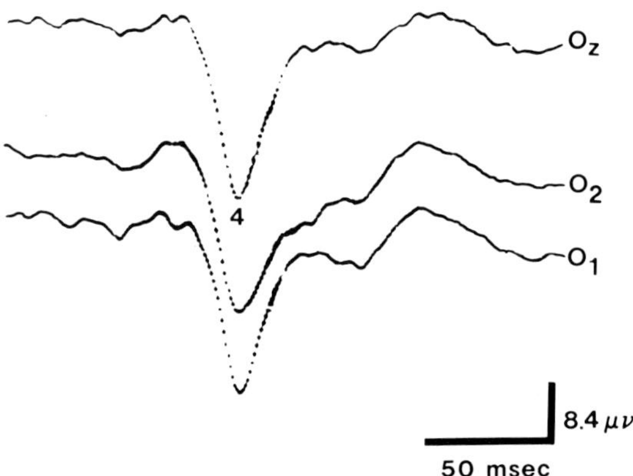

Fig. 2. *Normal transient pattern VER.* A transient pattern VER to a 1° white-black checkerboard stimulus is depicted to Oz, O₂, and O₁. The first major positive wave, wave 4, is the most consistent and clinically useful.

roanatomic substrate as the flash VER. A VER is highly sensitive to stimuli which contain contours and edges especially for pattern targets smaller than 30 minutes of arc. For targets of this magnitude refractive correction and patient cooperation are critical. Maximum VER amplitude occurs with checkerboard patterns that subtend angles between 10 and 20 minutes of arc and correspond to a visual acuity of 20/20. Since refractive changes as small as one diopter can reduce amplitude by as much as 30%, the VER can be used as an objective re-

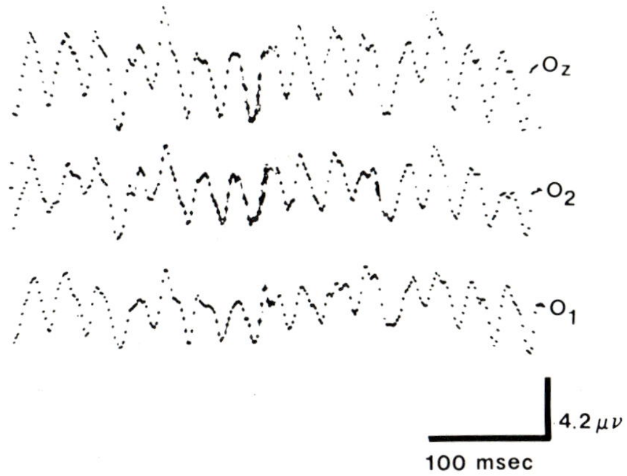

Fig. 3. *Normal steady-state pattern VER.* A normal VER to a 15-minute white-black checkerboard target alternating at 30 cps is depicted to O_z, O_2, and O_1. The frequency of the response, phase angle, and amplitude have all been clinically useful.

fractive technique.[7] It is generally believed that an infant's visual acuity does not resolve targets in the 20/20 range until approximately age five years. VER data would suggest that a neuroanatomic substrate capable of processing information between 10 and 20 minutes of arc, 20/20 visual acuity, exists as early as six months of age.[8] Thus, the VER has become a useful tool to determine visual acuity in a young child, amblyope, malingerer, mental retard, or aphasic adult.

CLINICAL APPLICATION OF THE VER

Macula and Retinal Disease

Since the VER primarily reflects the central 10 degrees of vision, macular degeneration for any reason will result in a significantly altered VER. VER amplitude can be severely attenuated while latency is relatively preserved; however, little data has been published. In disorders of the peripheral retina, such as retinitis pigmentosa, the VER can be normal while the electroretinogram (ERG) is grossly abnormal. The VER and ERG have been useful in evaluating several progressive neurometabolic storage diseases of childhood.[9] In Tay-Sachs disease the VER can be absent while the ERG is normal. In the late infantile form of amaurotic familial idiocy, Batten's disease, the VER will have an amplitude 12–20 times greater than normal and the ERG, early in the disease process, will be unrecordable.

Optic Neuritis

Perhaps the most heralded clinical application of the VER has been to detect a prolonged latency or increased optic nerve conduction velocity in cases of possible or probable multiple sclerosis.

The transient flash VER can be a sensitive indicator of prolonged optic nerve conduction,[10-12] others have found this method relatively insensitive.[13] In our laboratory the normal transient flash VER is inconsistent, and we therefore rely on transient pattern and steady state flash and pattern VER stimuli. Peak amplitudes for a steady state VER, utilizing Fourier analysis, occur at 10 Hz, 13–22 Hz, and 42–60 Hz.[14, 15] Selective changes, prolonged latency and/or decreased amplitude, of the midrange response, 13–22 Hz, have been observed in 100% of patients with multiple sclerosis.[14] This type of stimulus can be used when visual acuity is severely reduced and allows detection of prolonged optic nerve conduction when other stimuli have not uncovered a defect.[16]

The medium frequency VER steady state components are more color dependent than either the lower or higher frequency steady state components.[15] A separate neuroanatomic substrate for color vision can be postulated. This may partially explain the presence of poor color discrimination with normal visual acuity and fields in optic neuropathy.

Transient pattern VER's are usually performed with targets greater than 30 minutes of arc. Smaller targets have given inconsistent results, probably due to the reduced visual acuity frequently seen with optic neuritis. Large pattern stimuli have shown ipsilateral delayed optic nerve latencies, 67–96% of cases, in multiple sclerosis[17, 18] (Fig. 4). Interocular latency differences and the utilization of colored targets may document impaired optic nerve conduction when absolute latency values are statistically normal[19] (Fig. 5).

The steady state pattern VER amplitude can be severely attenuated on the affected side (Fig. 6). This is due to the inability of

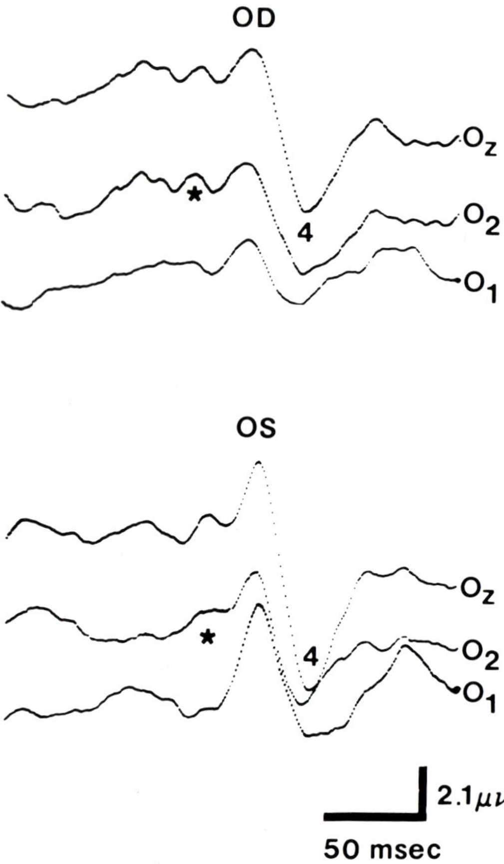

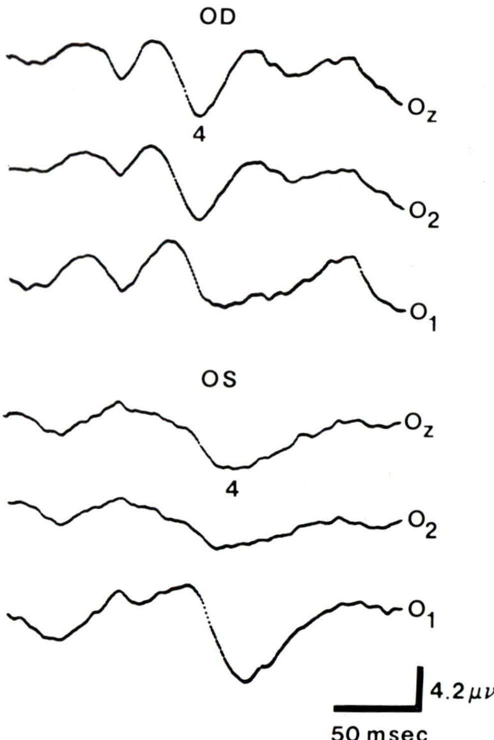

Fig. 4. *Transient pattern VER-bilateral optic neuritis.* Bilateral increased latencies to wave 4, from the normal mean of 104 msec*, for a 1° white-black target can be seen in a patient with definite multiple sclerosis.

Fig. 5. *Transient pattern VER-optic neuritis.* The transient pattern VER to a 1° white-black target gave normal latencies to wave 4 in a multiple sclerosis suspect. Utilizing a 1° red-black target uncovered an interocular prolongation of latency not revealed with the 1° white-black target. Visual acuity was normal.

the neural pathways to respond at the frequency of stimulation.

Ischemic Optic Neuropathy

Ischemic optic neuropathy is a frequent cause of monocular loss of vision after the fourth decade. The VER may be helpful in those instances where the etiology is questionable. Unfortunately, both normal and prolonged latencies have been observed.[20, 21] A significant reduction or attenuation of amplitude has been a consistent finding on the side of the ischemia. Since amplitude is not always reduced in a demyelinative optic neuropathy, a presumed diagnosis of ischemic optic neuropathy can be made, with the proper history, if latency is normal and amplitude is significantly reduced.

Orbital Tumor

An orbital tumor, with optic nerve compression, can selectively decrease amplitude prior to prolonging latency.[22] After decompression amplitude can improve (Fig. 7).

Other Optic Nerve Disorders

Papilledema and pseudopapilledema (without visual field defect) have normal VER's. A definite delay in VER latency has been documented in glaucoma patients by selective stimulation of the affected retinal area.[23] Localized retinal dysfunction is typically not detected with a wholefield transient stimulus but can be uncovered with sector steady state stimuli.

Optic Chiasm

Monocular stimulation may reveal a

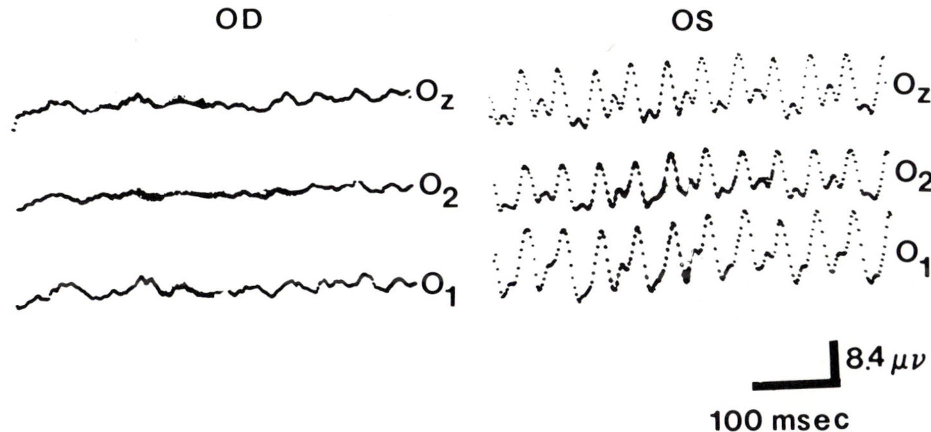

Fig. 6. *Steady state pattern VER-optic neuritis.* No response can be seen to a 1° white-black checkerboard target alternating at 20 cps on the right (OD). A normal response was obtained by stimulating the left (OS) with the same target. Visual acuity was 20/20 in each eye and the steady-state VER at 10 cps was normal.

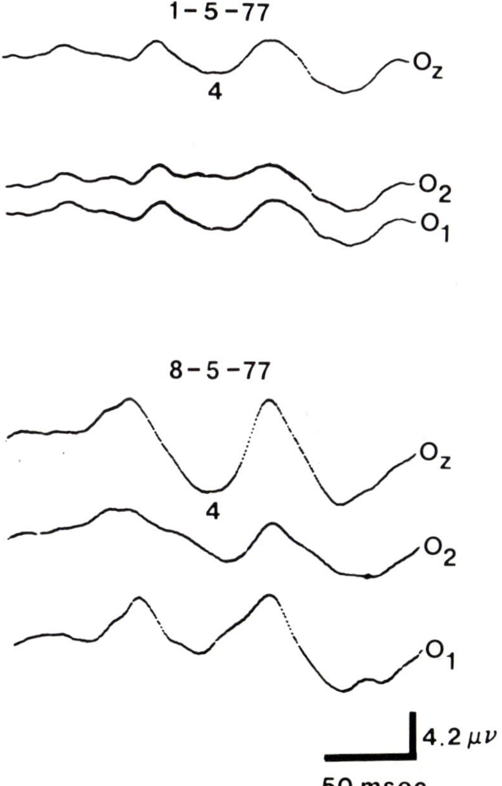

Fig. 7. *Transient pattern VER-orbital mass.* A definite increase in amplitude after surgery for an ophthalmic artery aneurysm is readily seen by comparing the pre-operative VER (1-5-77) to the post-operative VER (8-5-77) for a 1° white-black target alternating at 2 cps. The abnormally prolonged latency noted before surgery was not altered after surgery.

chiasmal lesion. With either a flash or pattern stimuli and referential electrodes, there will be preservation of the ipsilateral or uncrossed response and attenuation of the contralateral or crossed response[24-26] (Fig. 8). The early flash crossed components, wave 1, 2, 3, and the total crossed pattern response can be abolished. Halliday[22] reported prolonged latencies, abnormal waveshapes, and depressed amplitudes with parasellar tumors. The VER has been used to monitor optic nerve and chiasmal conduction during parasellar surgery. Almost instantaneous return of the VER waveshape has been observed at the moment of chiasmal decompression.[27]

In the normal human optic chiasm there is an equal proportion of decussating and nondecussating fibers. In the albino animal, the majority of optic nerve fibers decussate to the opposite hemisphere with only a small percentage of fibers going to the ipsilateral hemisphere. Asymmetrical flash VER's have been recorded in oculocutaneous albinism.[28] The early components are only prominent contralateral to monocular stimulation while the late components are observed bilaterally (Fig. 9). This would imply that the chiasm is composed predominantly of crossing fibers in oculocutaneous albinism.

Cortical Defects

Unpatterned transient VER's have revealed inconclusive data with central le-

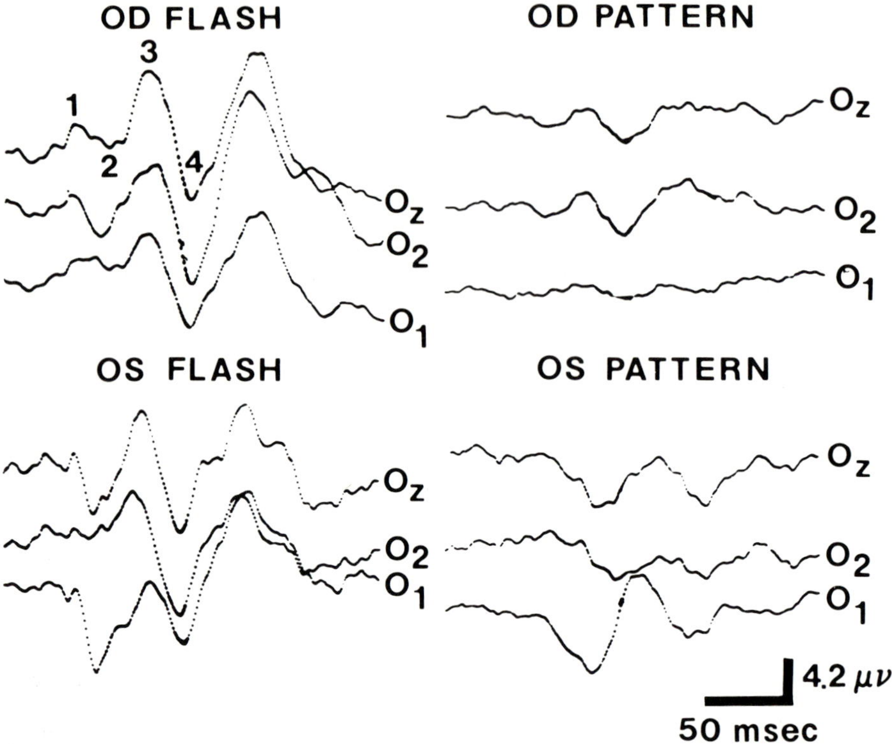

Fig. 8. *Transient flash and pattern VER-craniopharyngioma.* Both the transient flash and 1° white-black pattern VER in a patient with a dense bitemporal hemianopia and 20/20 vision OD and OS show a normal ipsilateral or uncrossed and an attenuated contralateral or crossed VER. Only the early components, waves 1, 2, 3, are contralaterally depressed with the monocular flashing stimulus.

sions.[29, 30] An abnormal primary or early response, ipsilateral to the lesion, with bilateral preservation of the late response, has been described with homonymous hemianopias.[31, 32] Similar flash VER findings have been observed in human subjects[33] and in experimental animals[34] after occipital lobectomy. Regan[35] simultaneously recorded from both occipital regions in normals and in a patient with an occipital infarct while stimulating each hemifield with steady state frequencies that differed by only 0.3 Hz. Narrow bandwidth Fourier analyzers localized the separate frequencies to the contralateral hemipheres in the normal. In the patient with the occipital infarct there was definite attenuation of the response ipsilateral to the lesion.

The normal major occipital waveshape, utilizing a transient pattern stimulus, appears ipsilateral to the hemifield stimulated with referential electrodes and contralateral to the hemifield stimulated with a bipolar electrode array.[36] By using a referential recording technique the transient pattern VER is most prominent over the involved occipital hemisphere.[37] Amplitude depression over an area of posterior occipital dysfunction has been observed with a steady state pattern VER.[38]

We have suggested that it is possible to separate a posterior cortical destructive lesion from one that is nondestructive or reversible by utilizing a combination of transient flash and pattern and steady state flash and pattern stimuli.[39] A posterior cortical destructive lesion, e.g., infarct or tumor, will show ipsilateral attenuation of the early components and bilateral preservation of the secondary or late components with a transient flash stimulus. Contralateral attenuation and ipsilateral preservation of the waveshape (over the region of dysfunction) will be seen with a transient pattern VER. Both steady state flash and pattern stimuli will show a subharmonic,

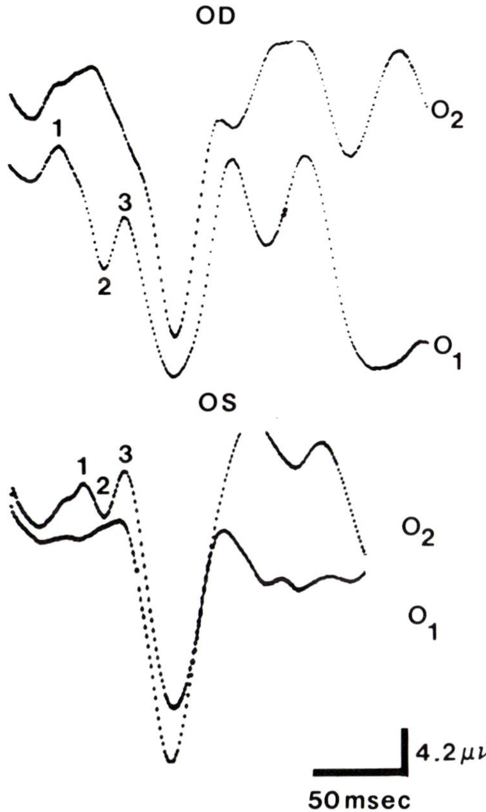

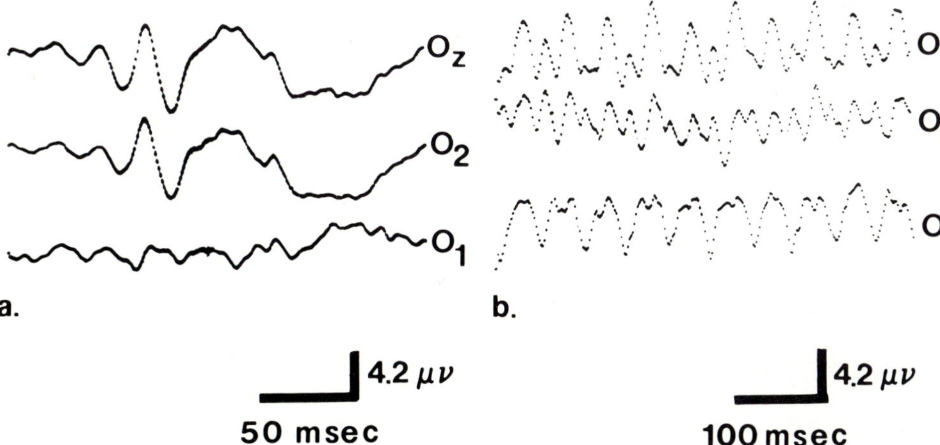

OD

OS

Fig. 9. *Transient flash VER-oculocutaneous albin-ism.* Monocular stimulation with a flashing light at 2 cps reveals an absent ipsilateral or uncrossed and an intact contralateral or crossed early response.

harmonic, and/or amplitude attenuation over the ipsilateral or involved hemisphere (Fig. 10). If the posterior cortical process is nondestructive, e.g., migraine or seizure, the transient pattern VER will show ipsilateral attenuation and contralateral preservation of the response (Fig. 11).

Cortical Blindness

Cortical blindness is characterized by a complete loss of vision with normal pupillary and funduscopic examinations. At times, it is difficult to differentiate true cortical blindness from malingering or functional blindness. In true cortical blindness the flash VER will reveal an absence of the early waveshape with preservation of the late components or total abolition of the waveshape in the occipital region.[40, 41] The integrity of the retino-geniculo-occipital pathways can be ascertained when there is a question of functional blindness. If the transient and flash VER to a 15-minute checkerboard pattern are normal, a psychological disorder should be suspected.[42]

Serial flash VER's in a patient with Jakob-Creutzfeldt disease initially showed an exaggerated response; however, as the dis-

This suggests that the optic chiasm in oculocutaneous albinism is almost totally crossed.

Fig. 10. *Transient and steady-state pattern VER-right occipital-parietal astrocytoma.* The transient pattern VER to a 1° white-black target alternating at 2 cps appears normal over the right involved hemisphere, O_2, and attenuated over the normal left hemisphere, O_1 (Fig. 10a). The steady-state response (Fig. 10b) to a 1° white-black target alternating at 20 cps reveals an increased frequency, harmonic, over the right involved hemisphere, O_2 and a linear or normal response over the left hemisphere, O_1. This combination of transient and pattern VER suggests a destructive process.

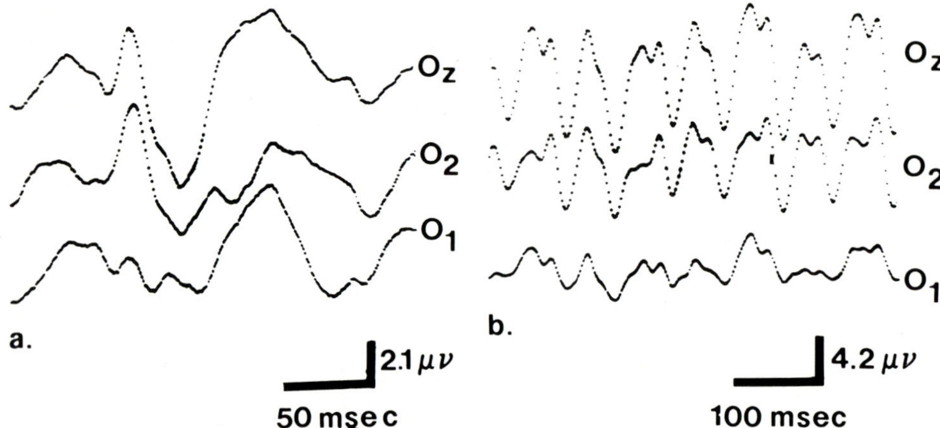

Fig. 11. *Transient and steady-state pattern VER-left occipital focal seizures.* The transient pattern VER to a 1° white-black target alternating at 2 cps revealed a normal VER over the intact right hemisphere, O_2, and a depressed or attenuated VER over the left hemisphere, O_1. A steady-state VER to a 1° white-black target alternating at 16 cps also revealed attenuation or depression of the VER amplitude over the left involved hemisphere, O_1. She had a normal neuro-ophthalmologic examination including Goldmann perimetry and EMI scan and complained of flashing lights in her upper right hemifield. The EEG showed a spike-wave focus in the left occipital region.

ease progressed, the early components decreased in amplitude and latency became prolonged. The attenuation of the early components was temporally related to the onset of cortical blindness.[43]

SUMMARY

The visual evoked response has been proven to be a valuable adjunct in the evaluation of disorders of the visual system. Despite multiple inherent variables, it is possible to differentiate and identify visual defects secondary to retinal, macular, optic nerve, chiasmal and posterior occipital lesions utilizing the appropriate mode of stimulation. The most common clinical application of the VER has been to detect subclinical optic nerve dysfunction in suspected multiple sclerosis.

In order to properly evaluate the functional integrity of the visual system, a laboratory must have the capacity to perform transient and steady state flash and pattern VER's.

EDITOR'S NOTE

I have personally seen only one case in which a visual evoked response gave me more information in an adult that a good

"OV" (office visit). By this I mean that a good history, a careful refraction, distance and near acuities, the pinhole test, and a careful set of visual fields—combined with a search for a Marcus Gunn pupil and careful assessment of the fundus—usually is much, much more valuable than any form of visual evoked response test. In small infants, however, the use of ERG and bright flash VER is at times quite helpful. Years ago, the ERG came in rather slowly in neuro-ophthalmology but has proven helpful so often that I think we should keep up with the workers in this field, and I am very thankful to Dr. Carlow for presenting this data for our review. To the practitioner, however, don't refer your patient off for a VER test to make the diagnosis of multiple sclerosis, unless you have done that careful office visit first. You'll then find that you usually don't need further testing. The history and clinical evaluation are still *THE* ways to make a diagnosis in medicine.

JLS

REFERENCES

1. Sokol, S. Visually evoked potentials: Theory, techniques and clinical applications. Sur. Ophthalmol. *21*:18–44 (1976).
2. Regan, D. New Methods for Neurological Assessment. In: *Overview: Proceedings of the San Diego*

Biomedical Symposium. J. I. Martin (Ed.), Academic, New York, London, 1977, pp. 55–62.

3. Ciganek, L. The EEG response (evoked potential) to light stimulus in man. Electroencephalogr. Clin. Neurophysiol. *13:*165 (1961).

4. Nakamura, Z. and Biersdorf, W. R. Localization of the human visual evoked response. Early components specific to visual stimulation. Am. J. Ophthalmol. *72:*988–997 (1971).

5. Jeffreys, D. A. and Axford, J. G. Source location of pattern-specific components of human visual evoked potentials. I. Components of striate cortical origin. Exp. Brain Res. *16:*1–21 (1972).

6. Jeffreys, D. A. and Axford, J. G. Source locations of pattern-specific components of human visual evoked potentials. II. Component of extrastriate cortical origin. Exp. Brain Res. *16:*22–40 (1972).

7. Millodot, M. and Riggs, L. A. Refraction determined electrophysiologically. Arch. Ophthalmol. *84:*272–278 (1970).

8. Millodot, M. Retinoscopy and the refraction of infants. Ophthalmol. Opt. *12:*1130–1132 (1972).

9. Harden, A. and Pampiglione, G. Visual evoked potentials, electroretinogram, and electroencephalogram studies in progressive neurometabolic "storage" diseases of childhood. In: *Visual Evoked Potentials in Man.* J. E. Desmedt (Ed.), Clarendon, Oxford, 1977, pp. 470–481.

10. Richey, E. T., Kooi, K. A., and Tourtellotte, W. W. Visually evoked responses in multiple sclerosis. J. Neurol. Neurosurg. Psychiatr. *34:*275–280 (1971).

11. Namerow, N. S. and Enns, N. Visual evoked responses in patients with multiple sclerosis. Arch. Neurol. *25:*269–275 (1972).

12. Feinsod, M., Abramsky, O. and Auerbach, E. Electrophysiological examinations of the visual system in multiple sclerosis. J. Neurol. Sci. *20:*161–175 (1973).

13. Halliday, A. M., McDonald, W. I., and Mushin, J. Visual evoked potentials in patients with demyelinating disease. In: *Visual Evoked Potentials in Man.* J. E. Desmedt (Ed.), Clarendon, Oxford, 1977, pp. 438–450.

14. Milner, B. A., Regan, D. and Heron, J. R. Differential diagnosis of multiple sclerosis by visual evoked potential recording. Brain *97:*755–772 (1974).

15. Spekreij, S. E. H., Estevez, O., and Reits, D. Visual evoked potentials and the physiological analysis of visual processing in man. *Visual Evoked Potentials in Man.* J. E. Desmedt (Ed.), Clarendon, Oxford, 1977, pp. 16–89.

16. Regan, D., Milner, B. A., and Heron, J. R. Slowing of visual signals in multiple sclerosis, measured psychophysically and by steady state evoked potentials. *Visual Evoked Potentials in Man.* J. E. Desmedt (Ed.), Clarendon, Oxford, 1977, pp. 461–470.

17. Asselman, P., Chadwick, D. W., and Marsden, C. D. Visual evoked responses in the diagnosis and management of patients suspected of multiple sclerosis. Brain *98:*261–282 (1975).

18. Halliday, A. M., McDonald, W. I., and Mushin, J. The visual evoked response in the diagnosis of multiple sclerosis. Br. Med. J. *4:*661–664 (1973).

19. Hoeppener, T. and Lolas, F. Visual evoked responses and visual symptoms in multiple sclerosis. J. Neurol. Neurosurg. Psychiatr. *41:*493–498 (1978).

20. Ikeda, H., Tremain, K. E., and Sanders, M. D. Neurophysiological investigation in optic nerve disease: combined assessment of the visual evoked response and electroretinogram. Br. J. Ophthalmol. *62:*227–239 (1978).

21. Wilson, E. B. Visual evoked response differentiation of ischemic optic neuritis from the optic neuritis of multiple sclerosis. Am. J. Ophthalmol. *86:*530–535 (1978).

22. Halliday, A. M., Halliday, E., Kriss, E., McDonald, W. I., and Mushin, J. The pattern evoked potential in compression of the anterior visual pathways. Brain *99:*357–374, (1976).

23. Cappin, J. and Nissim, S. Visual evoked response in the detection of field defects and glaucoma. Arch. Ophthalmol. *93:*9–18 (1975).

24. Kooi, K. A., Yamada, T., and Marshall, R. E. Field studies of monocularly evoked cerebral potentials in bitemporal hemianopsia. Neurology (Minneap.) *23:*1217–1225 (1973).

25. Holder, G. E. The effects of chiasmal compression on the pattern visual evoked potential. Electroencephalogr. Clin. Neurophysiol. *45:*278–280 (1978).

26. Borda, R. P. Visual evoked potentials to flash in the clinical evaluation of the visual pathways. *Visual Evoked Potentials in Man.* J. E. Desmedt (Ed.), Clarendon, Oxford, 1977, pp. 481–489.

27. Feinsod, M., Selhorst, J., Hoyt, W. E., and Wilson, C. B. Monitoring optic nerve function during craniotomy. J. Neurosurg. *44:*29–31 (1976).

28. Creel, D., Witkop, C. J., and King, R. A. Asymmetrical visually evoked potentials in human albinos: Evidence for visual system anomalies. Invest. Ophthalmol. *13:*430–440 (1974).

29. Cohn, R. Evoked visual cortical response in homonymous hemianopic defects in man. Electroencephalogr. Clin. Neurophysiol. *5:*922 (1963).

30. Vaughan, H. G., Katzman, R., and Taylor, J. Alterations of visual evoked responses in the presence of homonymous field defects. Electroencephalogr. Clin. Neurophysiol. *15:*737–746 (1963).

31. Kooi, K. A., Guvener, A. M., and Bagchi, B. K. Visual evoked potentials in lesions of the higher optic pathways. Neurology (Minneap.) *15:*841–854 (1965).

32. Biersdorf, W. R. Lateralization of visual evoked responses in normals and hemianopic patients. *Proceedings of the San Diego Biomedical Symposium.* J. I. Martin (Ed.), Academic, New York, London, 1977, pp. 177–182.

33. Corletto, F., Gentilomo, A., Rosadini, G., Rossi, G. F., and Vattoni, J. Visual evoked potentials as recorded from the scalp in the visual cortex before and after surgical removal of the occipital pole in man. Electroencephalogr. Clin. Neurophysiol. *22:*378–380 (1967).

34. Cohn, R. Visual evoked responses in the brain injured monkey. Arch. Neurol. *21:*321–329 (1969).

35. Regan, D. and Heron, J. R. Clinical investigation of lesions of the visual pathways. A new objective technique. J. Neurol. Neurosurg. Psychiatr. *32:*479–483 (1969).

36. Barrett, G., Blumhardt, L., Halliday, A. M., Halliday, E., and Kriss, A. A paradox in the lateralization of the visual evoked response. Nature *261:* 253–255 (1976).
37. Halliday, A. M., Barrett, G., Blumhardt, I. D., Halliday, E., and Kriss, A. The pattern evoked response in hemianopia. Communication in EEG. Electroencephalogr. Clin. Neurophysiol. *43:*537 (1977).
38. Goodwin, J. and Glaser, J. S. Visual evoked response studies in assessment of visual field defects. Trans. Am. Neurol. Assoc. *102:*153–157 (1977).
39. Carlow, T. J., and Rodriquez, M. Localization of cerebral dysfunction by visual evoked response (VER). Ann. Neurol. *4:*176 (1978).
40. Kooi, K. A., and Sharbrough, F. W. III. Electrophysiological findings in cortical blindness. Report of a Case. Electroencephalogr. Clin. Neurophysiol. *20:*260–263 (1966).
41. Spehlmann, R., Gross, R. A., Ho, S. U., Leetsma, J. E., and Norcross, K. A. Visual evoked potentials in post mortem findings in a case of cortical blindness. Ann. Neurol. *2:*531–534 (1977).
42. Kooi, K. A. and Yamada, T. Binocular and monocular visual evoked responses in the differential diagnosis of psychogenic and disease-related visual disorders. Int. J. Neurol. *9:*272–286 (1975).
43. Lee, R. G., and Blair, R. D. G. Evolution of EEG and visual evoked response changes in Jakob-Creutzfeldt disease. Electroencephalogr. Clin. Neurophysiol. *35:*133–142 (1973).

25 Elusive Lesions of the Cavernous Sinus

M. Judith Donovan Post, M.D.,
Joel S. Glaser, M.D.,
and Jonathan D. Trobe, M.D.

Mass lesions in the cavernous sinus are frequently difficult to diagnose, both clinically and radiographically. In a recent review of 21 patients with either cavernous meningioma or aneurysm, it was found that the pathology had not been initially appreciated in any individual. These misdiagnoses occurred despite multiple clinical and radiographic investigations conducted at many different institutions over long periods of time.[1-3]

To determine why these lesions had not been detected until late, the case records of these 21 individuals seen in referral at the Bascom Palmer Eye Institute were reviewed. In addition, the radiographic studies, consisting of plain skull films, complex motion tomograms, radionuclide brain scans, orbital venograms, CT scans, and angiograms were analyzed retrospectively.[1-3] From this review the clinical and radiographic criteria diagnostic for cavernous meningioma and aneurysm were established.

Of the 21 patients, nine had cavernous meningiomas and 12, intracavernous aneurysms. Diagnoses were made by surgery in two of the individuals in each group. In both the surgical and nonsurgical patients, angiography defined the pathology in seven meningioma and seven aneurysm cases.[1-3] Strong clinical and radiographic findings identified the etiology of the patients' cavernous sinus syndromes in the remaining individuals (two meningiomas and five aneurysms).

The symptoms which would have initially alerted the physician to the diagnosis of cavernous meningioma or aneurysm included diplopia, ptosis, trigeminal paresthesias, and (in those with aneurysms) trigeminal pain.[1-3] Mild proptosis, pupillary abnormalities, and ipsilateral deficits in ocular ductions were the physical findings which should have made the examiner suspect the presence of a chronic mass lesion in the cavernous sinus.[1-3]

Additional clues in the aneurysm group included the past history of significant systemic illnesses such as hypertension, diabetes, and cardiovascular disease.[1, 2] A later age of onset also favored the detection of intracavernous aneurysms—68.5 was the median age for the patients with aneurysms in this series, while it was 59 for those with meningiomas. Another nonspecific clue was a high female to male ratio. Females predominated in both classes (7:2 in the meningioma group, and 10:2 in those with aneurysms).

Initial clinical misdiagnoses in these patients presenting with chronic slowly progressive ophthalmoplegia included myasthenia gravis, diabetic or atherosclerotic neuropathies, dysthyroidism, orbital tumors, idiopathic ocular palsies, orbital pseudotumor, atypical facial pain, cranial arteritis, cluster headaches, Duane's retraction syndrome, maxillary sinus disease, hypertensive headache, posterior communicating artery aneurysm, and brain stem disease.[1, 2] Faulty clinical localization, aided by false positive neuro-ophthalmological tests, led to these incorrect clinical diagnoses.[1-3] Symptoms were felt to be related to orbital, brain stem, or intrinsic cranial nerve pathology, rather than to cavernous sinus disease.

Missed radiographic findings and the late performance of computed tomography added to these diagnostic delays. For example, despite the fact that abnormalities on plain skull films were present in eight of the nine meningioma cases, they were not initially recognized in four (Figs. 1 and 7).[1-3] Similarly, among the aneurysm patients whose first set of skull films were available for review (numbering 11), pathology was missed in seven (Fig. 4). Even on complex motion tomography, changes were not appreciated in a number of cases: in 25% of eight meningioma patients who were tomogrammed,[1-3] and in 55.6% of the nine aneurysm patients who were examined tomographically (Fig. 4).

Diagnostic delays also occurred with radionuclide brain scanning. Of the six meningioma patients who had nuclear studies, the findings on the initial scans were either missed (in 16.7%) or not classical (in 16.7%).[1,3] In another 33% the first examination was negative despite the presence of positive angiograms. In the remaining 33% the initial brain scans were classical, but they did not allow for early diagnosis—they were performed only late in the course of the patient's disease, after the presence of a cavernous sinus mass had already been established by CT.

Early diagnosis was not provided by radionuclide brain scanning in the aneurysm patients either. Ten of the 12 individuals with aneurysms had nuclear examinations. Abnormalities were, in fact, present in

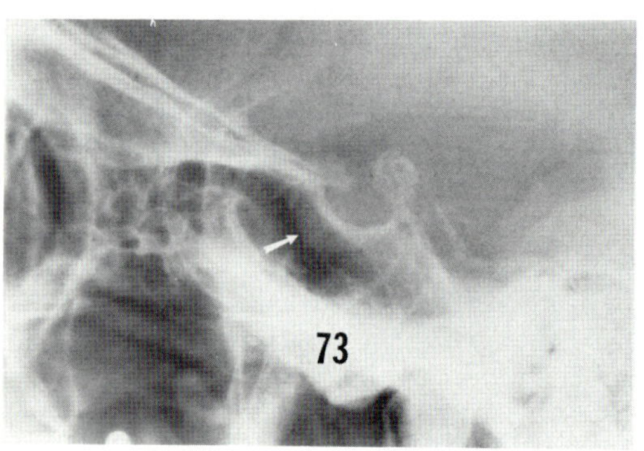

Fig. 1a

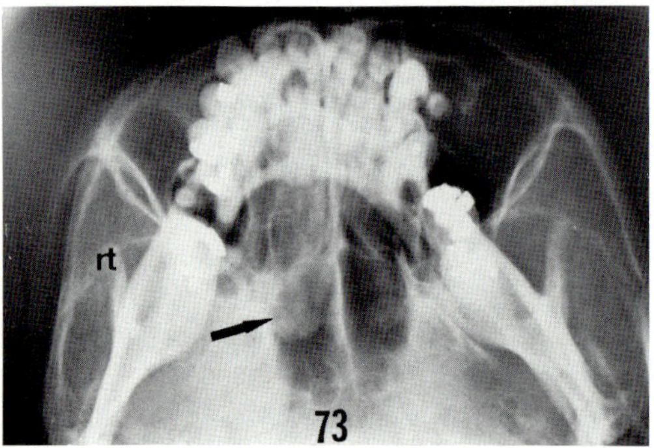

Fig. 1b

Figs. 1a–h. (Cavernous meningioma). A skull series in 1973 demonstrated no hyperostosis and no alteration in the configuration of the sella. However, in retrospect, on the lateral view a small soft tissue density was seen projecting into the sphenoid sinus (upper top row, left, 1a, arrow). A base view localized this density to the right sphenoid sinus (upper top row, right, 1b, arrow). Although an angiogram was performed at that time, a tumor stain in the right cavernous area was not appreciated. Without the benefit of subtraction, the arteriogram was misconstrued as being normal. Not until a CT scan was obtained in late 1975 was the diagnosis of a mass in the right parasellar region finally made. Subsequently in early 1976 a second angiogram was performed in order to establish a more specific diagnosis. The scout films for this study in lateral (upper top row, left 1c, arrow) and base (middle row, left, 1d, arrow) projections revealed that the entire right sphenoid sinus was now opacified. The subtracted films from the angiogram demonstrated a hypertrophied meningohypophyseal trunk and artery to the inferior cavernous sinus, and a tumor stain emanating from the right cavernous sinus (bottom row, left, 1e, arrows). These findings indicated the presence of a meningioma originating from the right cavernous sinus. Follow-up studies one year later in this man with only a very slowly progressive ophthalmoplegia revealed that hyperostosis had developed. Trispiral tomograms in the AP projection (upper top row, right, 1f, arrow) showed hyperostosis not only of the lateral wall of the right sphenoid sinus (small arrow), but also of the lateral wall of the superior orbital fissure (lower large arrow) and of the right anterior clinoid (upper large arrow). The opacification of the right sphenoid sinus was still evident on both the AP (1f) and lateral (middle row, right, 1g, arrows) tomograms. A nonenhanced CT scan at this time substantiated this involvement of the sphenoid sinus (lower bottom row, right, 1h, arrow) and the hyperostosis. The followup CT scan (Fig. 2a) again dramatically documented that this sphenoid sinus reaction was secondary to an adjacent enhancing mass centered in the cavernous sinus which was growing only very slowly.

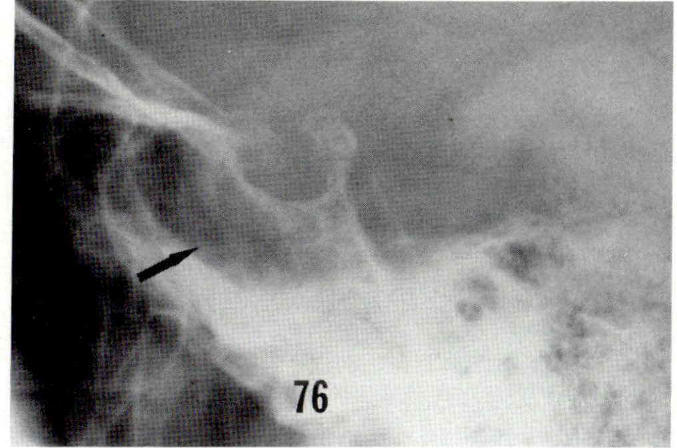

Fig. 1c

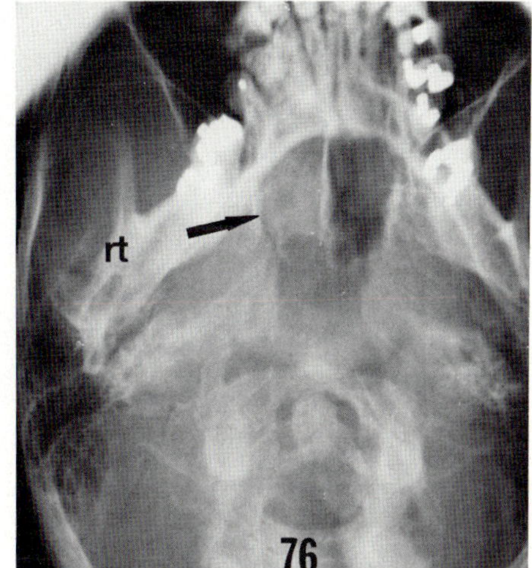

Fig. 1d

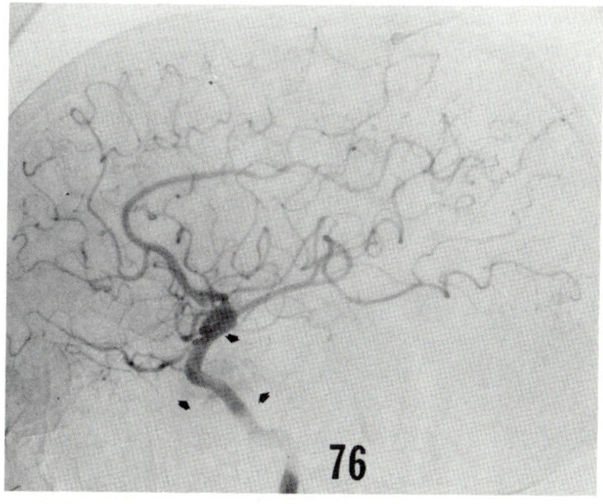

Fig. 1e

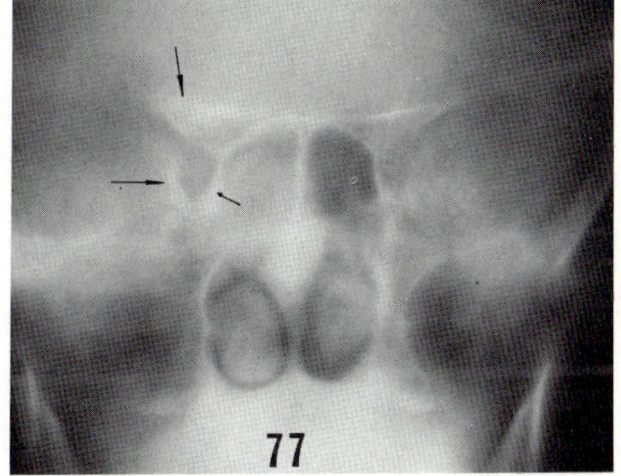

Fig. 1f

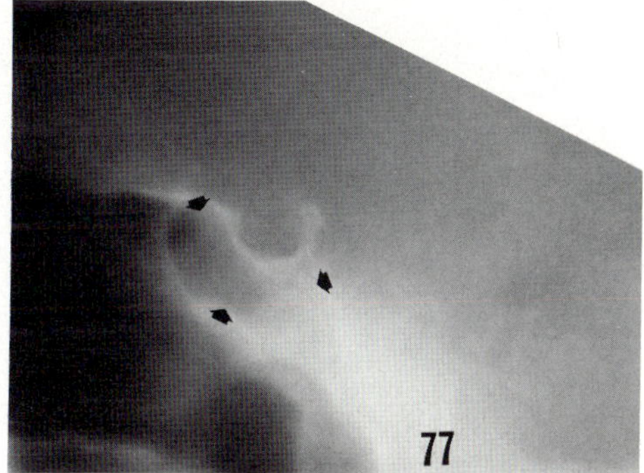

Fig. 1g

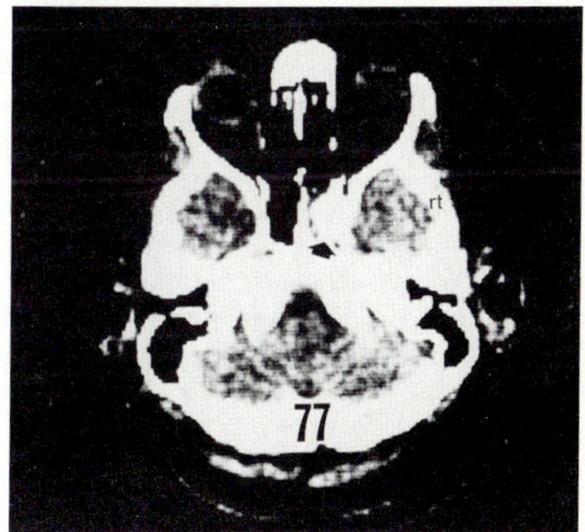

Fig. 1h

eight. However, in three of these eight cases the pathology was not initially evident. And in the remaining cases the scans were all performed late following computed tomography. These studies were obtained at that time for the purpose of distinguishing be-

tween cavernous meningioma and aneurysm.

Orbital venography was done in only two of the 21 patients in this series. This procedure was replaced by the advent of CT. Of the two orbital cavenograms which were performed, one was positive for a cavernous sinus mass but was not specific, while the other was a false negative.[1]

In seven of the nine meningioma patients

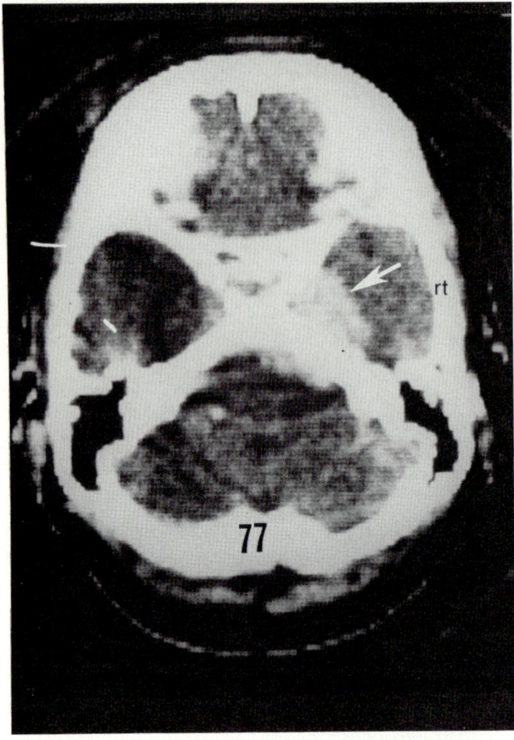

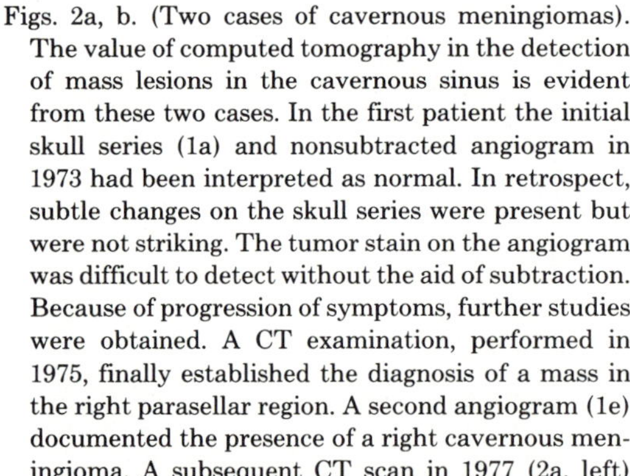

Fig. 2a

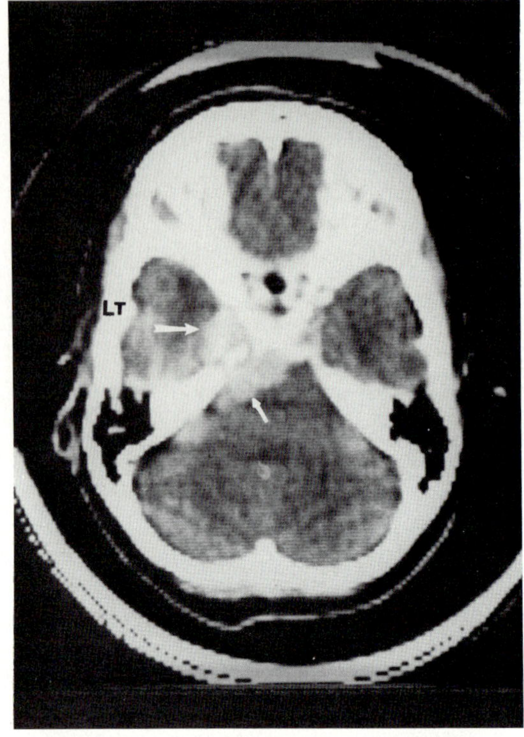

Fig. 2b

Figs. 2a, b. (Two cases of cavernous meningiomas). The value of computed tomography in the detection of mass lesions in the cavernous sinus is evident from these two cases. In the first patient the initial skull series (1a) and nonsubtracted angiogram in 1973 had been interpreted as normal. In retrospect, subtle changes on the skull series were present but were not striking. The tumor stain on the angiogram was difficult to detect without the aid of subtraction. Because of progression of symptoms, further studies were obtained. A CT examination, performed in 1975, finally established the diagnosis of a mass in the right parasellar region. A second angiogram (1e) documented the presence of a right cavernous meningioma. A subsequent CT scan in 1977 (2a, left) allowed for a relatively noninvasive and sensitive method of follow-up. A mild increase in the size of the tumor was found. Figure 2a shows this tumor. A large enhancing mass lesion, centered in the right cavernous sinus (arrow), extending laterally and posteriorly, is seen. Figure 2b represents another patient with slowly progressive ophthalmoplegia whose condition was undiagnosed until a CT scan was performed. The large arrow in Figure 2b, right, points to an enhancing parasellar mass. The small arrow indicates posterior extension. Angiography documented the presence of a meningioma centered in the cavernous sinus with secondary posterior fossa extension.

who were angiogrammed, abnormalities were found in all.[1,3] However, in 43% of cases, the pathological changes were not appreciated. In comparison, none of the angiograms performed on seven of the 12 aneurysm patients were misread. However, angiography was not chosen as a radiographic procedure early in the diagnostic evaluations.

Computed tomography, in contrast to the above studies, was not only positive in every case in which it was performed, but it was also never misinterpreted when the study was correctly performed.[1,3] The CT scan was the examination which finally established the presence of a mass lesion in the cavernous sinus in nine of the 9 meningioma patients (Figs. 2, 3, and 7), and in seven of the aneurysm cases (Figs. 5 and 8). (Angiography established the presence of a parasellar mass in the remaining five aneurysm patients. These patients, however, were studied before CT was available.) Diagnostic delays from CT occurred in only

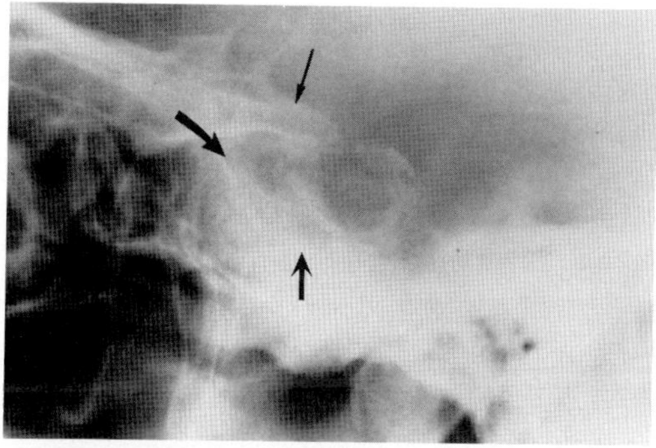

Fig. 3a

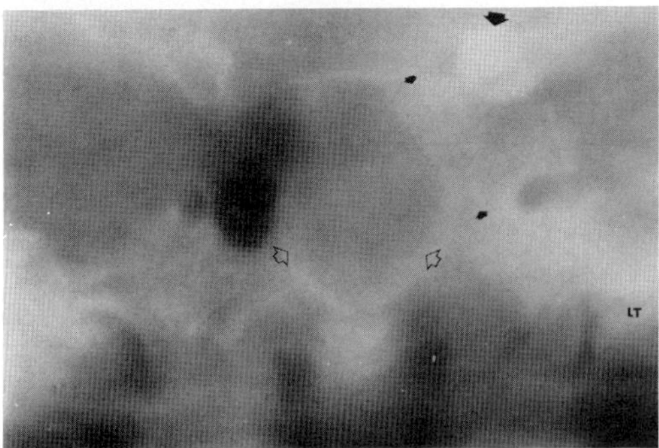

Fig. 3b

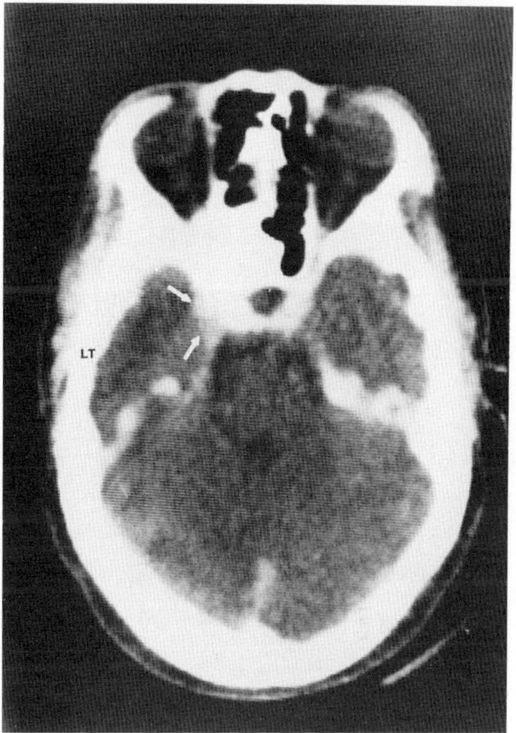

Fig. 3c

Fig. 3a–c. (Cavernous meningioma). Considerable hyperostosis of the sphenoid is seen in Figure 3a, left. Not only is the sphenoid sinus (lower two arrows) hyperostotic, but one of the anterior clinoids (highest arrow) is markedly thickened and dense from bony proliferation. An AP tomogram (3b, bottom) in this same patient documented these findings and revealed the exact location and extent of these changes. The enlarged and thickened left anterior clinoid is seen (highest arrow). In addition, left parasellar hyperostosis is demonstrated (the area between the two small black arrows). Soft tissue opacification and bony reaction is also visualized in the left sphenoid sinus (open arrows). A contrast CT scan (3c, right) not only verified the existence of this hyperostosis, but it also revealed the presence of an enhancing soft tissue mass in the left cavernous sinus (arrows). This combination of findings: hyperostosis on plain films and tomograms and enhancing mass on CT scan indicated that a parasellar meningioma was the most likely etiology of this patient's cavernous sinus syndrome.

one of the meningioma and one of the aneurysm cases. These delays resulted only because the cavernous sinus area was not included on the initial CT examination. When a repeat study was performed with base of the skull included, the enhancing cavernous sinus mass lesions were quickly recognized.

Because diagnostic delays occurred so frequently in this series of 21 patients due to missed radiographic findings, the abnormalities present on these examinations and their incidence are charted below. These statistics are listed because it is felt that familiarity with the changes that are commonly seen in the cavernous meningiomas and aneurysms will lead to an increased recognition rate of these two lesions.[1, 3] (Refer to Figs. 1, 3, and 7 for skull films on meningioma cases, and Figs. 4 and 5 for skull films on aneurysm cases. Refer to Figs. 1 and 3 for meningioma tomograms, and Fig. 5 for aneurysm tomograms. Refer to Figures 2, 3, and 7 for meningioma CT scans, and Figures 5 and 8 for aneurysm CT scans.)

The pathology present on either the initial or follow-up brain scans of patients with the meningiomas included abnormal flow studies in five of the six meningioma patients who were scanned.[1, 3] In three of these five positive cases, a pattern classical

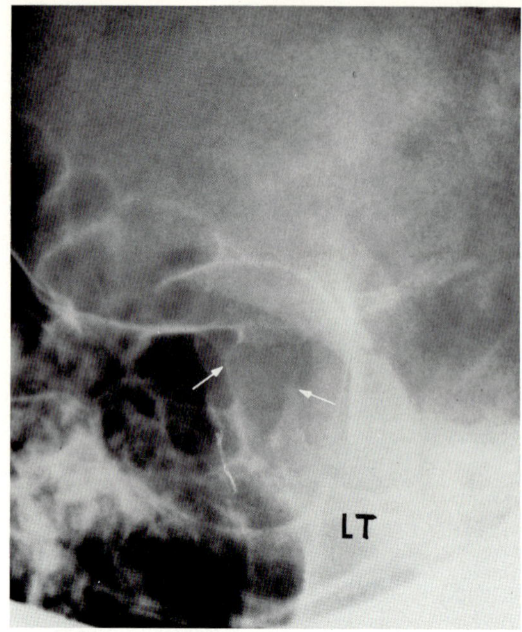

Fig. 4a

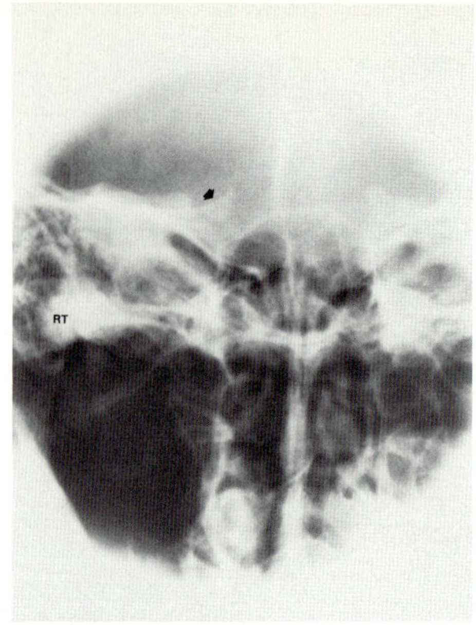

Fig. 5a

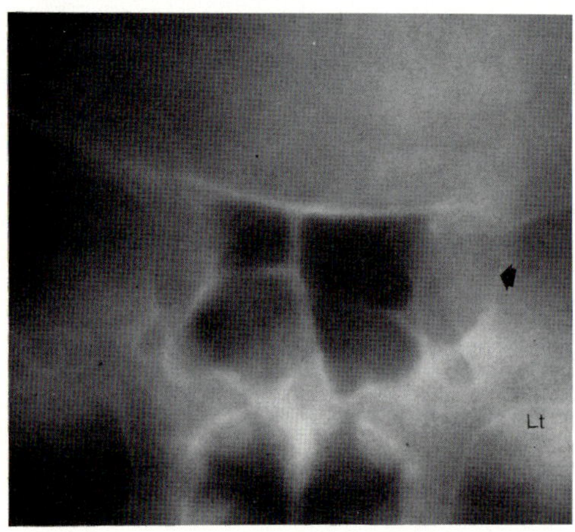

Fig. 4b

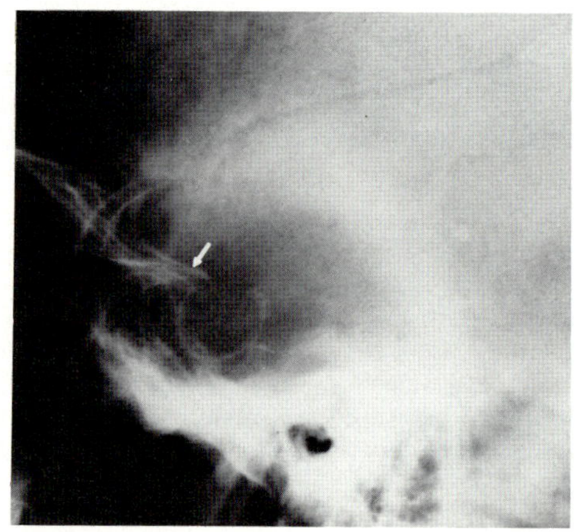

Fig. 5b

Figs. 4a, b. (Intracavernous aneurysm). The abnormalities on the plain skull films, Rhese views of the optic canals, and first set of tomograms were not initially appreciated in this patient with ophthalmoplegia. A delay in diagnosis, therefore, occurred until follow-up studies were performed. Erosion of the floor of the optic canal was evident in Rhese projection. (The higher arrow in Fig. 3a, left, points in the direction of the destroyed optical canal floor.) Enlargement of the left superior orbital fissure (SOF) was seen (lower arrow, 4a). Erosion of the SOF was also suggested. AP tomograms (4b, bottom) confirmed the enlargement of the SOF (arrow) and its eroded superior-lateral wall. An intracavernous aneurysm was documented as the cause of these abnormalities by the findings on a subsequent CT scan and radionuclide brain scan. (Prints reproduced through the courtesy of Masson Publishing, USA.)

Figs. 5a, b. (Intracavernous aneurysm). Undercutting and elevation of an anterior clinoid is a frequent radiographic finding in patients with intracavernous aneurysms. Figure 5a, top, demonstrates this anterior clinoid thinning and elevation (arrow) on the frontal projection of a plain skull film. These changes were also suggested on lateral views (5b, bottom, arrow). Complex motion tomography in lateral position confirmed these findings and demonstrated them to better advantage. The arrow in 5c, left, top row, points to the elevated and pencilled right anterior clinoid. A subsequent contrast CT scan (5d, bottom row, left, arrow) indicated that an enhancing mass lesion in the right cavernous sinus was the cause of this clinoidal erosion. A radionuclide brain scan was then obtained in order to differentiate between cavernous meningioma and aneurysm. The flow study (5e, right, top row) of this scan documented the presence of a right parasellar aneurysm by revealing immediate increased uptake

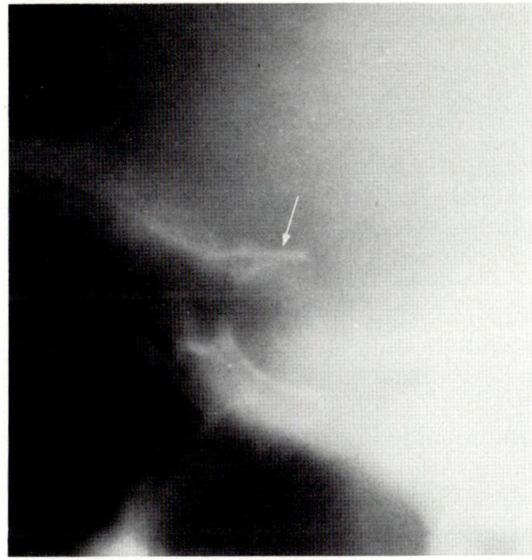

Fig. 5c

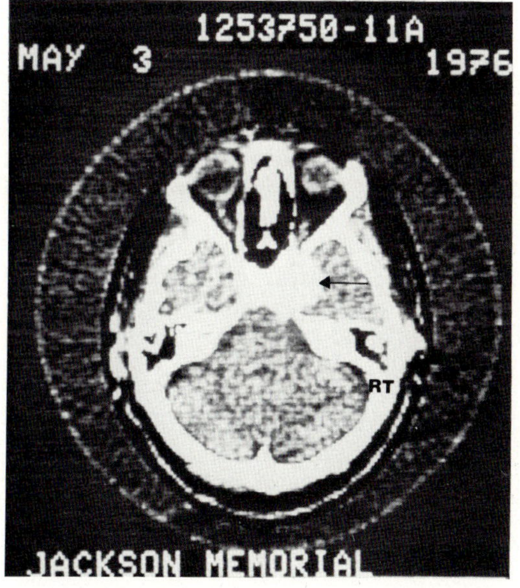

Fig. 5d

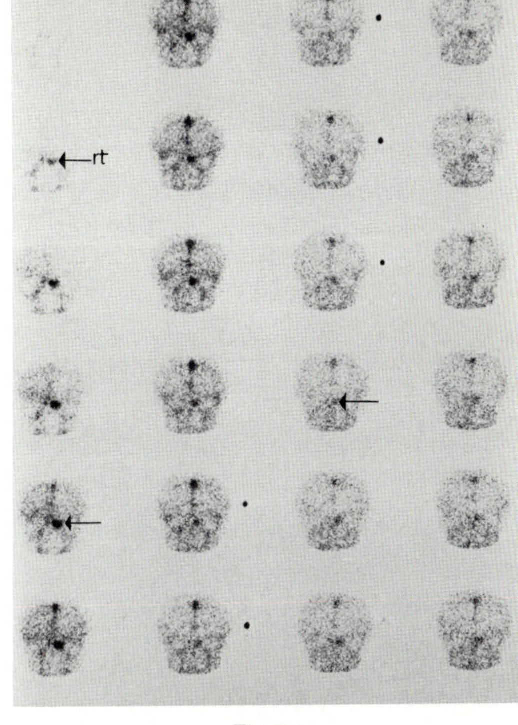

Fig. 5e

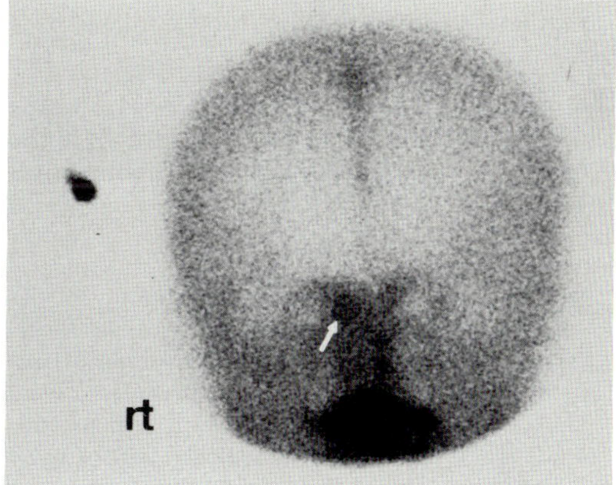

Fig. 5f

of technetium in the earliest arterial images (two arrows in the first row of this scan). Fading of this abnormal technetium accumulation was evident in the venous phase (arrows in the third row of this radionuclide flow study). Due to the large size of this lesion, the statics revealed increased isotopic uptake in the right parasellar region as well (5f, right, bottom row, arrow). (Prints reproduced through the courtesy of the Masson Publishing, USA.)

for cavernous meningioma was found. There was increased accumulation of technetium in the parasellar region appearing with increasing intensity in the venous phase. The static examinations, in contrast to the flow studies, were not dramatic at all. In three cases they were only questionably positive and in another two, negative.[1,3]

Radionuclide brain scans were more

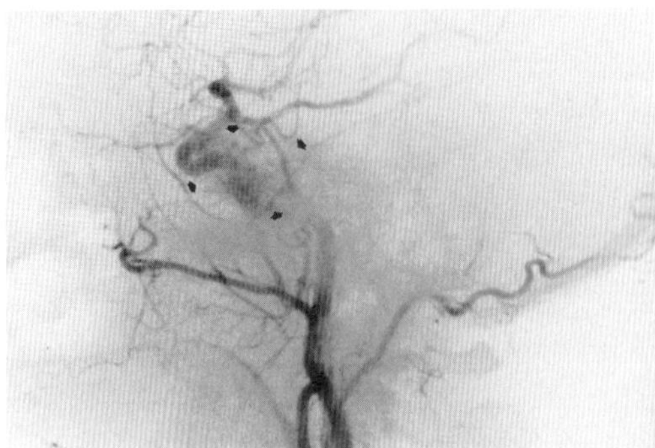

Fig. 6a

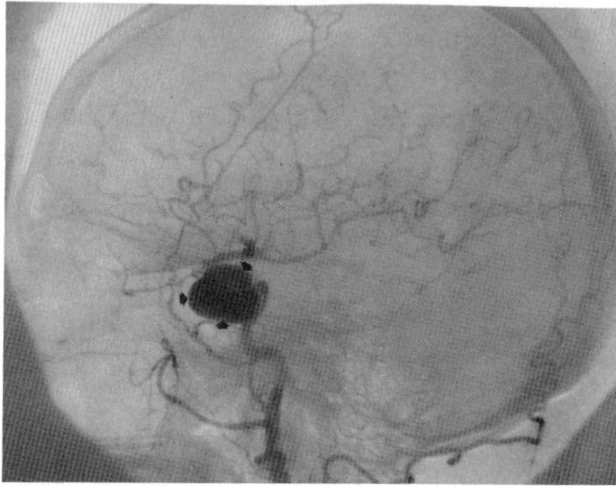

Fig. 6b

Figs. 6a, b. (Cavernous meningioma, case to left; intracavernous aneurysm, case to right). The value of angiography in differentiating between cavernous meningiomas and aneurysms is evident from the above two cases. On the left, a tumor blush (arrows, 6a) is seen emanating from the cavernous sinus on a right common carotid angiogram. Selective internal and external carotid injections, subsequently performed, demonstrated to better advantage that this tumor was being supplied by cavernous carotid and external carotid artery feeders. Surgery documented the presence of a right parasellar meningioma with posterior extent. In another patient with slowly progressive ophthalmoplegia, angiography also established the definitive diagnosis. A very large intracavernous aneurysm (arrows, 6b, bottom) was seen on this left common carotid angiogram.

helpful in the patients with aneurysms (Fig. 5).[1,3] Ten of the 12 individuals with aneurysms had nuclear studies. Of these 10, eight had dynamic studies which were positive. In contrast, the static phase was negative in five, equivocal in one, and positive in two. In the eight patients with abnormal flow studies, a pattern classical for aneurysm was present on the symptomatic side in seven, and on the nonsymptomatic side in one.* The immediate increased accumulation of technetium in the earliest arterial images in the parasellar area was diagnostic of intracavernous aneurysm. A gradual decrease in the intensity of this uptake in the venous phase was also characteristic. Because of the older age of the aneurysm patients and the added risk of angiography to these individuals, the radionuclide brain scan was felt to be invaluable in their diagnostic workup. When combined with CT, skull films, and tomograms, the radionuclide brain scan could establish the diagnosis of intracavernous aneurysm in a relatively noninvasive way.

In seven of the nine meningioma patients, angiography was performed (Figs. 1, 6, and 7). Subtraction and magnification was found necessary for optimal delineation of the abnormalities. Subtle changes at the skull base were missed without the aid of these techniques. Abnormalities found on review of the seven angiograms and their frequency included the following: (1) cavernous carotid arterial feeders: 100% (consisting of an enlarged meningohypophyseal trunk in 100% and hypertrophied artery to the inferior cavernous sinus: 86%); (2) tumor blush: 100% (relatively homogeneous although not sharply defined, centered in the cavernous sinus, and most intense in the late arterial and early capillary phase); (3) additional feeders: from newly formed cavernous and/or petrous carotid arteries: 29%; from external carotid: 29%; from basilar: 14%; (4) cavernous and/or petrous carotid arterial encasement: 71% (extreme: 20%, moderate: 40%, mild: 40%); (5) posterior extension anterior and lateral to brain stem: 86%.

The angiograms which were obtained in seven of the 12 aneurysms were all pathognomonic (Figs. 6 and 8). However, they were performed only late in the diagnostic work-up of these patients. The focal accumulation of contrast in the parasellar area, measuring 2.0 cm or over in transverse diameter in 71% of cases, was diagnostic.

* This patient had a clinically silent contralateral intracavernous aneurysm and an ipsilateral symptomatic intracavernous aneurysm with carotid-cavernous fistula.

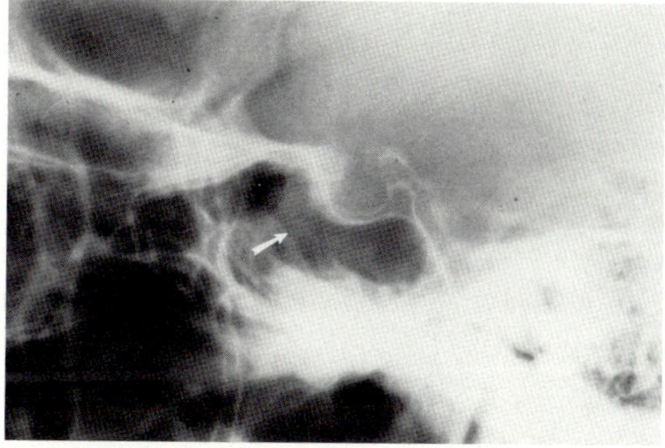

Fig. 7a

Figs. 7a–c. (Cavernous meningioma). A lateral view of the skull revealing a soft tissue density in the sphenoid sinus (left, 7a, arrow) was misinterpreted as normal. Computed tomography, performed at this same time, was not of aid since only a noncontrast study was obtained and since the cavernous area was not even included on the scan. One year later a nonenhanced CT study on the GE CT/T Scanner revealed a soft tissue density projecting into the sphenoid sinus. With contrast injection, a relatively small enhancing mass in the cavernous sinus was detected (upper right, 7b, large white arrow). Secondary sphenoid sinus reaction was also seen (small arrow). Since a radionuclide brain scan did not conclusively differentiate between a cavernous meningioma and aneurysm and since the patient was not elderly, an angiogram was performed. A left internal carotid injection documented the presence of a cavernous meningioma. Figure 7c shows encasement of the posterior cavernous and precavernous carotid (small arrows) and hypertrophied meningohypophyseal and inferior cavernous sinus arteries. A small tumor blush was shown best on the late arterial films. It was elected to follow the patient with serial CT scans. Surgical intervention is anticipated only if the tumor grows to such a size that brain stem or visual pathway compression develops.

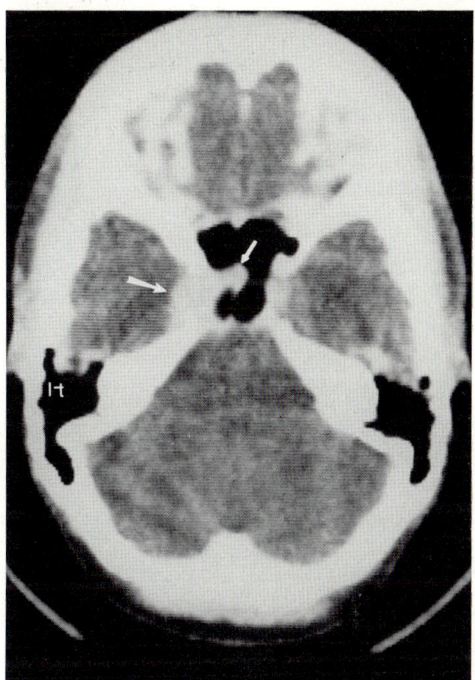

Fig. 7b

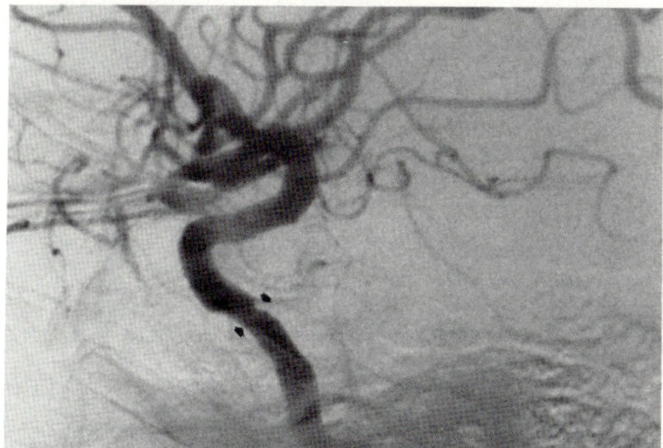

Fig. 7c

These aneurysms, always associated with local mass effect, filled the entire cavernous sinus in 86% of cases. Thrombus formation was indicated in 29% because of the discrepancy in the size of the mass effect and the contrast filled aneurysm sac. The cavernous carotid was irregular and narrowed in 57%, while the aneurysm sac was irregular in 100% and multilobulated in 43%.

That meningiomas and aneurysms of the cavernous sinus are relatively elusive lesions has been indicated by our review of 21 patients. A correct diagnosis was not made either clinically or radiographically in any patient. The infrequency of occurrence of these lesions, the lack of awareness of clinical symptomatology, and the incorrect assumption that meningiomas do not originate from the cavernous sinus all led to the clinical delays.[1-12] Incorrect clinical localization could have been avoided had meningiomas and aneurysms been included in the differential of those individuals presenting with slowly progressive ophthalmoplegia. And even in confusing cases in which radiographic findings were similar to those in other disease states, clinical correlation could have narrowed the differential (Figs. 9 and 10).

In retrospect, radiographic delays could

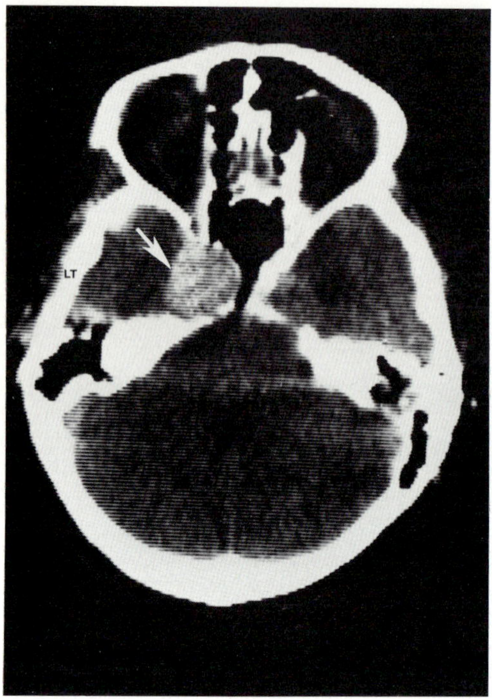

Fig. 8a

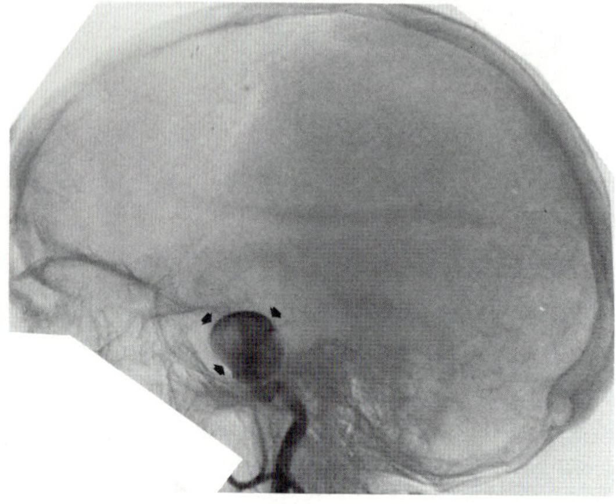

Fig. 8b

Figs. 8a, b. (Intracavernous aneurysm). In this 65-year-old white female with diplopia secondary to a chronic six nerve palsy, a CT scan established the presence of a mass in the cavernous sinus. The arrow in Figure 8a, left, points to the large enhancing parasellar lesion. Angiography, however, was needed in order to provide the specific diagnosis. The earliest arterial film of a left common carotid angiogram (8b, right) demonstrated a sizable intracavernous aneurysm (arrows). (CT scan courtesy of Donald Vining, M.D., Naples, Florida.)

have been avoided as well.[1, 3] The diagnosis of a chronic mass lesion in all 21 patients could have been made if complimentary radiographic studies with optimal techniques had been obtained at the onset of symptoms. Had CT in particular, because of its extreme sensitivity and low rate of misinterpretation, been obtained earlier in the course of each patient's disease, the presence of mass lesions in the cavernous sinus could have been established.

There is no doubt that a high index of clinical suspicion and thorough familiarity with the x-ray changes in these two pathological entities would have increased diagnostic accuracy.[1-3, 13] For example, had hyperostosis been noticed on many of the original skull films in the meningioma patients, and had sphenoid sinus and anterior clinoid erosion been observed in many of the aneurysm cases, the radiologic work-up would not have halted with the plain skull films. Complex motion tomograms would have been obtained to have documented and further characterized these abnormalities, and CT scans would have been performed to determine if these bone changes were caused by the presence of a mass lesion in the cavernous sinus. With visualization of an enhancing mass in the parasellar region, a radionuclide brain scan would have then been performed to differentiate in the elderly patient between cavernous meningioma and aneurysm. In younger patients, angiography would have completed the radiographic workup by documenting either the existence of a cavernous meningioma or aneurysm. A tumor blush contributed to by cavernous carotid feeders would have confirmed the presence of a meningioma, and a focally dilated arterial sac would have diagnosed the presence of an aneurysm.

TABLE I.

Radiographic Abnormality	Skull films		Complex motion tomograms	
	Meningiomas (performed on nine patients)	Aneurysms (performed on 12 patients)	Meningiomas (performed on eight patients)	Aneurysms (performed on nine patients)
a) Hyperostosis and/or b) Tumoral calcification	67% a) and b)	0%	a) 75% b) 63%	0%
Aneurysmal calcification	0%	33.3% (but striking in only 16.7%)	0%	33.3% (but striking in only 11.1%)
Soft tissue density in sphenoid sinus	44%	50%	88%	88.9%
Sphenoid sinus erosion	22%	50% (Unquestionable: 33.3%; further documentation by tomography: 16.7%)	50%	88.9%
Anterior clinoid erosion	22%	83.3%	25%	88.9%
Superior orbital fissure enlargement	0%	25%	0%	22.2%
Superior orbital fissure destruction	0%	16.7%	0%	11.1%
Sellar floor destruction	11%	25%	—	33.3%
Abnormal sellar configuration	11%	16.6%	0%	0%
Minimal sellar enlargement	0%	16.7%	0%	0%

TABLE II.

Computed scans Radiographic abnormality	Nonenhanced		Contrast	
	Meningiomas (performed on nine patients)	Aneurysms (performed on seven patients)	Meningiomas (performed on nine patients)	Aneurysms (performed on six patients)
Involvement of the sphenoid sinus (either of a soft tissue or hyperostotic nature)	100%	100%		
Hyperostosis	89%	0%		
Calcification		14.3%		
Undercutting of anterior clinoid	0%	57.1%		
Increase in soft tissue density of cavernous sinus on noncontrast study	78%	100%		
Tumoral calcification	44%	0%		
Contrast enhancement of cavernous mass	—	—	100% (dramatic: 56%; moderate: 11%; mild: 11%; minimal: 22.2%)	100% (dramatic: 66.7%; moderate: 33.3%)
Posterior extension of enhancing mass	—	—	89%	0%

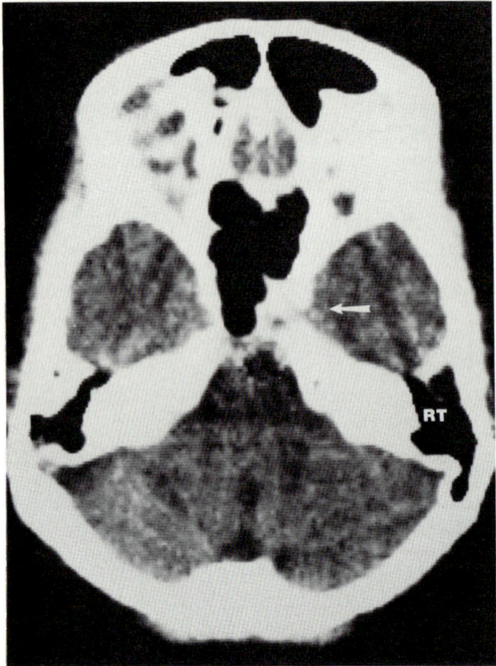

Fig. 9a

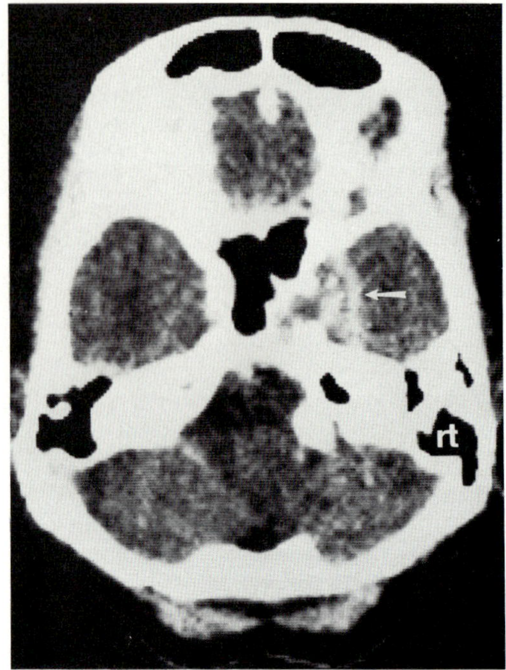

Fig. 9b

Figs. 9a–c. (Multiple melanoma). Although the CT scan is invaluable in establishing the presence of mass lesions in the cavernous sinus, the findings may be very subtle, especially early on in the course of a patient's disease. Abnormalities may, therefore, be missed resulting in diagnostic delays. A high index of clinical suspicion, high quality CT scans, and the use of other complimentary radiographic studies (plain skull films, complex motion tomograms, radionuclide brain scans, and angiograms) decrease the likelihood of misdiagnoses. Figures 9a–c illustrate this point. A contrast CT scan (9a, left) was originally read as normal although a subtle area of increased soft tissue density (white arrow) was present in retrospect. Right sphenoid sinus changes were also evident. Had complex motion tomography been performed at this point, bony abnormalities of the sphenoid bone would have been detected and the cause of this patient's cavernous sinus syndrome established. A contrast CT scan (9b, upper right) obtained one month later in this patient with a painful ophthalmoplegia revealed a large enhancing right parasellar mass (arrow). This lesion had increased dramatically in size since the prior study. The etiology of this patient's cavernous mass was not difficult to determine. The clinical history and the remainder of the CT scan made the diagnosis very evident. This middle-aged female had documented multiple melanoma. In fact, a prosthesis (9c, lower right, higher arrow) had been placed in the right orbit following surgery for orbital melanoma. Residual soft tissue tumor is seen on this same scan

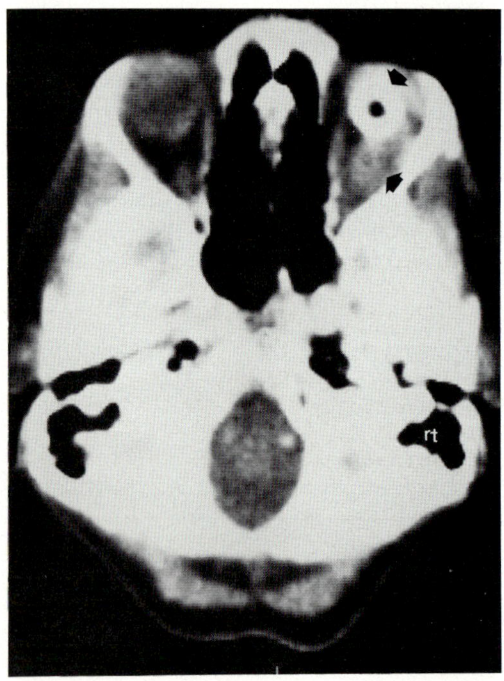

Fig. 9c

in the orbit laterally, (lower arrow, 9c). Diagnosis: metastatic melanoma to the cavernous sinus and orbit. (This patient was not one of the 21 cases reported in this paper.)

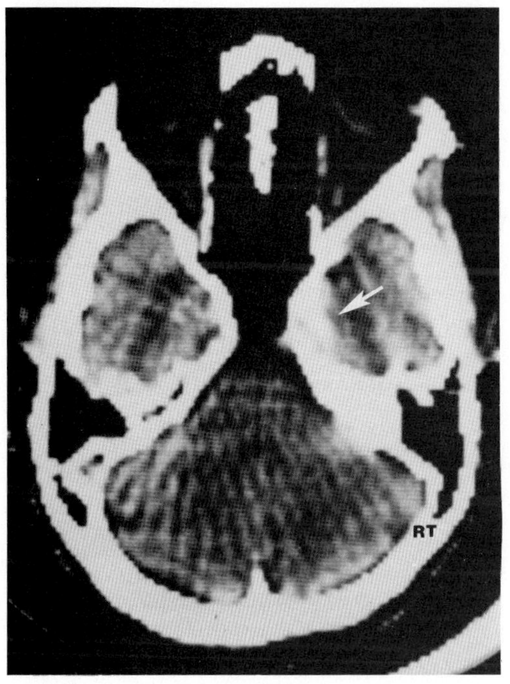

Fig. 10a

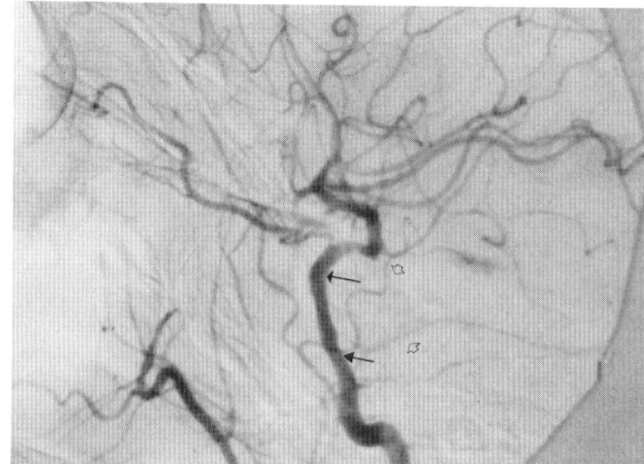

Fig. 10b

Figs. 10a, b. (Metastatic carcinoma to the right cavernous sinus). An abnormal area of enhancement was suggested on a contrast CT scan in the right cavernous sinus (Fig. 10a, left, arrow). Although similar in CT appearance to a cavernous meningioma, the clinical situation made the diagnosis of meningioma unlikely. The painful nature of this 38-year-old white female's ophthalmoplegia and the rapid onset of symptoms (three weeks) suggested the presence of a metastatic lesion. Angiography confirmed the presence of a parasellar mass by revealing encasement and displacement of the cavernous and petrous segments of the right internal carotid artery (arrows, 10b, right). A faint tumor blush supplied by cavernous carotid feeders (open arrows) indicated the presence of tumor. Subsequent mammography and breast biopsy revealed the presence of carcinoma, metastatic to the breast. Carcinoma, secondary to a metastasis to the cavernous sinus, was, therefore, confirmed. (This patient was not one of the 21 cases reported in this series.)

EDITOR'S NOTE

The authors have summarized 21 cases of intracavernous mass lesions well. Of this group there were nine cavernous meningiomas and 12 intracavernous aneurysms. My experience has been that the intracavernous aneurysms are considerably more common of the two. The sad part about this paper is that the plain skull films were abnormal in eight of the nine meningioma cases, but were not initially recognized in four. Furthermore, of 11 sets of routine skull films in the aneurysm patients, pathology was missed in seven. Now this does not tell me that we need more exotic tests as computed tomographic scans to diagnose such lesions. What it tells me is this: (1) everyone reading this chapter needs to re-read the classic paper by S. P. Meadows, M.D., "Intracavernous Aneurysms of the Internal Carotid Artery—Their Clinical Features and Natural History," which appeared in *Arch. Ophthalmol.* **62**:566–574, 1959. That is truly a classic paper and, although now 20 years old, it is loaded with red hot pearls that will enable you to suspect intracavernous aneurysms from the office visit. (2) The second point is that Meadows specifically mentions that special attention should be paid to the *optic foramina* and *superior orbital fissures* on plain skull films for diagnosis of these lesions. The dynamic radionuclide brain scan is also a helpful test for confirmation of the diagnosis of an intracavernous aneurysm, and can obviate the necessity for arteriography in many of these elderly patients.

In essence, if you see a middle-aged woman presenting over the age of 50 with often a slow and insidious onset of symptoms—with at times bouts of pain in and around the eye—and who then presents with a VI nerve palsy, and eventually a III nerve palsy usually with a rather small pupil, moderate unilateral exophthalmos, modest optic atrophy, and usually without a bruit, at times with some vascular hypertension, and who shows erosion of the optic foramen and widening of the superior orbital fissure on plain skull films—then you are dealing with an intracavernous aneurysm, in all probability. A dynamic carotid scan will show such a lesion, and arteriography can be avoided. Neither of the two lesions—meningioma or aneurysm—in the cavernous sinus should be considered surgical candidates—in most cases. As was noted years ago, these lesions spare the patient's life by causing loss of the eye. This is an important paper to help refresh our memory of these lesions, but is also a plea for a more careful look at the plain skull x-rays. The ophthalmologist will have to have those skull x-rays reviewed or he will miss the diagnosis in such cases.

JLS

Addendum: Dr. Norman Schatz has emphasized the development of aberrant regeneration of the III nerve in cases of intracavernous meningioma. The latter are rare lesions, but this is worth mentioning when one does encounter aberrant regeneration of III.

ACKNOWLEDGMENTS

Grateful appreciation is expressed to the following: (1) Ms. Hazel Garrett for the excellent typing of the manuscript; (2) The Biomedical Communications Department of the University of Miami School of Medicine for the fine photographic prints, and (3) Masson Publishing, USA, for permission to reproduce prints from Figures 4 and 5.

REFERENCES

1. Post, M. J. D., Glaser, J. S., and Trobe, J. D. The Radiographic Diagnosis of Cavernous Meningiomas and Aneurysms With a Review of the Neurovascular Anatomy of the Cavernous Sinus, In: *Critical Reviews in Diagnostic Imaging.* CRC Press, in press.
2. Trobe, J. D., Glaser, J. S., and Post, M. J. D. Meningiomas and aneurysms of the cavernous sinus, neuro-ophthalmologic features. Arch. Ophthalmol. *96*(3):457–469 (March 1978).
3. Post, M. J. D., Glaser, J. S., and Trobe, J. D. The radiographic recognition of two clinically elusive mass lesions of the cavernous sinus: Meningiomas and aneurysms. Neuroradiology *16*:499–503 (1978).
4. Locksley, H. B. Natural history of subarachnoid hemorrhage, intracranial aneurysms and arteriovenous malformation. J. Neurosurg. *25*:219–239 (1966).
5. Krayenbühl, H. Klassifikation and klinische Symptomatologie der zerebralen Aneurysmen. Ophthalmologica *167*:122–164 (1973).
6. Cushing, H. and Eisenhardt, L. *Meningiomas: Their Classification, Regional Behavior, Life History and Surgical Results.* Hafner, New York, 1962.
7. Zulch, K. J. *Brain Tumors: Their Biology and Pathology.* Springer, New York, 1957.
8. MacCarty, C. S. *The Surgical Treatment of Intracranial Meningiomas.* Charles C Thomas, Springfield, Ill. 1961.
9. Hoessly, G. F. and Olivecrona, H. Report on 280 cases of verified parasagittal meningioma. J. Neurosurg. *12*:614–626 (1955).
10. Harris, F. S. and Rhoton, A., Jr. Anatomy of the cavernous sinus. J. Neurosurg. *45*:169–180 (August 1976).
11. Sakalas, R., Harbison, J. W., Vines, F. S., and Becker, D. F. Chronic sixth nerve palsy, initial sign of basisphenoid tumors. Arch. Ophthalmol. *93*:186–190 (1975).
12. Thomas, J. E. and Yoss, R. E. The parasellar syndrome: problems in determining etiology, Mayo Clin. Proc *45*:617–623 (1970).
13. Baker, H. L., Jr. The angiographic delineation of sellar and parasellar masses. Radiology *104*:67–78 (July 1972).

26 Computed Tomography in the Evaluation of the Sella and Juxtasella Region

Jerome J. Sheldon, M.D.
Juan-Martin Leborgne, M.D.

Computed tomography has proven useful in evaluating patients with suspected sella and juxtasella pathology.[1-5] Lesions in this area often cause gross or subtle erosive and/or proliferative bony changes in the sella turcica. Because of volume averaging of the delicate bony structures and soft tissues in this area, these changes could be difficult to detect on the computed tomographic images. Consequently, the initial radiographic evaluation of patients with clinically suspected sella and juxtasella disease would include plain film radiographs and conventional tomography of the sella region. This is followed by computed tomography, which demonstrates the superior and lateral soft tissue extension of these lesions.

TECHNIQUE

The sella area is evaluated with axial images obtained at a 20° angulation to the canthomeatal plane (Fig. 1). Following this, images parallel to the canthomeatal plane are then obtained (Fig. 2). To decrease volume averaging from adjacent bony structures, and air-containing paranasal sinuses, the thinnest sections possible should be utilized. This would include 4-, 5-, or 6-mm sections on the new scanners, or 8-mm overlapping sections on the earlier model scanners. All of the above 20° and 0° images are repeated after the intravenous infusion of an iodine-containing contrast agent. (In our department, we use 100 cc of Vascoray containing 400 mg of organically bound iodine

per cc.) This allows for evaluation of the integrity of the blood brain barrier, and will enhance the soft tissue component of a lesion.[6]

The lowest image should be through the body of the sella and sphenoid sinus region. Sequential sections passing superiorly should demonstrate the sella turcica and its component bony structures, the suprasellar cistern, and the anterior portion of the third ventricle. In certain instances, to better delineate the pathological anatomy as to superior and inferior extension, direct coronal images through the sella region will be obtained (Fig. 3). With this projection, the plane of the imager is 90° to the canthomeatal reference plane.[7]

NORMAL ANATOMY

Computed cranial tomography, which includes evaluation of the sella and suprasellar cistern, demonstrates these anatomical areas in the axial projection.[8] These structures will have a slightly different appearance, depending upon the degree of angulation (Figs. 1, 2, and 4). Our routine evaluation of the sella region includes thin section images at 20° (Figs. 1, 4A, and 4C) and at zero degrees (Figs. 2, 4B, and 4D). In the lower images of the sella, the anterior clinoid processes, tuberculum sella, and dorsum sella are routinely identified. The soft tissue structures of the sella turcica are difficult to evaluate because of computer overshoot and volume averaging of the bony structures, air-filled sphenoid sinus,

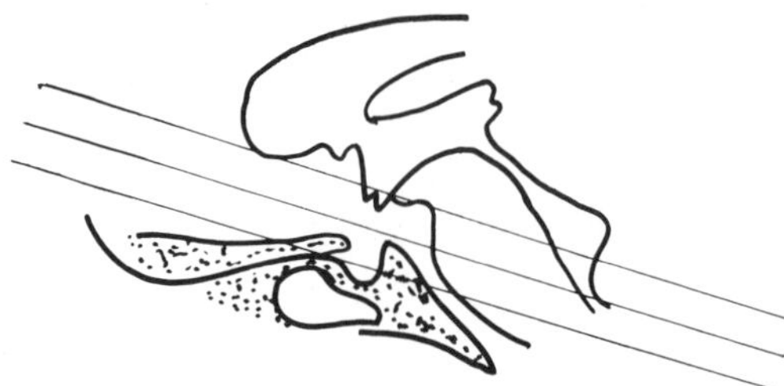

Fig. 1. Schematic diagram demonstrating the 8 mm thick images taken at the canthomeatal reference plane. The inferior level corresponds to the level of the image demonstrated in Figure 4A. The superior level corresponds to the level of the image in Figure 4C.

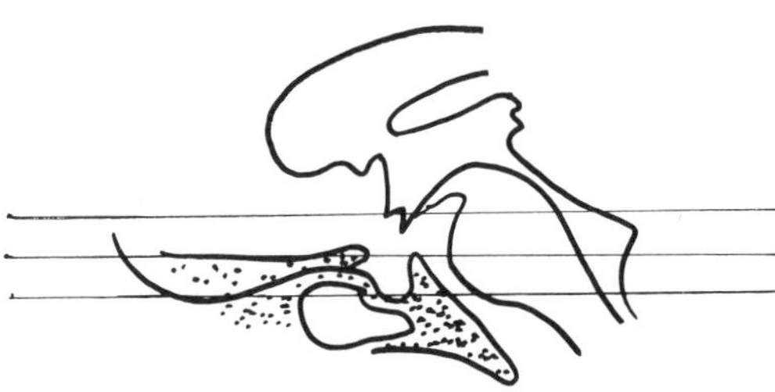

Fig. 2. Schematic diagram demonstrating the 8 mm thick images taken at 0° angulation to the canthomeatal reference plane. The inferior level corresponds to the image demonstrated in Figure 4B. The superior level corresponds to the level of the image in Figure 4D.

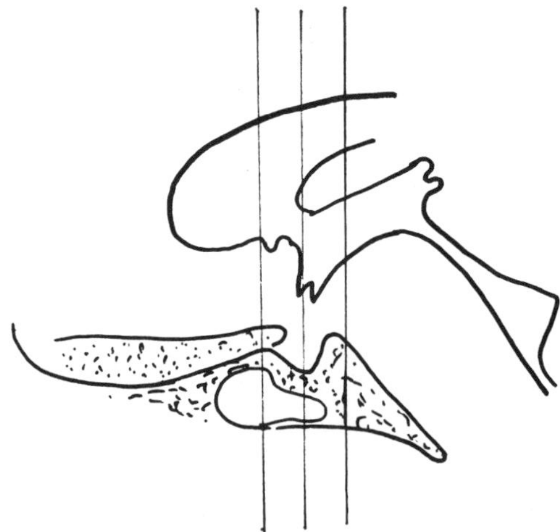

Fig. 3. Schematic diagram demonstrating the coronal projection with the plane of the images at approximately 90° to the canthomeatal reference plane. This corresponds to the images demonstrated in: Figures 7E, F, G, H; Figures 10C, D, E, F; Figures 12D, E, F; Figures 13E, G; Figures 14C, D; Figures 15C, D.

and adjacent soft tissues. The suprasellar cistern will have a pentagonal appearance on the image at 20 degrees (Fig. 4C). The anterior portion of the cistern is bordered by the subcalossal gyri, the lateral borders by the uncus, and the posterior margin by the pons on the 20° image, and the mesencephalon on the 0° image. The suprasella cistern contains spinal fluid and consequently has a more radiolucent appearance with absorption numbers in the spinal fluid range (0–24 Hounsfield units on the ±1,000 scale). A horizontal density occasionally can be seen within the cistern, and this represents the optic chiasm.

The 0° and 20° images are repeated after the intravenous infusion of an iodine-containing contrast agent. This allows evaluation of the blood brain barrier, and by extending extravascularly into a lesion will enhance its visibility.[6] It normally can be seen to outline blood vessels and the circle of Willis can be identified, outlining the suprasellar cistern[9] (Fig. 5).

SELLA AND JUXTASELLA PATHOLOGY

Computed tomography can directly demonstrate the different pathological entities that involve the sella and juxtasella region. Prior to the advent of this relatively safe, noninvasive technique, these lesions were indirectly diagnosed by arterial, cisternal, or ventricular displacements demonstrated on the more invasive neuroradiological modalities of cerebral arteriography and pneumoencephalography. In current practice, computed tomography will demonstrate the lesion, and the more invasive studies are used to aid in the differential diagnosis and in patient management.

The following presentation includes examples of a variety of lesions of the sella area examined in the computed tomography section of the department of Radiology of the Mount Sinai Medical Center, Miami Beach, Florida, from February 1976 to January 1979. These include examples of pituitary adenomas, craniopharyngiomas, meningiomas, giant aneurysms, sphenoid sinus mucoceles, metastasis, chiasmal gliomas, and colloid cysts.

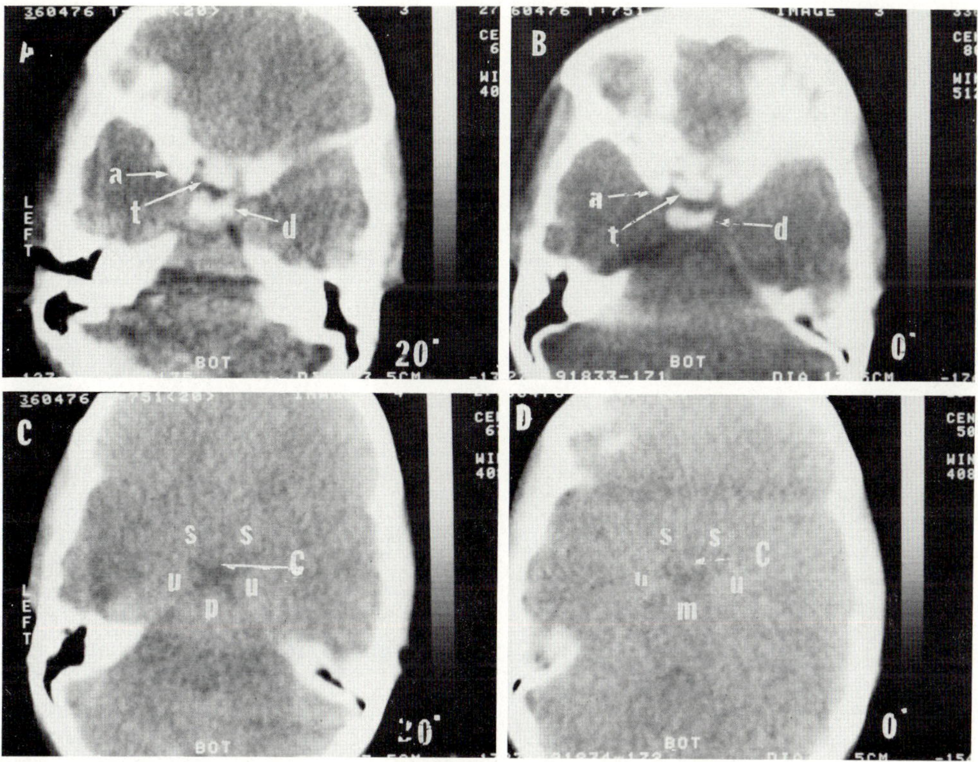

Fig. 4. A. CT image taken at 20° to the canthomeatal reference plane at the level of the sella turcica. The anterior clinoids (a), tuberculum sella(t), and dorsum sella (d) are identified. B. Image taken at 0° to the canthomeatal reference plane at the level of the sella turcica. The anterior clinoid (a), tuberculum sella (t), and dorsum sella (d) are identified. Because of the 0° angulation, the roof of the orbits are included in this plane of section, while they were angled inferior to the plane of section on the 20° images. C. Image taken at 20° to the canthomeatal reference plane at the level of the suprasellar cistern. The cistern has a pentagonal appearance. The anterior margins are formed by the subcollosal gyri (S), the lateral margins by the uncus (U) of the temporal lobes, and the posterior border being formed by the pons (P). A horizontal density in the anterior aspect of the suprasellar cistern corresponds to the optic chiasm (C). D. Image taken at 0° with the canthomeatal reference plane through the level of the suprasellar cistern. At this angulation, the suprasellar cistern has an oval appearance. The anterior margin is formed by the subcollosal gyri (S), the lateral borders by the uncus (U), and because of the more shallow angulation, the posterior margin is formed by the mesencephalon (M). The optic chiasm (C) can faintly be seen in the anterior portion of the suprasellar cistern.

PITUITARY ADENOMAS

Pituitary adenomas are lesions arising in the anterior lobe of the pituitary within the sella turcica.[10, 11] They can extend laterally, displacing or invading the cavernous sinus, superiorly into the suprasellar cistern (Fig. 6) or inferiorly through the body of the sphenoid into the nasopharynx (Fig. 7). Symptoms may be produced by direct pressure on the pituitary, causing hypofunction, or on the optic chiasm, causing a bitemporal field defect. The tumor may be a hormone secreter, causing specific endocrine symptoms, i.e., an eosinophilic adenoma causing acromegaly or giantism, a basophilic adenoma causing hyperadrenalism, or a prolactin secreting tumor causing galactorrhea (Fig. 8). In general, the hormone producing tumors, because of their endocrine related symptoms, are usually diagnosed earlier, and hence are usually smaller when first discovered, and may even be confined to the sella[10] (Fig. 8). The chromophobe adenoma occasionally may endocrine secrete, but is usually inert and produces symptoms

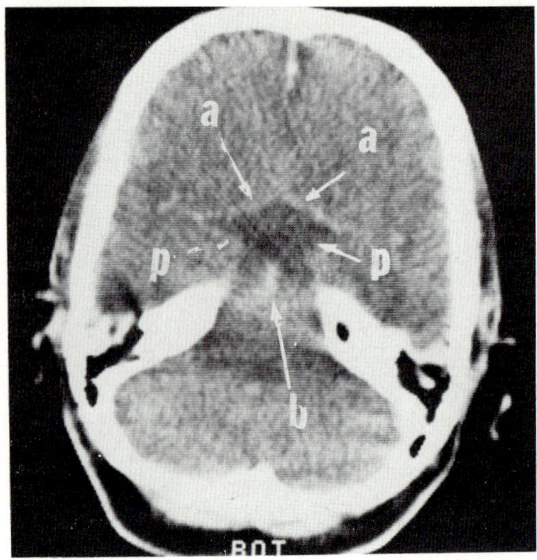

Fig. 5. Image taken with 20° angulation to the canthomeatal reference plane at the level of the suprasellar cistern after the intravenous infusion of contrast. The anterior cerebral arteries (a), the posterior cerebral arteries (P), and the basilar artery (b) are demonstrated, filled with contrast outlining the pentagonal cerebral spinal fluid filled suprasella cistern. The pentagonal appearance of this cistern is easily seen on this image. From the lateral margins of the pentagon the middle cerebral arteries can be seen extending into the sylvian fissures.

by pressure on surrounding structures. These lesions may be quite large when first seen.

The intrasella and suprasella component of the pituitary adenoma may be demonstrated by computed tomography.[12] IV contrast infusion may be necessary to directly demonstrate the intrasella component (Figs. 8A and 8B). However, erosive changes demonstrated either on conventional roentgenograms or on the CT may indicate its presence. Obliteration of the normal low absorption number CSF containing suprasellar cistern by a mass, usually isodense with brain, indicates suprasellar extension (Figs. 6A and 6B). Intravenous contrast infusion will homogeneously enhance the mass, increasing its absorption numbers and consequently its radiodensity[12] (Figs. 6C and 6D). The margins, while lobulated, are usually well defined. Occasionally, a mottled lucency will be present, after enhancement, indicating areas of necrosis and cyst formation.[2]

In summary, pituitary adenomas cause enlargement of the sella on conventional radiography. On computed tomography they present as an isodense mass, which most frequently will homogeneously enhance after the intravenous infusion of an iodine-containing contrast agent. The margins are sharp and usually polylobulated. The intrasellar component, as well as suprasellar, parasellar, or nasopharyngeal extension, can be directly demonstrated.

CRANIOPHARYNGIOMAS

Craniopharyngiomas account for two to three percent of all intracranial tumors, with a peak incidence in childhood and adolescence, and a second peak in the fifth decade.[10, 11, 13, 14] The lesion most often arises in the suprasellar cistern or, less commonly, inside the sella turcica. It is thought to originate from remnants of Rathke's pouch.[10, 11] The neoplasm may be solid or cystic, and is composed of squamous epitheleum or low columnar epitheleum, having the appearance of the basilar epidermoid cells.[10] The cystic lesion will contain a straw- to brown-colored fluid, which may contain cholesterol crystals. Calcifications will occur in approximately 70–80%[11, 14] and will be either solid in the solid lesions or curvelinear in the cystic lesions. The tumor produces symptoms by causing pressure on surrounding structures, especially the pituitary and optic chiasm. It can extend superiorly and obstruct the foramen of Monro (Fig. 9).

On computed tomography the lesion most commonly presents as a suprasellar calcification (Fig. 9A), which will enhance on the contrast portion of the examination[14] (Figs. 9C and 9D). The enhancement in the solid lesions will usually be homogeneous. Mottled lucencies will occur if microcyst formation occurs. The cystic lesions will have a ringlike pattern of enhancement, with central area of decreased absorption, which may be either isodense with brain, or less dense than brain, if there is a high content of cholesterol.

If the lesion arises inside the sella, it may extend inferiorly, destroying the sella and the base of the skull (Figs. 10A and 10B).

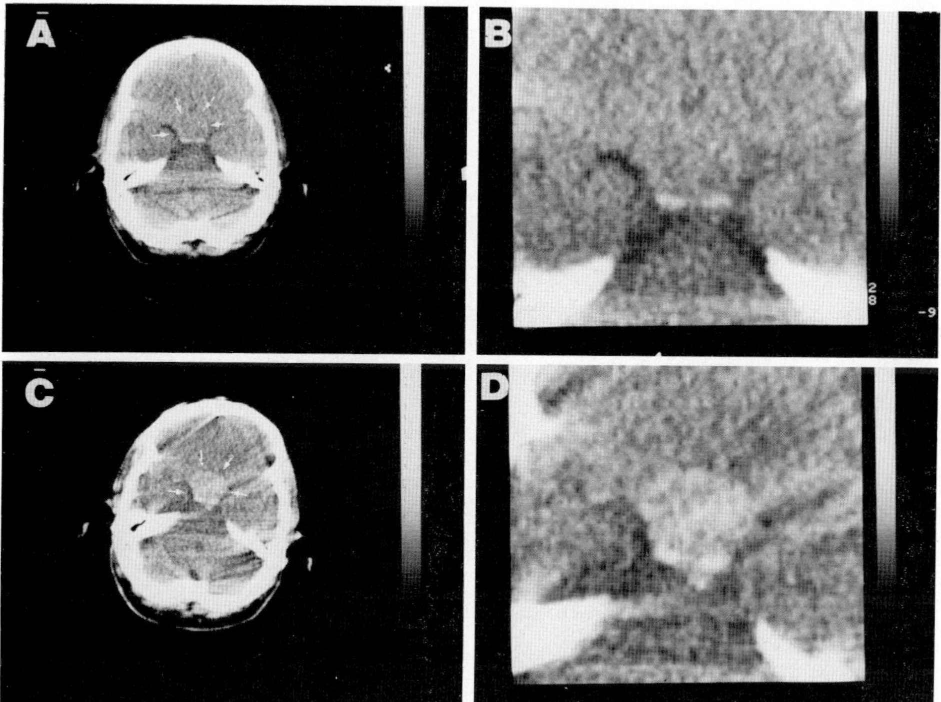

Fig. 6. A. Noncontrast CT scan through the suprasellar region, showing the obliteration of the suprasellar cistern by an isodense mass (arrows). B. Magnification of the same, demonstrating that the suprasellar cistern is occupied by a tumor. C. The contrast examination at the same level showing an enhancing homogeneous tumor. D. Magnification of the same tomographic cut. This represents a chromophobe adenoma with suprasellar extension. The sella turcica was enlarged on plain films.

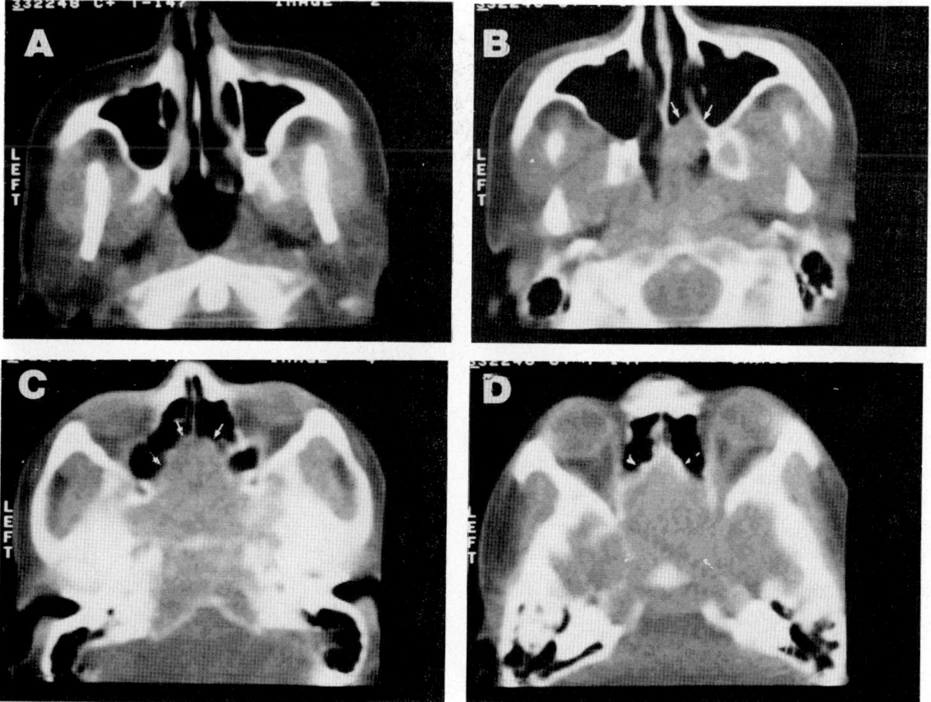

Fig. 7. A, B, C, and D, are consecutive computed tomographic cuts from the nasopharynx to the base of the skull. A. Shows a normal nasopharynx; however, the arrows of B, C, and D are demonstrating a large chromophobe adenoma protruding into the choana and nasopharynx.

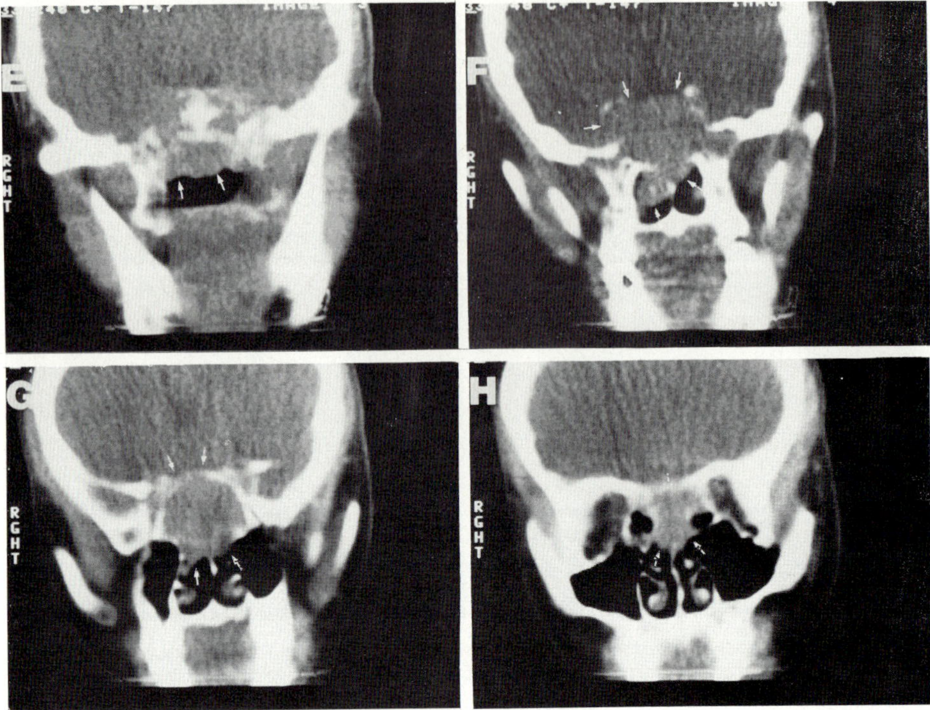

Fig. 7. E, F, G, H. Computed tomographic sections in the coronal projections demonstrate to advantage the sella tumor with predominant extension into the nasopharynx (Lower arrows of E, F, G, H).

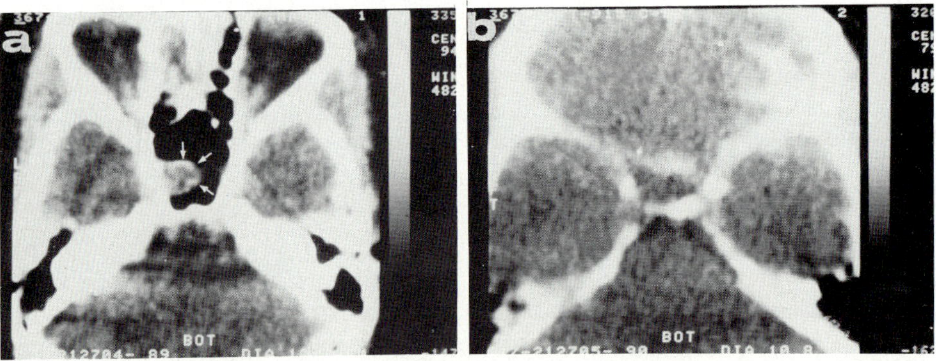

Fig. 8. Computerized axial cut through the sphenoid sinus showing an asymmetrically enlarged sella protruding into the sinus (arrows). B. Shows asymmetric enlargement of the sella turcica on the left side. This patient had a purely intrasellar prolactin producing adenoma.

Computed tomography in the axial projection (Figs. 10C and 10D) will confirm the destruction and demonstrate the isodense lesion. Coronal computed tomography (Figs. 10E and 10F) more clearly demonstrates the superior and inferior extent of these lesions.

The diagnosis of craniopharyngiomas on computed tomography would depend upon the demonstration of juxtasella calcifications, cyst formation, and contrast enhancement. Any two of these three findings leads to a strong possibility of a craniopharyngioma as the etiology of the juxtasellar mass.[14]

MENINGIOMAS

Meningiomas comprise about 15% of intracranial neoplasms.[11, 13] Approximately

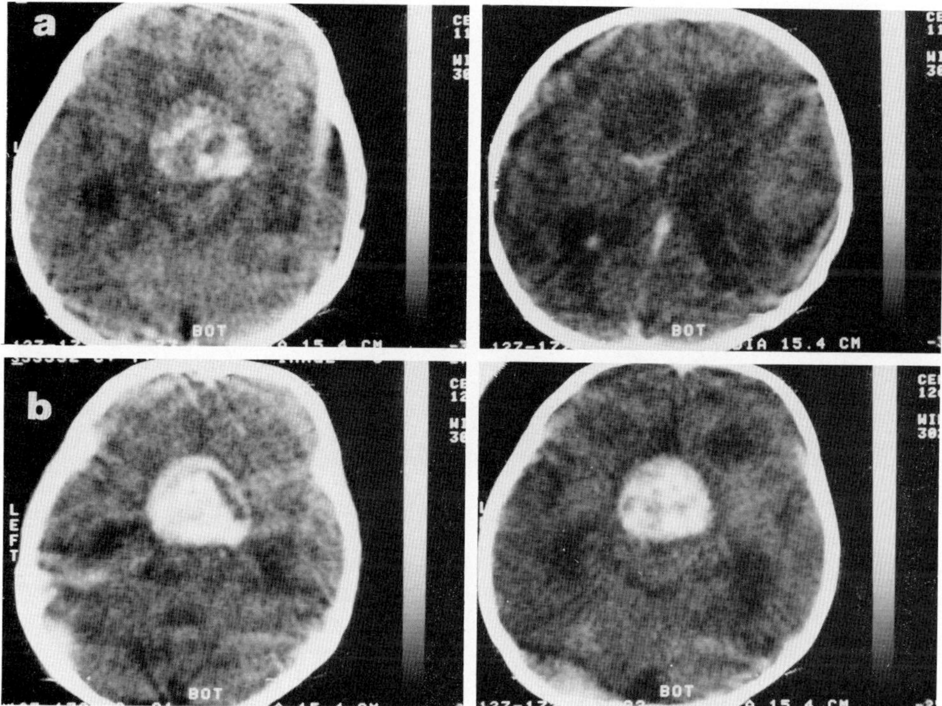

Fig. 9. A. Shows a nonhomogeneous suprasellar calcified lesion, which enhances after contrast administration. B. The third ventricle is effaced and enlargement of the lateral ventricles is noted. The study is somewhat limited due to patient motion artifact. This lesion represented a suprasellar craniopharyngioma.

10% will occur in the juxtasellar region[11] (Fig. 11), arising from the diaphragm sella (Fig. 12), the tuberculum sella, and adjacent planum sphenoidale (Fig. 13), the anterior clinoid and adjacent medial one third of the lesser sphenoid wing (Fig. 14), or the posterior clinoid and adjacent anterolateral margin of the tentorial incisura (Fig. 15). Because of the geographically small anatomic area, extension to more than one of the above locations, including the dural margins of the cavernous sinus, is not uncommon. Clinical symptoms are due to pressure on the adjacent structures, including the optic nerve and chiasm as well as the third, fourth, ophthalamic division of the fifth, and the sixth cranial nerves.

Conventional roentgenograms may demonstrate hyperostosis, blistering of the planum sphenoidale (Fig. 13A), or calcification in the tumor. Computed tomography may also show these findings (Fig. 13B). In addition, an isodense or slightly hyperdense mass will be seen deforming or filling the suprasellar cistern and displacing the adjacent third ventricle or frontal horns. On the contrast examination, there is dense homogeneous enhancement of the isodense mass seen on the plain computed tomographic examination. Because of its adequate blood supply, it is uncommon for meningiomas to have central necrosis and hence it is very unusual for meningiomas to have a ringlike or mottled pattern of enhancement.

In summary, sclerosis of the bony sella margins and/or blistering of the planum sphenoidale on conventional roentgenograms, associated with a contiguous juxtasellar mass which may or may not contain calcium and which homogeneously enhances on the contrast examination, are the radiographic findings that would suggest a meningioma.

ANEURYSMS

Juxtasella aneurysms most frequently involve the cavernous portion (Fig. 16) or the supraclinoid portion (Fig. 17) of the internal carotid artery.[15] The etiology is unknown, but is thought to be either congenital or

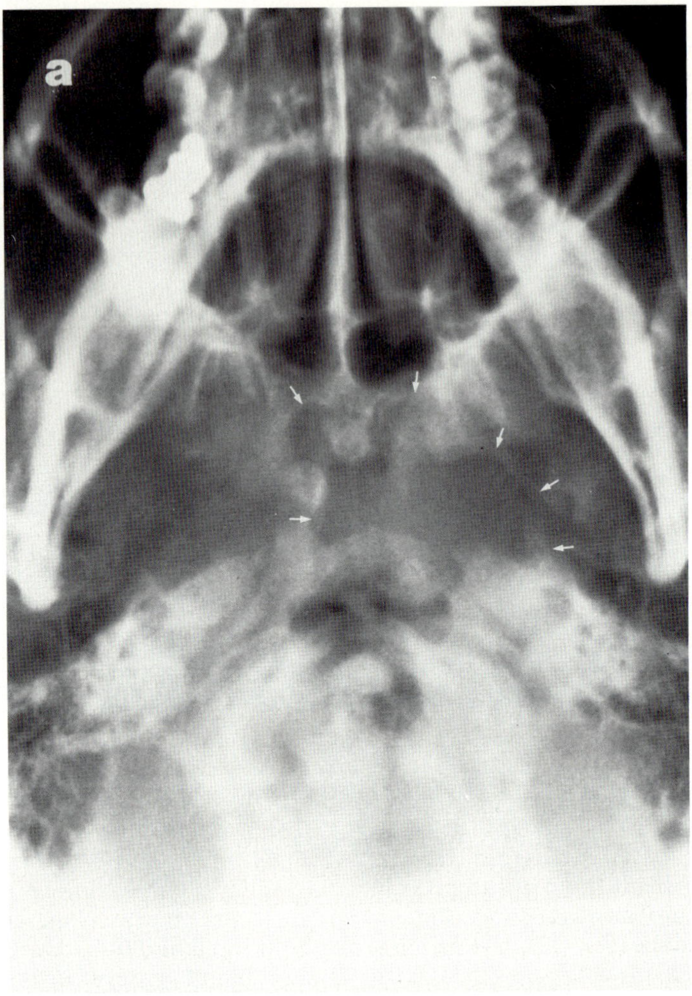

Fig. 10A

Fig. 10. A. Base projection which shows a lytic destructive lesion involving the base of the skull at the level of the clivus and extending towards the left middle fossa, with erosion of the left petrous tip (arrows). B and C again demonstrate the same base of the skull destruction in the axial computed tomogram (arrows). D and E are computed tomograms in coronal projection through the sella turcica, demonstrating a large mass which is extending to the nasopharynx (lower arrows) destroying the base of the skull, and extending to the left middle fossa in parasellar extension (E). F is a lateral view of the skull, with the patient in supine position outlining a cystic craniopharyngioma after instillation of air and contrast material. Note the air fluid level (upper arrows) and the contrast material layering posteriorly (lower arrows).

arteriosclerotic in origin. Symptoms are usually due to the expanding aneurysmal mass. The patient can present with headache and cranial nerve signs. Patients with an aneurysm of the cavernous portion of the internal carotid artery can show signs of pressure on the third, fourth, ophthalamic division of the fifth, and the sixth cranial nerves. A supraclinoid aneurysm can press on the third nerve, and ipsilateral cerebral peduncle, causing a Weber syndrome. If large enough, it can cause pressure on the optic chiasm.

The plain CT findings will be that of an isodense or hyperdense mass (Fig. 17A), which may have a rim of calcium (Figs. 16A and 16B). On the contrast portion of the examination, there may be homogeneous enhancement (Fig. 17B) of the entire mass in the case of a thin-walled aneurysm. If

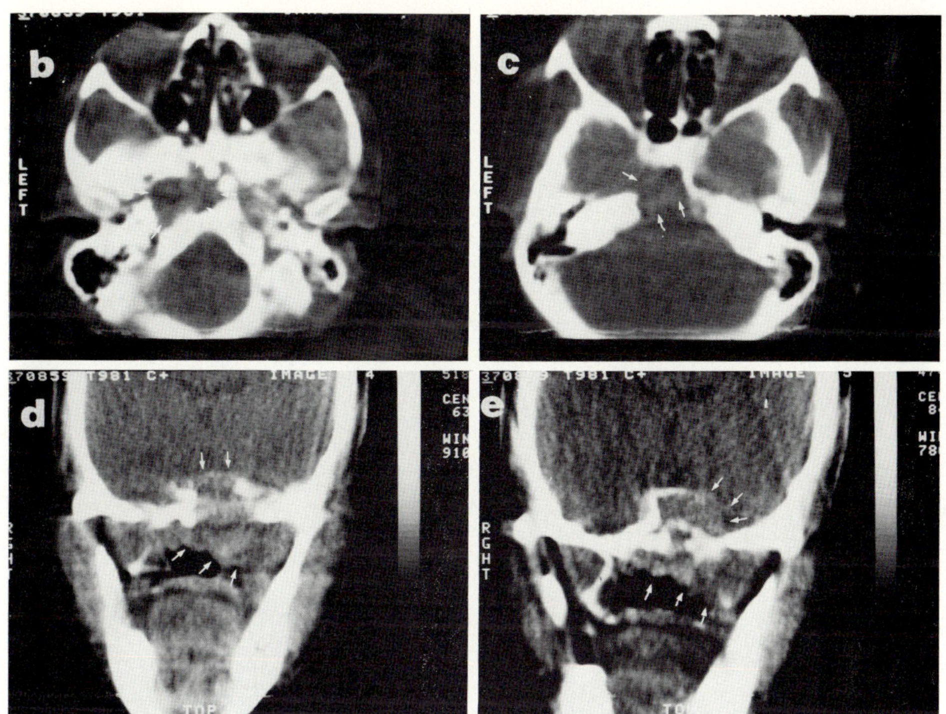

Fig. 10B–E

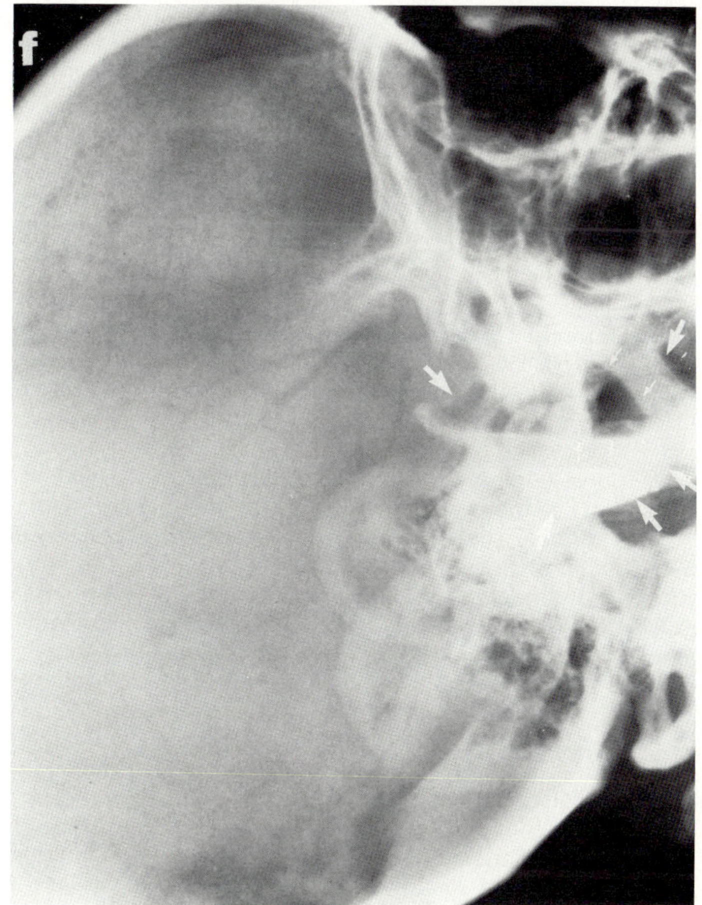

Fig. 10F

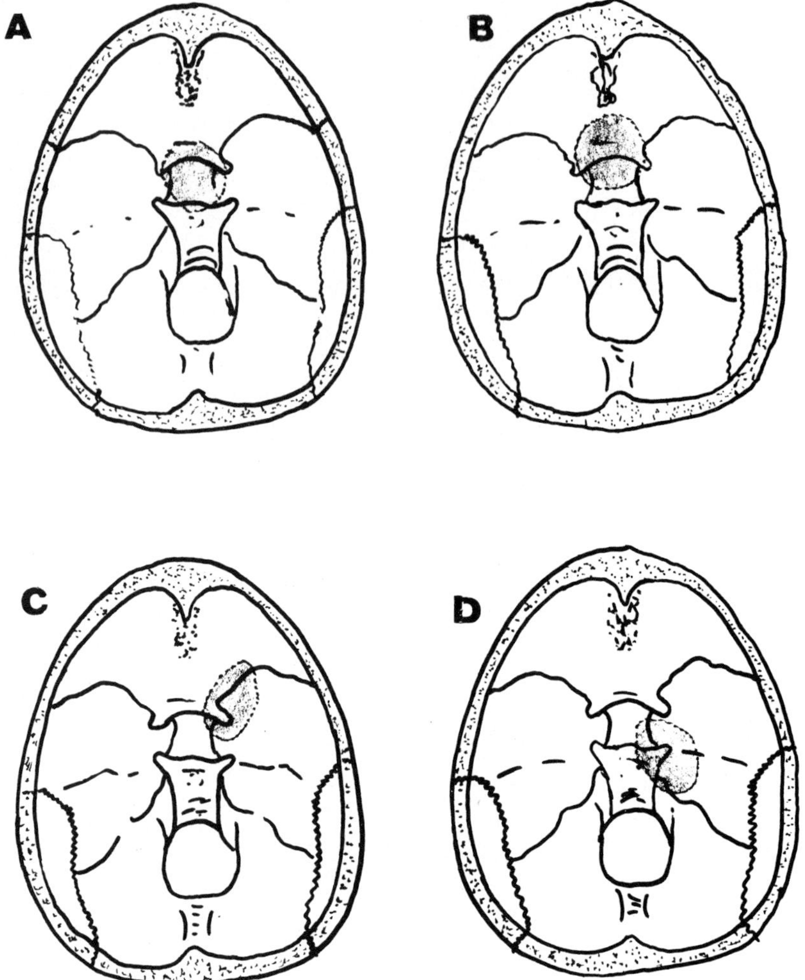

Fig. 11. Schematic diagram demonstrating the more common locations of juxtasellar meningiomas. A. Diaphragm sella meningioma, corresponding to that demonstrated in Figure 12. B. Tuberculum sella meningioma, corresponding to that demonstrated in Figure 13. C. Lesser sphenoid wing, and anterior clinoid meningioma corresponding to that demonstrated in Figure 14. D. Posterior clinoid incisural meningioma, corresponding to that demonstrated in Figure 15.

there is a mural thrombus, only the lumen may enhance (Fig. 16C). In some instances, the wall of the aneurysm and the central lumen will enhance, but will be separated from each other by a hypodense mural thrombus. Inasmuch as all of these computed tomographic findings can also be seen with neoplasms, the diagnosis of a juxtasellar aneurysm is confirmed with arteriography (Figs. 16E and 17C).

SPHENOID SINUS MUCOCELE

Mucoceles of the sphenoid sinus are rare. It is formed by blockage of the draining ostia of the sinus.[16] The resultant accumulation of mucous (or pus in the case of a pyocele) under pressure expands the sinus. The septa within the sinus are destroyed, and then the walls of the sinus, including the sella floor, are expanded and ballooned outward. The ballooned side walls can bulge into the middle fossa (Fig. 18). On computed tomography the thick mucous or pus will appear isodense or have a slightly greater density than surrounding brain. This will be surrounded by a rim of increased density, having absorption numbers in the range of calcium or bone. On the plain computed tomography examination,

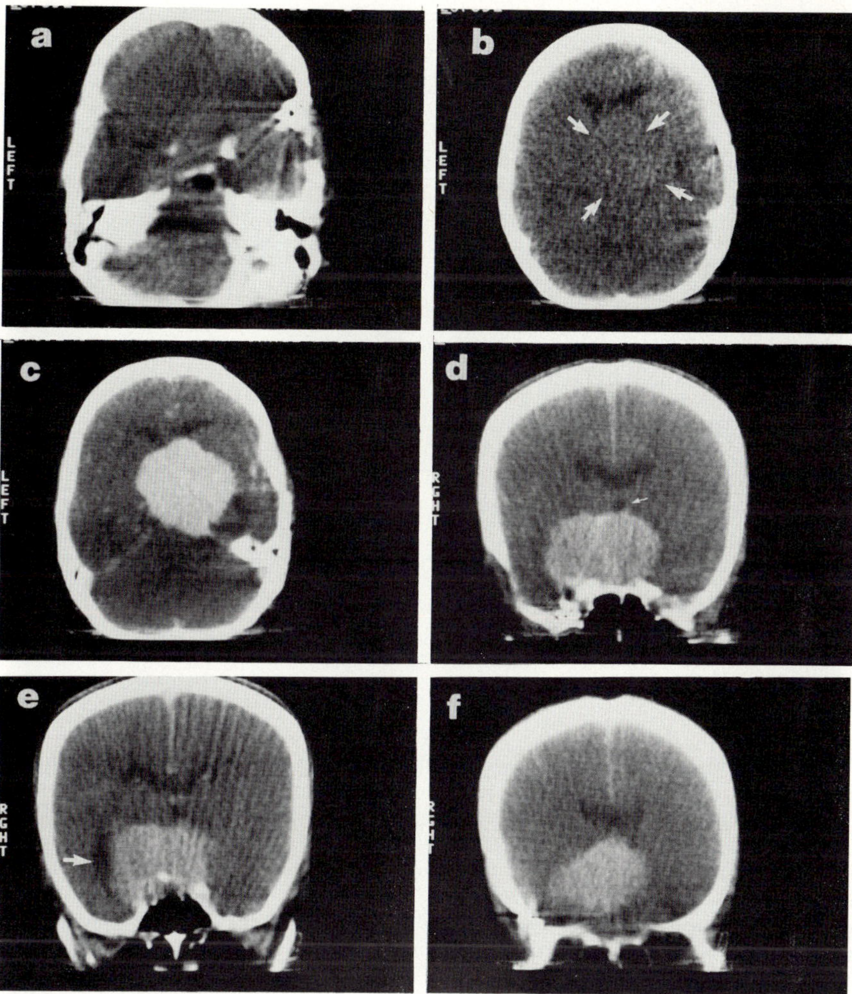

Fig. 12. A and B. The noncontrast axial computed tomogram, demonstrating an homogeneous mass effect, effacing the third ventricle and part of the right frontal horn (arrows). C. The contrast CT scan at the same level of B, demonstrating intense homogeneous enhancement typical of a meningioma, occupying the suprasellar region. E and F. Coronal sections through the suprasellar region demonstrating this huge suprasellar meningeoma elevating the third ventricle (small arrow) and extending to the right middle fossa and parasellar region (large arrow) and projecting anteriorly into the anterior fossa (F).

they may be difficult to differentiate from juxtasella giant aneurysms or craniopharyngiomas. On the contrast examination, enhancement of the central lumen of an aneurysm or the walls of a craniopharyngioma will aid in the differentiation. If there has been surgical manipulation of the mucocele, an air fluid level may be present (Fig. 18B) further differentiating these lesions.

METASTASIS

The pituitary and adjacent hypothalamus is not a common site for metastatic deposits. When metastasis does occur, there is usually evidence of carcinomatosis elsewhere.[17] The plain CT will usually show an isodense suprasellar mass. The usual edema associated with metastatic foci may or may not be recognized. After contrast infusion, the mass can homogeneously enhance (Fig. 19). If there is central necrosis, a ring pattern may result. The lesion on CT has the appearance of other juxtasellar masses.[2] However, because of the usually known carcinomatosis, the etiology is determined on a clinical basis.

Metastasis to the bony sella, either blood

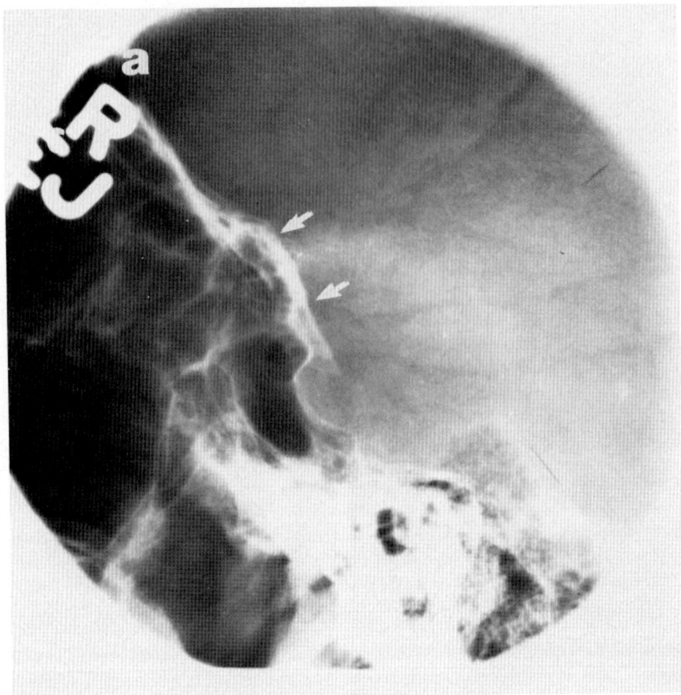

Fig. 13A

Fig. 13. A is a coned down lateral view of the sella turcica demonstrating sclerosis and blistering of the planum sphenoidale (arrows). B and C. Axial computed tomograms through the suprasellar region without contrast. B shows the sclerosis and blistering of the planum sphenoidale (large arrows) and the distortion and filling of the suprasellar cistern by an isodense mass effect (small arrows). D and E are the equivalent contrast CT scans demonstrating the homogeneous enhancement in the topography of the planum sphenoidale and suprasellar region, typical of a meningioma. F. Coronal section through the sella, demonstrating the suprasellar extension and effacement of the third ventricle, while G is demonstrating the thickened planum sphenoidale (arrows) and the anterior component of the meningioma.

borne or via contiguity from the nasopharynx or sphenoid sinus, causes bone destruction which can be diagnosed on the conventional roentgenograms as well as computed tomography. Computed tomography can exclude suprasella and middle fossa extension, and the histological diagnosis, if not already known from the known primary, may be determined by transnasal biopsy.

CHIASMAL GLIOMAS

Chiasmal gliomas usually occur in childhood, most often between the ages of two to nine years. A 24% incidence of associated neurofibrosis has been reported. A tumor may be confined to the optic chiasm and adjacent hypothalamus. However, involvement of one or more optic nerves is not uncommon and has been reported in as high as 55%.[18]

On computed tomography, an optic glioma appears as an isodense mass, filling the suprasellar cistern[2] (Fig. 20). Images at the level of the orbit can demonstrate optic nerve involvement if present. These lesions infrequently enhance after the intravenous injection of contrast.

COLLOID CYSTS

Colloid cysts arise from the roof of the third ventricle, anteriorly, at the level of the foramen of Monro. It is thought to arise either from the paraphysis, which is a pouch in the embryo at the telencephalon-diencephalon junction, which disappears before birth, or from the neuroepithelium,

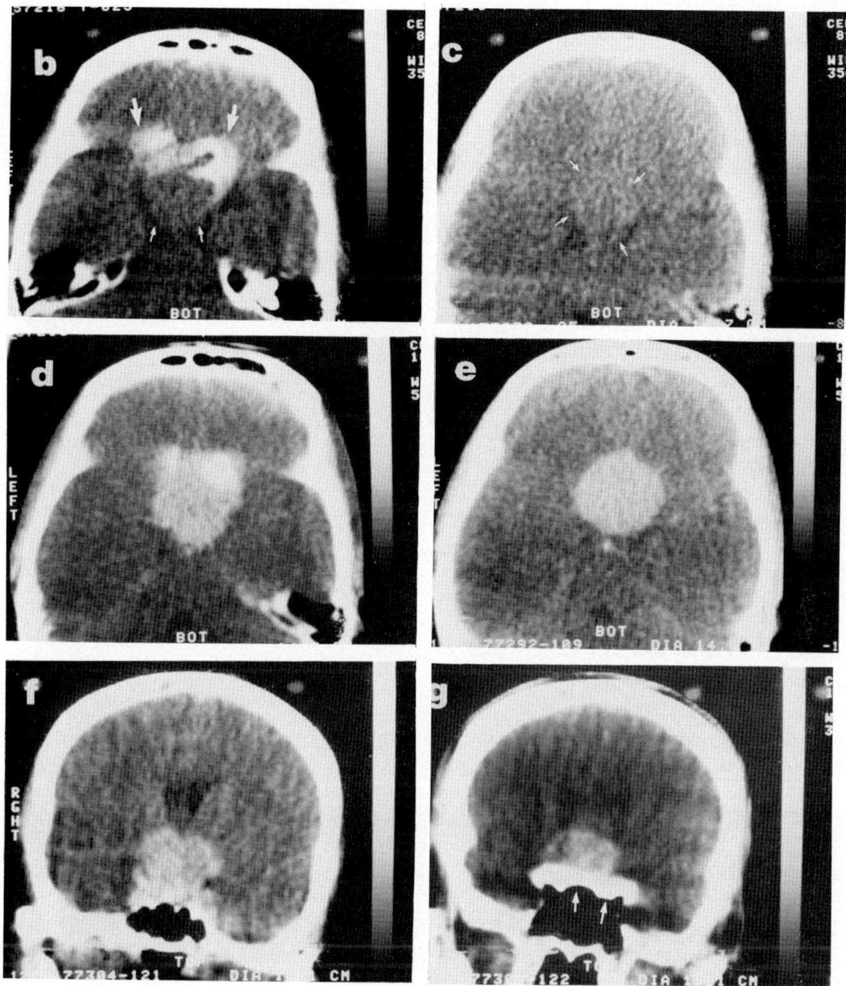

Fig. 13B–G

hence the synonyms paraphyseal or neuroepithelial cysts.[10, 19] The cyst is usually smooth, lined by cuboidal epithelium, and is filled with colloidal, gelatinous, gray- to green-colored material with high mineral content.[1, 17] Its fibrous capsule is attached to the choroid plexus as it passes through the foramen of Monro.[10, 19] They are found mostly in early adult life, and cause symptoms related to intermittent hydrocephalus, due to intermittent obstruction of the lateral ventricles at the foramen of Monro (Fig. 21). The superior border may extend through the foramen of Monro and appear in the floor of one or both lateral ventricles.

On computed tomography, the cyst is round, sharply contoured, located in the anterior portion of the third ventricle, and, because of its high mineral content, is usually hyperdense on the plain examination[2] (Fig. 21). Intravenous contrast may or may not enhance the lesion. Obstructive hydrocephalus is usually present.

DISCUSSION

Patients with a suspected sella or juxtasella mass should have as their original roentgenographic evaluation conventional skull films and computed tomography. The conventional skull films will yield information as to sella size, erosions, hyperostosis, and calcifications. This can be supplemented by polytomography to evaluate

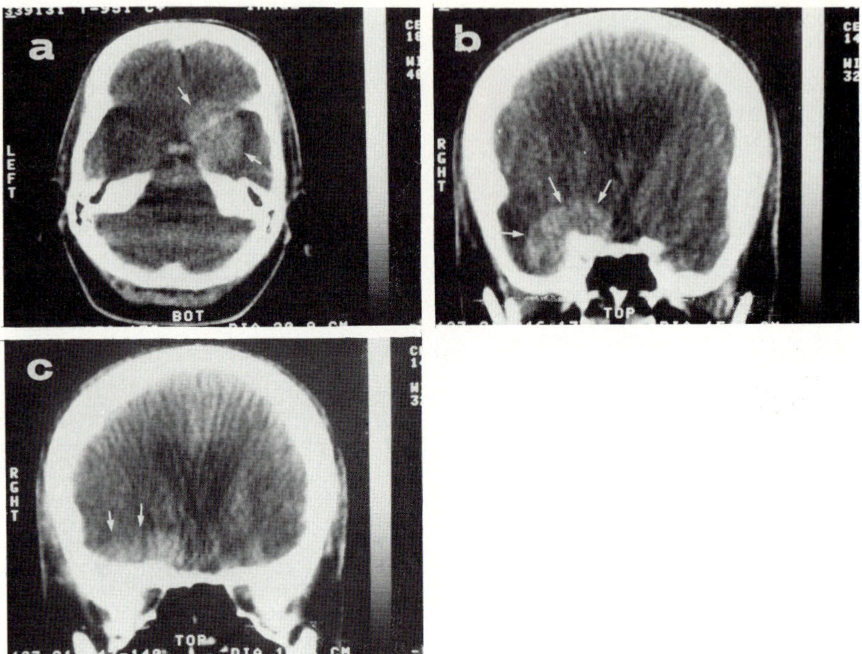

Fig. 14. A. Axial contrast CT scan showing a right parasellar meningioma extending to the anterior and middle fossa, typical of a sphenoid ridge meningioma. B. Showing the parasellar extension into the right middle fossa, in coronal section, and partial obliteration of the suprasellar cistern. C demonstrates the extension of the meningioma into the anterior fossa (arrows), over the lesser wing of the sphenoid.

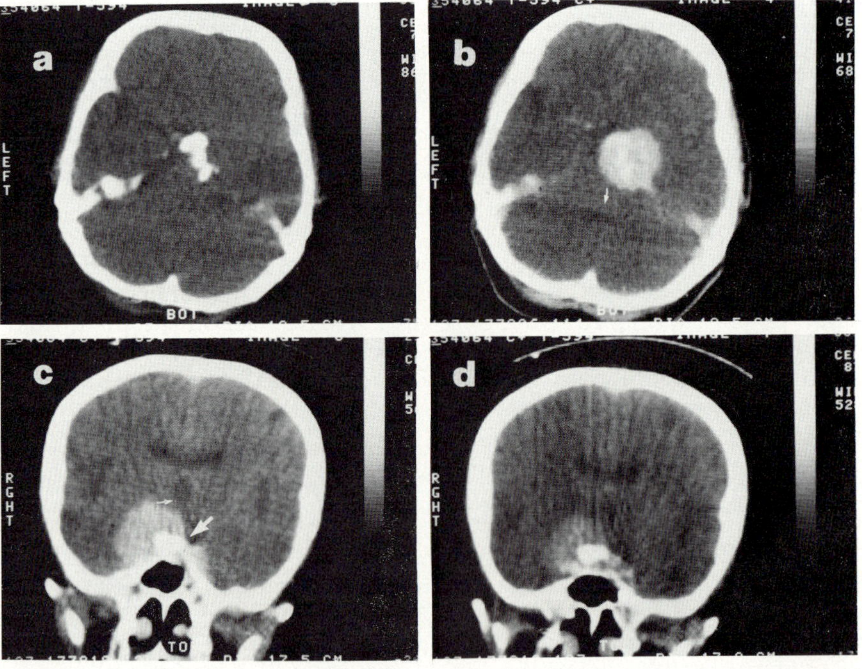

Fig. 15. A. A noncontrast examination through the suprasellar region, demonstrating amorphous calcifications. B. Axial tomographic cut after the contrast administration, demonstrating an enhancing meningioma around the calcifications. The fourth ventricle is slightly flattened (small arrow) due to pressure upon the brain stem. C and D. Coronal projections through this lesion demonstrating the effect upon the third ventricle (upper small arrow) and partial filling of the suprasellar cistern (large arrow).

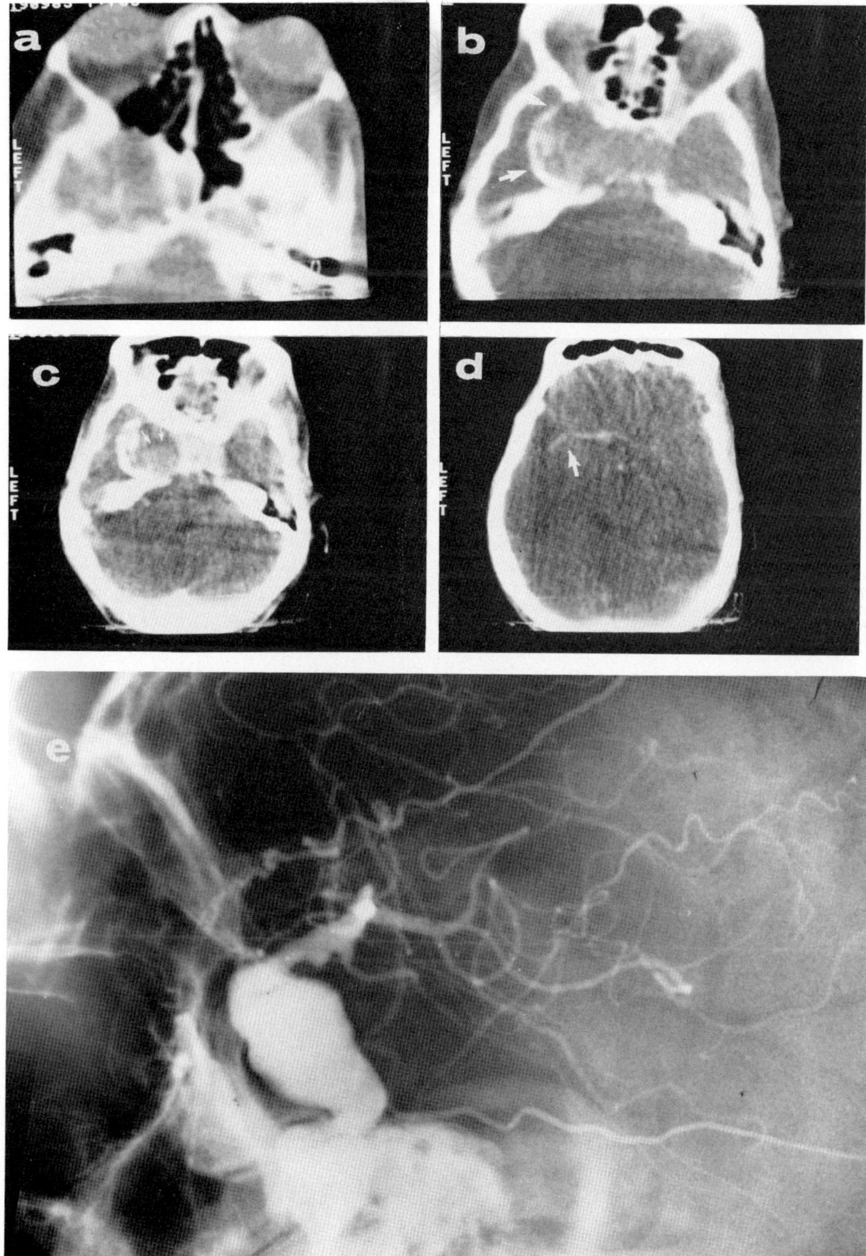

Fig. 16. A and B demonstrate vascular ringlike calcifications in the left middle fossa (arrows). C. The enhanced examination demonstrating partial enhancement of the lesion (arrows). D shows the displacement and elevation of the left middle cerebral artery (arrows). This represents the large carotid siphon aneurysm with peripheral calcification and mural clot. E Is the corresponding angiogram.

double floors, to determine the presence of scalloping and if there is undermining of the tuberculum. The computed tomogram examination will demonstrate most sella and juxtasella lesions. The etiology of these lesions may be suggested correlating the clinical findings, the CT observations, and statistical probabilities. However, there is wide overlap in the computed tomographic findings of these different lesions, and further neuroradiological investigation is warranted. Neuroangiography should be per-

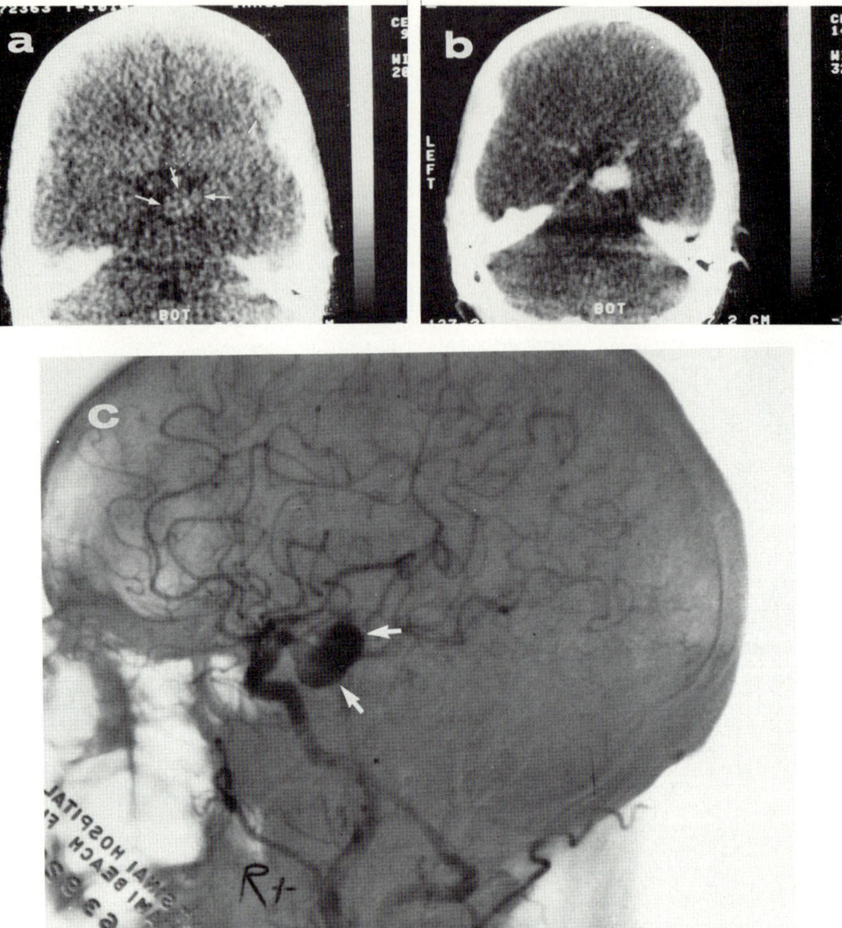

Fig. 17. A. Shows an isodense suprasellar nodule partially obliterating the suprasellar cistern (arrows). B is the contrast CT scan showing intense enhancement of the lesion. C. Angiogram demonstrating a large aneurysm arising from the supraclinoid portion of the internal carotid artery (arrows).

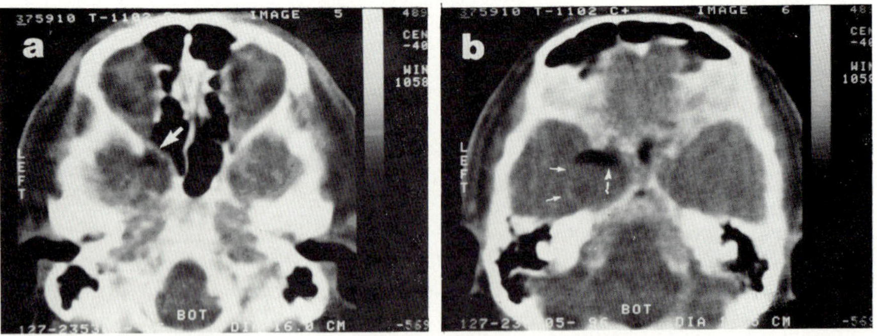

Fig. 18. A and B. Two low axial tomographic sections demonstrating a left parasellar mass with a mucous fluid level (vertical arrow) characteristic of a mucocele of the sphenoid sinus, extending into the left middle fossa. It is protruding into the sphenoid sinus on the left (Fig. A) and displacing the enhanced dura laterally (Fig. B) (small arrows).

formed to rule out an aneurysm and to demonstrate the vascular displacements and encasements secondary to the mass. A blood supply to the tumor may be demonstrated. Pneumoencephalography is performed when it is desired to obtain better anatomical detail of suprasellar extension of a lesion. This is particularly important in patients with a microadenoma, where a transphenoidal surgical approach is being considered. Patients with endocrine abnormalities, or subtle visual changes indicating dysfunction of the optic chiasm and a normal computed tomographic examination, should also have pneumoencephalography to determine the presence of a small lesion beyond the resolution of the computed tomogram.

EDITOR'S NOTE

There is no question but that carefully done computed tomographic scans with enhancement have been a great asset in evaluating mass lesions in and near the sella turcica. Dr. Sheldon and associates are expert with their Delta machine and turn out very nice pictures for us which help us many times with our patients, and they also are kind enough to send us an extra set of the pictures for our own files—and that is very important in helping us to learn, too!

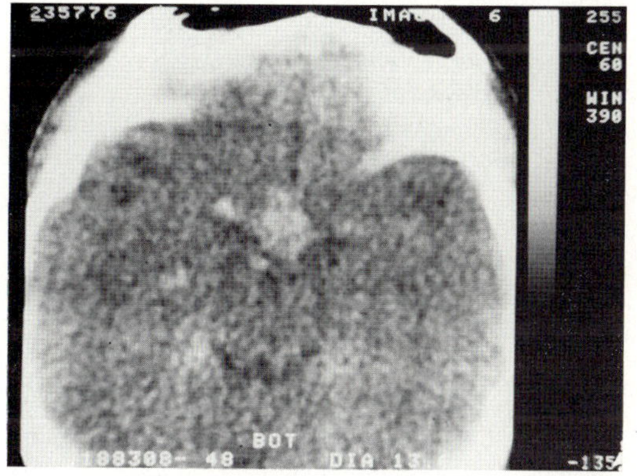

Fig. 19. Contrast CT scan through the suprasellar region reveals an enhancing nodule occupying the suprasellar cistern, which proved to be a metastasis.

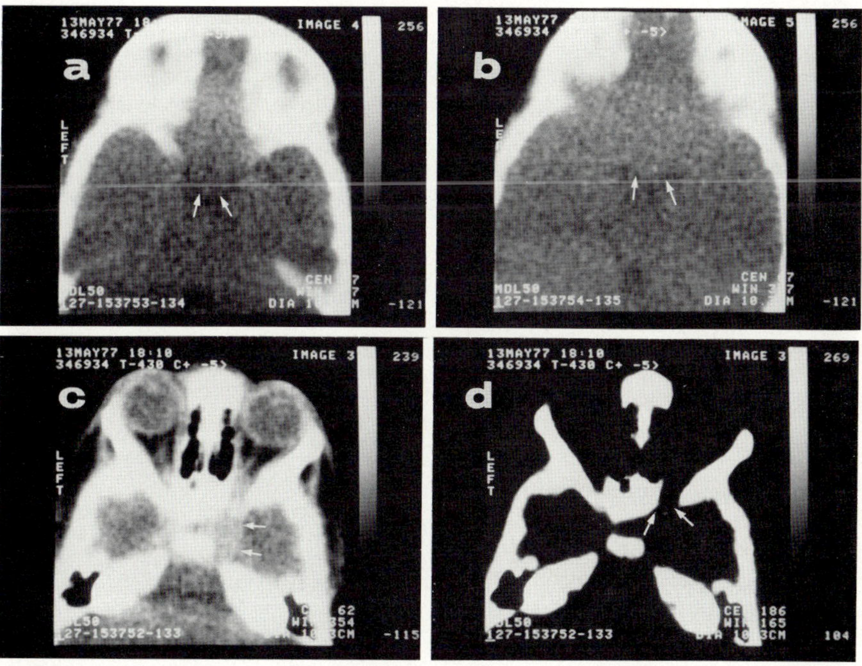

Fig. 20. A and B. CT scans demonstrating the impingement upon the suprasellar cistern by an anterior isodense lesion (arrows). C. The contrast CT scan shows lateral extension into the right parasellar region (arrows). D shows widening of the optic canal, indicating extension to the optic foramen. This represents a chiasmatic glioma with optic nerve extension on the right.

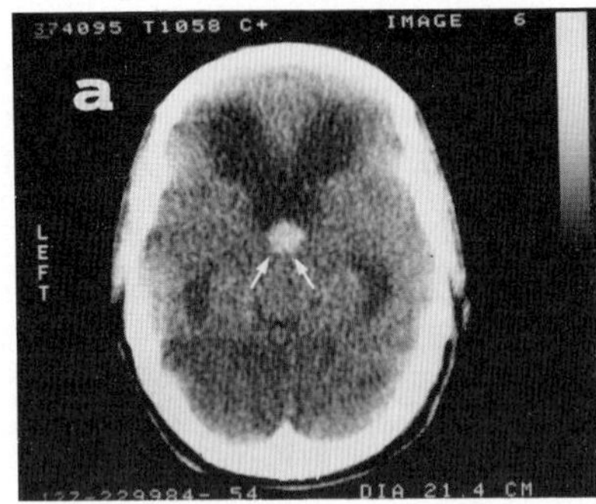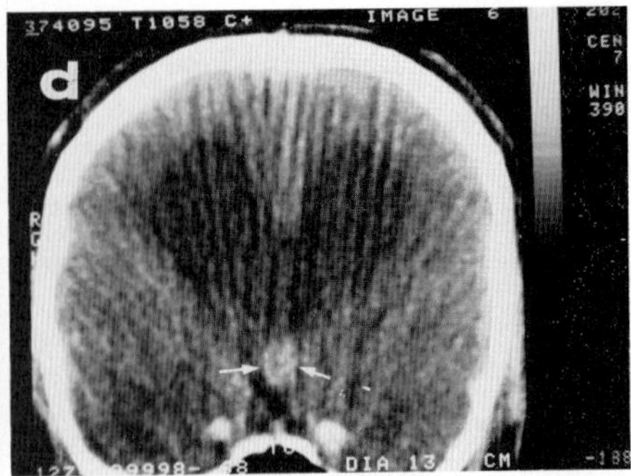

Fig. 21. A. Noncontrast examination showing a dense nodular lesion within the third ventricle, producing obstructive hydrocephalus. The coronal section (D) confirms position of the lesion within the third ventricle. This is quite characteristic of a colloid cyst of the third ventricle.

However, I simply want to emphasize that one *MUST* get a *good* set of *routine skull films* FIRST in evaluating the sella. Bony detail of the clinoids, demineralization of the dorsum, undermining of the planum, and the like, usually are seen BETTER on plain films than on CT scans. I believe that a good set of visual fields (after good plain films) and a carefully done history and, if indicated, some endocrine evaluation, will pay off in diagnosis of a chromophobe adenoma EARLIER than a CT scan.

Dr. Sheldon also gave us a "pearl" in that the biggest artefact in good *CORONAL* computed tomographic scans is the presence of *FILLINGS* in the teeth! So, if you look in the patient's mouth, and see a lot of fillings, you might as well not get good coronal cuts (even though coronal cuts are very, very helpful—particularly with planum meningiomas). Dr. Lester Mount's chapter will illustrate that to better advantage. Therefore, again computed tomography is excellent—but a good HISTORY and a good set of VISUAL FIELDS are even better. I teach the residents as follows: "Be sure to get a *CF* before a *CT!*" This says—"Be sure to get a confrontation field before a computed tomographic scan." You'll often pick up parachiasmal mass lesions YEARS AND YEARS before the CT scan is abnormal. Again, have the pictures reviewed carefully!

JLS

REFERENCES

1. Hammerschlag, S. B., Wolpert, S. M., and Carter, B. L. Computed tomography of the skull base. J. Comput. Asst. Tomography *1*:75–80 (1977).

2. Leeds, N. E. and Naidich, T. P. Computerized tomography in the diagnosis of sellar and parasellar lesions. Semin. Roentgenol. *12*(2):121–135 (April 1977).

3. Naidich, T. P., Pinto, R. S., Kushner, M. J., Lin, J. P., Kricheff, I., Leeds, N. E., and Chase, N. E. Evaluation of sellar and parasellar masses by computed tomography. Radiology *120*:91–99 (July 1976).

4. Nakagawa, H. and Wolf, B. S. Delineation of lesions of the base of the skull by computed tomography. Radiology *124*:75–80 (July 1977).

5. Reich, N. E., Zelch, J. V., Alfidi, R. J., Meany, T. F., Duchesneau, P. M., and Weinstein, M. A. Computed tomography in the detection of juxtasellar lesions. Radiology *118*:333–335 (February 1976).

6. Gado, M. H., Phelps, M. E., and Coleman, R. E. An extravascular component of contrast enhancement in cranial computed tomography. Radiology *117*:595–597 (December 1975).

7. Wolfman, N. T. and Boehnke, M. The use of coronal sections in evaluating lesions of the sellar and parasellar regions. J. Comput. Asst. Tomography *2*:308–313 (July 1978).

8. Wiggli, U. and Benz, U. F. Normal computed tomography anatomy of the suprasellar subarachnoid space. Radiology *128*:65–70 (July 1978).

9. Weinstein, M. A., Duchesneau, P. M., and Weinstein, C. E. Computed Angiotomography. Am. J. Roentgenol. *129*:699–701 (October 1977).

10. Newton, T. H. and Potts, G. D. Radiology of the skull and brain. In: *Anatomy and Pathology*. C. V. Mosby Co., St. Louis, 1977, Vol. III, pp. 2787–3821.

11. Taveras, J. M. and Wood, E. H. *Diagnostic Neuroradiology*. Williams & Wilkens Co., Baltimore, 1964, pp. 1–960.

12. Citrin, C. M. and Davis, D. O. Computerized tomography in the evaluation of Pituitary adenomas. Invest. Radiol.: 27–35 (January-February 1977).

13. Zimerman, H. M. The ten most common types of brain tumor. Semin. Roentgenol. *6*(1):48–58 (January 1971).

14. Fitz, C. R., Wortzman, G., Harwood-Nash, D. C., Holgate, R. C., Barry, J. F., and Boldt, M. B. Computed tomography in craniopharyngiomas. Radiology *127*:687–691 (June 1978).

15. Byrd, S. E., Bentson, J. R., Winter, J., Wilson, G. H., Joyce, P. W., and O'Connor, L. J. Computer Asst. Tomography 2:303–307 (July 1978).
16. Newton, T. H. and Potts, O. G. Radiology of the skull and brain. In: *The Skull,* C. V. Mosby Co., St. Louis, 1971, Vol. 1, Bk. 1, pp. 1–459.
17. Minckler, J. In: *Nervous System. Pathology.* 4th ed. W. A. D. Anderson (Ed.), C. V. Mosby Co., St. Louis, 1961, pp. 1286–1384.
18. Harwood-Nash, D. C. Optic Gliomas and Pediatric Neuroradiology. Radiol. Clin. North Am. *10*:83–100 (1972).
19. Thompson, W. L., Swenson, N. L., and Buell, H. *Radiologic Pathologic Work Book.* C.N.S., American Registry of Pathology, A.F.I.P., Washington, D.C., 1967, pp. 62–64.

27 The Amenorrhea-Galactorrhea Syndrome

Ronald L. Young, M. D.

Despite the relatively low incidence of abnormal galactorrhea and amenorrhea, a growing interest in the neuroendocrine system in general and in prolactin-related studies specifically has led to increased attention to this problem.

We have traditionally classified amenorrhea-galactorrhea into three syndromes: the Chiari-Frommel syndrome, the Forbes-Albright syndrome, and the Ahumada-del Castillo syndrome. This classification system is based on whether the amenorrhea-galactorrhea is related to recent pregnancy or puerperium, to a pituitary tumor, or is unrelated to either of these conditions.

The Chiari-Frommel syndrome, described in 1852 by two investigators working independently, refers to inappropriate lactation and amenorrhea following pregnancy. In 1932 Ahumada and del Castillo described a similar clinical entity that occurred without recent pregnancy, i.e., as an idiopathic event. About 20 years later, amenorrhea-galactorrhea secondary to a pituitary tumor was introduced as the Forbes-Albright syndrome.[1]

As our knowledge of neuroendocrine pathophysiology expands and hypothalamic-pituitary interrelationships are characterized, specific delineation of the syndromes becomes less clear. For example, patients with suspected Ahumada-del Castillo syndrome have been shown to harbor an occult microadenoma; the tumor-associated Forbes-Albright syndrome has been known to occur during pregnancy and also in the postpartum period. Cases have been reported that evolved through all three syndromes.[2] There are some marked discrepancies in the literature concerning symptomatology, as well as conflicting laboratory data regarding circulating levels of gonadotropins, thyroid hormones, and prolactin.

There has been within the past five years an active controversy about the use of eponyms at all. Some investigators, supporting the view that the syndromes are just different expressions of the same disorder, propose that the names be dropped in favor of a functional classification.[3] Quite possibly, in dealing with the syndrome of amenorrhea and galactorrhea, we are confronting a single condition evolving from adenomatous hyperplasia through microadenoma to macroadenoma. It is also possible that arbitrary classification or clinical diagnosis alone might preempt some diagnostic workup considerations or periodic monitoring of the patient and possibly result in an oversight of an insidious tumor. Many more reasons supporting either a clarification or total revision of the terminology have been cited, including the point that drug-induced amenorrhea-galactorrhea, the most commonly occurring form, is not even a part of the classical terminology. Also deserving mention as etiologic factors are hypothalamic neoplasms and inflammations, other prolactin secreting neoplasms, endocrine and metabolic disorders including hypothyroidism and Cushing's disease, and neurogenic stimulation of the breasts or chest brought about by inflammation, trauma, or surgery.

BREAST DEVELOPMENT AND LACTATION

The amenorrhea-galactorrhea syndrome(s) cannot be understood without some knowledge of breast development and

TABLE I. *Causes of amenorrhea-galactorrhea*

1. Central
   A. Functional
      1. Postpartum (Chiari-Frommel)
      2. Idiopathic (Ahumada-del Castillo)
   B. Organic
      1. Pituitary
         a. Prolactin-secreting tumor (Forbes-Albright)
         b. Other tumors
         c. Inflammatory
         d. Stalk secretion
      2. Hypothalamic
         a. Neoplasm
         b. Inflammatory
   C. Drug Action
2. Peripheral
   A. Metabolic/endocrine disorders
      1. Hypothyroidism
   B. Neoplasm
      1. Ectopic prolactin producing tumor
   C. Neurogenic
      1. Chest wall trauma, surgery, or herpetic lesion
      2. Breast lesion
3. Pregnancy

lactation, as well as the physiology of prolactin, the common denominator for both.

Breast development and function is a complex evolution of events depending on many hormonal factors. Estrogen and progesterone are the primary stimuli for breast development during the prepubertal and pubertal periods. In turn, their function is dependent on adequate levels of growth hormone, insulin, cortisol, and thyroxine (T_4). Prolactin, an adenohypophyseal polypeptide, may compensate partly for deficient functioning of any of these hormones and is itself responsible for maturation of the mammary secretory cells and subsequent production of milk protein. Estrogen specifically stimulates ductal development and growth in conjunction with growth hormone and adrenal corticosteroids. Lobuloalveolar growth in turn is dependent on progesterone plus estrogen as well as prolactin, growth hormone, and the adrenal steroids. Lactogenesis and milk secretion are stimulated by prolactin with adrenal steroids playing an additional role.

Pregnancy

During pregnancy, levels of estrogen, progesterone, and prolactin are greatly elevated. In addition, high levels of human chorionic somatomammotropin are synthesized in the placenta. But in spite of these high levels of prolactin and somatomammotropin, lactation is not a normal event of the antepartum, probably because sex hormones inhibit lactation at the level of breast tissue. This may be viewed as a local inhibition of prolactin effect. Following delivery, the rapid decrease in levels of circulating sex steroids, concomitant with increased levels of cortisol, prolactin, and oxytocin, is usually associated with the initiation of milk production. Suckling results in sharp elevations of prolactin and oxytocin levels. Oxytocin causes contraction of the myoepithelial cells in the breast, and milk is ejected from the nipple. At the same time, prolactin secretion restores the milk supply.

Control of Prolactin Secretion

Prolactin secretion from the pituitary gland appears to be under tonic inhibition rather than stimulation. The hypothalamus produces the polypeptide prolactin-inhibitory factor that is antagonistic to both prolactin synthesis and release. Control of prolactin-inhibitory factor is mediated in higher central nervous centers and in the hypothalamus itself via catecholamine metabolites and through a series of transducer neurons. Specifically, dopamine, which is released from hypothalamic neurons, acts on an α-adrenergic receptor of certain hypothalamic cells causing them to secrete prolactin-inhibitory factor. Another thesis holds that dopamine itself, acting without an intermediary, may function as the prolactin-inhibitory factor.[4] Interference with any of these dopaminergic metabolic or neuronal pathways results in decreased prolactin-inhibitory factor production and increased secretion of prolactin. Various pharmacologic mechanisms for this have been described including catecholamine depletion via interference with reuptake or storage, metabolic substrate competition, and blockage of hypothalamic alpha-adrenergic receptors.[5]

Although no specific prolactin-releasing factors have yet been identified in the human, several investigators have identified a distinct prolactin-releasing effect attributable to the thyroid-hormone-releasing factor.[6, 7] In turn, that appears to have a feedback effect on the hypothalamus that results in stimulation of prolactin-inhibitory factor as well as inhibition of the gonadotropin-releasing factor. Much work needs to be done before the complexities of these interlacing hormonal-feedback phenomena have been completely unravelled.

PATHOPHYSIOLOGY

Chiari-Frommel Syndrome

Since the postpartum-associated amenorrhea-galactorrhea syndrome was first described, several hypotheses for its pathophysiology have been set forth. Frommel (1882) attributed the amenorrhea to a wearing-out process and resultant uterine atrophy. In 1923, Schiller reported that lactation atrophy of the uterus resulted from hormones produced by the mammae which eventually inhibited ovarian function.[8] Recently, however, more emphasis has been placed on an altered hypothalmic-pituitary relationship that results from pregnancy. Prolonged inhibition of the hypothalamus leads to disarrangement of the control mechanisms that coordinate pituitary and ovarian function. This may be exacerbation of a previously present, albeit subclinical, condition.

Forbes-Albright Syndrome

In the case of the tumor-associated amenorrhea-galactorrhea, there are basically two hypothetical mechanisms. Increased prolactin levels might be due to large amounts of prolactin secreted autonomously by the tumor; or, alternatively, the tumor may mechanically interfere with either the secretion or delivery of prolactin inhibitory factor. It is possible that the two mechanisms may be at work together to produce the elevated prolactin levels.

Ahumada-del Castillo Syndrome

Pathoyphysiologic considerations here are still somewhat complicated. Many cases of so-called idiopathic amenorrhea-galactorrhea have, in retrospect, been shown to be actually drug-related. Many others are not, however, and still are without plausible etiologic explanation. Abdominal and thoracic trauma or surgery as well as herpes zoster of the chestwall have been associated with galactorrhea and, at least in part, have been explained by a neurogenic mechanism. These may or may not be associated with amenorrhea. Hypothyroidism, with associated general metabolic depression, has also been indicted as a cause of prolactin inhibitory factor inhibition and consequent elevation of prolactin levels.

Amenorrhea

Hypotheses for the pathophysiology of amenorrhea have been comparatively scarce. Amenorrhea is associated with galactorrhea in about 60% of cases. Thompson and Kempers thought that the amenorrhea was due to low levels of pituitary gonadotropins and decreased ovarian function.[9] Other investigators have suggested that the antigonadal action of prolactin results in secondary atrophy of the endometrium, hence amenorrhea. Although their antagonism has been well described, the exact relationship between prolactin and the gonadotropins is still not clear, and this fact is further complicated by recent evidence that prolactin may play a vital role in steroidogenesis at the ovarian level.[10] Gonadotropins are suppressed in lactating mothers. Suppression of prolactin during therapy for amenorrhea-galactorrhea usually results in resumption of normal menstruation. Indeed, hyperprolactinemia has been described in some series of amenorrhea alone with an occurrence rate as high as 15–20%.[11]

DRUG-INDUCED AMENORRHEA-GALACTORRHEA

Drugs can both stimulate and inhibit lactation. Actually, the most common kind of amenorrhea-galactorrhea is thought to be drug-induced. Numerous recent review articles on this subject have continued to expand the list of associated drugs.[12] Complicated interactions mediated by agonism or antagonism to dopamine and serotonin have been described. Drugs may interfere with catecholamine synthesis or block the transducer neuronal pathway, inhibiting prolactin-inhibitory factor and producing an elevation of circulating prolactin.[12, 5] For instance, phenothiazines, the largest category of drugs found to cause galactorrhea, interfere with the action of catecholamines and α-adrenergic receptor sites. Methyldopa inhibits the transformation of dopa into dopamine. Reserpine depletes the hypothalamic neurons of catecholamines. Some of the psychotropic drugs have been shown to cause hyperprolactinemia in almost 100% of patients. Not all, however, develop galactorrhea.

The effects that estrogen and progesterone-containing oral contraceptives have on lactation are even more complex. Postpill amenorrhea-galactorrhea is not an uncommon occurrence, and, pathophysiologically, it may not be unlike its postpartum counterpart. In fact, the presence of galactorrhea in a patient taking oral contraceptives may be an ominous sign of excessive hypothalamic suppression. This possibility, along with recent suggestions that oral contraceptives may exacerbate or even induce microadenomata of the pituitary gland, should dictate an immediate cessation of oral contraceptive therapy for patients who exhibit amenorrhea and galactorrhea, or galactorrhea alone, while taking birth-control pills. A workup of the patient should immediately follow pill discontinuation.

CLINICAL PRESENTATION

The only normal physiological breast secretion occurs during pregnancy, during the puerperium, and for a varying time thereafter, depending on how long the mother nurses. Otherwise, any secretion of milk is to be considered abnormal. True galactorrhea, a composition of milk and colostrum, is usually unlike the nipple discharges associated with mastitis or neoplastic disorders. These must be ruled out in the normal course of any workup of abnormal galactorrhea. The discharge associated with the galactorrhea syndrome is either a continuous and spontaneous lactation or can easily be induced manually.

Postpartum Amenorrhea-Galactorrhea

The typical postpartum amenorrhea-galactorrhea patient is a primipara between the ages of 19 and 35. Her breasts usually remain enlarged and show continuous or easily induced lactation. She is amenorrheic and may complain of a variety of additional symptoms, including headaches, lassitude, abdominal discomfort, vaginal dryness, and depression. She may be poorly nourished and frequently is obese. There need not be a continuity between nursing and galactorrhea; galactorrhea may appear suddenly, weeks after nursing has been discontinued. The syndrome, obviously, may arise in the non-nursing mother or even in one who has had some therapy to suppress puerperal lactation.

Examination may reveal dryness or even atrophic changes of the vulva and vagina. Laboratory findings usually include elevated prolactin level, low thyroid hormones, and low levels of urinary gonadotropins or estrogens. A biopsy may show endometrial atrophy. Neurologic exam is generally without specific findings, and there is no radiologic evidence of changes in the sella turcica.

Polycystic ovaries, Cushing's syndrome, and primary hypothyroidism have been shown to occur concomitantly with postpartum amenorrhea-galactorrhea. Kinch *et al.* support the view that pregnancy and its metabolic stresses may result in a deterioration of thyroid function, and that a decrease in serum T_4 is the first sign of the uncoupling of the hypothalamic-pituitary control system.[13]

Tumor-Associated Amenorrhea-Galactorrhea

The clinical presentation of the tumor-associated amenorrhea-galactorrhea is somewhat different from that associated with the postpartum period. The patient is usually about 10 years older than her postpartum counterpart. Because of the slow growth of the associated tumor, it is uncommon for the patient to have headaches, visual disturbances, or specific neurologic deficit along with her amenorrhea and galactorrhea. Extensive examination, however, may reveal some loss of visual acuity, a frank visual field deficit, optic atrophy, diplopia, and cranial nerve palsy, along with genital atrophy, decreased libido, changes in sex-related hair distribution, and general hypopituitarism. Most adenomata, when discovered, have been neurologically asymptomatic.[14]

Radiographic examination of the sella turcica may reveal sellar abnormalities caused by an adenohypophyseal tumor. Very small tumors may escape x-ray detection, especially by the conventional x-ray methods.

WORKUP AND DIAGNOSIS

Once amenorrhea-galactorrhea is diagnosed, two questions must be answered: (1) Is a tumor present? and (2) Is the syndrome drug-induced or drug-related? A thorough and directed history ought to reveal whether or not drugs or medications are involved. Unfortunately, the detection of the tumor, often a microadenoma, may present more difficult problems. It has long been known that simple anterior and lateral views of the sella turcica are usually inadequate in detecting the smaller tumors. Therefore, it should be remembered that a radiologically normal sella does not rule out the presence of a microadenoma. A planar or hypocycloid tomogram is a great deal more helpful, and here it may be suggested that lateral views be employed more extensively where possible due to fear of excessive radiation to the lens in anterior/posterior views. The neurosurgeon may also request even more sophisticated tests such as pneumoencephalography or angiography. Computerized axial tomography, unfortunately, has failed to be of much benefit in detecting pituitary microadenomas.

A workup of the amenorrhea-galactorrhea patient includes a thorough history and physical examination with neurologic and visual field testing, thyroid function tests, sellar tomography, and measurement of serum prolactin levels. Arbitrarily, one may include numerous other hormone measurements, such as levels of gonadotropins, sex steroids, and growth hormone. These frequently serve only academic interest.

Although it is safe to conclude that the basic abnormality in the amenorrhea-galactorrhea patient is an increased output of prolactin, the levels of serum prolactin in patients with the syndrome may vary greatly.[15] Hyperprolactinemia is seen initially in 70% of patients with galactorrhea. The highest prolactin levels are seen in patients with pituitary tumors, but several investigators have reported marked elevations of prolactin in patients with postpartum-associated conditions. Friesen and Hwang pointed out that some patients with significant galactorrhea may have only modest prolactin elevations, and, conversely, some patients with great elevations of prolactin do not evidence any galactorrhea.[16] A further complication is that many women with persistent galactorrhea may eventually experience a return to normal prolactin levels. Thus, in such cases, the therapeutic dilemma is whether or not specific drugs effective against hyperprolactinemia would be of any value.

TABLE II. *Drugs which increase circulating prolactin or stimulate lactation*

1. Phenothiazines
   Alpha-adrenergic receptor blockers
2. Rauwolfia
   Catecholamine storage depletion and receptor blockage
3. Tricyclic antidepressants
   Receptor blockers
4. Opiates (codein, morphine, methadone)
   Block catecholamine reuptake
5. Methyldopa, carbidopa
   Inhibit metabolism of dopa to dopamine
6. Haloperidol (butyrophenone)
   Receptor blockage
7. Thioxanthenes
   Receptor blockage
8. Thyroid releasing factor
   Prolactin release
9. Sex steroids
   Stimulate prolactin secretion (locally inhibit lactation)
10. Corticosteroids
    Action similar to sex steroids
11. Spironolactone
    Action similar to sex steroids
12. Piperoxane
    Alpha-adrenergic antagonist
13. Metoclopramide
    Dopamine antagonist
14. Neutral amino acids (alpha-methylotyrosine, alpha-methyl dopa)
    Catecholamine metabolism inhibition
15. Pimozide, clonidine, phenoxybenzamine, phentolamine, propanolol

There are also some conflicts as to exactly what normal prolactin levels are.[15, 17] Not only have studies shown that there may be wide prolactin fluctuations in normal women in the course of a single day or in the course of the menstrual cycle, but they have also shown that normal levels may vary from laboratory to laboratory. The clinician ought not to fall into the trap of arbitrarily setting a specific prolactin level (e.g., a minimum of 100 ng/ml) that he feels would indicate the presence of a pituitary tumor, and thus fail to look for a tumor if the patient's prolactin is below this minimum. As much as possible, the microadenoma ought to be ruled out in all cases, even in those patients whose amenorrhea-galactorrhea appears to be drug-related.

Unfortunately, the apparent success of clinical differentiation between autonomic tumor production of prolactin and functional hyperprolactinemia by means of various stimulatory or inhibitory tests is not standing the test of time. Thyroid-hormone-releasing factor stimulation, chlorpromazine stimulation, levodopa (L-dopa) suppressions, and water or glucose loading have all been used in the past to diagnose the presence of a tumor by its autonomic or ectopic production of prolactin.[18] Recent reports have shown that these tests produce inconsistent and sometimes ambiguous results.

TREATMENT

Historically, most therapeutic approaches to the amenorrhea-galactorrhea patient have been less than satisfactory. In those conditions where drugs are implicated, discontinuation of the drug will be followed by a reduction in circulating levels of prolactin, cessation of galactorrhea, and, generally, resumption of the menses within a few months. Early pregnancies have been reported in infertility cases of many years standing. In instances where discontinuation is impossible, it is often beneficial to reassure the patient. Probably no attempt should be made to treat galactorrhea in patients for whom the continuation on lactogenic drugs is a necessity.

Tumor-associated amenorrhea-galactorrhea has been treated surgically most successfully. Radiotherapy has proved to be relatively ineffective. In addition, with the exception of a few isolated cases, none of the drugs effective in lowering circulating prolactin levels have been shown to have any particular chemotherapeutic value in treating the tumor. They may suppress even drastically elevated levels of prolactin associated with tumor growth without bringing about a reduction in tumor size.

Many compounds have been used in the medical management of galactorrhea and hyperprolactinemia, few with any significant effect. Estrogen and progesterone, clomiphene citrate, apomorphine, and oral contraceptives have been employed with various degrees of success in both clinical and laboratory conditions. None has generated any lasting enthusiasm.

Three drugs, however, have been tested more extensively in clinical situations and have won some degree of acceptance. Pyridoxine (vitamin B_6), a coenzyme in the catecholamine metabolic pathway, has proved to be an effective inhibitor of puerperal lactation and, in some studies, has also been useful in inhibiting the lactation associated with the amenorrhea-galactorrhea syndromes. Effective dose, length of therapy, and rebound all need additional study before this drug can be totally accepted. Indeed, some recent reports deny any significant clinical use for this drug.

L-dopa, a catecholamine precursor, has also been used effectively to treat lactation and hyperprolactinemia. Its clinical limitations are secondary to the severity of its side effects, and it generally is not an acceptable drug for use in the gynecologic patient with amenorrhea and galactorrhea.

The most promising of the new drugs is

TABLE III. *Drugs which decrease circulating prolactin or inhibit lactation*

1. Dopamine receptor agonists
    Bromocryptine
    Levodopa
    Apomorphine
    Lergotrile mesylate
2. Pyridoxine
    Catecholamine metabolism coenzyme
3. Monoamine oxidase inhibitors
4. Barbituarates
5. Sex steroids (lactation inhibition)

2-α-Br-ergocryptine. This drug appears to act directly on the pituitary gland and has been extremely effective in treating hyperprolactinemia, with rapid cessation of galactorrhea and restoration of menses. In most studies, it was given in doses of 2.5 mg three times daily for periods of up to six months. Few side effects of any significance were reported in these studies, but galactorrhea recurrence, following cessation of therapy, is known to occur. This drug has recently been released for general use in treating nontumor related galactorrhea and hyperprolactinemia (Parludel[R]), but remains under study for use in acromegaly, parkinsonism, amenorrhea, and other conditions.

EDITOR'S NOTE

The amenorrhea-galactorrhea syndrome is of great interest because we went from NEVER seeing such cases in neuro-ophthalmologic practice to a virtual epidemic of them. I don't believe they were always missed before. I suspect that the widespread use of "the pill" has caused microadenomas to grow until they are "crawling out of the bushes"! The practical point is that when you see a case of amenorrhea-galactorrhea you need a careful history, particularly with emphasis on prior use of "the pill" or other estrogen-like substances, a good set of visual fields, and then *laminograms of the sella. Plain skull films, cone down stereos of the sella,* and *sellar laminograms are needed.* A *CT scan* is *NOT needed* for these cases. Dr. Young has given a good review of this syndrome in this chapter!

JLS

REFERENCES

1. Forbes, A. P., Henneman, P. H., Griswold, G. C., and Albright, F. Syndrome characterized by galactorrhea, amenorrhea and low urinary FSH: Comparison with acromegaly and normal lactation. J. Clin. Endocrinol. Metab. *14:*265 (1964).
2. Young, R. L., Bradley, E. M., Goldzieher, J. W., Meyers, P. W., and Lecocp, F. R. Spectrum of nonpuerperal galactorrhea: Report of two cases evolving through the various syndromes. J. Clin. Endocrinol. Metab. *27:*461 (1967).
3. Daughaday, W. H. *The adenohypophysis.* In: *Textbook of Endocrinology.* R. H. Williams (Ed.), Saunders, Philadelphia, 1974, pp. 33–79.
4. MacLeod, R. M. H., Kimura, H., and Login, I. Inhibition of prolactin secretion by dopamine and piribeoit (ET-495). In: *Growth Hormone and Related Peptides.* A. Pecile and E. E. Muller (Eds.). Elsevier, New York, 1976, pp. 443–453.
5. Lu, K. H., Amenomori, Y., Chen, C. L., and Meites, J. Effects of central acting drugs on serum and pituitary prolactin levels in rats. Endocrinology *87:*667 (1976).
6. Keye, W. R., Jr., Ho Yuen, B., Knoph, R., and Jaffe, R. B. Amenorrhea, hyperprolactinemia and pituitary enlargement secondary to primary hypothyroidism. Obstet. Gynecol. *48:*697 (1976).
7. Snyder, P. J., Jacobs, L. S., Utiger, R. D., and Daughaday, W. H. Thyroid hormone inhibition of the prolactin response to thyrotropin-releasing hormone. J. Clin. Invest. *52:*2324 (1974).
8. Schiller, H. Lactation atrophy of uterus. Am. J. Obstet. Gynecol. *6:*333 (1973).
9. Thompson, J. P. and Kempers, R. O. Amenorrhea and galactorrhea. Am. J. Obstet. Gynecol. *93:*65 (1965).
10. McNatty, K. P. and Sawers, R. S. Relationship between the endocrine environment within the grafian follicle and the subsequent secretion of progesterone by human granulosa cells in culture. J. Endocrinol. *66:*391 (1975).
11. Franks, S. M. A., Murray, A. F., Jecqvier, A. M., Steele, S. J., Nabarro, J. D. N., and Jacobs, H. S. Incidence and significance of hyperprolactinemia in women with amenorrhea. Clin. Endocrinol. (Oxf) *4:*597 (1975).
12. Dickey, R. P. and Stone, S. C. Drugs that affect the breast and lactation. Clin. Obstet. Gynecol. *18*(2):95–109 (1975).
13. Kinch R. A., Plunkett, E. R., and Delvin, M. C. Postpartum amenorrhea-galactorrhea of hypothyroidism. Am. J. Obstet. Gynecol., *105:*766 (1969).
14. Young, R. L. The amenorrhea-galactorrhea syndrome. Compr. Ther. *4*(9):40 (1978).
15. Archer, D. F., Hankin, H. R., Gabos, P. F., Maroon, J., Nosetz, S., Wadhwa, S. R., and Josimovich, J. B. Serum prolactin in patients with inappropriate lactation. Am. J. Obstet. Gynecol. *119:*466 (1974).
16. Friesen, H. and Hwang, P. Human prolactin. Ann. Rev. Med. *24:*251 (1973).
17. Yen, S. S. C. Galactorrhea-amenorrhea syndrome. In: *Reproductive Endocrinology.* S. S. C. Yen and R. B. Jaffe (Eds.), Saunders, Philadelphia, 1978, pp. 353–359.
18. Kase, N., Andriole, A., and Sobrinho, L. Endocrine diagnosis of pituitary tumor in galactorrhea syndromes. Am. J. Obstet. Gynecol. *114*(3):321–328 (1972).

28 Transsphenoidal Microsurgery in the Management of Acromegaly

Edward Raymond Laws, Jr., M.D.

The revival of the transsphenoidal approach to the pituitary gland has revolutionized the current day management of patients with acromegaly. Along with improvements in the surgical technique, advances in endocrinology and neuroradiology have allowed much more accurate preoperative diagnosis of such patients and have influenced the entire spectrum of pituitary disease. The diagnosis of acromegaly is now being made more frequently when the disease is in its early stages. The proportion of the patients having large tumors with accompanying visual field defects is smaller than in the past, and it is already evident that early surgical intervention when tumors are small will result in much more satisfactory long term management. At this time, 95% of all pituitary tumors being treated surgically at our institution are approached transsphenoidally rather than by craniotomy.

This report describes a personal experience with 100 consecutive patients with acromegaly treated by transsphenoidal microsurgery during a period from November 1972 until December 1978. Accurate follow-up information including basal growth hormone levels and visual field examinations were available in virtually every patient and have been analyzed.

MATERIALS AND METHODS

The case records of 100 consecutive patients with acromegaly operated upon by the same surgeon were reviewed with regard to presenting symptoms and signs, preoperative endocrine evaluation, findings at surgery, postoperative endocrine evaluation, and over-all results of neurosurgical management. In addition, pre- and postoperative visual field examinations were performed on all patients with visual complaints and a majority of those who had no disturbance of vision. Human growth hormone levels and serum were determined by quantitative radio-immuno-assay. Because the normal basal value for serum growth hormone in females in our laboratory is less than or equal to 10 ng/ml, and, because this level is commonly utilized in reports of the results of treatment of acromegaly, it was used as the "normal" postoperative growth hormone value. More precise assessment requires the use of dynamic endocrine testing and results of glucose or insulin tolerance tests were not available in all the patients.

The study group consisted of 59 men and 41 women whose ages ranged from 16 to 75 years with an average of 42 years. Complete follow-up review including growth hormone determinations was available in 98 of the 100 cases. In one patient tumor removal (diffuse adenoma) was not completed because of hemorrhage; one patient (microadenoma) lives abroad and has not returned for followup examination. At the time of analysis the follow-up period ranged from 2 to 74 months following surgery with a mean of 24 months. Previous therapy had been given in 22 of the 100 cases; radiation therapy in 19; radio-frequency thermocoagulation in two; and craniotomy and two courses of radiotherapy in one case of gigantism and acromegaly. Two of the patients had been treated unsuccessfully with heavy particle radiation therapy via the proton beam.

Tumors were classified on the basis of radiologic findings and appearance at surgery. *Microadenomas* were those tumors less than or equal to 10 mm in diameter that could be demarcated from normal pituitary gland. *Diffuse adenomas* were those tumors that filled the sella but remained confined by the dura though some of these had suprasellar extension. *Invasive adenomas* were those tumors that had invaded dura or both dura and bone, and some of these also had suprasellar extension.

PREOPERATIVE AND OPERATIVE OBSERVATIONS

Clinical Presentation

All of the patients had hormonally active acromegaly and presented with a wide spectrum of symptoms and signs characteristic of this disease. Four of the patients had gigantism with disease of long standing, and one teenage girl had gigantism and acromegaly. Associated visual complaints were present in seven of the 100 patients, all of whom had bitemporal visual field defects when examined. Headache, osteoarthritis, and arthralgia were common complaints. Diabetes mellitus was present in approximately 50% of the cases, and many patients had histories of thyroid disease or menstrual irregularity. Four patients had multiple endocrine neoplasia syndromes.

Two of the patients who had undergone prior therapy (one radio-frequency thermocoagulation, one craniotomy) presented with associated cerebrospinal fluid rhinorrhea.

Laboratory Studies

Preoperative basal growth hormone values ranged widely. Among patients with active acromegaly, there were some who had "normal" baseline values as well as those who had markedly elevated levels. By tumor category, there were 24 cases of microadenoma with mean basal preoperative growth hormone level of 25.4 ng/ml, 52 cases of diffuse adenoma with a mean preoperative growth hormone level of 52.4 ng/ml, and 24 cases of invasive adenoma with a mean of 69.7 ng/ml. Preoperative prolactin values were elevated in 12 of the 60 patients in whom it was measured.

The presence of a pituitary adenoma was confirmed by polytomography of the sella or carotid angiography with magnification and subtraction in each case.

Surgical Considerations

All patients were operated upon by a standard transseptal transsphenoidal route. Enlargement of the features and bony structures made the surgical approach difficult in some cases, with the depth of the sella occasionally being 11 cm or more. Abandonment of the procedure was thought advisable in one case where excess hemorrhage occurred from a large intracavernous sinus.

RESULTS

Transsphenoidal surgery produced improvement in the signs and symptoms of acromegaly in all but eight of the 100 patients. No significant postoperative change occurred in any of the four acromegalic giants, in the patient whose operation was abandoned because of excessive bleeding, in one patient whose persistent postoperative growth hormone elevation was eventually cured by craniotomy, in one patient who developed a recurrent tumor, and finally in the single patient who is not alive at this time. He died of an adenocarcinoma of the colon, and his growth hormone was higher than when determined preoperatively.

All seven patients who presented with visual field defects had improvement in vision both subjectively and objectively following surgery. No patient had vision worsened by the surgical procedure.

On the basis of findings at surgery, 24 tumors were characterized as microadenomas (less than or equal to 10 mm in diameter), 52 as diffuse adenomas (including 13 with suprasellar extension), and 24 as invasive adenomas (including four with suprasellar extension). Total removal of the tumor with preservation of normal gland was the goal in most cases. Total hypophysectomy was purposely performed in two patients, one who was an acromegalic giant with diabetic retinopathy.

Follow-up basal growth hormone values were available in 98 of the 100 cases and are presented in Table I along with the results of postoperative assessment of remaining anterior pituitary function. Radiation therapy has been given or recommended to 37 of the 87 patients who had not received it previously, the recommendation usually being based on the invasiveness or extent of the tumor or the postoperative growth hormone value.

There was no operative mortality in this series. Surgical complications consisted of one case with transient cerebrospinal fluid rhinorrhea, four cases of partial anterior pituitary insufficiency, and 14 cases of complete anterior pituitary insufficiency. Permanent diabetes insipidus occurred in one case and transient diabetes insipidus which lasted more than one month occurred in two other patients. Perforation of the nasal septum developed in one patient. One patient suffered subdural hemorrhage and decrease of vision as a complication of her postoperative radiation therapy three months following surgery.

Four patients underwent more than one operation. One man initially thought to have a microadenoma had a diffuse adenoma at his second transsphenoidal operation which resulted in control of a persistently elevated growth hormone level. Another patient whose tumor activity remained uncontrolled after radio-frequency thermocoagulation and a transsphenoidal operation was ultimately cured by crani-

TABLE I. *Results of transsphenoidal surgery in 100 patients with acromegaly*

	N	Postop growth hormone			Postop pituitary function			Visual field defect	Elevated prolactin[b]	MEN syndrome
		≤10	>10	?	Unimpaired	Impaired	Suprasellar extension			
Microadenoma										
TS surgery only[a]	20	19 (95%)	1	0	20	0			1	1
Prior Rx	1	0	1	0	1	0			0	0
Surgery and radiotherapy	3	1	1	1	2	1			1	1
Total microadenoma	24	20	3	1	23	1	0	0	2	2
Diffuse adenoma										
TS surgery only	27	22 (81%)	4	1	25	2	6	2	4	2
Prior Rx	8	7	1	0	5	3	1	0	1	
Surgery and radiotherapy	17	8	9	0	15	2	6	3	1	
Total diffuse adenoma	52	37	14	1	45	7	13	5	6	2
Invasive adenoma										
TS surgery only	7	4	3	0	5	2	2	0	1	
Prior Rx	4	1	3	0	0	4	0	0	0	
Surgery and radiotherapy	13	8	5	0	9	4	3	2	3	
Total invasive adenoma	24	13 (54%)	11	0	14	10	5	2	4	0
Total acromegalics	100	70	28	2	82	18	19	7	12/60	4

[a] Includes two invasive microadenomas.

[b] Preoperative prolactin levels available in a total of 60 patients.

otomy and removal of an extrasellar tumor nodule. One of the patients with gigantism and acromegaly had a postoperative growth hormone level of 22 and was reexplored transsphenoidally one year after the initial procedure. Additional tumor tissue in the wall of the left cavernous sinus was removed, but the growth hormone values continued to be abnormal. One patient required reexploration for repair of postoperative CSF rhinorrhea. There has been one recurrence of an intrasellar diffuse adenoma in a patient whose growth hormone values initially fell and then progressively rose during an 18-month period of observation. She has been referred for proton beam therapy.

Five of the seven young women with amenorrhea have resumed menstruating and three of the five have become pregnant. Postoperative prolactin values are normal in all of the patients whose values were abnormal preoperatively, and galactorrhea has not persisted in any of the patients who had this symptom preoperatively.

DISCUSSION

Because the follow-up period is relatively short, the effects of successful surgery upon the natural history of the disease cannot be evaluated fully. It is anticipated, however, that long-term control will be better and that the recurrence rate will be lower than those resulting from other forms of therapy.

Classification of tumors into categories of microadenoma, diffuse adenoma, and invasive adenoma appears to be validated by the postoperative growth hormone values. Clearly, the most favorable results occur in those patients with microadenomas. That persistent fraction of uncured patients in every series of acromegalics is probably best accounted for by tumors that involve the sellar dura or parasellar structures and therefore cannot be resected totally. It is important to note that our over-all plan of management does include radiation therapy postoperatively for a significant number of patients, and the results of postoperative endocrine evaluation are the most accurate means of determining the success of the surgery and the possible need for follow-up radiation therapy. The results in

terms of preservation of normal anterior pituitary function have been most encouraging, and represent a significant advance over previous systems of therapy for acromegaly.

Transsphenoidal microsurgery currently has an excellent potential for achieving ideal results—the removal of the pituitary adenoma with preservation of normal pituitary function. Every effort should be made to treat acromegalics at the earliest possible phase of the disease, when the selective removal of a small microadenoma is most readily accomplished.

EDITOR'S NOTE

The classic indication for surgery of a parachiasmal mass lesion has always been loss of vision or visual field. Dr. Laws has operated on 100 cases of acromegaly via the transsphenoidal route with no operative mortality at all. I heard him present some of this data at the Harvey Cushing Society and believe the results are sufficiently impressive to have asked him to give this larger total series. It is evident that transsphenoidal surgery now allows earlier operation in acromegaly with less morbidity for the patient. The endocrine aspects of this diagnosis are now more important in following the patients. In the old days, only about half of the acromegalics were found to have visual field defects. This percentage is now much smaller, due to earlier detection of the cases. Of course, all of these patients should have quantitative perimetry, both before and after surgery.

There is much excitement in the literature about medical therapy for acromegaly and this should be mentioned here. Bromocriptine is a drug that has allowed some women with amenorrhea or galactorrhea to get pregnant—and they *may* suddenly develop visual loss, field defect, or cranial nerve palsies if they have an undetected pituitary tumor that swells during the pregnancy. Two recent papers should be mentioned here, however. Spark, R. F., Dickstein, G., and Pallotta, J. reported "Complete Remission of Acromegaly with Medical Treatment" in *J. Am. Med. Assoc.* **241**(6):573–575, Feb. 9, 1979. They reported a 40-year-old woman with a 10-year history of acromegaly despite prior treatment with irradiation and two transsphenoidal operations. She was treated with bromocriptine and within three months ovulatory menses resumed for the first time in ten years. The soft-tissue changes of acromegaly were also said to have improved.

A very impressive paper is by McGregor, A. M., *et al.*, entitled "Reduction in Size of a Pituitary Tumor by Bromocriptine Therapy" in *New Engl. J. Med.* **300**(6):291–293, Feb. 8, 1979. This patient presented at age 24 with a three-month history of impotence, loss of libido, headache, nausea, and diplopia. A complete right third nerve palsy was found, but acuity and fields were found to be normal. Right frontal craniotomy showed a pituitary adenoma and 4,500 rads of external megavoltage irradiation was given postoperatively. He was hospitalized three years later and now had 20/20 vision in the right eye and 20/50 vision in the left eye. A left temporal hemianopia and a right upper nasal quadrantanopia were present. The fantastic thing is that a computed tomographic scan is shown at this point showing a large, enhancing tumor with suprasellar and right lateral extension. It is obvious that the lesion was involving the right optic tract from this scan and the visual field defects reported. The patient was treated medically with bromocriptine and within three months was virtually asymptomatic. Vision was now 20/20 in both eyes, the fields are said to be full, and a repeat computed tomographic scan was virtually normal! This is extremely impressive radiographic documentation of regression of a known pituitary tumor on bromocriptine therapy. It is obvious that this is going to

have more study. This is an exciting field as new information continues to come in!

JLS

REFERENCES

1. Giovanelli, M. A., Motti, E. D. F., Paracchi, A., *et al.* Treatment of acromegaly by transsphenoidal microsurgery. J. Neurosurg. *44:*677–686 (1976).
2. Guiot, G. and Thibaut, B. L'extirpation des adénomes hypophysaires par voie trans-sephénoïdale. Neurochirurgia (Stuttg.) *1:*133–150 (1959).
3. Hardy, J. Transsphenoidal surgery of hypersecreting pituitary tumors. Excerpta Medica International Congress Series No. 303: 179–194 (1973).
4. Hardy, J., Robert, F., and Somma, M., *et al.* Acromegalie-gigantisme: traitement chirurgical par exerese transsphenoidale de l'adenome hypophysaire. Neurochirurgie 19 Suppl 2:1–184 (1973).
5. Kjellberg, R. N. and Kliman, B. Treatment of acromegaly by proton hypophysectomy. In: *Current Controversies in Neurosurgery.* T. P. Morley (Ed.), Saunders Philadelphia, 1976, pp. 392–405.
6. Laws, E. R., Jr. Transsphenoidal approach to lesions in and about the sella turcica. In: *Current Techniques in Operative Neurosurgery.* Schmidek HH, Sweet WH (Eds.), Grune & Stratton, New York, 1977, pp. 161–172.
7. Laws, E. R., Jr., Trautmann, J. C., and Hollenhorst, R. W., Jr. Transsphenoidal decompression of the optic nerve and chiasm: visual results in 62 patients. J. Neurosurg. *46:*717–722 (1977).
8. Lüdecke, D., Kautzky, R., Saeger, W., *et al.* Selective removal of hypersecreting pituitary adenomas? An analysis of endocrine function, operative and microscopial fundings in 101 cases. Acta Neurochir. (Wien) *35:*27–42 (1976).
9. U, H. S., Wilson, C. B., and Tyrrell, J. B. Transsphenoidal microhypophysectomy in acromegaly. J. Neurosurg. *47:*840–852 (1977).
10. Vezina, J. L., and Maltais, R. La selle turcique dans l'acromégalie: étude radiologique. Neurochirurgie 19 Suppl 2:35–56 (1973).
11. Williams, R. A., Jacobs, H. S., Kurtz, A. B., *et al.* The treatment of acromegaly with special reference to transsphenoidal hypophysectomy. Q. J. Med. *44:*79–98 (1975).

29 The Meningiomas of the Planum Sphenoidale and Tuberculum Sellae

Gerald N. Kadis, M.D.
Lester A. Mount, M.D.

HISTORICAL ASPECTS

Parasellar meningioma was first reported in the literature in 1897. Stirling[1] described the post mortem findings of an "endothelioma" arising from the meninges in the vicinity of the sella in a patient with blindness in one eye and contralateral temporal field defect developing over a period of six years. Other cases followed in the literature (Stewart,[2] 1899, Archibald,[3] 1908, and Heinrichsdorff,[4] 1914). All of these cases were discovered at post mortem examination. Cushing[5, 6] pointed out that these lesions appeared to arise from the tuberculum sellae and sulcus chiasmaticus. Prophetically he went on to say[7] "...few appear to have a better prognosis when surgically removed: and few promise in the future to be as easily recognized while still of small size." Neurosurgeons since the time of Cushing have noted that the opportunity to make an early diagnosis usually rests with the ophthalmologist. We are still striving to make the diagnosis "while the tumor is still of small size."

SEX AND AGE CHARACTERISTICS

In most of the series in the literature there is a female predominance: Gregorius,[8] 21 women/2 men; Cushing,[7] 20 women/8 men; Kadis and Mount,[9] 74 women/31 men. The average age on admission to the hospital tends to be 50 years.

CLINICAL PRESENTATION

Essentially all of our 105 patients presented with the complaint of painless impairment of vision. Rarely did they complain of headache, and when they did it was not of localizing value. Only in the very large tumors was there a history of change of mentation or endocrine dysfunction. The time to make the diagnosis is when the symptomatology is limited to one eye alone, before symptoms extend to the second eye, and while the tumor is of small size. Unfortunately, the time from the onset of visual symptoms to the time of admission to the hospital for surgery has in the past been quite long varying from six months to seven years. This will change when a CT scan is performed on all patients who have unexplained impairment of vision.

PHYSICAL EXAMINATION

Most of the patients in our experience of 105 cases had visual acuity of 20/200 or worse in at least one eye and all of the patients had impairments in the visual fields preoperatively. We have seen many different varieties of visual field defects; all but one had some variety of temporal field cut. A point worth emphasizing is that in the most recent group of patients visual complaints were present in only one eye although with careful testing subtle defects were often found in the second eye. As has been pointed out, symptoms and findings in the visual fields are not as uniform as previously thought to be.[10]

Relative afferent pupillary defects as demonstrated by the swinging light test and relative dimness of red test objects either in one eye compared to the other or in portions of the field helps in the detection of the subtle defects.

All of the patients in our experience had abnormal discs which probably means that they were not diagnosed sufficiently early. The most common abnormality was disc pallor alone. An occasional patient had Foster-Kennedy Syndrome. An occasional patient with a huge tumor was found to be anosmic or to have testable changes consistent with bilateral frontal lobe dysfunction.

LABORATORY FINDINGS

Thyroid studies, 17-ketosteroids, and ketogenic steroids were occasionally abnormal, again only in the very large tumors. Cerebrospinal fluid protein was elevated in about one-half of the patients in whom it was measured. Electroencephalography was not very useful but results were interpreted as abnormal in about one-half of the patients with these tumors.

NUCLEAR BRAIN SCANNING

In patients in whom the test is interpreted as abnormal the test is useful; however, in our experience false negatives were reported approximately one-third of the time. Most of our isotope scans are HG^{197}, only a few are RISA I^{131}. In all of the

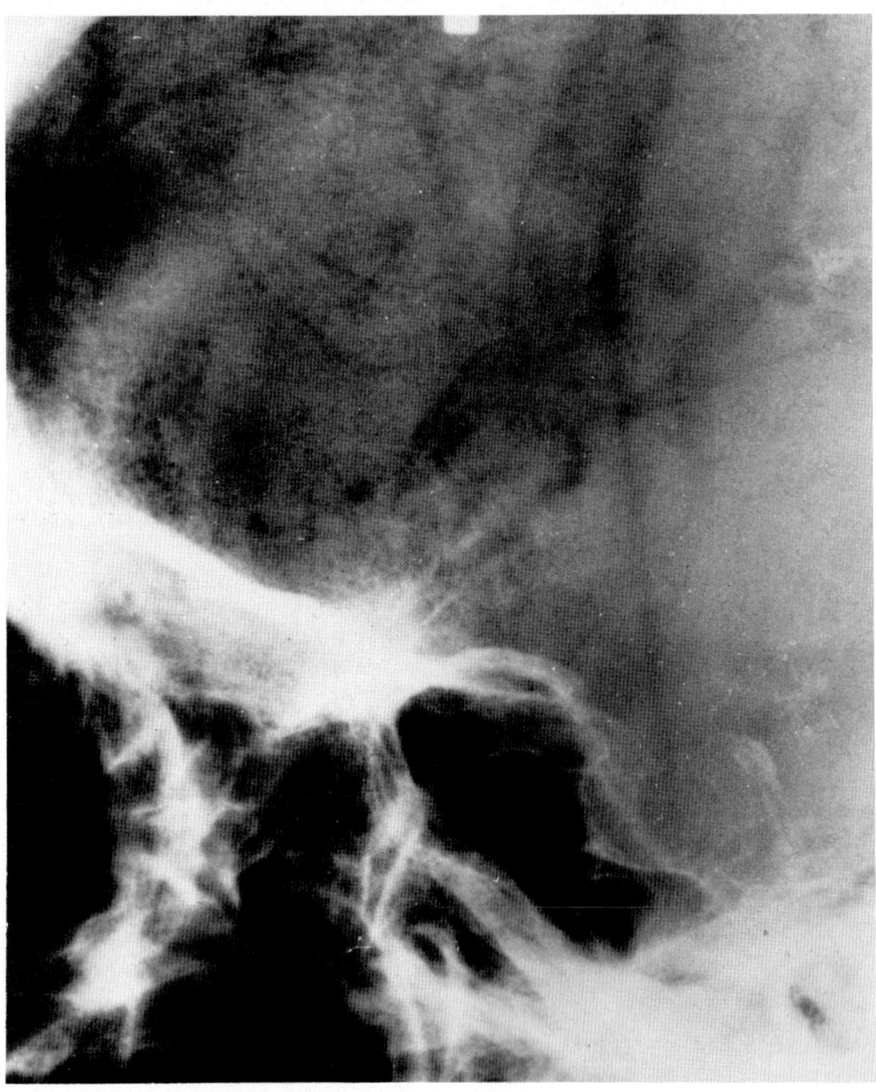

Fig. 1. Skull x-ray 1. Blistering of planum sphenoidale.

patients that had negative isotope scans who subsequently underwent computed tomography scanning the tumors were detected 100% of the time

SKULL X-RAYS

In patients with these tumors definite evidence of meningioma will be seen approximately two-thirds of the time as blistering of the planum or tuberculum (Fig. 1). However, again one-third of the skull films will show false negatives. Optic foraminal views and tomograms will occasionally pick up subtle hyperostosis not seen in the plain films.

COMPUTED TOMOGRAPHY

Computed tomography in our experience will show the mass successfully provided sufficiently low cuts are obtained and contrast medium is given. In several cases the mass was not at all appreciated until contrast material was given (scans 1 and 2 in Fig. 2). Coronal cuts further define the masses (scan 3 in Fig. 3) and in one case showed the mass when it had not been properly appreciated on axial cuts or angiography (scans 4 and 5 in Fig. 4 and Angiogram 3 in Fig. 7). Computed tomography has shown itself useful in the early detection of all sorts of tumors.[12, 13] We feel that it should play an expanded role in the early workup of failing vision of unexplained etiology.

ANGIOGRAPHY

In all of our cases angiography has been

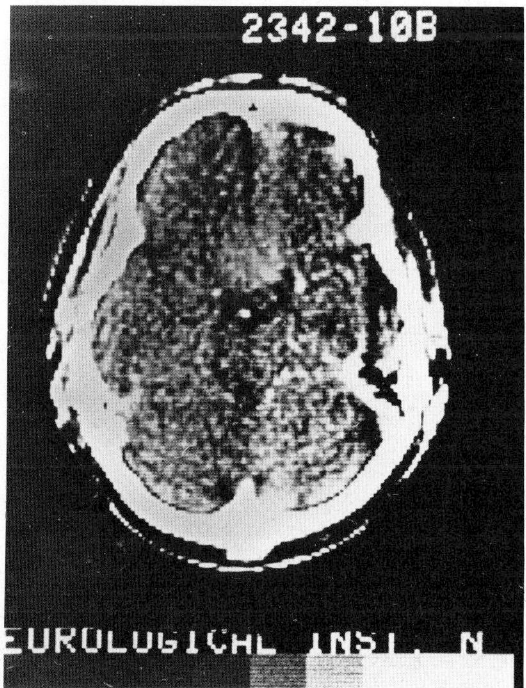

Fig. 2. Scan 2

Fig. 2. Scans 1 and 2. These scans show the importance of administering contrast material when doing the scan.

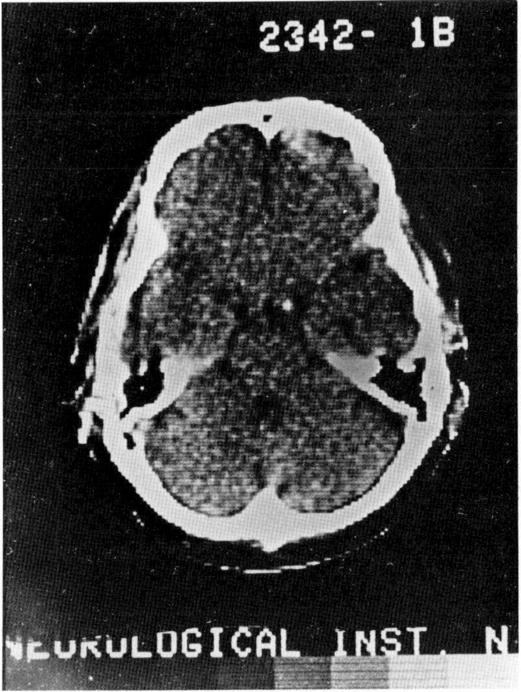

Fig. 2. Scan 1

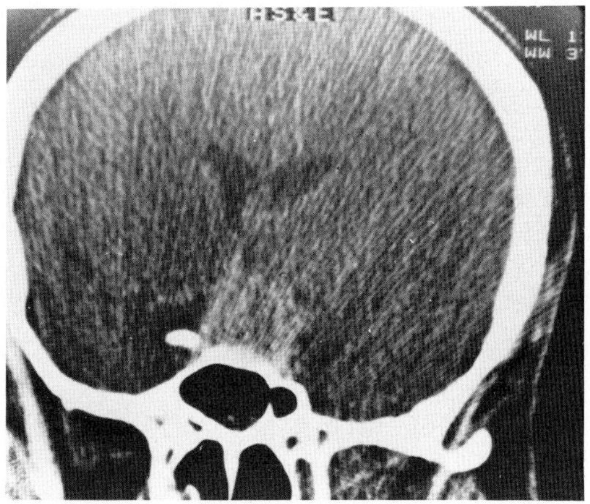

Fig. 3. Scan 3 clearly outlines the tumor in the coronal sections.

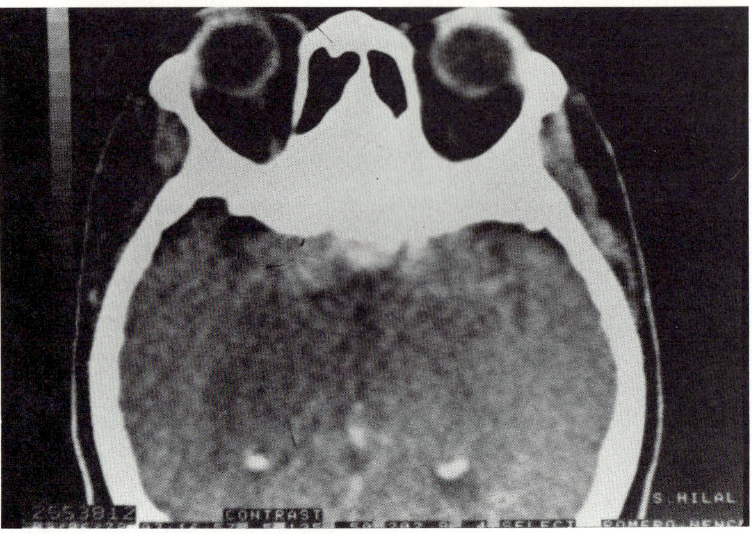

Fig. 4. Scan 4

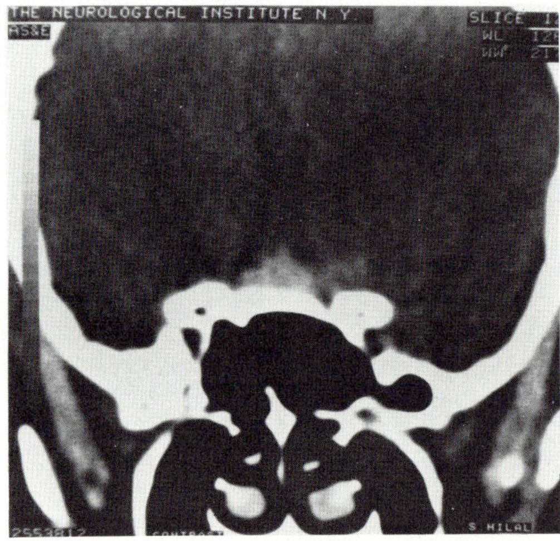

Fig. 4. Scan 5

Fig. 4. Scans 4 and 5 show the better demonstration of the tumor in the coronal sections.

performed preoperatively. In all but one case the angiogram clearly showed the mass either through stain or vascular displacement (angiograms 1 and 2 in Figs. 5 and 6). In the one case that failed to show the mass the coronal computerized tomogram clearly showed the mass (angiogram 3 in Fig. 7 and scans 4 and 5 in Fig. 4).

SURGERY

We prefer to approach the tumors via a bifrontal craniotomy because it allows bet-

ter visualization and, hence, less risk to important structures. Microsurgical technique is indispensable. In most cases the optic nerves will be displaced by the tumors although in occasional cases the nerves and even the chiasm will be encased in the tumor as may be the carotid arteries and anterior cerebral arteries. In rare cases the tumor actually invaded the chiasm and was inseparable from it. Encasement of a major artery is the most common reason for incomplete removal. One patient had an adenocarcinoma that had metastasized to the

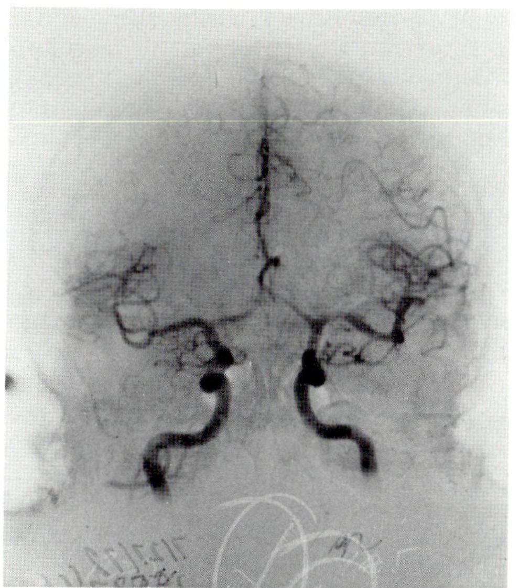

Fig. 5. Angiogram 1 shows the tumor elevating and compressing the anterior cerebral arteries.

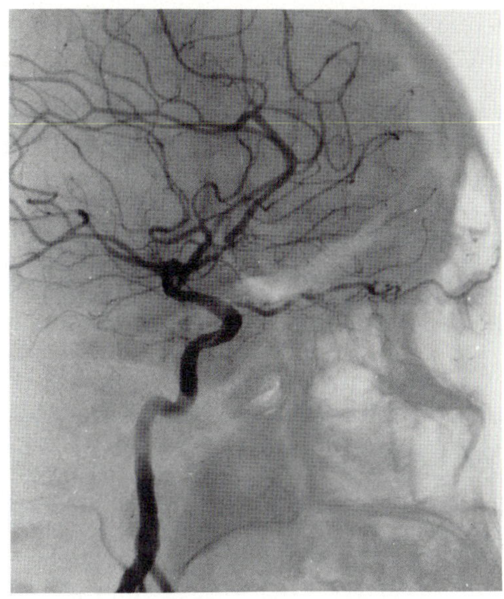

Fig. 7. Angiogram 3. This shows how easily the tumor, well shown in Scan 5, Fig. 4, could have been missed in the arteriogram, which was almost normal.

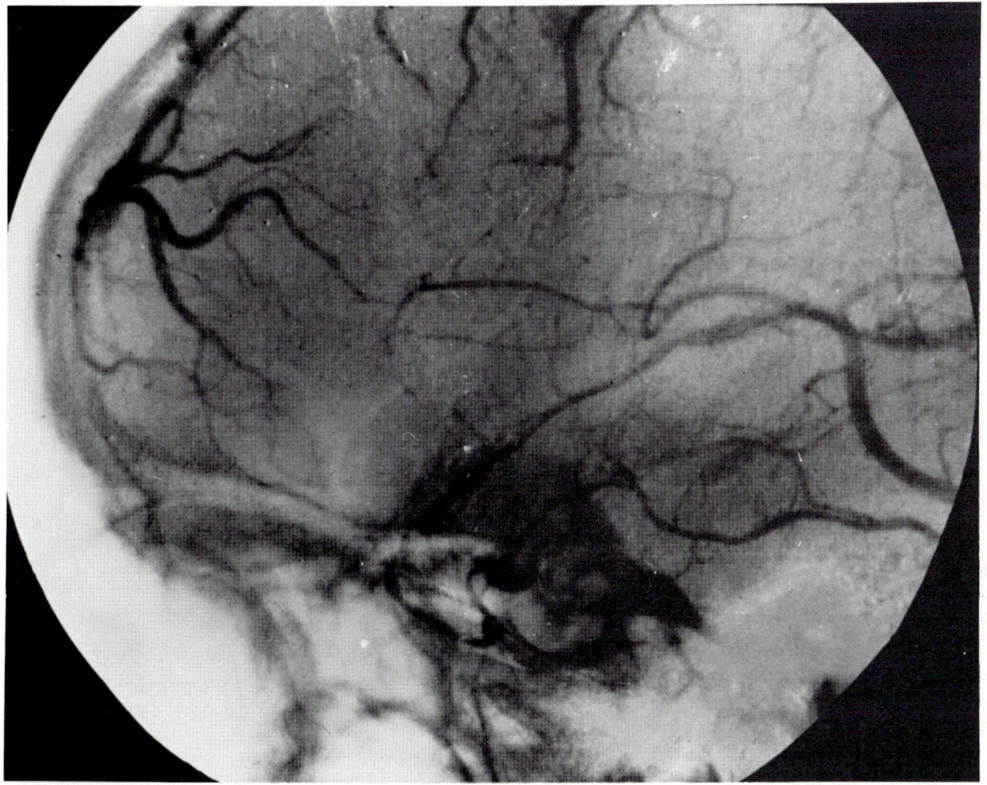

Fig. 6. Angiogram 2. The venous phase shows the tumor stain in the suprasellar region.

meningioma without evidence of metastasis elsewhere in the cranial vault. The primary later turned out to be in the lung and was of very small size. As noted by other authors difficulty was often encountered in correlating precisely in all cases the preoperative deficits with the placement of the tumor purely on a compressive basis. Compromise of the central chiasmic blood supply may help to explain some of these discrepancies.[14]

MORTALITY AND MORBIDITY

Operative mortality and morbidity is clearly related to the size of the tumor at the time of attempted removal. In patients with tumors larger than 3 cm in diameter 10.4% died. In those with tumors less than 3 cm in diameter there were no postoperative deaths. In our experience all of the deaths occurred (nine prior to 1972 and one since 1972) because a major vessel which had been encased was damaged. We have not had a single death in an individual with a tumor of 3 cm in diameter or smaller. Serious complications occurred in approximately 10% of the patients undergoing surgery for these tumors such as cerebrospinal fluid leak, cerebral edema, and permanent neurological deficits other than visual loss. Again the complication rate in patients with tumors greater than 3 cm in diameter is much greater than in patients with the smaller tumors.

VISUAL RESULTS

In nine patients with tumors larger than 3 cm in diameter follow-up data were not available; of the remaining 75 patients, in 39 (52%) acuity improved, in 14 (19%) worsened, and in 22 (29%) it remained the same.

In those patients with tumors less than 3 cm in diameter, 9/10 (90%) improved and one had not improved at the time of discharge from the hospital.

It is clear that delay in diagnosis and treatment of these meningiomas is detrimental to the patient in terms of visual recovery, morbidity, and mortality. Early accurate diagnosis is possible through the use of computerized tomography and its use is extremely useful in the workup of patients with unexplained impairment of vision so that early operative treatment can be performed.

EDITOR'S NOTE

Drs. Kadis and Mount have done an excellent job in emphasizing the diagnostic difficulties encountered with planum and tuberculum meningiomas. The diagnosis of such cases really rests primarily on the one examining the patient's eyes! Three good rules in these cases are: (1) do a *good confrontation field* on *every new patient* you see; (2) *review* those *plain skull films* carefully; and (3) don't forget *coronal cuts* on *CT* scans when you are thinking of tuberculum or planum meningiomas. If the patient has a lot of dental fillings, you can just about forget the coronal cuts, however, as they cause horrible artefacts on the coronal views. The best rule, however, is—"Always get a *CF* before a *CT!*" This says—"Always get a CONFRONTATION FIELD before a COMPUTED TOMOGRAPHY!"

JLS

REFERENCES

1. Stirling, J. W. Tumor of the meninges in the region of the pituitary body, pressing on the chiasm. Ann. Ophthalmol. *6:*15–16 (1897).
2. Stewart, J. The symptomology of tumors involving the phypophysis. Trans. Assoc. Am. Physicians *14:*282 (1899).
3. Archibald, E. Surgical affections and wounds of the head. In: *American Practice of Surgery.* Bryant and A. Buck (Eds.), William Wood and Co., New York, 1908.
4. Heinrichsdorff, P. Ein Psammom im vorderen chiasmawinkel. Klin. Monatsbl. Augenheilkd. *16:* 185–187.
5. Cushing, H. The meningiomas (Dural Endotheliomas): Their source and favored seats of origin. Brain *45:*282 (1922).
6. Cushing, H. and Eisenhart, L. Meningiomas arising from the tuberculum sellae. Arch. Ophthalmol. *1:*168 (Jan. 1929).
7. Cushing, H. and Eisenhart, L. *Meningiomas: Their classification, regional behavior, life history and surgical end results.* Charles C. Thomas, Springfield, Ill., 1938.
8. Gregorius, F. K., Helper, R. S., and Stern, W. E. Loss and recovery of vision with suprasellar meningiomas. J. Neurosurg. *42:*69–75 (1975).
9. Kadis, G. N. and Mount, L. A. The importance of

early diagnosis and treatment of the meningiomas of the planum sphenoidale and tuberculum sellae—a retrospective study of 105 cases. Submitted for publication.

10. Finn, J. E. and Mount, L. A. Meningiomas of the tuberculum sellae and planum sphenoidale. Arch. Ophthalmol. *92:*23–27 (1974).

11. Knight, C. L., Hoyt, W. F., and Wilson, C. B. Syndrome of incipient prechiasmal optic nerve compression. Arch. Ophthalmol. *87:*1–11 (1972).

12. New, P. F. J., Scott, W. R., and Schnur, J. A., *et al.* Computed tomography with the EMI scanner in the diagnosis of primary and metastatic intracranial neoplasms. Radiology *114:*75–87 (1974).

13. Davis, K. R., Taveras, J. M., and Robertson, G. H. Some limitations of computed tomography in the diagnosis of neurological diseases. Am. J. Roetgenol. *127:*111 (1976).

14. Bergland, R. and Ray, B. S. The arterial supply of the human optic chiasm. J. Neurosurg. *31:*327–334 (1969).

30 Innovations in CT Technology

Clark Watts, M.D.

The introduction of computerized tomography (CT) has been considered the greatest advance in radiology since the introduction of the roentgen ray created the specialty.[1] The head unit has certainly revolutionized neuroradiology. While the initial reports of its use electrified the medical profession and indeed the world, advances which have been made in the past few years have predictably greatly enhanced the use of the technology by the medical profession and suggest that future advances await only more imaginative application of the technology with time. Since computerized tomography images are created by computer, they are inherently amenable to computer image processing techniques. A majority of the advances alluded to above have been made as the result of the application by computer sciences of this concept. This paper will review some of these advances. Although a basic understanding of the principles of computer tomography is assumed, the reader is referred to the literature for a review of these principles.[2, 3]

GENERATIONS OF SCANNERS

The basic CT unit contains a source for x-rays which are detected after they pass through the body, a computer system which analyzes the x-rays, and a display unit. The detectors are placed at 180° from the x-ray source. Following each emission the x-ray unit is rotated a certain distance and another pulse is generated. This is continued until the x-ray source has rotated 180° giving a 360° examination. The unit is then moved to another level and this process repeated. Usually eight to nine "slices" of 8–13 mm thick are obtained. The slices are usually referenced to a routine plane, 25° to Reads line. At each point on the slice a certain number of transmissions are detected, each adding to the total bank of information the computer must analyze. For example, if 160 readings of photon transmissions are obtained with each degree of rotation, then 28,800 (160 × 180) absorption readings are analyzed at each slice. Following these analyses the computer's output is then displayed either on a paper printout or on an oscilloscope. The size of the displayed matrix (and therefore the resolution of the scanner) will depend upon the number of calculated absorption values within each slice. Thus a 160 × 160 matrix requires at least 25,600 observations, while reconstruction of a 320 × 320 matrix will require at least 102,400 observations.

The initial CT scanner design, or first generation unit, which produced an 80 × 80 matrix utilized a single pencil x-ray beam source and a single sodium iodide crystal detector coupled to a photomultiplier tube. The gantry (containing the x-ray source and the detectors at 180° from each other) was rotated 1° at a time and each scan took approximately 4½ min to complete. A water bag head cap was used to reduce distortion created at the air-head interface.

The second generation units eliminated the use of the water bag. Multiple beams of x-rays were utilized with simultaneous recording from multiple crystal detectors. A narrow angle fan beam x-ray allowed the rotation of the scanner gantry at 10° increments instead of 1° increments, thus, markedly reducing scan time to about 20 sec or less. This also resulted in greater resolution which permitted, for example, the identification of intra-orbital structures (Fig. 1).

Third generation scanning units utilize a

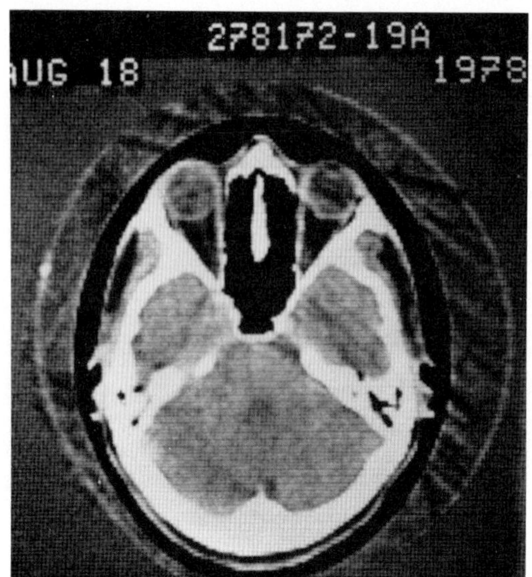

Fig. 1. CT scan demonstrating intra-orbital contents including the globe, optic nerve, and extra-occular muscles.

very wide angle fan beam of x-rays which is divided into a large number of individual pencil beams recorded simultaneously by high pressure xenon gas detectors. Much more rapid scanning (as short as 2 or 3 sec) is obtained.

The fourth generation scanners utilize a large number of crystal detectors which are stationary and arranged in a 360° circular ray around the patient. The x-ray source rotates within the detector ring, and the wide angle fan beam encompasses multiple detectors within its arc. This results in rapid scanning speed, lack of vibration of the unit, and very high spatial resolution. The fourth generation unit utilizes bismuth germinate crystal detectors.

These improvements in the basic technology have thus resulted in more rapid scanning with higher resolution and simplification of patient management (with the elimination of the water bag). This latter improvement resulted for the first time in the application of body scanner techniques.

CONTRAST ENHANCEMENT

At the time of its introduction, CT scanning was heralded as a major advance in the noninvasive examination of the patient. It became obvious, however, that this con-

cept placed distinct limitations on the use of the technology. Investigators quickly became aware of the fact that much more information was available as a result of the use of intravenous and subarachnoid contrast agents for enhancement.

Intravenous contrast enhancement is imperative if the maximum information is to be realized in the examination for brain tumors and vascular lesions such as infarctions and arteriovenous malformation. Indeed this technique has permitted, on occasion, the identification of intracranial arterial aneurysms (Fig. 2).

The utilization of CT scanning with the subarachnoid injection of metrizimide, a water soluble contrast agent, permits better delineation of the subarachnoid spaces and the study of cerebrospinal fluid dynamics. This has clinical applicability in the identification of the subarachnoid blocks of hydrocephalus (Fig. 3) and the site of cerebrospinal fluid leaks which heretofore have fallen in the domain of nuclear medicine and its use of isotope cisternography.

Therefore, it is clear that CT scanning has passed from the realm of a completely safe, noninvasive, diagnostic tool of good accuracy to that of a diagnostic tool of excellent accuracy that has invasive characteristics. Thus, it must be presumed that certain risks do exist. Indeed complications such as renal failure and death have been reported.[4, 5]

ALTERNATE PLANNER RECONSTRUCTIONS

It became obvious to computer scientists early that there exists within CT technology the potential of significantly increasing the viewer's ability to further locate and identify diseased areas by providing the capability to view any angle plane desired simply by making multiple transverse scans. If these scans are performed by overlapping slicing techniques, thin slices in the order of 2-mm thickness can be produced (Fig. 4). An excellent review of this process has been written by Larsen *et al.* to which the reader is referred.[6]

The most clinically useful reconstructed planes are the coronal and sagittal planes. However, any plane parallel to the sagittal or coronal planes can be reconstructed. In addition, any plane within the angle subtended by the transverse and coronal planes, the transverse and sagittal planes, or the sagittal and coronal planes can be reconstructed (Fig. 5). The computer is asked to construct a plane by extracting absorption values from each of the transverse overlapping cuts which lie on that plane. The data values in the constructed matrix represent the x-ray absorption for each point in that matrix.

As a result of total multiplane reconstruction a regular 3-dimensional matrix of data is obtained. Each point is assigned a rotational unit (0–180) and a density unit (for example, −500–+500). A pseudo-three-dimensional view can be formed in the image plane and displayed in a 2-dimensional manner on a display screen by scanning along the line of sight for a preselected density range.[7]

The technology has practical application to the operating neurosurgeon and to the radiation therapist. The neurosurgeon can obtain a better appreciation of the contour and volume of the mass. This same information may allow the radiation therapist to more accurately calculate isodense curves thus permitting the more accurate delivery of radiation to the volume of tissue required. Although as yet unreported (to the knowledge of the author), such 3-dimensional reconstructions of the orbit should be possible.

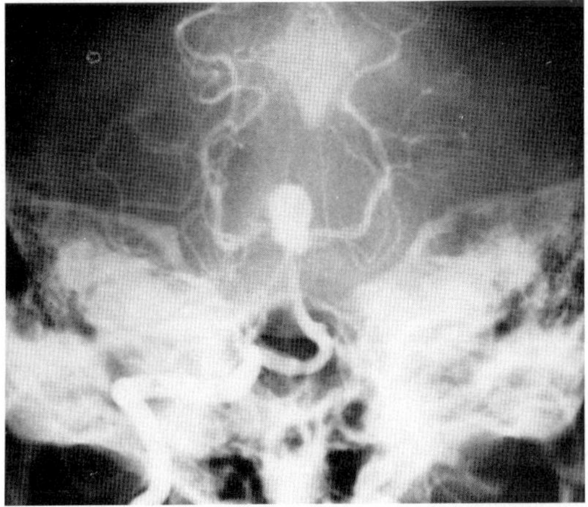

Fig. 2A. Vertebral artery angiogram revealing basilar artery aneurysm.

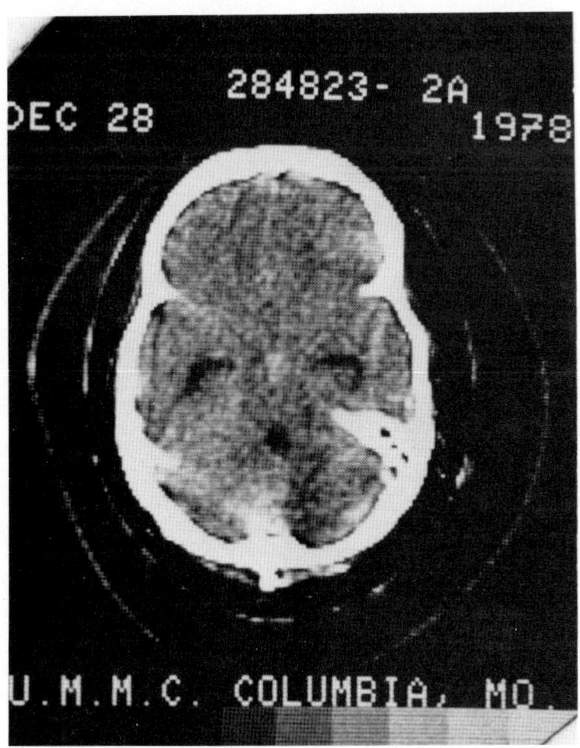

Fig. 2B. Contrast enhanced CT scan revealing basilar artery aneurysm in the center of the scan.

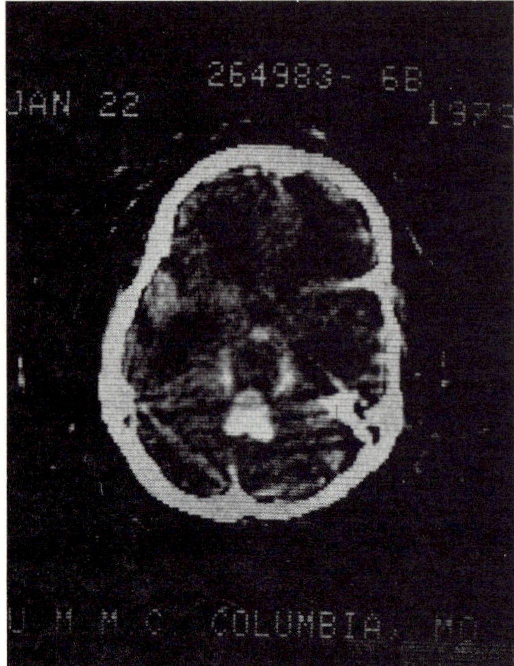

Fig. 3. Metrizimide has refluxed into the fourth and third ventricles and is outlining the cisterns surrounding the brain stem in a patient with communicating hydrocephalus secondary to basilar arachnoiditis following surgery and irradiation for a medulloblastoma.

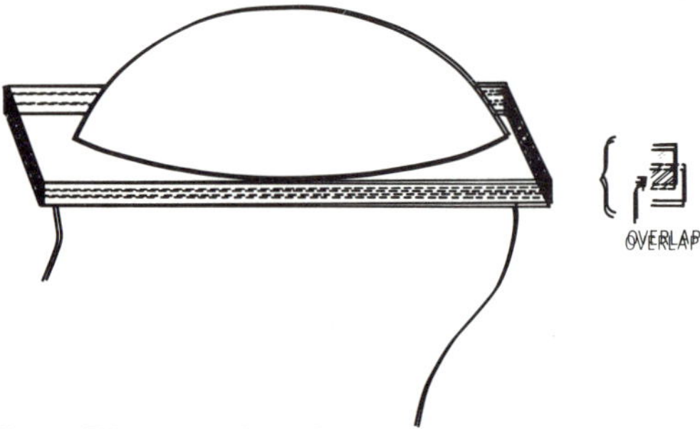

Fig. 4. The area of overlapping scan is contained between the dotted lines (see text for detail).

COMPUTER IMAGE ENHANCEMENT

Advances have been made in image enhancement by applying digital filtering techniques to reconstructed CT images in an attempt to enhance borders and clearly delineate areas of different densities. This is for the purpose of improving, by the use of the computer, feature extraction and the analysis of the extracted information. Several computer analytic systems have been investigated. The standard method has

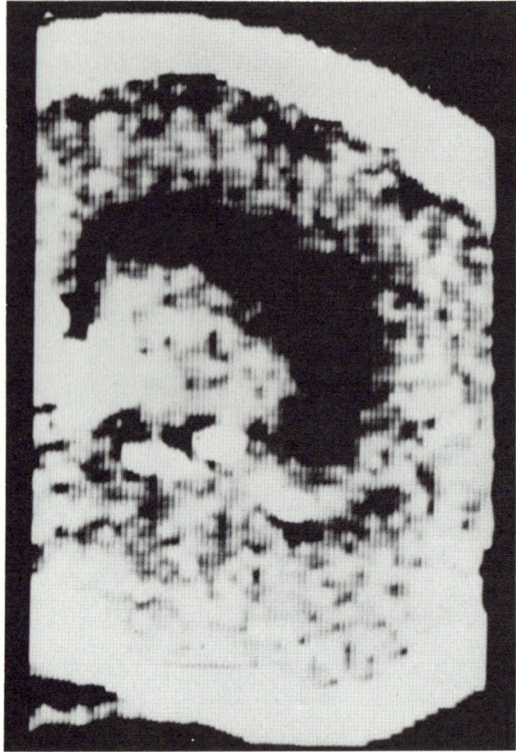

Fig. 5A. A reconstructed CT scan in the sagittal plane demonstrating the body, trigone, and temporal horn of the lateral ventricle.

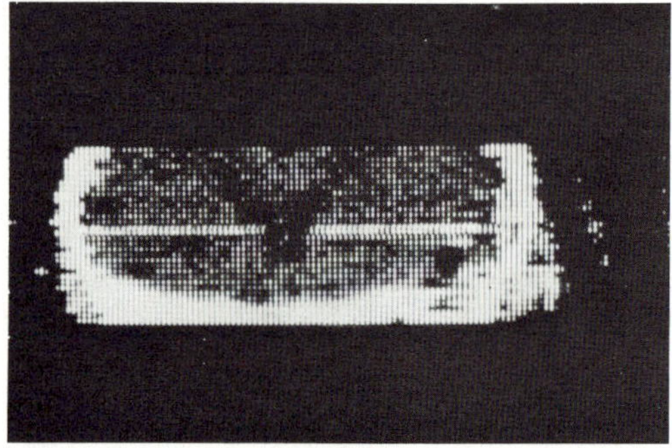

Fig. 5B. A reconstructed scan in the coronal plane showing the frontal horns of both lateral ventricles at the region of the foramen of Monroe. The horizontal white lines are demonstration artefacts.

been that of simple linear filtering (or "windowing"). This involves isolation of areas of similar density (Fig. 6). However, these techniques do not fundamentally change the nature of the transformation of information from the x-ray density value as seen in the brightness and contrast indication of a cathode ray tube. They merely define an

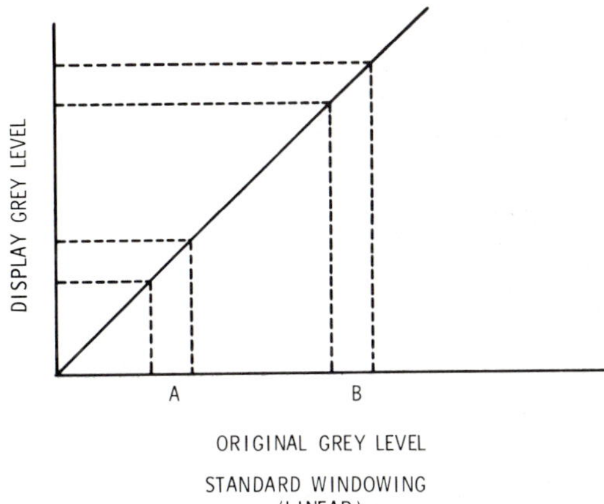

Fig. 6. By proper windowing filtration the densities within area A can be viewed separately from the densities within area B, but their relationships to each other remain the same.

information window for the observation of preselected densities (Fig. 7).

A system that holds more promise of success interactively alters the information window to provide alternative perspective. That is, it enhances the brightness of one density relative to another similar density. For example, the standard windowing examination may look at densities 5–10, which the viewer perceives as one density because the subtleties of the transition from one grey level to the next are not recognized by the individual. However, if the densities 5–7 are combined as one and 8–10 are combined as another and displayed, the viewer may then be able to view the transition as two separate densities. This technique is called nonlinear grey level "windowing" (or mapping).

The isodense subdural hematoma (subacute) is a clinical problem to which this technology has been applied.[8] The acute subdural hematoma is readily visable on the CT scan largely due to the concentration of hemoglobin and calcium as clotting occurs (Fig. 8A). As the hematoma ages the attenuation coefficients gradually fall such that the chronic hematoma appears hypodense with lower attentuation coefficients than brain (Fig. 8B). It is during the time when the attenuation coefficients of the aging subdural hematoma is similar to those of brain (14–24 units), when it is termed isodense, that diagnostic accuracy with computerized axial tomography falls

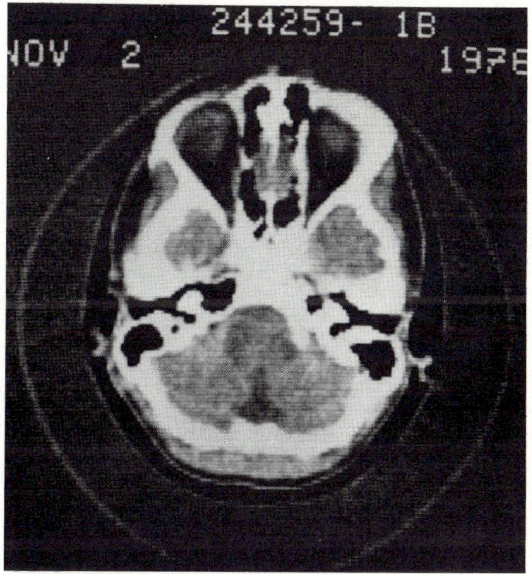

Fig. 7A. Normal CT scan display.

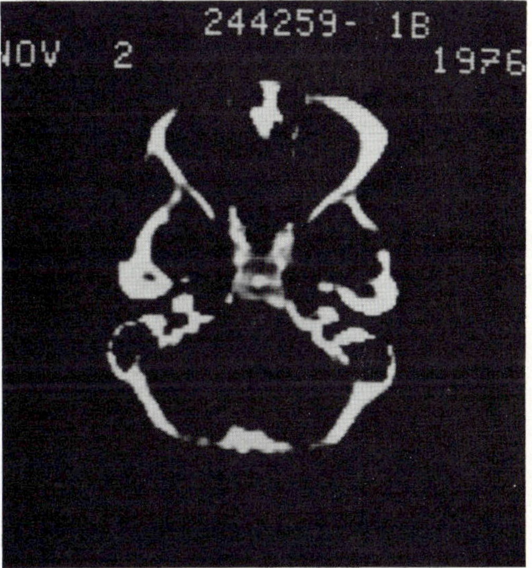

Fig. 7B. A selected set of grey levels are examined and displayed corresponding to area B in Figure 6.

(Fig. 8C). The problem is to separate the attenuation coefficients (densities, or grey levels) of the hematoma from those of the adjacent brain and enhance their perspective.

Two techniques are employed. In one, adjacent small groups of densities are compressed to form single density patterns which, when viewed collectively, are recognized by the computer as separate individual densities and are displayed with a clarity recognizable to the human eye (Fig.

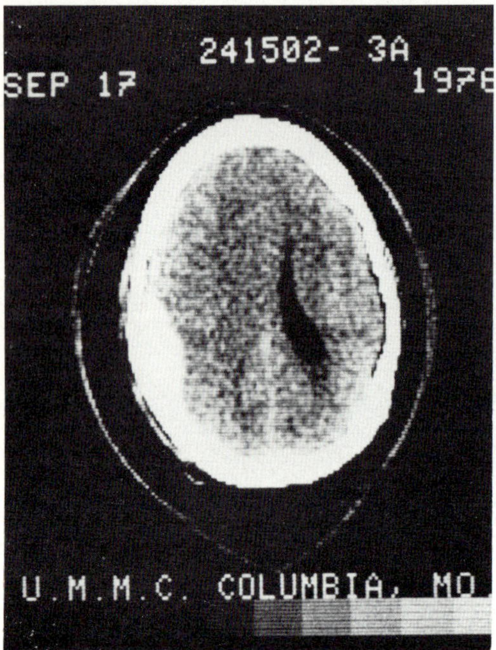

Fig. 8A. Acute subdural hematoma.

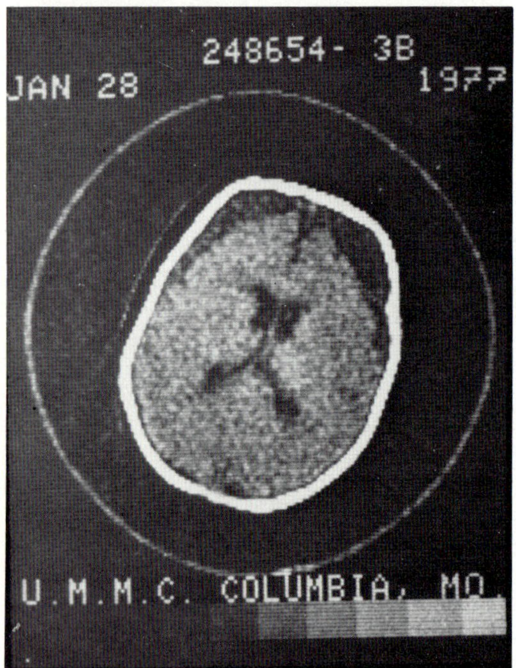

Fig. 8B. Bilateral chronic subdural hematoma.

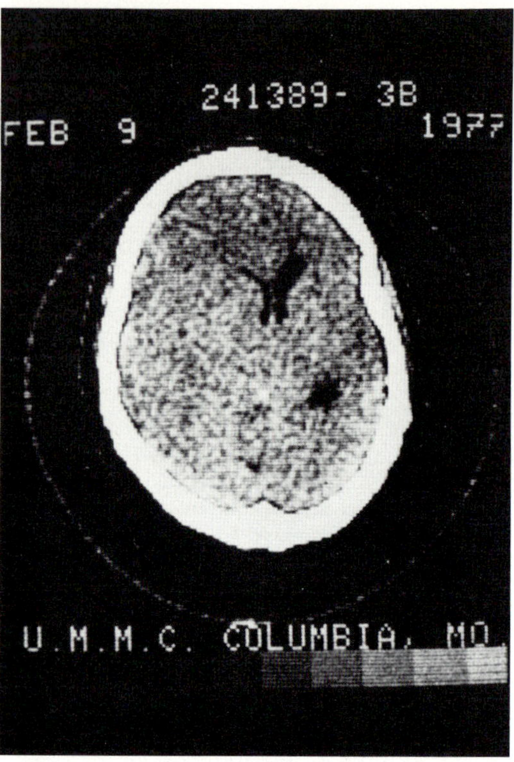

Fig. 8C. Left-sided isodense subdural hematoma perceived indirectly by ventricular shift.

from those at the upper end of the scale by a greater magnitude to enhance their visualization by the viewer (Fig. 10). An example of the visualization of an isodense subdural hematoma by these techniques is seen in Figure 11.

Similar attention to the concept of improved feature extraction and visualization by computer manipulation of CT data is seen in the attempts to predict tumor histology on the basis of density identification. This investigation has taken several tacks. One is the quite simple modality of analyzing the results of intravenous contrast enhanced CT scans and comparing these data with the histopathology of the tumors. In looking at malignant astrocytomas it has been shown that the histopathologic findings of vascularity and necrosis showed the best correlation with contrast enhancement in supratentorial astrocytomas whereas vascularity and cellularity correlated significantly with the scan in cerebellar astrocytomas.[9] It was concluded that the degree of malignancy of supratentorial astrocytomas

9). The second technique is to enhance the difference between individual density units and stretch these differences out separating the densities at the lower end of the scale

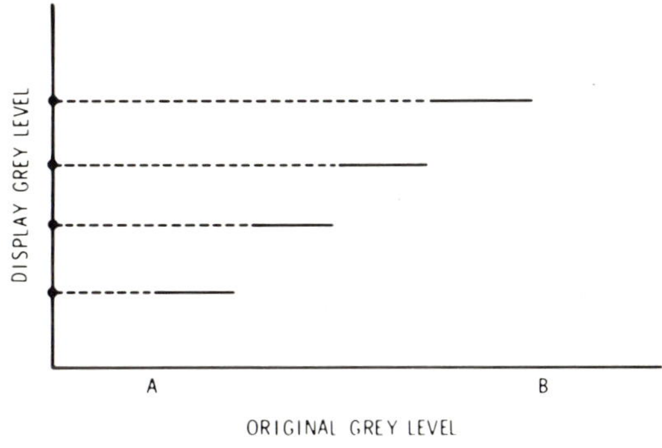

Fig. 9. The grey levels between A and B are selectively divided, compressed and then displayed as separate images.

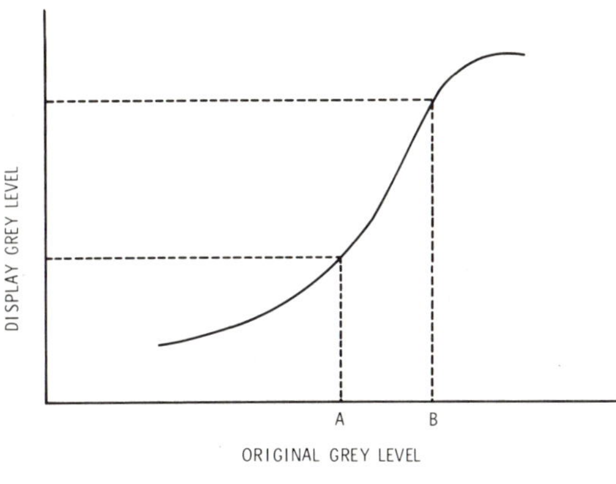

Fig. 10. Original grey levels between A and B are stretched and displayed in a less compact relationship.

could be infered from the contrast enhanced CT scan; however, this was not possible with astrocytomas located in the posterior fossa.

In a more complex study several parameters were analyzed to determine the reliability of computer tomography for the diagnosis and differential diagnosis of meningiomas, gliomas, and brain metastases, namely: absorption in the plain scan, intravenous contrast enhancement, the border lines of the tumor, expansion as evaluated from the deviation of the ventricles and cisterns, peritumoral areas of decreased absorption, interrupted edema, and the presence of calcification. The investigators found that using their algorithm they were

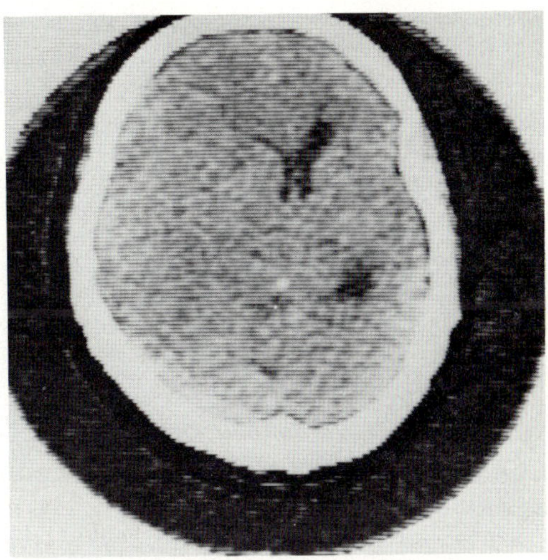

Fig. 11A. Isodense hematoma (see Fig. 8C).

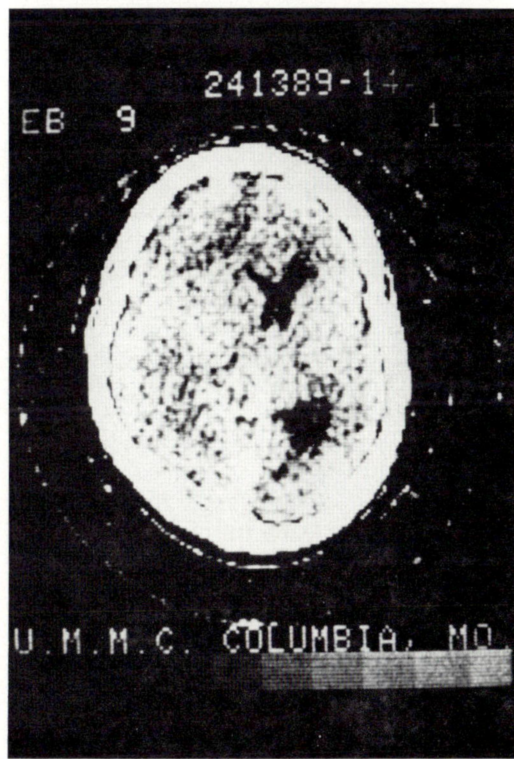

Fig. 11B. Membrane of isodense subdural in left frontal temporal area identified by intravenous contrast enhancement.

extremely successful in predicting from the CT scan the ultimate histopathology of the tumor.[10]

The studies referred to above indicate imaginative attempts to analyze standard

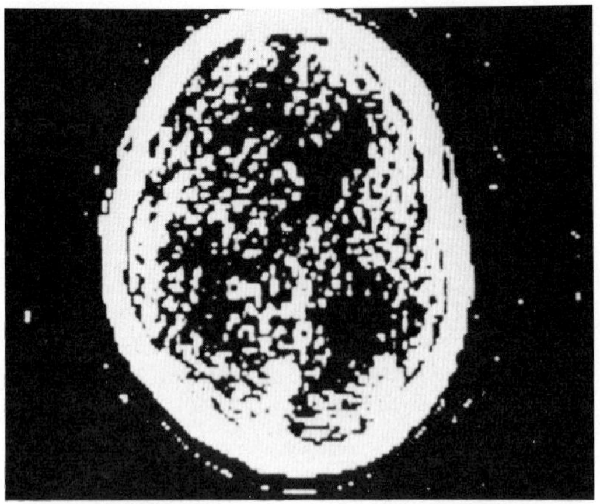

Fig. 11C. Left fronto-temporal isodense subdural hematoma demonstrated by nonlinear windowing enhancement without intravenous contrast enhancement.

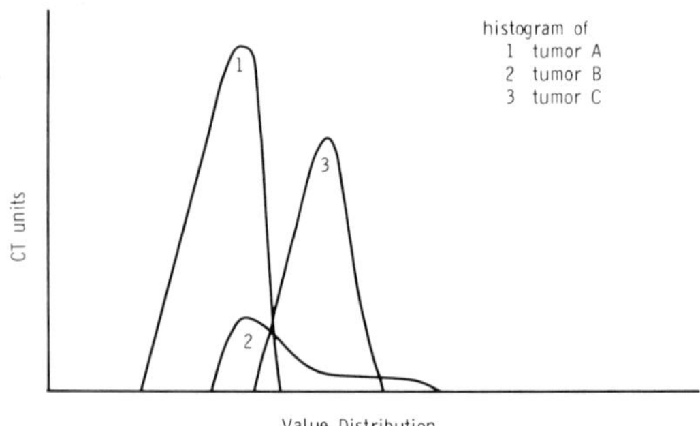

Fig. 12. Theoretical histograms of three tumor types (derived from data reported by Naidich, *et al.*[11])

CT data more critically for the purpose of improving preoperative diagnostic acumen without the use of interactive computer manipulation of the data. Such manipulation has been successful, however, in the evaluation of sellar and parasellar masses.[11] After the routine CT scan has been obtained, an area of interest is identified. The digital data of the CT scan, which are stored on tapes or disks, are further analyzed. To avoid the partial volume phenomenon, only the central region of the lesion is evaluated. The location of the central zone is fed into the unit computer and a frequency profile, or histogram, of the absorptive values contained within the central zone is obtained. This results in a bar graph of the actual number of times each individual value appears within the lesion. A curve is then generated by connecting the tops of the bars to reflect the relative frequency or distribution of the absorption values within the lesion by constructing similar histograms of the lesion with data obtained from both pre- and post-intravenous contrast scans. A profile is generated which suggests the histologic nature of the lesion (Fig. 12). It was shown that the evaluation of small regions of interest were more successful in differentiating pathology than the evaluation of an entire hemisphere. This technique emphasizes that in the evaluation of the density and homogeneity of a lesion it is the analysis of the digital data generated by the unit computer algorithm and not the observation of the "shades of grey" on the polaroid image which yields the greatest information.

BODY SCANNING

Following the introduction of computerized tomography of the head, it was soon obvious that this might be a tool for examination of the rest of the body. Significant advances were not made, however, until the elimination of the water cap and the improvement in detection analysis, resulting in more rapid scanning. Thus, the artifacts caused by breathing and cardiac action were minimized. The state of the art is such that the accuracy of CT is equal to that of nuclear medicine and ultrasound in the diagnosis of hepatic, pancreatic, and renal diseases, especially tumors.[12] Optimism exists for its value in thoracic and extremity disorders.[13]

From the standpoint of the clinical neuroscientist some of the most exciting advances in the application of CT technology to the body have been in the realm of vertebral spine scanning.[14] This is especially true in the lumbar spine where body defects are readily demonstrated with diagnostic clarity (Fig. 13).[15] Although current technology does not permit the satisfactory delineation of soft tissue disease within the canal, such as noncalcified tumors and syringomyelia, present recent advances suggest that breakthroughs will soon be forthcoming. The combination of newer instrumentation resulting in faster and more detailed discrimination coupled with such techniques as nonlinear window-

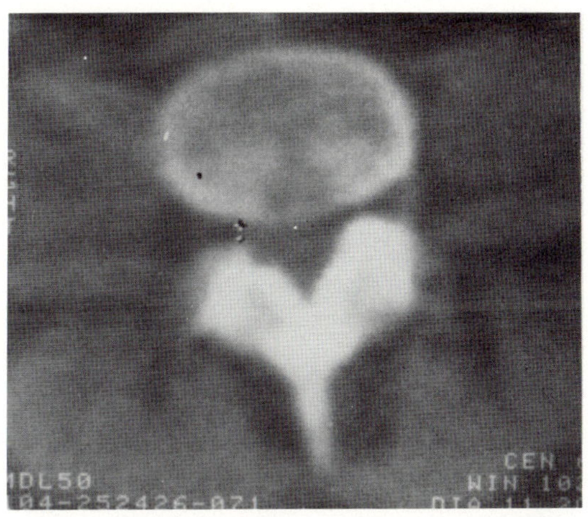

Fig. 13. Transverse body scan of lumbar spine revealing narrowed intervertebral foramen by spondylosis and facet joint hypertrophy.

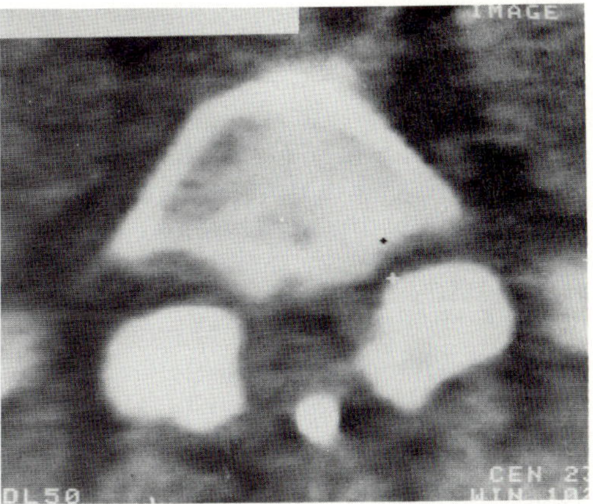

Fig. 14. Ventral boney and soft tissue densities seen in a transverse body scan of a lumbar vertebra in a patient with ventral spondylosis and soft disc herniation.

ing mapping for image enhancement (see above) speak to this possibility.

Indeed the extruded disc fragment in the lumbar spine is serving as a model for this investigation (Fig. 14). The utilization of the more refined feature extraction techniques suggests that eventually soft tissue densities can be separated to the extent that individual nerve roots and disc fragments can be identified. One does not have to look far to see that this technology could result in the termination of the need for myelography as a routine tool in the evaluation of a patient for intraspinal pathology.

The evaluation of the patient with spine trauma lends itself as an ideal use for scanning of the vertebral spine. It results in much less manipulation of the patient, and coupled with alternate planer reproduction (see above), offers the attending physician the possibility of a much clearer picture of the site of trauma.

FUTURE TECHNOLOGY

It would seem somewhat presumptuous to attempt to predict the future developments of a technology that is as complex and changing as rapidly as that of computerized tomography. That which is considered to be in the future at the time this paragraph is being written may very well be a standard of the present at the time that it is read, so rapid are the changes. It appears the future is limited only by the imagination of the investigators and the sophistication of the science of computer processing.

Nevertheless, there are developments worth commenting on at this time. Because the CT scan can so accurately localize and depict lesions within the intact body and because the computer technique of alternate planer reproduction is with us, it would seem that the procedure of computerized tomographic-assisted biopsy is feasible. In fact, initial reports are very encouraging not only with the body scanner[16] but also with the use of the head scanner for intracranial biopsies.[17]

Even computer tomographic-assisted stereotactic surgery is almost here as a standard procedure.[18] This makes use of standard computerized tomographic data from which extraneous data have been eliminated by further computer processing. Thus 3-dimensional information is obtained giving precise location of the target. Phantom testing of the technique has shown accuracy to be better than 0.5 cm.

EDITOR'S NOTE

Dr. Watts has given a nice historical review of the development of computed axial tomography from inception with the first EMI machine to the more recent and sophisticated pieces of equipment now available. There is one innovation, however, that will constantly require more and more emphasis—no matter what type of machine is developed. The innovation I want to emphasize is that it is absolutely essential that the *machine* be *aimed by* the patient's *history*! If one has a meticulous study of the orbits and orbital optic nerves on both sides, yet has had no optic canal polytomography, quite a few cases of intracanalicular optic nerve sheath meningiomas are going to be missed. Worse than that is to get an ordinary CT scan study of a patient presenting with downbeat nystagmus and not recalling that the foramen magnum level is a very difficult area to assess with CT scan and that the best study in that patient would be a pneumoencephalogram with PA and lateral tomography with emphasis on posterior fossa and cervicomedullary junction region. The metrizamide CT scan may also be helpful in such cases. Dr. Hoyt and I agree that the problem today with the CT scan—and it has been truly a TERRIFIC advance—is *not* with the *positive* scan. The problem in the office practice of neuro-ophthalmology today is the patient who had already had three CT scans which are called *negative*—and the patient has a classic history of migraine, or shows typical fundi of Leber's optic nerve disease, or has euthyroid eye disease, or something that should have been knocked out of the ball park by a good history in the first place. There is no way that a meticulous CT scan can make the diagnosis of convergence insufficiency in the graduate student complaining of headaches when he reads. Again, the importance of a careful history and complete physical examination FIRST of all is emphasized, or the CT scan will reveal only that the patient has had a *"wallet-ectomy"* with nothing else of real value.

JLS

REFERENCES

1. Hounsfield, G. N. Computerized transverse axial scanning (tomography): I. Description of system. Br. J. Radiol. *46:*1023–1047 (1973).
2. Marshall, C. H.: Principles of computed tomography. Postgrad. Med. *60:*105–109 (1976).
3. Brooks, R. A. and Di Chiro, G. Theory of image reconstruction in computed tomography. Radiology *117:*561–572 (1975).
4. Hanaway, J. and Black, J. Renal failure following contrast injection for computerized tomography. J. Am. Med. Assoc. *238:*2056 (1977).
5. Warren, S. E., Bott, J. C., Thornfeldt, C., Thornfeldt, C., Swerdlin, A.-H., and Steinberg, S. M. Hazards of computerized tomography: renal failure following contrast injection. Surg. Neurol. *10:*335–336 (1978).
6. Larsen, G. N., Glenn, W., Kishore, P. R. S., Davis, K., McFarland, W. and Dwyer, S. J.: Computer processing of CT images: advances and prospects. Neurosurgery *1:*73–79 (1977).
7. Glenn, W. V., Jr., Johnston, R. J., Morton, P. E., and Dwyer, S. J. Image generation and display techniques for CT scan data. Thin transverse and reconstructed coronal and saggital planes. Invest. Radiol. *10:*479–489 (1975).
8. Watts, C., Larsen, G., and Tully, R. Image enhancement of isodense subdural hematomas with computed tomography. Presented at the Annual Meeting of the American Association of Neurological Surgeons, New Orleans La., 1978.
9. Butler, A. R., Horii, S. C., Kircheff, I. I., Shannon, M. B., and Budzilovich, G. N. Computed tomography in astrocytomas. Radiology *129:*423–439 (1978).
10. Amundsen, P., Dugstad, G., and Syvertsen, A. H. The reliability of computer tomography for the diagnosis and differential diagnosis of meningiomas, gliomas, and brain metastases. Acta Neurochirugia *41:*177–190 (1978).
11. Naidich, T. P., Pinto, R. S., Kishner, M. J., Lin, J. P., Kircheff, I. I., Leeds, N. E., and Chase, N. E. Evaluation of sellar and parasellar masses by computed tomography. Radiology *120:*91–99 (1976).
12. Alfidi, R. J. and Haager, J. R. Computed tomography of the body. Postgrad. Med. *60:*133–136 (1976).
13. Schellinger, D. Computerized body tomography with the ACTA scanner. J. Am. Med. Assoc. *234:*314–317 (1975).
14. Hammerschlag, S. B., Wolpert, S. M., and Carter, B. L. Computer tomography of the spinal canal. Radiology *121:*361–367 (1976).
15. Resjo, I. M., Harwood-Nash, D. C., Fitz, C. R., and Chuang, S. J. Comput. Assist. Tomog. *2:*549–558 (1978).
16. Haaga, J. R. and Alfidi, R. J. Precise biopsy localization by computed tomography. Radiology *118:*603–607 (1976).
17. Maroon, J. C., Bank, W. O., Drayer, B. P., and Rosenbaum, A. E. Intracranial biopsy assisted by computerized tomography. J. Neurosurg. *46:*740–744 (1977).
18. Penn, R. D., Whisler, W. W., Smith, C. A., and Yasnoff, W. A. Stereotactic surgery with image processing of computerized tomographic scans. Neurosurgery *3:*157–163 (1978).

31 Pitfalls in CT Scanning in Patients with Head Injuries

Edward Tarlov, M.D.,
Kenneth R. Davis, M.D.

Computerized tomography is the most important advance in head injury diagnosis and management since recognition of the importance of the unilaterally dilated pupil. This valuable method has greatly improved accuracy of diagnosis and effectiveness of head injury management. Although the diagnosis of intracranial hematoma or mass effect is obvious in the majority of cases, our five years experience with CT scanning of head injured patients shows that common sense, care in the execution and interpretation of the scan, and close clinical correlation are necessary to avoid serious errors in diagnosis.

This chapter outlines, with clinical examples, fourteen areas in which difficulty in arriving at the correct diagnosis has arisen (Table I).

I. ISODENSITY OF HEMATOMAS

The subacute to chronic intracranial hematoma whose absorption is close to that of normal cerebral tissue may present problems in CT diagnosis.

The photon absorption of intracranial hematomas initially increases slightly. Whole blood with a hematocrit of 45% has a density of about 28 EMI units. With clot retraction serum is extruded bringing the absorption of a one- to two-day-old clot into the range of 30–40 units, well above the 16–18 EMI unit absorption of cerebral tissue. With progressive breakdown of red cells and removal of the protein fraction of hemoglobin by phagocytic activity the absorption of the hematoma progressively diminishes beginning at its periphery. By one to four weeks, depending on its size, the hematoma's absorption continues to decrease but during the phase when the hematoma is isodense, careful analysis of scan and clinical data may be necessary for detection. There is thus a period in the natural history of a hematoma when its photon absorption is the same as normal brain. At this time, when the hematoma is isodense with brain, otherwise unexplained mass effect or ventricular distortion can be the only clue to the presence of a subacute chronic subdural hematoma. If the hematoma is bilateral, no midline shift may be apparent and the diagnosis may be even more difficult. Although contrast enhancement of subdural membranes, facilitating diagnosis, has been seen occasionally, contrast enhancement has not, in our experience, been sufficiently helpful to warrant its routine use in the evaluation of head injuries. Contrast enhancement may, however, be useful in selected cases when chronic subdural hematoma is a consideration.

Case 1. A 76-year-old man on anticoagulants because of previous pulmonary embolism became confused and lethargic following a fall four weeks previously. When initially seen in the emergency room, there were no localizing neurological findings, and he was sent home after CT scanning was felt to have failed to reveal any significant pathology. When he returned to the hospital on the following day, more confused, the possibility of subdural hematoma was considered on clinical grounds. CT scanning was repeated at this stage (Fig. 1). His ventricles appeared compressed. Large bilateral subdural hematomas were removed on the evening of admission to the hospital.

In numerous other cases the only obvious

clue on CT scan was the presence of an otherwise unexplained ventricular shift.

Case 2. A 62-year-old man, severely incapacitated by pain in the left arm due to metastatic carcinoma, developed a left hemiparesis and confusion. A clinical suspicion was metastatic cerebral involvement. CT scanning demonstrated no absorption abnormality. A slight right to left midline shift was present. At autopsy large bilateral subdural hematomas, larger on the right side, were visualized.

TABLE I. *Pitfalls in CT scanning in head injury*

1. Isodense intracranial hematoma	6. Intracranial gas
2. Movement artifact	7. Ring sign
3. Posterior fossa extraaxial hematoma	8. Low middle fossa lesion
4. Foreign bodies Intracranial pressure equipment Bullets Metallic cranial plates	9. Intraventricular hemorrhage 10. Side reversal 11. Vermian artifact 12. Plane problem 13. Shape of margins of hematoma
5. Chronic subdural hematoma vs. atrophy	14. Size of high lesion

II. MOVEMENT ARTIFACT

The scanning artifact created by movement of the patient during scanning can cause both false negative and false positive results. With the newer, faster scanners this problem diminishes, but, particularly with the earlier scanning equipment, immobilizing the patient with anesthesia has sometimes been necessary in order to obtain satisfactory scans. Although a suboptimal scan which excludes the presence of a very large acute intracranial hematoma may help in management, it is worthwhile to consider sedation, or anesthesia if necessary, to obtain satisfactory scans in restless patients.

III. DIFFERENTIATION OF LONG-STANDING EXTRACEREBRAL HEMATOMA FROM CEREBRAL ATROPHY

As chronic subdural hematomas liquefy, their CT absorption values drop below that of brain tissue. This may take several weeks, depending on the size of the hema-

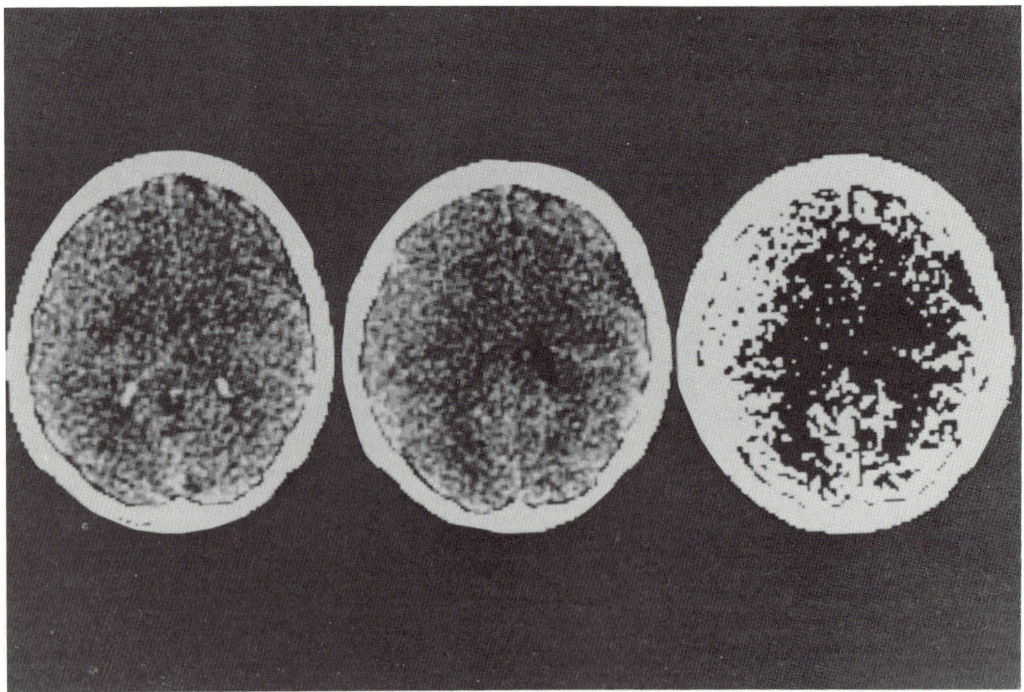

Fig. 1. Large bilateral isodense chronic subdural hematomas (Case 1). Failure to visualize the ventricular system, which is compressed, is a clue to the diagnosis in a patient of 76 years in whom the ventricles would be expected to be somewhat dilated.

toma. At very late stages when the absorption approaches that of CSF, radiological differentiation from cerebral atrophy depends mainly on the presence or absence of sulcal and ventricular enlargement signifying atrophy, or mass effect, suggesting intracerebral hematoma (Fig. 3). Only occasionally does intravenous contrast material enter the subdural collection on delayed scans, or does the use of intrathecal metrizamide CT scanning clearly differentiate the compartments.

Case 3. A 76-year-old man, confused after head injury six weeks earlier, was felt on CT scan to have evidence of bilateral subdural hematoma. At operation only atrophic changes were found (see Fig. 3).

IV. LOW-LYING TEMPORAL OR INFRA-TEMPORAL HEMATOMA

In the horizontal plane of CT scanning the significance of low-lying lesions in the middle fossa may not be readily apparent, particularly if their density approaches that of adjacent cerebrum. A partial volume effect when the lesion is near bone may contribute to the difficulty in diagnosis. Visualization of the scan data in the coronal plane can diminish the difficulty of recognizing low-lying middle fossa lesions. In the coronal plane, the section is at right angles to the lesion and the smaller dimension of the volume element in this plane provides spatial resolution and eliminates partial volume averaging.

Case 4. This 66-year-old lady had had very severe headache, confusion, and the evolution of a left hemiparesis on the day prior to CT scanning. Cerebral angiography was felt to be normal. A low-density change in the right posterior temporal region was felt to be present, thought to represent cerebral contusion. Her level of consciousness waxed and waned. The scan was repeated six days later when consciousness worsened and again 12 days later. No new significant abnormality was recognized (Figs. 4 and 5).

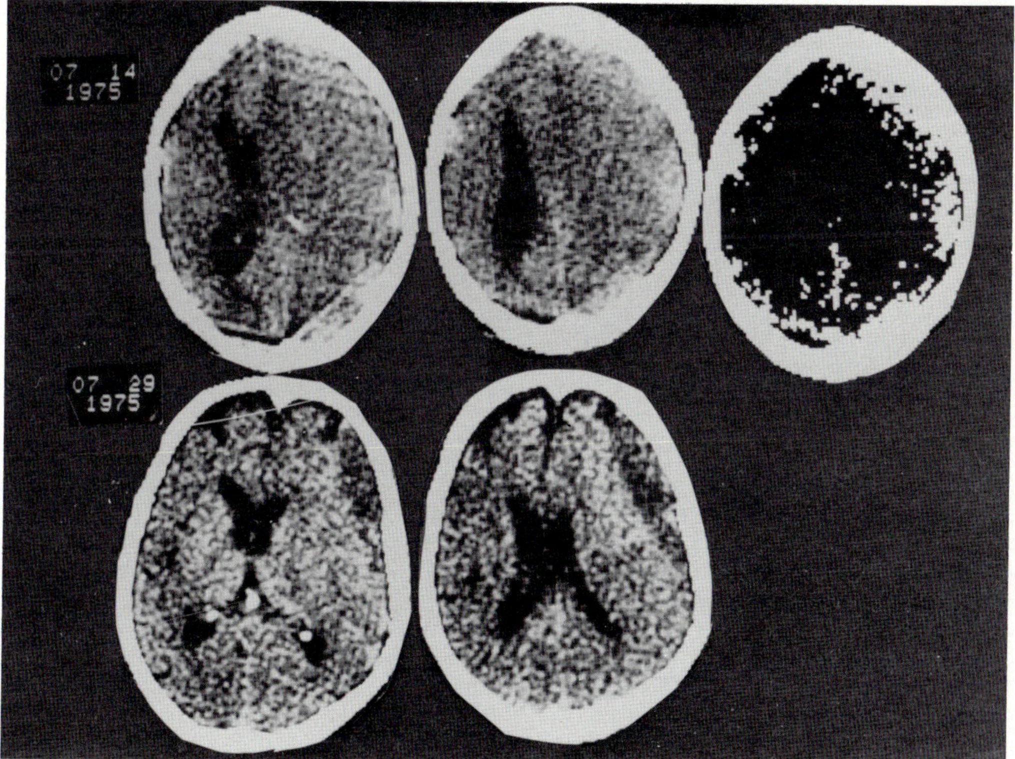

Fig. 2. Large right subdural hematoma. Initial scan (upper row) shows massive ventricular shift due to isodense hematoma. Fifteen days later postoperative scan shows decreased attenuation of residual hematoma, now less dense than brain tissue.

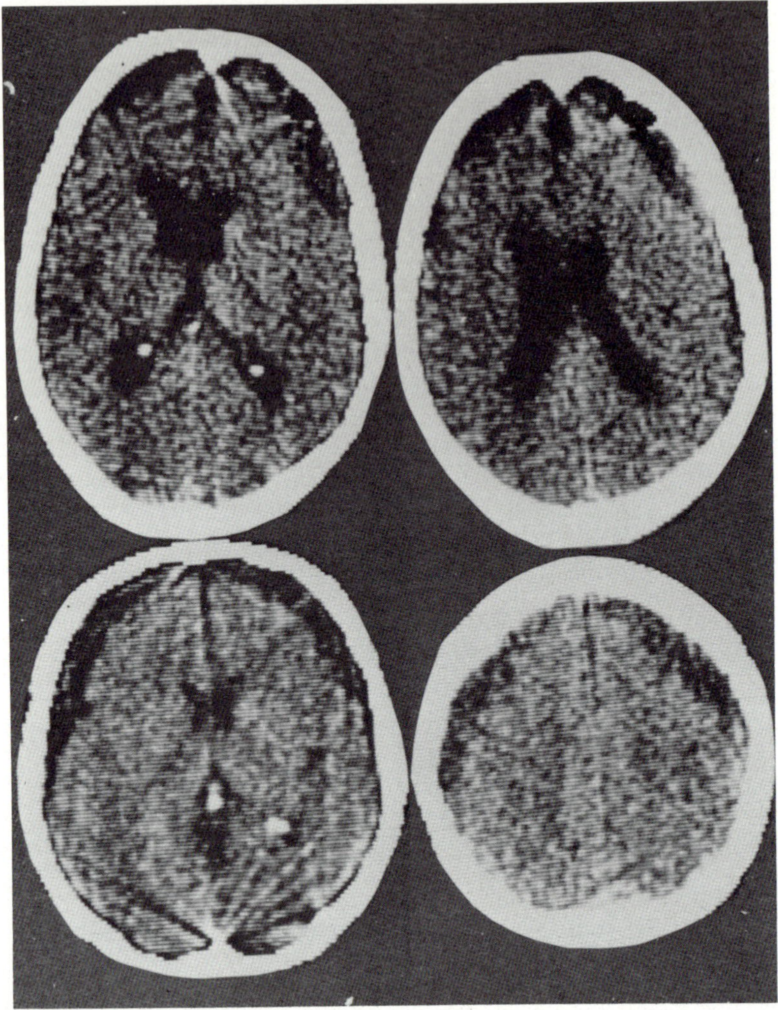

Fig. 3. Typical examples of atrophy and chronic subdural hematoma. In the upper pair of images, enlargement of the sulcal pattern and ventricles is seen. In the lower tier of images, the sulcal pattern is not significantly enlarged and the ventricles are somewhat compressed. In intermediate forms between these two typical examples, the differentiation can rest on clinical grounds.

Angiography, however, with special views (Fig. 6) showed the presence of an inferior temporal or infratemporal mass which at operation proved to be a very large subpial hematoma on the inferior temporal surface, removal of which effected a very good recovery.

V. POSTERIOR FOSSA EXTRAAXIAL MASSES

Although posterior fossa hematomas are usually easily apparent on CT scanning, we have seen several patients in whom the presence of a large postoperative epidural hematoma found at operation was not recognized on CT scanning. Both these instances occurred under emergency circumstances. The postoperative changes in this region complicated interpretation.

Case 5. A 23-year-old man was making smooth recovery two days following posterior fossa craniotomy for suspected tumor. Over a six-hour period he became obtunded at first, then his pupils became fixed, and respiratory arrest occurred. His physicians carried out a CT scan (Fig. 7) and because no posterior fossa clot was recognized, con-

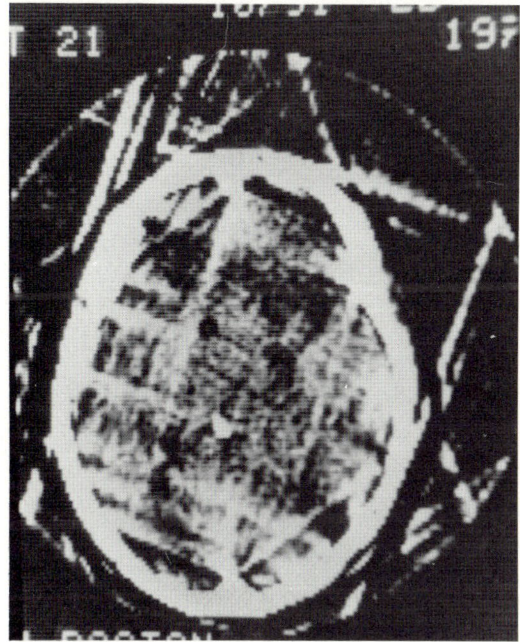

Fig. 4. Initial CT scan (Case 4). Movement artifact. Question of right posterior temporal contusion was raised.

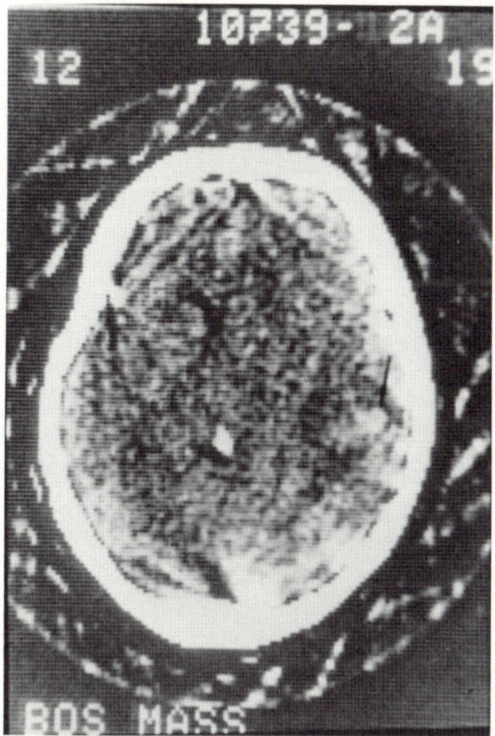

Fig. 5. Subsequent CT scan (Case 4) six days after scan in Figure 4. Evidence of right-sided mass effect. Difficult to appreciate on this scan is the large size of lesion or the fact that it lies on the inferior temporal surface of the brain as shown on the angiogram (Fig. 6).

sidered shunting his somewhat enlarged ventricles. After reconsideration the wound was reopened and a large epidural hematoma removed. He made a good recovery.

VI. NONSPECIFICITY OF THE "RING SIGN"

A rim of dense tissue or tissue enhancing with contrast surrounding an intracerebral lesion may give an appearance midleadingly suggestive of abcess formation or tissue cavitation. Peripheral contrast enhancement is a nonspecific change which can surround regions of infarction, contusion, neoplasm, inflammation, or even giant aneurysm.

Case 6. A drug addict, struck over the head by a shovel, had suffered a depressed skull fracture with dural laceration. He was aphasic early in the course of his recovery. A CT scan (Fig. 8) several days after his fractures had been elevated, with his history of self-injections with narcotics and the potentially contaminated nature of his wound, was felt suggestive of abscess. Its clinical course and resolution, however, indicated it to be an area of contusion.

Case 7. This young carpenter accidentally suffered a penetrating injury from a broken drill bit involving the deeper parts of the left frontal lobe. The evolution beginning in a hematoma of an area of ring enhancement is demonstrated in Figure 9. Again, although abscess was considered, the clinical course rather indicated this to be an nonspecific change surrounding an area of injury.

VII. PNEUMOCEPHALUS

Intracranial gas-tissue interfaces may obscure detail, but the availability of improved scanners is decreasing this problem.

Case 8. A young man developed recurrent meningitis following surgery on the frontal sinuses. Pneumocephalus was present. Gas-tissue artifact obscured visualization of the base of the frontal lobes (Fig. 10). Subsequent to repair of cerebrospinal

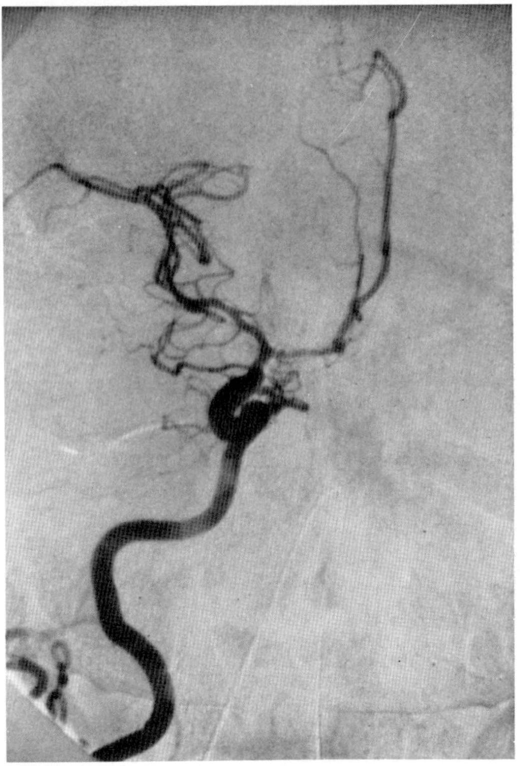

Fig. 6. Right carotid angiogram (Case 4) the same day as the CT scan in Figure 5. Large inferior temporal or subtemporal mass effect with upward displacement of middle cerebral group. The lesion proved to be a very large subpial hematoma.

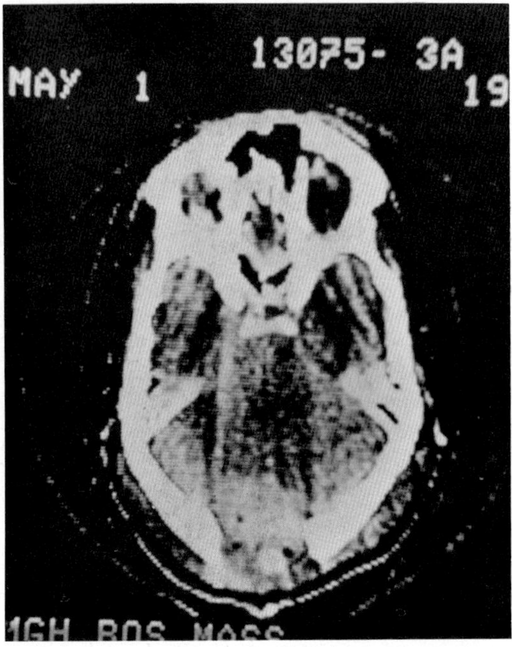

Fig. 7. CT scan (Case 5). A large postoperative epidural hematoma in posterior fossa was evacuated.

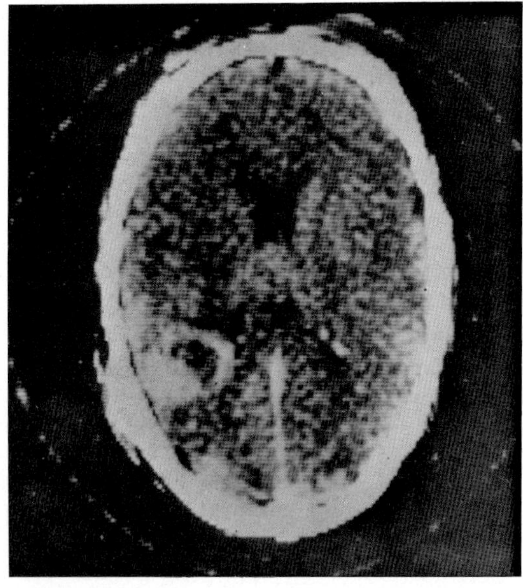

Fig. 8. CT scan (Case 6) showing "ring sign" here due to left posterior temporal contusion. This was not a brain abscess.

fluid fistula when the gas had absorbed, an area of abnormality where an otological curet had probably entered the frontal lobe was apparent, previously obscured by gas (Fig. 11).

VIII. ARTIFACTS DUE TO METALLIC OBJECTS

Metallic cranial plates, bullets, intracranial pressure monitoring equipment, and other foreign objects can obscure intracranial detail. Scanner improvements have also diminished this problem.

Case 9. A young woman had extensive frontal contusions on initial CT scan at admission. An intracranial pressure measurement device was placed. A CT scan 11 days later showed extensive metallic artifact. Four days later when the device had been removed, the presence of a subdural hematoma could be recognized (Figs. 12 and 13).

IX. CONFIGURATION OF EXTRACEREBRAL HEMATOMA

The shape of the margins of an extracerebral hematoma are not always clearly diagnostic of its location. Although the ma-

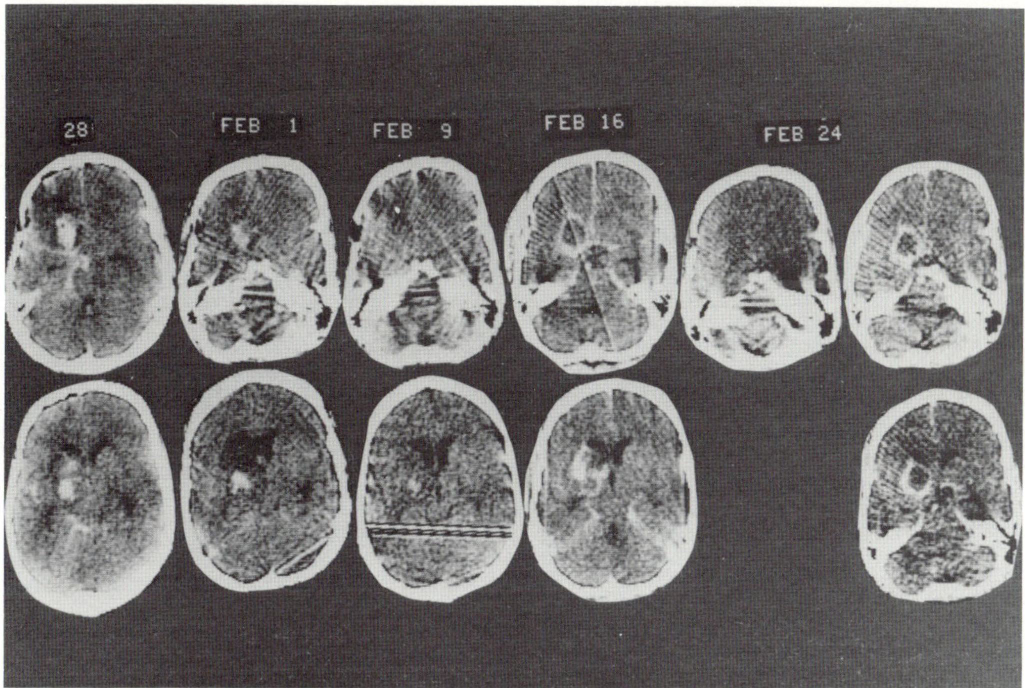

Fig. 9. Evolution of "ring sign" following penetrating injury left deep frontal region (Case 7). Over the January 28 to February 16 period, a ring-like rim of increased attenuation around contusion has developed. No clinical evidence of abscess formation.

jority of subdural hematomas had a concave appearance, these not infrequently had convex margins, the appearance more usual with epidural hematoma. Although the CT differentiation may not necessarily be of major therapeutic significance, the configuration of extracerebral collections does not always permit accurate prediction of sub- or extradural location.

X. INTRAVENTRICULAR HEMORRHAGE NOT NECESSARILY A POOR PROGNOSTIC SIGN

Although intraventricular hemorrhage has been considered a very poor prognostic sign, the routine use of CT scanning has shown that intraventricular hemorrhage may be present acutely in patients with minimal neurological deficits following head injury. Cases such as the following one indicate that hemorrhage into the ventricular system may be an epiphenomenon in head injury, not necessarily of any significance, and may occur more frequently than was recognizable prior to CT scanning. It might be an error to give a poor prognosis on the basis of this finding alone, as in the following case.

Case 10. A 23-year-old man suffered a cerebral concussion while intoxicated. At the time of his CT scan (Fig. 14) he was only slightly lethargic. Although intraventricular hematoma in his lateral third and fourth ventricles was present four days after trauma, the hematoma had absorbed. Lumbar puncture demonstrated bloody fluid with only slightly elevated pressure. In follow-up outpatient visits no intellectual impairment has been obvious. It is clear that intraventricular blood disappears more rapidly than blood in the cerebral parenchyma, subdural or epidural space.

XI. PLANE PROBLEM

In occasional instances a bone flap has been malpositioned because of error in interpreting the precise location of a traumatic lesion from the usual plane on CT scanning. Several methods for localizing the lesion are available. One of these is to measure from the lesion to the top of a Polaroid picture of the scan. The measurement can

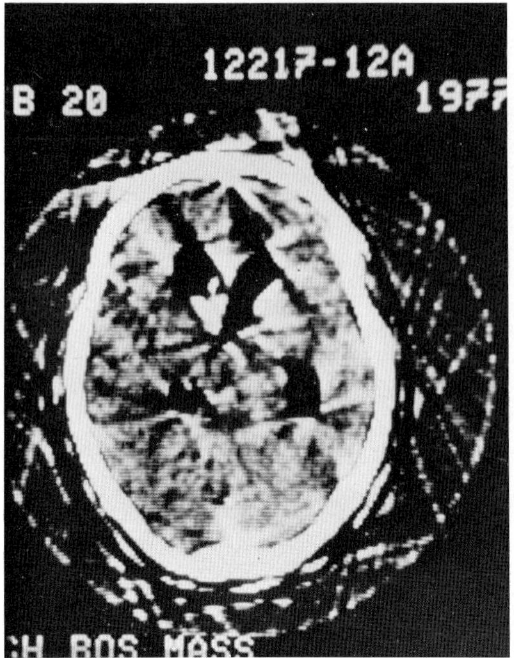

Fig. 10. Gas-tissue interface artifact (Case 8), obscuring detail.

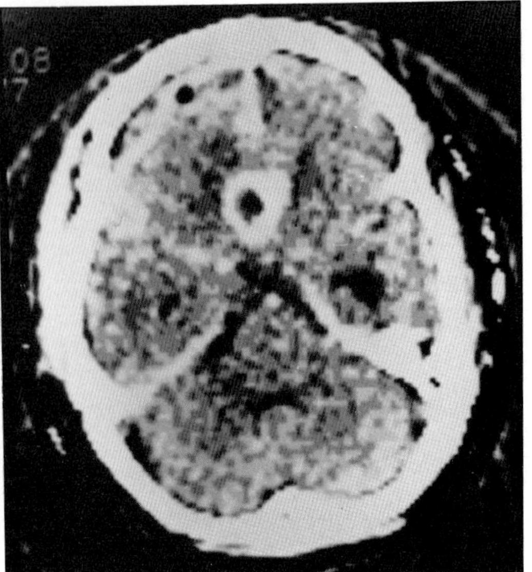

Fig. 11. Ring sign, site of inferior frontal contusion (Case 8). This region obscured by gas-tissue interface artifact on previous scan.

then be superimposed on a lower slice containing a landmark such as the ventricular trigone or petrous apex. This method gives the location of the lesion in relation to a landmark.

XII. THE HIGH CONVEXITY LESION—MISLEADING SIZE

Because of the partial volume effect with overlying bone, high convexity extraaxial hematomas may be considerably larger than might be suspected from the CT scan.

XIII. REVERSAL OF IMAGE

Certain CT scanning equipment including many of the body scanners display an image of the intracranial cavity with right and left sides reversed. Unless the surgeon is aware of this feature, confusion as to the side of a hematoma may arise.

XIV. VERMIAN ARTIFACT

An occasional artifactually increased density in the region of the cerebellar inferior vermis may misleadingly suggest the presence of a hematoma in this location.

SUMMARY

The pitfalls in the execution and interpretation of CT scans in head injury which we have enumerated in no way detract from the value of this study in head injury management. The isodense chronic subdural hematoma can be the most difficult of the pitfalls mentioned in obscuring the correct diagnosis on CT scanning. Patient movement artifact will be less of a problem as faster scanning becomes more widely available. Low-lying middle fossa lesions, high-convexity lesions, artifacts due to metallic foreign bodies, the nonspecificity of the ring sign, pneumocephalus, the differentiation of long-standing subdural hematoma from

Fig. 12. Metallic artifact due to intracranial pressure measurement device (Case 9). Left scan shows bifrontal contusions at admission. Middle scan shows extensive metallic artifact. Right scan shows subdural hematoma on the left side, obscured on previous scan by artifact.

Fig. 13. Extensive artifact caused by metallic cranial plate.

Fig. 14. Intraventricular hemorrhage (Case 10). Absorption nearly complete at four days. No neurological deficit in follow-up.

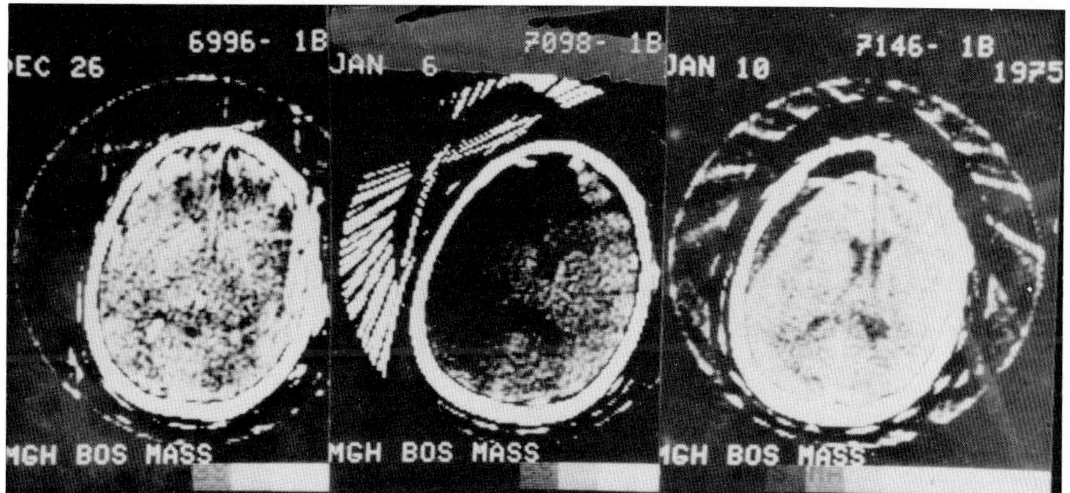

Fig. 12

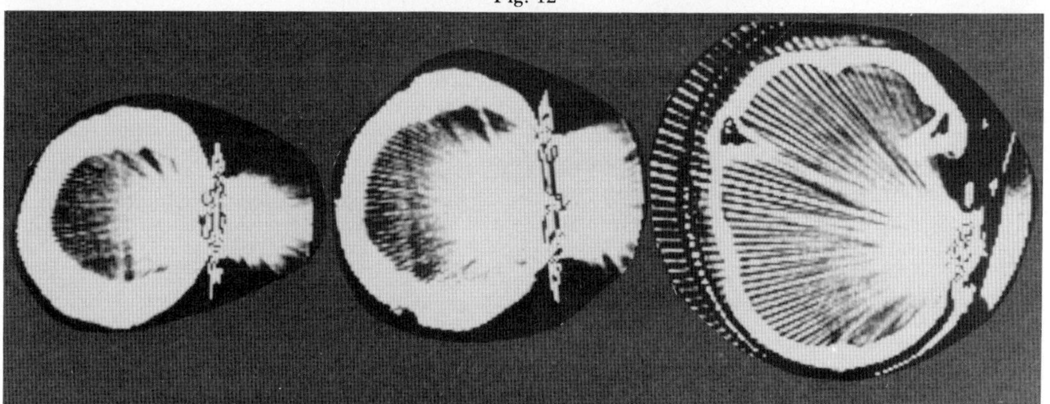

Fig. 13

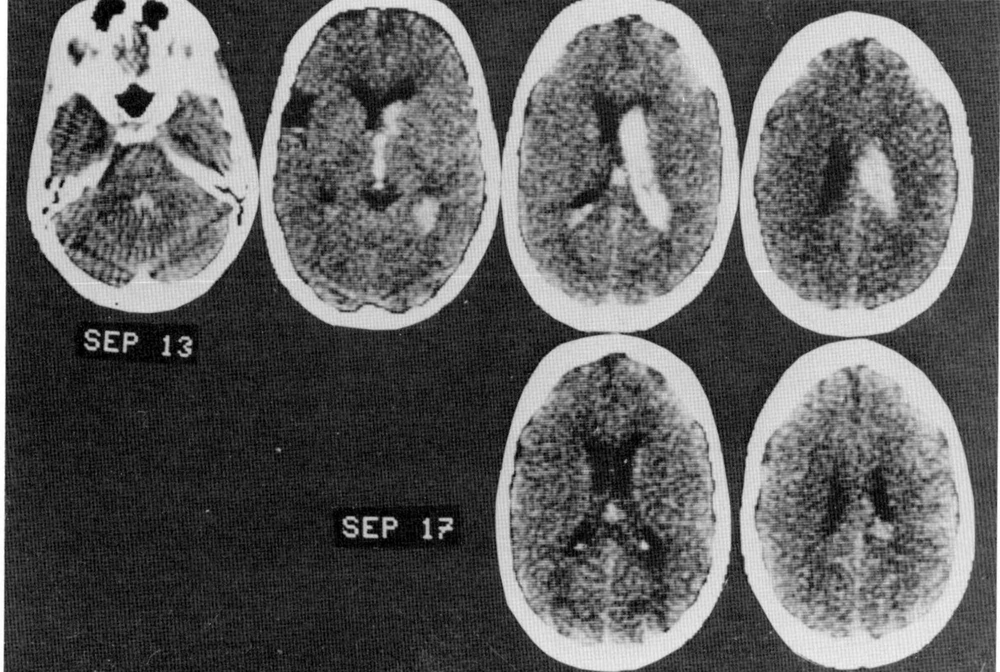

Fig. 14

atrophic changes, difficulties arising from interpretation of a plane of a lesion, and reversal of the CT image are all sometimes potential problem areas. The technological development of CT scanning has in no way supplanted the need for common sense in correlating and interpreting the findings.

EDITOR'S NOTE

Drs. Tarlov and Davis have given us *14* "CT pearls" about head injury cases. They obviously have learned these the hard way. Their point #13 is *reversal of image*. I am used to looking at x-rays with the patient's right on the right side of the film as I look at it, and with the patient's left on the left side of the film as I look at it. Some of the CT pictures do this "backwards," however, and one must be on the lookout for this. Hopefully, this could be agreed upon by convention that all the CT machines would label their pictures the same way, and it should be in the way we are used to looking at x-rays. This may seem like a small point, but good medicine usually consists in being more attentive to small details!

JLS

REFERENCES

1. Ambrose, J., Gooding, M. R., Uttley, D. EMI Scanning in the management of head injuries. Lancet *1*:847–848 (April 17, 1967).
2. Bergstrom, M. Computerized tomography of cranial subdural and epidural hematomas: Variation of attenuation related to time and clinical events such as rebleeding. J. Comput. Assist. Tomogr. *1*(4):449–455 (October 1977).
3. Bradach, G. B., *et al.* Limitations of computed tomography for diagnostic radiology. Neuroradiology *13*(5):243–247 (July 29, 1977).
4. Dublin, A. B., French, B. N., and Renick, J. M. Computerized tomography in head trauma. Radiology *122*:365–369 (February 1977).
5. Forbes. CAT scanning in subdural hematoma. Radiology *126*(1):143–148 (January 1978).
6. French, B. N. and Dublin, A. B. The value of computerized tomography in the management of 1000 consecutive head injuries. Surg. Neurol. *7*:171–183 (1977).
7. Kramer, R. N. Vermian pseudotumor: A potential pitfall of CT with contrast. Neuroradiol. *13*(5):229–230 (July 29, 1977).
8. New, P. F. J. and Aronow, S. Attentuation Measurements of Whole Body and Blood Fractions in Computed Tomography. Radiology *121*:635–640 (1976).
9. Scotti, G., *et al.* Evaluation of the age of subdural hematomas by computed tomography. J. Neurosurg. *47*:311–315 (September 1977).
10. Zhilka, B. E., Kendall, Low, *et al.* Diagnosis of subdural hematoma by computed axial tomography: Use of xenon inhalation for contrast enhancement. J. Neurol. Neurosurg. Psychiatr. *41*:370–373 (1978).
11. Zimmerman, R. A. Cranial computed tomography in the diagnosis and management of acute head trauma. Am. J. Roentenol. *131*(1):27–34 (July 1978).

32 Cerebral Radionuclide Angiography

Barbara D. Barnes, M.D.

Radionuclide angiography (RA) is a dynamic study of cerebral perfusion performed following an intravenously injected radiopharmaceutical. The arterial, capillary, and venous phases of the cerebral circulation can be seen. Neither computerized axial tomography (CT) scans nor static radionuclide scans assess cerebral perfusion. RA is safe, noninvasive, and can be performed rapidly. It is clinically useful because areas of the brain with either increased or decreased perfusion can be identified. Knowledge of changes in cerebral perfusion aids the clinician to establish the proper diagnosis by defining the location of a lesion and its vascularity.[1-7]

DESCRIPTION OF THE METHOD

The patient is positioned under a scintillation camera (Pho/Gamma IV Model 6-106, G. D. Searle and Co., Des Plaines, Ill.) for anterior Townes, lateral, or vertex views. A bolus of the radionuclide ^{99m}technetium-diethylene-triamine pentaacetic acid (^{99m}Tc-DPTA) is injected rapidly into the antecubital vein. Scintillation data on the passage of the nuclide through the cerebral intra- and extracranial circulation can be collected on Polaroid or other photographic film or fed into a computer for replay and manipulation. In our laboratory at San Francisco General Hospital Medical Center, the data are collected both on photographic film and by computer (DEC PDP-11/45) in 1.25-sec histograms (64 × 64 matrix) for 50 sec following injection. The process by which the computer acquires and subtracts imaging data has been described previously.[8]

The clinical value of radionuclide angiography is enhanced by computer processing of the data, which permits flow studies to be performed in two different projections of the head during a single laboratory visit. Without computerization, only a single view can be done on each day because background radioactivity from the first injection interferes with the resolution of the image from the second injection.[8] The value of two projections is discussed in the section on detection of ischemic lesions (below).

With the computer, flow data can be replayed as a cinematic presentation, showing the arterial and venous phases of the cerebral circulation. Patterns of vascular filling and emptying of a lesion can be visualized, and feeding or draining vessels may be identified. A color video screen coupled to the computer displays the "movie" in color scale. In my opinion, this enhances the recognition of abnormalities.

Quantitative comparisons of relative flow to the two hemispheres can be computed for predesignated regions of interest in each hemisphere. For example, the right hemisphere might receive 50% less blood flow than the left hemisphere. Serial studies on an individual patient can be used to follow the course of an abnormality. An infarcted hemisphere might initially receive 50% less blood than the uninvolved side, but, after several weeks, blood flow may return toward normal. It should be noted, however, that the RA study cannot be standardized to yield cerebral blood flow in absolute terms (e.g., ml/100 g brain/min).

VALUE OF RA IN DETECTING ISCHEMIC AND VASCULAR LESIONS

Detection of Ischemic Lesions

Cerebral Infarction. RA is very useful

in identifying an area of ischemia within the distribution of the anterior circulation: anterior cerebral artery (ACA) and middle cerebral artery (MCA). As soon as the patient has symptoms of cerebral infarction, an ischemic area can be seen; there is no 7–10-day delay in the appearance of the lesion, as in a static scan. Therefore, a combination of a normal static brain scan or CT with the RA showing an ischemic region helps the clinician to diagnose cerebral infarction.[5, 6]

In order to achieve the greatest diagnostic accuracy, the RA should be performed in two projections of the head. One of the two views should simultaneously visualize both hemispheres to allow a comparison of the relative blood flow to each hemisphere. Either a vertex or an anterior Townes projection can be used for this purpose. We routinely use the anterior Townes projection because the flow in both common carotid arteries can be assessed with this view, and high-grade stenosis or occlusion can be recognized. However, low-grade stenosis or ulcerative plaques at the carotid bifurcation require cerebral arteriography for definition. (Although we believe that two views should be performed, this concept is not yet widely practiced; either an anterior Townes or a vertex projection is most often employed.)

The choice of the second projection should be based on the patient's clinical symptomology. For example, a patient with a right hemiparesis and aphasia should be studied with a left lateral projection because the lateral projection evaluates primarily the MCA distribution. Ischemia of the whole or a part of the MCA distribution may be seen. Branch occlusion of the superior or inferior division correlates well with the clinical symptomology. Ischemic areas of the posterior frontal or parietal regions may be seen only if a lateral projection is performed, and can be missed on an anterior Townes projection alone (Fig. 1). Multiple ischemic areas within the MCA distribution, e.g., multiple emboli, are best seen in a lateral projection.

The resolution of the RA study is approximately 2–3 cm; therefore lacunar infarcts cannot be detected. In addition, lesions that are deep, near-midline structures, such as hypertensive hemorrhage in the striatum, may be missed because normal blood flow to the overlying cortex may mask the lesion.

Although a nonperfused area of the brain is characteristic of cerebral infarction on RA, the finding is nonspecific, and can occur with many lesions of the CNS. A knowledge of the patient's clinical presentation and neurologic examination is essential in order to arrive at a reasonable differential diagnosis. Other avascular lesions include: edematous brain (secondary to trauma, tumor, or infection) or focal areas of loss of brain parenchyma (due to operation, trauma, or congenital malformation). The occasional appearance of a vascular blush following cerebral infarction is discussed below.

Postsubarachnoid Hemorrhage. Serial RA studies have been proposed as a method of assessing vasospasm following subarachnoid hemorrhage from rupture of an intracranial aneurysm.[9-11] The anterior Townes projection is used to compare the flow to the two hemispheres. Decreased blood flow on the side of the ruptured aneurysm suggests vasospasm in the vessels adjacent to the aneurysm; symmetrical flow suggests a lack of significant vasospasm. In the series reported by Kelly,[10] serial RA studies showed changes in the relative flow to each hemisphere, e.g., decreased perfusion correlated with vasospasm and normal perfusion correlated with the resolution of the vasospasm.

The presence of severe vasospasm is considered a risk factor for development of postoperative cerebral infarction if surgery is performed during the period of the severe spasm. Decreased flow on the RA study correlated more strongly with the patient's outcome than did the assessment of vasospasm by arteriography.[10] Delaying the operation until the spasm disappeared decreased the risk of operative infarction. Therefore, Kelly *et al.* suggest postponing surgery if the patient has evidence of vasospasm by the RA study. The risk of rebleeding from the aneurysm would be an obvious concern in considering delay in operation.

Detection of Posterior Superior Sagittal Sinus Occlusion. Sagittal sinus oc-

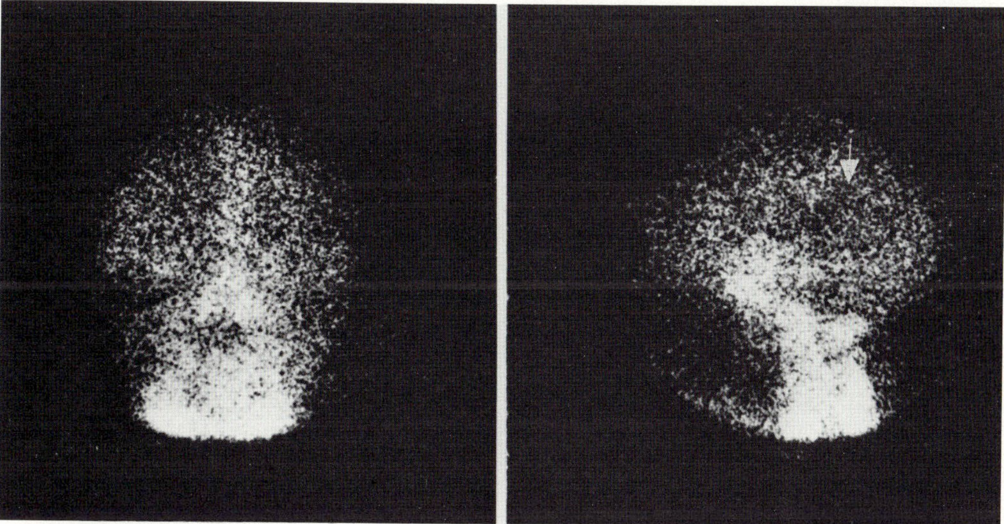

Fig. 1. RA, midarterial phase. Anterior Townes projection (left) is normal. Left lateral projection (right). There is a small ischemic region in the infrasylvian division of the left MCA (arrow).

clusion is difficult to diagnose clinically because of the variation of the clinical presentation. Until recently, definitive diagnosis has relied on contrast arteriography or sinography to visualize the occlusion. RA clearly visualizes the posterior sagittal sinus and can be substituted for arteriography as a screening procedure.[12] However, the sinus can be seen adequately, *only* in the posterior oblique projection (Fig. 2). In a straight anterior or posterior view, the anterior and posterior portions of the sagittal sinus are overlapped, so that a partial occlusion may be overlooked. The clinician must specify that sinus occlusion is suspected to ensure that the flow study can be properly performed. Patients at risk for sagittal sinus occlusion include those with pseudotumor cerebri syndrome, thromboembolic disorders, and elderly patients having pulmonary emboli or unexplained deterioration of mental status.

Detection of Vascular Lesions

RA readily detects most arteriovenous malformations (AVM's) in the cerebral hemispheres.[4, 13] An AVM appears very early in the arterial phase of the RA study, and large feeding vessels can often be identified (Fig. 3). The lesion persists throughout the venous phase and draining vessels may also appear. The RA study visualizes

the lesion more intensely than the routine static nuclide scan. The static image of the blood brain barrier is not as bright as the perfusion image. AVM's of the posterior fossa are more difficult to detect than those of the cerebral hemispheres but may be seen if they are sufficiently large. Lesions under 1–2 cm in diameter may not be apparent.

Cerebral arteriography remains the definitive test for detecting aneurysms. Cerebral berry aneurysms generally are too small to be seen by nuclide angiography. Giant aneurysms that are not extensively thrombosed may be seen.

Major vascular fistulas, such as a carotid-cavernous fistula, can be seen by RA.[14–16] In one of the cases in our laboratory, the fistula filled from both carotids.[17] Relative blood flow to the hemispheres was assessed and revealed that an asymptomatic cerebral steal occurred when the carotid ipsilateral to the fistula was manually compressed. Preoperative serial RA studies helped to plan the operative approach which avoided a permanent vascular steal. A postoperative study confirmed obliteration of the fistula and preserved blood flow to both cerebral hemispheres.

Other lesions, such as primary (or occasionally metastatic) tumors, may appear as a vascular blush on RA. The blush tends to occur later in the arterial phase than with

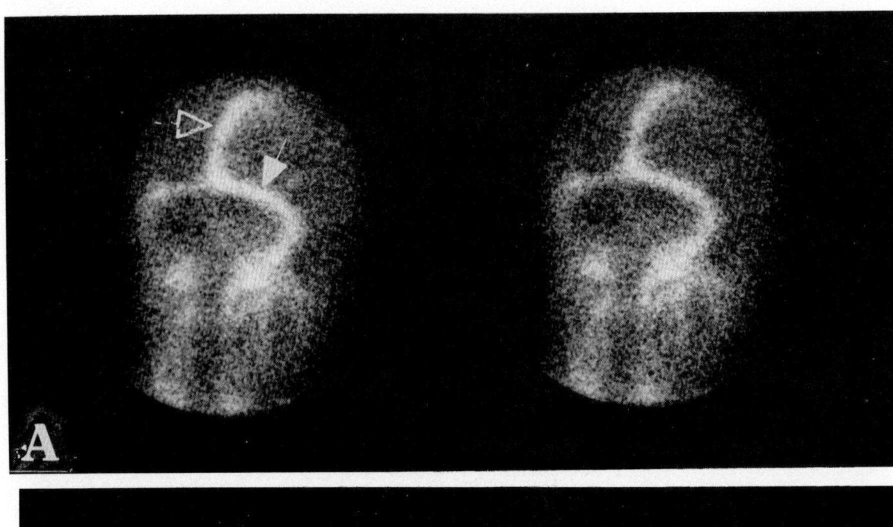

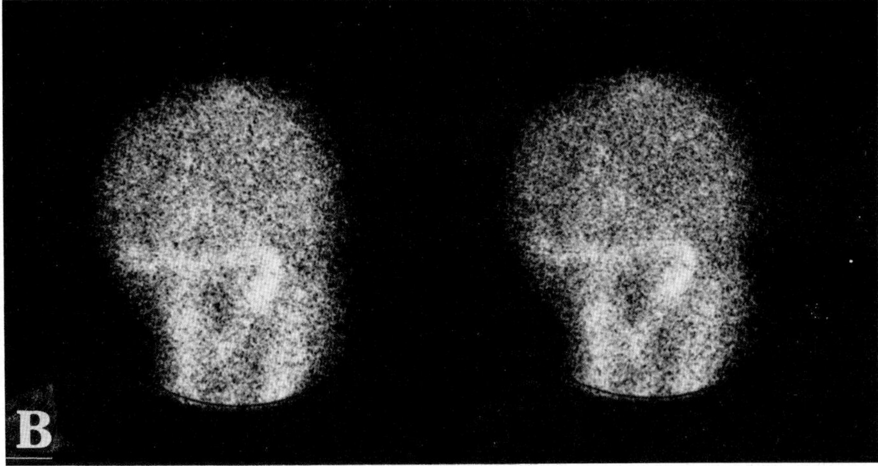

Fig. 2. RA, right posterior oblique projection, venous phase. (A) Normal patient. The posterior sagittal sinus (open arrow) is seen emptying into the transverse sinus (solid arrow). The slightly larger right transverse sinus is a common variation. (B) Patient with posterior sagittal sinus occlusion. The transverse and right sigmoid sinus can be identified. The posterior sagittal sinus does not appear.

an AVM, and tends to be less intense than with an AVM. It may persist throughout the venous phase and gain in intensity late in the study. In contrast to the AVM, a neoplasm is usually more intense in the static radionuclide scan than in the flow study, reflecting the breakdown of the blood brain barrier.

Cerebral infarction paradoxically may appear as a vascular blush. This phenomenon, termed "a hot stroke," is thought to be analogous to luxery perfusion seen on ^{133}Xe CBF studies.[18, 19] The blush most typically occurs in the first few days following infarction, and later studies may show normal or decreased flow to the same region.

In some patients with ischemic lesions on initial studies, follow-up studies several weeks later may show a prominent blush, probably due to capillary proliferation during the reparative changes in the brain.

Patients with focal status epilepticus, either clinical (e.g., continual left-sided focal motor seizures) or electrical (EEG paroxysmal activity without clinical seizures), often have asymmetric perfusion with the greater flow to the hemisphere with the seizure.[20] The hyperperfusion of this hemisphere may persist for a variable period of time following cessation of the clinical or electrical seizures. The duration of the asymmetry of flow has not been well defined, but it is my impression that it may persist for at least 24 hours. Subsequent flow alteration may appear, depending on the pathology of the lesion initiating the seizures. Most typical of my experience has been the change from hyperfusion to ischemia of the affected hemisphere, reflecting the underlying pathology of cerebral infarction or contusion.

COMPARISON OF RA TO OTHER NEURODIAGNOSTIC STUDIES

CT Scan. Combining CT and RA helps to better define the nature of a lesion because RA depicts cerebral perfusion while CT scanning does not. For example, a high density lesion on the CT scan, having increased perfusion on RA, supports the diagnosis of a vascular neoplasm or AVM. A high-density lesion with decreased perfusion suggests a cerebral infarction, intraparenchymal hemorrhage, or avascular tumor (Table I). A low-density lesion on CT with decreased perfusion could be a cyst, edema, or cerebral infarction.

Contrast enhancement of the CT scan occurs when a lesion has blood-brain barrier breakdown (analagous to uptake seen on the static radionuclide scan) or has a large vascular component. A contrast en-

TABLE I. *Differential diagnosis of cerebral lesions by CT and RA*

CT	RA	Diagnosis
CT, high density	Decreased perfusion	Intraparenchymal hemorrhage, Cerebral infarction, Avascular neoplasm
	Increased perfusion	AVM Vascular neoplasm

hancing lesion may have normal, increased, or decreased blood flow. For example, a low-density lesion following cerebral infarction may have decreased blood flow and show contrast enhancement due to an abnormal blood-brain barrier. Vascular lesions show contrast enhancement on the CT and increased blood flow on the RA.[21-24]

CT scanning is preferred over RA when bleeding within the intracranial cavity is suspected; subarachnoid, intraparenchymal, or intraventricular hemorrhage can be identified by the CT scan. The existence of intracranial bleeding cannot be detected by the RA (or by the static nuclide scan); however, blood flow alterations may occur in patients with any of these sites of hem-

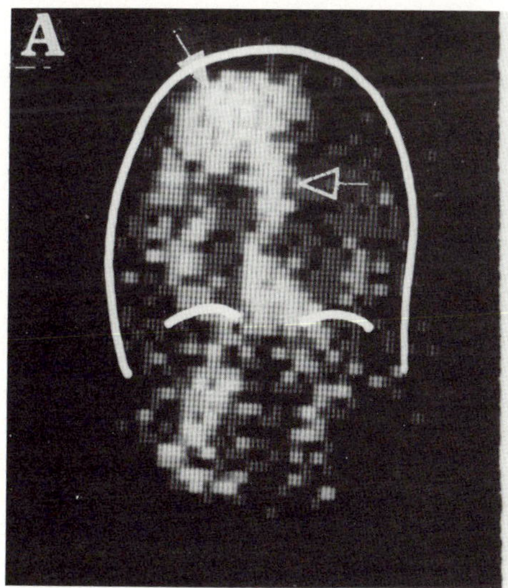
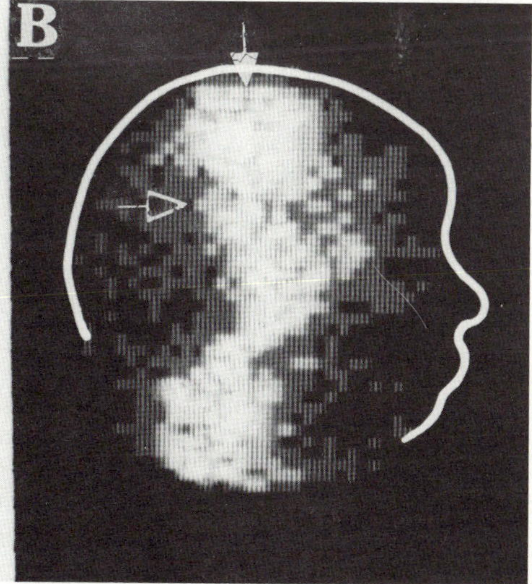

Fig. 3. RA, early arterial phase. Patient with AVM. (A) Anterior Townes projection. A large vascular blush appears in the right hemisphere (closed arrow) and prominent blood supply derived from the ACA is seen (open arrow). (B) Right lateral projection. The vascular lesion is in the fronto-parietal region (closed arrow) and receives blood supply from the MCA (open arrow).

orrhage. Frequently, the RA is normal in subarachnoid hemorrhage, but brain ischemia may be apparent if significant vasospasm is present. Intraparenchymal hemorrhage in the cortex may appear ischemic on RA, but if the hemorrhage is located deep in the brain (e.g., a small hypertensive basal ganglia hemorrhage), the nuclide flow study may be normal. Intraventricular hemorrhage cannot be identified in the RA.

Cerebral Contrast Arteriography. Cerebral contrast arteriography visualizes the anterior and posterior intracranial circulation, but it is an invasive procedure which requires arterial puncture. RA is often used as a screening procedure prior to arteriography to help identify the site of a lesion or its vascularity. Although the carotid arteries in the neck may be seen in the RA study (anterior Townes projection), cerebral arteriography is needed to evaluate the carotid arteries prior to vascular surgery. Low grade carotid stenosis and ulcerative plaques at the carotid bifurcation cannot be resolved by RA.

RA is primarily limited to evaluation of the anterior circulation (ACA and MCA) but occasionally may be used to examine the posterior circulation (vertebral basilar and posterior cerebral arteries). Ischemic posterior circulation lesions are seldom visible. Arteriography is needed to define the vascularity of most posterior fossa lesions. Ischemic lesions of the occipital cortex can be identified by RA, using the vertex projection.

[133]Xenon Regional Cerebral Blood Flow and Emission Computerized Tomography. Regional cerebral blood flow (rCBF) studies utilizing inhalation or intracarotid injection of [133]Xenon (^{133}Xe) are performed for research purposes and provide quantitative blood flow data (ml/100 g brain/min).[18, 25] Quantitative rCBF measurements are determined by analyzing the washout of ^{133}Xe from the brain for several minutes following injection. Multiple determinations can be performed during a single examination under different physiological conditions, such as varying blood pressure or arterial CO_2 pressure. These studies have not been used routinely although they have provided important physiological information. Further discussion of the differences between RA studies and the Xe rCBF studies can be found in the references.[17, 25]

To evaluate cerebral perfusion, the RA study can be performed more economically and rapidly than other methods. In addition, the radionuclide, scintillation camera, computer, and computer software required for the RA study are widely used in nuclear medicine laboratories throughout the United States and are readily available to the clinician without additional expense for equipment.

Emission computerized tomography is an exciting new research tool utilizing short-lived cyclotron produced radiopharmaceuticals to study a variety of physiological parameters.[26] This tecnique has much potential value.

EDITOR'S NOTE

Radionuclide angiography still has a definite place in the clinician's armamentarium. It is very helpful in detecting a high-grade carotid stenosis when a dynamic flow study is ordered. It is the best test to order when you suspect an intracerebral arteriovenous malformation after looking at the plain films and may allow one to avoid an invasive procedure in such a patient. Dr. Barnes has given us an extra "pearl" in this chapter in that this test should also be considered when the diagnosis of superior sagittal sinus thrombosis is suspected. I don't know enough about emission computered tomography to make a reasonable comment. But, with the exceptions listed, in my opinion I'd advise a computed tomographic scan first—rather than a radionuclide scan—in most neuro-ophthalmological situations. However, the exceptions noted above are specific, and important!

JLS

REFERENCES

1. Fish, M. D., Pollycove, M., O'Reilly, S., *et al.* Vascular characterization of brain lesions by rapid sequential cranial scintiphotography. J. Nucl. Med. *9:*249–259 (1968).
2. Fish, M. D., Barnes, B., and Pollycove, M. Cranial scintiphotographic blood flow defects in arteriographically proven cerebral vascular disease. J. Nucl. Med. *14:*558–564 (1973).
3. Cowan, R. J., Maynard, C. D., Meschan, I., *et al.* Value of the routine use of the radioisotope cere-

bral dynamic study: Analysis in over 1,000 patients. Radiology *107*:111–116 (1973).

4. Deland, F. H. *Cerebral Radionuclide Angiography*. Saunders, Philadelphia, 1976.

5. Barnes, B. D., Parker, H., and Anger, H. O. Neurologic diagnosis using the 80-lens optical camera. Neurology (Minneap.) *27*:26–31 (1977).

6. Barnes, B. D., Finklestein, S., and Winestock, D. P. Radionuclide angiography: a sensitive diagnostic test for anterior circulation ischemia. Neurology (Minneap.) *28*:775–781 (1978).

7. Mishkin, F. S. Cerebral radionuclide angiography. Angiology *28*:261–275 (1977).

8. Barnes, B., Parker, H. G., and Nohr, M. L. Technique for multi-view radionuclide angiography. Stroke *9*:566–569 (1978).

9. Goodman, S. J. and Hayes, M. Value of cerebral isotope flow studies in timing of surgery for ruptured aneurysms when there is vasospasm and neurologic deficit. J. Nucl. Med. *15*:1113–1116 (1974).

10. Kelly, P. J., Gorten, R. J., Grossman, R. G., et al. Cerebral perfusion, vascular spasm, and outcome in patients with ruptured intracranial aneurysms. J. Neurosurg. *47*:44–49 (1977).

11. Nilsson, B. W. Cerebral blood flow in patients with subarachnoid haemorrhage studied with an intravenous isotope technique. Its clinical significance in the timing of surgery of cerebral arterial aneurysm. Acta Neurochir. *37*:33–48 (1977).

12. Barnes, B. D. and Winestock, D. P. Dynamic radionuclide scanning in the diagnosis of thrombosis of the superior sagittal sinus. Neurology (Minneap.) *27*:656–661 (1977).

13. Gates, G. F., Fishman, L. S., and Segall, H. D. Scintigraphic detection of congenital intracranial vascular malformations. J. Nucl. Med. *19*:235–244 (1978).

14. Curl, F. D., Harbert, J. C., Luessenhop, A. D., et al. Radionuclide cerebral angiography in a case of bilateral carotid-cavernous fistula. Radiology *102*: 391–392 (1972).

15. Matin, P., Goodwin, D. A., Nayyar, S. N. Radionuclide cerebral angiography in diagnosis and evaluation of carotid-cavernous fistula. J. Nucl. Med. *15*:1105–1109 (1974).

16. Tully, T. E., Shafer, R. B., Reinke, D. B., et al. Radionuclide angiography in the diagnosis of carotid cavernous sinus fistula. J. Nucl. Med. *15*:797–800 (1974).

17. Barnes, B. D., Rosenblum, M. L., Pitts, L. H., et al. Carotid-cavernous fistula. J. Neurosurg. *49*:49–55 (1978).

18. Paulson, O. B. Cerebral apoplexy (stroke): Pathogenesis, pathophysiology and therapy as illustrated by regional blood flow measurements in the brain. Stroke *2*:327–360 (1971).

19. Yarnell, P., Burdick, D., and Sanders, B. The hot stroke: A clinical, radioisotopic angiographic correlation of increased relative perfusion to the area of cerebral infarction. Arch. Neurol. *30*:65–69 (1974).

20. Yarnell, P. R., Burdick, D., Sanders, B., et al. Focal seizures, early veins, and increased flow: A clinical angiographic, radioisotopic correlation. Neurology (Minneap.) *24*:512–516 (1974).

21. Chiu, L. C., Christie, J. H., and Schapiro, R. L. Nuclide imaging and computed tomography in cerebral vascular disease. Sem. Nucl. Med. *7*:175–195 (1977).

22. Campbell, J. K., Houser, O. W., Stevens, J. C., et al. Computed tomography and radionuclide imaging in the evaluation of ischemic stroke. Radiology *126*:695–702 (1978).

23. Fordham, E. W. The complementary role of computerized axial transmission tomography and radionuclide imaging of the brain. Sem. Nucl. Med. *7*:137–159 (1977).

24. Alderson, P. O., Gado, M. H., and Siegel, B. A. Computerized cranial tomography and radionuclide imaging in the detection of intracranial mass lesions. Sem. Nucl. Med. *7*:161–173 (1977).

25. Holman, B. L. Concepts and clinical utility of the measurement of cerebral blood flow. Sem. Nucl. Med. *6*:233–251 (1976).

26. Grubb, R. L., Raichle, M. E., Higgins, C. S., et al. Measurement of regional cerebral blood volume by emission tomography. Ann. Neurol. *4*:322–328 (1978).

33 Demeclocycline HCL in the Treatment of Chronic Siadh Syndrome in Children

Joan L. Venes, M.D.
John Forest, Jr., M.D.

Chronic diabetes insipidus occurs more commonly than chronic inappropriate secretion of antidiuretic hormone in patients with hypothalamic lesions. However, when chronic inappropriate antidiuretic hormone secretion occurs in the pediatric age group, it often presents a significant management problem. Fluid restriction may be difficult to regulate in the child attending school. Prolonged fluid restriction for the hospitalized child may lead to hypovolemia and secondary hyperaldosteronism with its attendant problems. Demeclocycline HCL is a relatively nontoxic antibiotic that produces a reversible nephrogenic diabetes insipidus in normal persons in doses of 600–1200 mg. daily.[1] Both Demeclocycline HCL and Lithium interfere with the cellular action of antidiuretic hormone and both agents have been recommended as therapy for chronic inappropriate antidiuretic hormone secretion syndrome. A comparison between Demeclocycline HCL and Lithium in the treatment of chronic inappropriate antidiuretic hormone secretion syndrome was conducted by the Nephrology Department at Yale and the University of Pennsylvania School of Medicine. Their conclusion was that Demeclocycline was clearly superior to Lithium therapy.[2] This experience led us to consider the use of Demeclocycline HCL in the treatment of a severely ill child admitted to the Pediatric Neurosurgical Service at the Yale-New Haven Hospital in August 1975.

This 5⁶⁄₁₂-year-old girl first presented in October 1973 at the age of two years with severe optic atrophy, marked hydrocephalus, and a large avascular mass in the parasellar region. Subtotal resection of a cystic hypothalamic glioma was carried out. The histology was consistent with the diagnosis of spongioblastoma polare. Because of her age it was elected to defer radiation. Several months later the child moved from the area, was irradiated, and apparently continued to do well until the summer of 1976 when she had several admissions with repeated attempts to drain a large cystic cavity in the right frontal area. She was transferred to Yale-New Haven Hospital for a second opinion after the parents were informed that the child was unsalvageable and advised that therapy should be terminated.

On admission she was noted to be obtunded with a left hemiplegia and blood and urine chemistries consistent with the diagnosis of inappropriate antidiuretic hormone secretion syndrome (Table I). Twenty-four hours after the institution of fluid restriction, she was alert and following simple commands but with a persistent left hemiparesis. Her hospital course was stormy and complicated by attempts to control persistent hyponatremia and hypoosmolarity. By her third hospital week she was on a one-third fluid restriction, and her course was complicated by the secondary effects of hyperaldosteronism including hypertension and hypokalemia.

Although the use of tetracycline is generally contraindicated in children under eight years of age because of the effect on developing tooth enamel, it was felt that the gravity of the situation warranted its use in this case. Therapy was instituted on

"

TABLE I. *Urine and serum electrolytes in a 5⁵/₁₂-year-old girl with hypothalamic glioma (Case 1) indicate persistence of hyponatremia with fluid restriction alone. The arrow marks initiation of Demeclocycline therapy. Note the prompt improvement of electrolyte balance and the liberalization of fluid intake*

	Sept			Oct	
	15	20	8	16	21
Serum					
urea nitrogen (mgm%)	7	4	10	13	15
sodium (mEq/L)	130	130	131	141	143
osmolarity (mOsm/L)	264	266	262	286	—
Urine					
sodium (mEq/L)	139	151	50	57	—
osmolality (mOsm/L)	—	470	—	316	—
Intake	—	485 cc	419 cc	685 cc	1100 cc

9 October and as can be seen (Table I), within one week her serum electrolytes became normal in spite of increased fluid intake. Although her chemistries remained stable, the patient's neurological condition waxed and waned. In spite of various therapeutic maneuvers her condition steadily deteriorated and by 27 October it was elected to discontinue all therapy. She died a short while later.

Our initial satisfaction with the drug was strengthened with its use in the treatment of a 16-year-old boy who initially presented in late 1975 at the age of 14 years. Subfrontal craniotomy and biopsy confirmed the clinical impression of hypothalamic glioma. He had some mild transient hyponatremia postoperatively but this cleared rapidly and he tolerated his radiation well. For the next several months he did rather well save for some declining visual acuity which was stabilized by the institution of Dexamethasone. In September 1976, he was seen complaining of lethargy and polydipsia. Serum and urine electrolytes indicated overhydration (Table II) and the patient was placed on a mild fluid restriction. Over the next several weeks his pediatrician continued to increase his fluid restriction in an attempt to maintain serum sodium at 130 mEq/L. As his fluids were restricted below 1000 cc. daily he became increasingly despondent. He was admitted on 19 November for evaluation of increasing memory loss, lethargy, and depression. At that time he was rigidly adherent to his fluid restriction of 800 cc. daily. Serum and urine electrolytes were now consistent with the diagnosis of inappropriate secretion of antidiuretic hormone

TABLE II. *Urine and serum electrolytes in a 16-year-old boy (Case 2) with a hypothalamic glioma. Note the increasing urine osmolarity and salt-wasting consistent with the evolution of inappropriate secretion of antidiuretic hormone*

	Sept. 1976	Nov. 1976
Serum		
urea nitrogen (mgm%)	10	12
sodium (mEq/L)	127	132
osmolarity (mOsm/L)	258	261
Urine		
sodium (mEq/L)	53	125
osmolarity (mOsm/L)	270	860

(Table II). He was begun on Demeclocycline HCL, 300 mg. b.i.d. and increased to 900 mg. daily, by which time he was on an unrestricted fluid intake. Over the next six months some improvement was noted in his school performance, and he appeared to be doing fairly well. In June 1977, he presented with a two-week history of increasing malaise, weight loss, polydipsia, polyuria, and positional syncope. His rapid weight loss and symptoms were consistent with the laboratory evidence of severe dehydration (Table III) found on admission. Demeclocycline HCL was stopped, and within 48 hours he began to feel better. His condition appeared to stabilize, and a limited dehydration test ten days after the cessation of Demeclocycline HCL showed resolution of his diabetes insipidus (Table IV). He maintains normal kidney function one year later save for a transient mild episode of hyponatremia associated with shunt malfunction.

The efficacy and safety of Demeclocycline HCL in the management of the syn-

TABLE III. *Urine and serum electrolytes (Case 2) on admission confirm marked dehydration noted clinically. Cessation of Demeclocycline therapy (arrow) was followed by prompt clinical improvement and normalization of laboratory values*

June 1977	16	19	21	25
Serum				
urea nitrogen (mgm%)	36	26	14	10
sodium (mEq/L)	159	152	151	147
osmolarity (mOsm/L)	322	306	301	295
Urine				
sodium (mEq/L)	28	14	33	
osmolarity (mOsm/L)	328	326	474	
Weight	45.6 kg		51 kg	

TABLE IV. *Limited dehydration test (Case 2) demonstrates the resolution of nephrogenic diabetes insipidus induced by demeclocycline*

Weight (−1.0 kg)	Urine sodium (mEq/L)	Urine osmolarity (mOsm/L)
6 AM	107	377
7 AM	153	520
8 AM		514

drome of chronic inappropriate ADH secretion has been well demonstrated in the adult population.[2] These two cases indicate a similar potential in the pediatric age group. The only significant side effects reported with Demeclocycline HCL at the dosages used have been nausea and photosensitivity. In the young child the effect on dentition must also be considered. Careful drug titration and frequent clinical and laboratory evaluations for dehydration are necessary, particularly in the small child in whom large fluid shifts are less well tolerated. Demeclocycline HCL must be used with caution in patients in whom tumor growth has affected the normally operating thirst mechanisms and may be contraindicated in this group. Although the use of Demeclocycline HCL in very young children may be limited by the adverse effect on dentition, the guarded prognosis for lengthy survival makes this a less important consideration in those children with hypothalamic tumors in whom chronic inappropriate secretion of antidiuretic hormone occurs.

EDITOR'S NOTE

If *Declomycin* is useful in the treatment of inappropriate section of antidiuretic hormone, it might be worth considering as a routine postoperative antibiotic following craniotomy for conditions where this syndrome might arise. Remember the problem that the medication can cause with the teeth, however, in youngsters! This is worthy of trial by others, I believe.

JLS

REFERENCES

1. Cherrill, D. A., Stole, R. M., Birge, J. R., and Singer, I. Demeclocycline treatment in the syndrome of IADH. Ann. Intern. Med. *83*:654–56 (1975).
2. Forrest, J. N., Jr., Cox, M., Hong, C., Morrison, G., Bier, M., and Singer, I. Demeclocycline versus Lithium for inappropriate secretion of antidiuretic hormone. New Engl. J. Med. *298*:173–177 (1978).

34 Supratentorial Arachnoid Cysts

Frank M. Anderson, M.D.

Supratentorial arachnoid cysts are congenital lesions which probably arise from entrapment of CNS between layers of embryonic arachnoid membranes.[4] This process causes the formation of thin-walled globular masses which may be responsible for serious brain damage and lead to permanent mental and physical defects, especially in infants and children. Usually these cysts do not communicate with ventricles or subarachnoid spaces, but they probably expand slowly by absorption of water from their environs. Such cysts may be large at birth, causing distortion of the brain and compression of ventricles resulting in early elevation of intracranial pressure. Occasionally pressure is further raised by bleeding into the cysts[5]; at other times the lesion produces no problems until middle age or later, and rarely a cyst which has remained silent during life is discovered at autopsy.[7]

CLINICAL FEATURES

The characteristic symptoms and signs of arachnoid cysts in infants and young children are basically caused by pressure and the presence of a large mass, factors which may cause the infant's head to be large at birth and maintain accelerated growth later. Poor feeding, vomiting, irritability, and perhaps somnolence are also commonly noted. Examination shows the head to be larger than average with full fontanels and wide sutures similar to a patient with conventional hydrocephalus. Often, however, the vault is asymmetrical because the cyst tends to cause one-sided bulging of the overlying skull (Fig. 1). There may be developmental delays, impaired nutrition, and mild spasticity of extremities, all of which are increased by head trauma

or recent bleeding into the cyst. Adults and children older than about three years may complain of headache and dullness and exhibit papilledema, strabismus, unilateral proptosis, visual field defects, memory impairment, and occasionally mild hemiparesis.

RADIOLOGY

Plain x-rays of the skull in patients with supratentorial arachnoic cysts frequently show some outward protrusion and thinning of parietal bone over the lesion, or deepening of the middle fossa with elevation and forward displacement of the sphenoid wing.[6] Radionuclide scans show displacement of the longitudinal sinus away from a large, clear area, and angiography similarly defines an avascular lesion of large size displacing cerebral arterial branches, veins, and venous sinuses to the opposite side. Ventriculography, as formerly used, gave good definition of cysts in certain cases.

Computerized tomography has proven very helpful for diagnosis and follow-up care of patients with cysts and is to be recommended for any patient with symptoms suggesting an intracranial mass lesion or raised intracranial pressure.[2, 3] In CT scans supratentorial cysts appear as relatively large, nonenhancing, unencapsulated lesions exhibiting no apparent communication with ventricles or subarachnoid spaces (Fig. 2). The fluid content is usually of water density, but is denser in occasional cases because of increased protein from bleeding. Indentation and distortion of the brain may be severe; ventricles are usually displaced and somewhat dilated. Bulging of the overlying skull is often obvious.

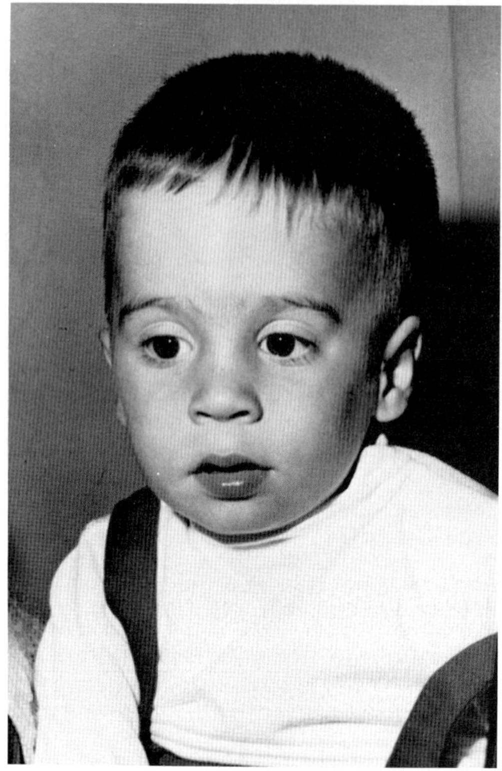

Fig. 1. This two-year-old child has a left parasagittal arachnoid cyst. Note cranial asymmetry with protrusion of skull over the lesion. Such deformity even in an asymptomatic patient should alert the clinician to the possible presence of a large space-taking lesion such as cyst.

Differentiation of cysts from other lesions is usually not unduly difficult. Chronic subdural hematomas are generally lens shaped rather than globular, and their contents are considerably more opaque than water; hematomas older than about two weeks usually show a capsule which enhances with contrast solution. Cystic neoplasms can be identified by the presence of an enhancing solid mass; if a liquified part is present, this will appear much smaller than the usual arachnoid cyst. Porencephalic defects are somewhat irregular in configuration, usually exhibit obvious communication with ventricles or subarachnoid spaces, and do not cause mass effects such as displacement of ventricles.

DIAGNOSIS

Differentiation of lesions which cause pressure symptoms may require careful thought and investigation. When the physician is confronted with an infant who shows undue head growth or an older patient with pressure signs, he should consider all types of mass lesions, such as hydrocephalus, cerebral tumor, and infections including meningitis and abscess. Complete history and examination are essential in such patients after which x-rays of skull and chest and perhaps spinal fluid examination may be appropriate. In infants, illumination of the head is a useful screening test (Fig. 3); subdural taps are often valuable for demonstrating or excluding chronic subdural hematomas. Angiography may have a place at any age if CSF is bloody or history indicates previous intracranial hemorrhage. CT scan is the most valuable test because it is risk-free, provides a means of distinguishing various space-taking lesions, and also can show or exclude traumatic or toxic brain swelling or on occasion reveal an apparently normal but oversized brain—megalencephaly. Finally, if CT scan shows a large and strange-looking space within the cranium, especially in a child, the observer must not be misled into concluding that this is a hopeless brain defect. It may

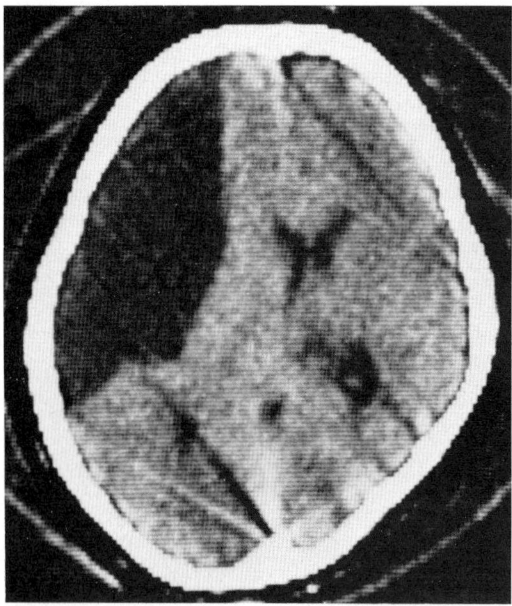

Fig. 2. CT scan in a patient similar to Case 1. The large arachnoid cyst has severely distorted the left hemisphere and displaced the ventricles; cortex is intact. Left side of skull is larger than right.

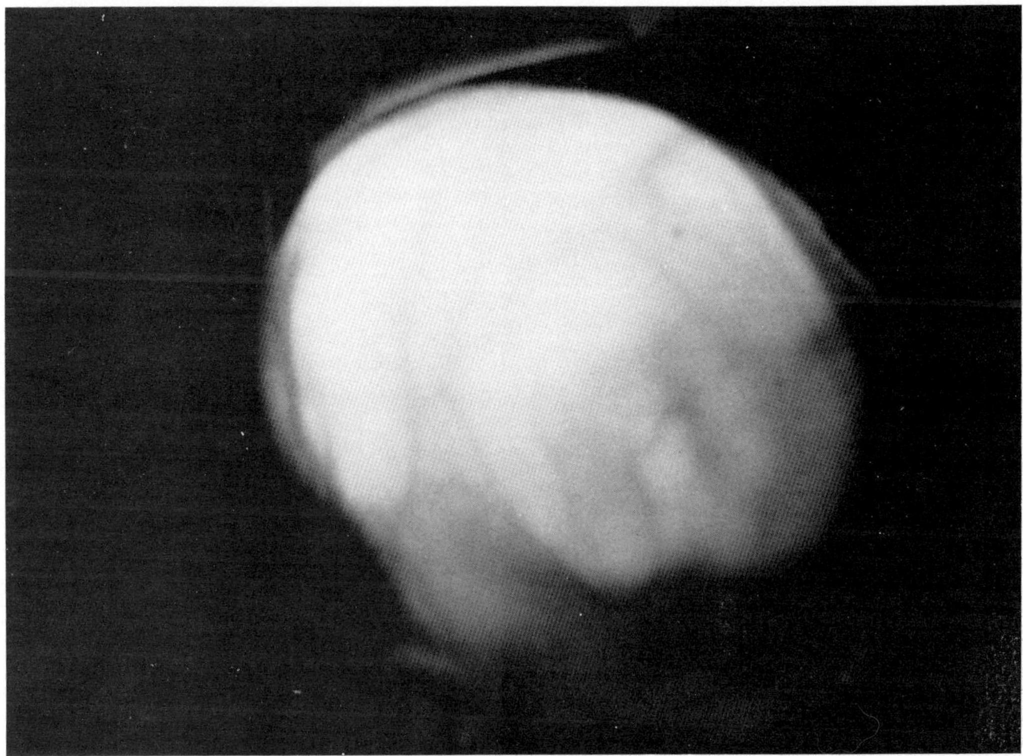

Fig. 3. Transillumination in a three-month-old infant whose head was large at birth and continued relatively rapid growth. Excessive illumination shown over right side of the head was due to a large arachnoid cyst occupying two-thirds of the hemicranium (see Case 1).

in fact be a benign arachnoid cyst which can be treated and cured.

REPORT OF CASES

Case 1, Male, Three Months. This patient's head was larger than average at birth, and excessive growth continued. The head was large (47 cm), fontanels full, and sutures widened. Vault was mildly asymmetrical with expansion of right parietal region, and the entire right side of the head transilluminated markedly (see Fig. 3). The patient was alert and active, but vision was poor. Skull x-rays showed some enlargement of the right hemicranium and needle ventriculogram revealed a cystic space displacing the distended ventricles. Craniotomy (Fig. 4) disclosed a huge loculated arachnoid cyst which was subtotally resected; later a cystoperitoneal shunt was required to control pressure. The patient's progress was good, and 10 years later he appeared normal except his head was somewhat larger than average; vision was good and there were no neurological defects, but some difficulties were observed in reasoning and behavior. CT scan showed overgrowth and dysplasia of the brain with irregular contouring of ventricles. Cyst remnant was small.

Case 2. This 51-year-old man believed he had observed a visual field defect and mild diminution in acuity of his left eye for six months. Examination showed an upper nasal quadrantanopsia and slight elevation of pressure in this eye, as well as mild proptosis. Fundus examination was negative, eyes were otherwise normal, and general and neurologic examinations were negative. X-rays of the skull showed expansion of the left middle fossa with bulging of the temporal squama and forward displacement of the left posterolateral orbital wall. CT scan showed these changes plus left proptosis and a water density defect ante-

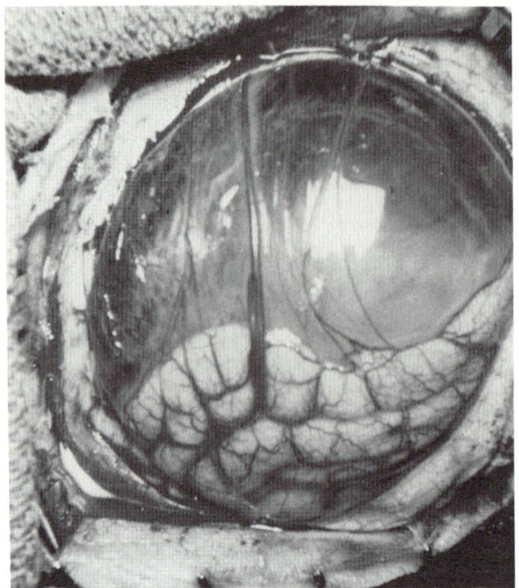

Fig. 4. (Case 1). Operative view of extensive cyst elevating and distorting, but not invading, the right temporal, frontal, and parietal lobes. The attenuated vein of Labbe is seen in outer layer of the cyst.

rior to the foreshortened temporal lobe (Fig. 5). Left frontotemporal craniotomy disclosed a 6-cm middle fossa arachnoid cyst, the small anterior end of which extended forward, wedging between the left optic nerve and carotid artery. The membranous cyst wall was subtotally removed. In the eight months since operation the patient has continued to show gradual lessening of visual defects.

TREATMENT

After investigation has confirmed the probable presence of cyst, surgical treatment is advisable without undue delay. This is recommended because of the possibility of relatively abrupt increase in intracranial pressure, perhaps with transverse shift of the brain caused by the large unilateral mass. A bone flap centered over the lesion provides good access for incision of the dura mater, identification of the cyst, and opening of its membranous outer wall. Nonadherent portions of cyst are then removed from the cerebral cortex and dura, avoiding important blood vessels. All bleeding points should be meticulously controlled with bipolar cautery and the large

residual space filled with physiologic solution before closure. In debilitated or elderly patients and those with rapidly increasing headache, lethargy, or other signs of rising pressure, it may be wiser to place only a burr hold, aspirate some fluid from the cyst, and install a cystoperitoneal shunt.[5] This procedure may give permanent relief without additional operations.

Extended postoperative observation is very important in all cases; CT scan should be obtained after about one month and periodically thereafter depending upon the patient's course and CT findings. In occasional cases additional surgery may be required for subdural hematoma, or for traumatic or spontaneous hemorrhage into the cyst bed.

SUMMARY OF RESULTS

In general the prognosis for an older child or adult with supratentorial cyst is favorable if diagnosis and proper treatment are

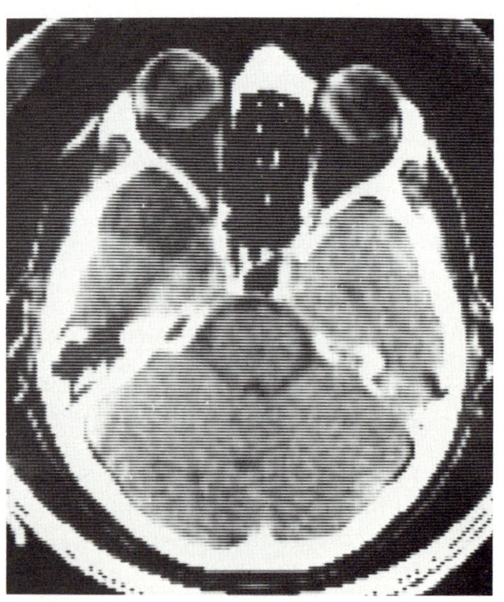

Fig. 5. (Case 2). Male, 51 years, with nasal visual field defect and slightly elevated intraocular pressure in left eye only, plus mild left proptosis. CT scan shows an arachnoid cyst in the anterior end of left middle fossa; the temporal squama protrudes and the posterior wall of orbit is pushed forward. The cyst has a narrow anterior extension which was found at surgery to lie between the carotid artery and optic nerve.

accomplished, and there may be no serious sequelae. However, if the lesion is not identified with reasonable promptness, continuing cerebral compression and elevated intracranial pressure may lead to progressive brain damage with resultant hemiparesis, stupor, and even death.[1]

In infants and young children having large cysts additional problems sometimes develop because of interference with normal growth of the brain leading to permanent defects in mental and physical functions. In a recently reported series,[2] seven infants with greater than normal head size at or soon after birth were found to have unusually large arachnoid cysts and underwent surgical treatment before the age of 12 months. When these patients were reexamined six to nineteen years later six of the group were found to have personality defects or learning difficulties of varying severity without notable physical limitations. Appearance was good except the patients' heads appeared large and measured at or above the 98th percentile. Their recent CT scans disclosed moderate overgrowth of brain, and irregularities in structure with uneven configuration of ventricles and some widening of sulci. Cyst remnants were relatively small.

The situation presented by these rather unusual patients suggests that in some individuals having arachnoid cysts there may be other embryonic errors in cerebral structure which account for functional defects in later life. It is clear, however, that the detrimental pressure effects of large cysts may be controlled if patients are afforded the benefits of prompt diagnosis and treatment. This is particularly important in infants, whose brain growth is rapid and myelination incomplete.

With wider knowledge of these complicated factors, and advance in technical skills, the long-term prognosis for such patients may with good fortune improve.

EDITOR'S NOTE

I heard Dr. Anderson give a paper on this topic at the Harvey Cushing Society and was impressed with his radiographs and surgical pictures. The big point he makes is that just because a small infant has a massive transillumination defect of the skull (see his Fig. 3 in this chapter)—this does not necessarily mean that the neurological prognosis is hopeless. Rather than writing the child off as hydranencephaly, careful study with computed tomography may reveal an arachnoid cyst which can be operated with dramatic improvement in some cases. That is a good point to the clinician!

JLS

REFERENCES

1. Aicardi, J. and Bauman, F. Supratentorial extra-arachnoid cysts in infants and children. J. Neurol. Neurosurg. Psychiatr. *38*:57–68 (1975).
2. Anderson, F. M., Segall, H. D., and Caton, W. L. Use of CT scan in supratentorial arachnoid cysts. A report of 20 children, 4 adults. J. Neurosurg., to be published.
3. Banna, M. Arachnoid cysts on computed tomography. Am. J. Roentgenol. *127*:979–992 (1976).
4. Ghatak, N. R. and Mushrush, G. J. Supratentorial intra-arachnoid cyst. Case report. J. Neurosurg. *35*:477–482 (1971).
5. Geissinger, J. D., Kohler, W. C., Robinson, B. W., and Davis, F. M. Arachnoid cysts of the middle cranial fossa: surgical considerations. Surg. Neurol. *10*:27–33 (1978).
6. Smith, R. A. and Smith, W. A. Arachnoid cysts of the middle cranial fossa. Surg. Neurol., *5*:246–252, 1976.
7. Starkman, S. P., Brown, T. C., and Linell, E. A. Cerebral arachnoid cysts. J. Neuropath. Exp. Neurol. *17*:484–500 (1958).

35 Clinical Approach to Dementia

Robert Katzman, M. D.

There has been a rapidly growing interest in the dementias on the part of neurologists and psychiatrists, both as a result of the increasing public health importance of this group of diseases and because of improved knowledge and understanding of them. The dementias are, for the most part, age-related diseases, and, as a consequence, the number of patients afflicted has increased with the aging of the population. Thus, using the rough figure that 5% of those over 65 have dementia, there were approximately 150,000 cases in 1900, one million cases in 1975, and one can project that there should be over three million cases in the year 2050. Over half of the beds in our nursing homes are filled with patients suffering from dementia. At the same time, there has been improvement in our ability to diagnose the etiology of many cases of dementia and to pick out those who may have a treatable form of this disorder.

Dementia is characterized by a chronic, usually progressive, deterioration of memory and other intellectual and cognitive functions. Haase[4] has described approximately 50 diseases that may produce dementia. For our purposes, these diseases may be considered in ten classifications, as shown in Table I. The diseases listed on this table account for over 99% of the cases of dementia described both in the clinical series reported by Wells[10] and in the extensive autopsy series reported by Jellinger.[5] Although there are other diseases that may produce dementia that are not listed, these remaining entities are so infrequent as to be medical curiosities, often only single case reports.

The diseases listed in Table I are arranged in descending order of frequency. The most frequent cause of dementia, both in the presenium and in the senium, is Alzheimer's disease. Alzheimer's disease is characterized by widespread degeneration of cortical and hippocampal neurons with development of neurofibrillary tangles and senile plaques. Ultrastructurally, the most striking feature is the replacement of the normal neurofilament by pairing of two neurofilaments in a helical array and the overproliferation of these abnormal subcellular organelles in cortical and hippocampal cells. There has been a recently described and authenticated finding that the enzyme, choline acetyltransferase, the biosynthetic enzyme for acetylcholine, is decreased by about 90% early in the course of this disorder.[3] Thus, Alzheimer's is a disease that is well characterized pathologically with beginning biochemical characterization. Clinically, it presents as a slowly insidious, progressive dementia, usually with few focal neurological findings; sometimes it is associated with slowing in the basic frequencies of the EEG. In both the senium and presenium, Alzheimer's disease accounts for approximately 50–55% of all cases of dementia.

The second most common etiology of dementia, accounting for about 20–25% of cases, is vascular. Cerebral arteriosclerosis does not, by itself, produce dementia, even if quite severe. However, if there are multiple areas of dead tissue, usually amounting to over 50 g of tissue destruction as may occur in patients with multiple strokes, then dementia may begin to occur; when over 150 g of brain tissue are destroyed throughout the cerebral hemispheres, then dementia is almost always present. In many instances of vascular dementia, one may expect to find some evidence of either a history of a stroke or of focal neurological

TABLE I. *Classification of diseases producing dementia in descending order of frequency*

1. Alzheimer's disease (synonyms: senile dementia of the Alzheimer type; senile brain disease; progressive idiopathic dementia)
2. Vascular or multi-infarct dementia
    Multiple strokes
    Cortical microinfarcts
    Lacunar state
    Binswanger's disease
3. Alcoholic—Korsakoff's psychosis
4. Normal pressure hydrocephalus
5. Intracranial masses
6. Other degenerative diseases
    Huntington's chorea
    Parkinson's disease
    Pick's disease
    Olivopontocerebellar disease
    Steele-Richardson-Olszewski syndrome
7. Infectious or inflammatory diseases
    Creutzfeldt-Jakob disease
    Neurosyphilis
    Chronic meningitis, especially cryptococcal
    Postencephalitic
    Multiple sclerosis
8. Post-traumatic (and post-subarachnoid hemorrhage)
9. Chronic drug toxicity
10. Metabolic
    Pernicious anemia (B_{12} deficiency)
    Hypothyroidism
    Hyperthyroidism
    Hepatic insufficiency

findings suggesting a past stroke, but the individual strokes may be so small or located in silent areas so that it may be difficult to differentiate Alzheimer's and vascular disease clinically in a few cases.

The group of patients who develop dementia after a prolonged history of alcoholism usually present with primarily memory loss as in Korsakoff's psychosis, but, in some instances, seem to have a more generalized cognitive disorder. Normal pressure hydrocephalus is a potentially treatable syndrome,[6] characterized by gait disturbance which usually precedes cognitive changes, a usually mild dementia manifested more by psychomotor retardation and mild memory loss without language or constructional difficulties, and sometimes by incontinence. Intracranial masses, including subdural hematomas and tumors, especially those in so-called "silent" areas, may produce a clinical picture of dementia.

In Huntington's chorea, the presence of a family history and a movement disorder permits diagnosis, whereas, in Pick's disease, the syndrome is similar to that of Alzheimer's and cannot be differentiated clinically. However, Pick's disease is quite rare, and, in our experience, occurs in relationship to Alzheimer's at a ratio of one to fifty. An important syndrome is that of progressive supranuclear palsy or the Steele-Richardson-Olszewski syndrome which is characterized by extrapyramidal features, impairment of eye movements, especially vertical eye movements, and a dementia which is often similar to the dementia of normal pressure hydrocephalus, a so-called subcortical dementia. Among the infectious and inflammatory diseases, Creutzfeldt-Jakob is, by far, the most common. This disease has a more subacute course than the other dementias being considered; the initial presentation is often that of unusual psychiatric disturbances, frequently with visual illusions or hallucinations, with the subsequent development of dementia, myoclonus, cerebellar signs, periodic EEG, and, finally, coma vigil. Dementia is a frequent feature of late, progressive multiple sclerosis, and has been reported in as many as 20% of those with multiple sclerosis, although it occurs in only 1–2% of patients presenting with dementia. The categories of post-traumatic dementia and chronic drug toxicity are self-evident. Metabolic causes of dementia are surprisingly uncommon, perhaps because of the excellent diagnoses today of the metabolic disorders in general. In the Wells'[10] series of 222 patients with dementia, there was only one case with pernicious anemia, one with hepatic failure, and one each with hypothyroidism and hyperthyroidism. Thus, all of these metabolic disorders constitute only 2% of the patients with dementia. Nevertheless, because these disorders are eminently treatable, their diagnosis becomes a prime element in dementia workup.

THE DEMENTIA WORKUP

Does the Patient Have Dementia?

A surprisingly large percentage of patients referred to neurologists for the differential diagnosis of dementia do not have dementia. In the Marsden and Harrison series[8] of 106 patients referred to The National Hospital, Queen Square, for diagnosis of dementia, 12 were found to have other psychiatric conditions or not be demented. Two conditions, in particular, need to be identified. One is the depression that presents as dementia, and the other are instances of normal memory loss in the aged which is overinterpreted by the patient or his physician.

Depression or Dementia

The differential diagnosis of depression and dementia in the elderly is usually straightforward, since most depressed patients do not show changes on ordinary mental status examination. However, if a physician fails to take a mental status examination, the fact that a depressed person becomes increasingly less able to interact with his family or physician, becomes slow in all of his activities, does not care for himself or dress appropriately, etc., may be misinterpreted as dementia. In these cases, the standard mental status examination will lead to the discovery that the patient is blue and depressed and is not primarily demented. There are, however, a small number of patients who are depressed and give the appearance of being demented on mental status examination, so-called "pseudodementia." This is a difficult group to diagnose, because many patients with dementia understandably have a secondary depression. According to McHugh and Folstein,[9] a patient with a dementia secondary to depression may have a history of the onset of loss of memory and cognitive skills, but the onset is usually fairly rapid and then plateaus. Also, there is usually a past history of depression that has been treated by psychiatrists prior to the episode of pseudodementia. If there is any question, however, the patient should be given a vigorous trial of antidepressant medication to determine whether this will affect their cognitive ability.

Normal Aging (Benign Senescent Forgetfulness) versus Dementia

The normal aging process as distinct from Alzheimer's disease may include a mild, nonprogressive impairment of memory that has been called "benign senescent forgetfulness." Kral[7] has shown that this mild memory defect seen in some normals is not progressive and does not foreshadow a generalized intellectual decline. Benign senescent forgetfulness is characterized clinically by some impairment of recollection of details of an event, but not recollection of the event itself as often occurs in Alzheimer's disease. Occasionally, a normal elderly individual will seek neurological advice, fearing the approach of a senile dementia, and needs to be reassured. In a few instances, formal psychological testing may be required to confirm the fact that the memory defect is not the beginning of a more generalized decline in cognitive function.

History and Mental Status Examination

The presence of dementia is established by a history of loss of memory or cognitive functions and by confirmation of this history with a *mental status examination.* While obtaining a history from the patients, the examiner already has some idea as to whether the patient is able to speak in a normal coherent fashion. However, early in a dementia, patients may give what is apparently a rational description of themselves and a few symptoms and yet show marked defects on mental status examination. The formal part of the mental status examination involves testing of orientation, memory, calculations, information and comprehension, speech and constructional ability. A very useful test is the ability of the patient to do reversals, for example, by asking him to count from one to twenty and then from twenty to one, to give the months from January to December and then backwards, and to spell "world" backwards. Patients with dementia will frequently perceive only their face being touched when the examiner simultaneously touches their face and hand; this is termed the "facehand test," and it is a confirmatory test in demented patients.

In taking the *history*, look for:

Insidious onset; slow, relentless progression; personality changes—suggesting Alzheimer's disease.

Past history of hypertension or cardiac arrhythmias; prior "strokes" or "blackout spells"—suggesting multi-infarct dementia.

Prior history of alcoholism, especially with complications; unsteady gait; peripheral neuropathy—suggesting Korsakoff's psychosis.

Gait disturbance; general slowing; occasionally, incontinence—suggesting normal pressure hydrocephalus.

Headaches; progressive hemiparesis—suggesting a tumor.

Rapid, nonrhythmic movements of extremities or face—suggesting chorea.

Paresthesias in hands and feet together with gait disturbance—suggesting subacute combined degeneration.

Visual disturbances followed rapidly by memory disturbances, myoclonus, unsteady gait—suggesting Creuzfeldt-Jakob disease.

Physical, Neurological, and Neuro-ophthalmological Examination

Look for:

Arrhythmia, hypertension, and retinal hypertensive vascular changes predisposing to multi-infarct dementia.

Changes in skin texture and hair; slow relaxation of deep tendon reflexes—suggesting hypothyroidism.

Peripheral sensory loss and absent reflexes—suggesting nutritional deficiency or subacute combined degeneration.

Magnetic gait—suggesting normal pressure hydrocephalus.

Visual field defects; hemiparesis; reflex asymmetries—suggesting multiple strokes.

Absence of vertical eye movements; rigidity—suggesting progressive supranuclear palsy.

Argyll Robertson pupils—suggesting general paresis.

Papilledema—suggesting intracranial mass lesion.

Extensor flap or asterixis—suggesting hepatic insufficiency.

Special Tests (See Table II)

The most important test used today in the differential diagnosis of dementia and the one with the highest yield is the CT scan. It should be emphasized that the CT scan is used specifically for the diagnosis of hydrocephalus (and if hydrocephalus is present, additional tests such as isotope cisternography must be used to determine the nature of the hydrocephalus), intracranial mass lesions, and old infarcts. Rarely, the CT scan may be diagnostic of the plaques of multiple sclerosis. In the instances described above, the CT scan is of great importance. The remaining group of diseases, however, which includes Alzheimer's disease, other degenerative and inflammatory diseases, drug toxicities, and metabolic diseases, cannot be diagnosed on CT scan. It should be emphasized that although there is probably a small degree of overall atrophy of the cerebral cortex in Alzheimer's disease, the brain does change in size with normal aging, and a report of mild atrophy in an older individual is not, by itself, diagnostic of Alzheimer's. The EKG listed in Table II is a recent addition to our tests required for the differential diagnosis of dementia. It has been demonstrated recently that cardiac arrhythmias unequivocally predispose towards cerebral emboli and quite probably towards multi-infarct dementia.[1] The features on the EKG therefore of interest are those of an arrhythmia or those of a bundle branch block or other changes suggesting the possibility of a conduction defect sufficiently grave to lead to paroxysmal bradycardia. The electroencephalogram is a potent tool in the

TABLE II. *Workup for the differential diagnosis of a dementia*[a]

By the examiner
History
Mental status examination
Physical examination
Neurological examination
(including neuro-ophthalmological examination)
Special tests
CT scan
Chest x-ray
EKG
EEG
Blood
CBC; metabolic screen; thyroid profile; B_{12} level; VDRL
Psychometric evaluation

[a] Modified from Wells.[10]

diagnosis of dementia. In conditions such as Creutzfeldt-Jakob disease, very characteristic changes, including the occurrence of periodic complexes, are almost diagnostic. In Alzheimer's disease, there is usually a slowing of the EEG, with the normal 10/sec rhythm decreasing in frequency and with the appearance of 5–7/sec activity as the disease progresses. In a follow-up of a series of Alzheimer patients whom we had published in 1973,[2] we discovered two misdiagnoses among our 20 reported patients; in both instances, these were patients with normal EEG's, whereas the other 18 patients all had some evidence of slowing in their EEG's.

The blood examination permits the determination of the presence of neurosyphilis, B_{12} deficiency, thyroid abnormality, hepatic or renal insufficiency, or other metabolic changes that may predispose to dementia.

Finally, psychometric examination is often useful in difficult cases in establishing the presence, for example, of a primary memory defect as in Korsakoff's, in separating the cortical from the subcortical dementias, and in following the course of a dementia over a period of time.

EDITOR'S NOTE

Dr. Katzman has given us a very useful outline of the clinical approach to a patient with dementia. I'd like to simply add three points: (1) a serum FTA-ABS test is advisable as well as a routine VDRL, in my opinion, to detect cases of seronegative late syphilis; (2) Jakob-Creutzfeldt disease is one of those diseases that is so rare that when you diagnose it, you can rest assured you'll usually be wrong! However, there are two pearls about Jakob-Creutzfeldt that should be mentioned: (1) Dr. Goldhammer told me that in Jakob-Creutzfeldt disease— "The *EEG* turned into an *EKG!*" In other words, his mnemonic for remembering that a rather specific change in the electroencephalogram occurred in this disease is that the EEG can actually look like the appearance of the routine electrocardiogram. The second point is that Jakob-Creutzfeldt disease has been transmitted in man by corneal transplantation so that one should not

use corneal or ocular material from patients dying with dementia for eye surgery. The final point is that patients with progressive supranuclear palsy nearly always have inability to look down as one of their first complaints. Thus, they have difficulty reading, eating, walking down stairs, and the like. A helpful thing to try in these patients is a pair of "Bed-Specs." Have the patient make out a check for $19.80 to Selsi Company, Inc., 40 Veterans Blvd., Carlstadt, N. J. 07072 and ask them to send him a pair of their catalog #228 "Bed-Specs" and these will be forthcoming in about six weeks. The patient can look out straight ahead through these glasses and can see what they are eating below. Many patients with progressive supranuclear palsy like them, and if they don't, they still haven't been hurt too much financially. The price listed was that given in the Selsi Catalog I received in September 1978 and obviously may change a bit later. That is a helpful point to patients who cannot look down, however.

JLS

REFERENCES

General References

Katzman, R. Dementias. Postgrad. Med. *64:*119–125 (1978).

Katzman, R. (Ed.). *Congenital and Acquired Cognitive Disorders.* Research Publications, Association for Research in Nervous and Mental Disease, Vol. 57. Raven Press, New York, 1979.

Katzman, R., Terry, R. D., and Bick, K. L. (Eds.). *Aging, Vol. 7: Alzheimer's Disease: Senile Dementia and Related Disorders.* Raven Press, New York, 1978.

Wells, C. E. (Ed.). *Dementia.* 2nd ed. F. A. Davis Co., Philadelphia, 1977.

Bibliography

1. Abdon, N.-J. Unrecognized intermittent bradycardias in patients treated for senile dementia. In: *Cardiac Pacing,* Proc. of the Symp., Excerpta Medica. Y. Watanabe (Ed.), Elsevier, Amsterdam, The Netherlands, 1977, pp. 93–101.

2. Coblentz, J. M., Mattis, S., Zingesser, L. H., Kasoff, S. S., Wisniewski, H. M. and Katzman, R. Presenile Dementia. Clinical Aspects and Evaluation of Cerebrospinal Fluid Dynamics. Arch. Neurol. *29:* 299–308 (1973).

3. Davies, P.: Biochemical changes in Alzheimer's disease-senile dementia: Neurotransmitters in senile dementia of the Alzheimer's type. In: *Congenital and Acquired Cognitive Disorders.* Research Publications, Association for Research in Nervous and Mental Disease, Vol. 57. R. Katzman, (Ed.), Raven Press, New York, 1979, pp. 153–160.

4. Haase, G. R. Diseases Presenting as Dementia. In: *Dementia*. 2nd ed. C. E. Wells (Ed.), F. A. Davis Co., Philadelphia, 1977, pp. 27–68.
5. Jellinger, K. Neuropathological aspects of dementia resulting from abnormal blood and cerebrospinal fluid dynamics. Acta Neurol. Belg. 76:83–102 (1976).
6. Katzman, R. Normal pressure hydrocephalus. In: *Dementia*. 2nd ed. C. E. Wells (Ed.), F. A. Davis Co., Philadelphia, 1977, pp. 69–92.
7. Kral, V. A. Senescent forgetfulness: Benign and malignant. Can. Med. Assoc. J. 86:257–260 (1972).
8. Marsden, C. D. and Harrison, M. J. G. Outcome of investigation of patients with presenile dementia. Br. Med. J. 2:249–252 (1972).
9. McHugh, P. R. and Folstein, M. F. Psychopathology of dementia: Implications for neuropathology. In: *Congenital and Acquired Cognitive Disorders*. Research Publications, Association for Research in Nervous and Mental Disease, Vol. 57. R. Katzman (Ed.), Raven Press, New York, 1979, pp. 17–30.
10. Wells, C. E. Diagnostic evaluation and treatment in dementia. In: *Dementia*. 2nd ed. C. E. Wells (Ed.), F. A. Davis Co., Philadelphia, 1977, pp. 247–276.

36 Recent Advances in Thyroid Disease

Norman G. Schneeberg, M. D.

We owe much of our recent knowledge of thyroid physiology and thyroid disease to the application of radioimmunoassay (RIA), which permits the accurate and rapid determination of blood levels of thyroid-stimulating hormone (TSH), thyroxine (T_4), and triiodothyronine (T_3). The recent availability of injectable thyrotrophic releasing hormone (TRH) has offered a further refinement in thyroid diagnosis.

THYROID STIMULATING HORMONE (TSH)

There is a sensitive homeostatic feedback relationship between TSH, the pituitary hormone that maintains thyroid function, and T_4 and T_3, the thyroid hormones whose synthesis and secretion depend upon TSH. The sensitivity of this control mechanism is so exquisite that even a minimal reduction of T_4 and T_3 results in a reciprocal increase of TSH. In patients whose thyroid effective mass has been reduced by subtotal thyroidectomy, radioiodine irradiation, or chronic thyroiditis, T_4 and T_3 may be so minimally reduced as to remain within the normal range, but TSH becomes elevated. The patient remains clinically euthyroid. This sequence of events has been called "progressive thyroid failure," the inference being that the elevated TSH is a warning that a clinical state of hypothyroidism is probably inevitable. Opinion is divided as to the ultimate fate of these patients. Some thyroid experts would immediately institute substitution therapy with sodium l-thyroxine whereas others would prefer to withhold therapy until the serum T_4 becomes subnormal and the patient exhibits some clinical evidence of hypothyroidism.

Serum TSH is now regarded as the most sensitive laboratory test of hypothyroidism, being unequivocally elevated in hypothyroidism due to primary thyroid insufficiency, and low or indeterminant in hypothyroidism from anterior pituitary insufficiency (i.e., TSH deficiency). The determination of TSH has also proved of great value in screening programs for the detection of congenital hypothyroidism.[1] Infant heel-stick blood is absorbed on filter paper and tested for T_4 and TSH. The yield in North America has been one hypothyroid newborn per 6,000 live births, a frequency more than twice that for phenylketonuria.

THE THYROTROPHIN-RELEASING HORMONE (TRH) TEST

One of the more momentous achievements of modern endocrinology has been the elucidation of the structure of TRH reported almost simultaneously in 1962 by Guillemin *et al.*[2] and Bøler *et al.*[3] TRH proved to be an unexpectedly simple compound; it is a weakly basic tripeptide, L-pyroglutamyl–L-histidyl–L-proline amide. Synthesis was therefore readily accomplished, and large amounts of TRH became available for research. Roger Guillemin and Andrew Schally shared half the 1977 Nobel Prize in Medicine for their role in this endocrine saga.

TRH* has recently been released for clinical use.

Naturally occurring TRH is concentrated principally in the median eminence of the hypothalamus, traverses the pituitary portal circulation and stimulates the pituitary thyrotrophes to synthesize and secrete

* Protirelin (Thypinone-Abbott Labs.).

TSH. It is employed in a test to gauge endogenous stores of pituitary TSH. A bolus of 500 μg of TRH is injected intravenously and serum TSH is measured at intervals thereafter. A 30-min TSH value usually suffices, but TSH can be measured at 60 and 120 min in addition, as illustrated in Fig. 1. In normal subjects TSH rises 5–30 uU/ml to a peak value in 15–45 min whereas there is no rise in anterior pituitary insufficiency. In thyroid insufficiency the TSH increase is quantitatively large and proceeds from an already elevated baseline value. It is clearly superfluous in obvious cases of primary hypothyroidism, but in a situation where the T_4 is subnormal and the TSH is in an equivocal range, i.e., 5–10 uU/ml a brisk reponse to TRH stimulation will clearly indicate primary hypothyroidism; failure to respond will be typical of pituitary insufficiency. The TRH test has revealed a third variety of hypothyroidism, namely that from a TRH deficiency or "hypothalamic hypothyroidism." The TSH rise is usually adequate but delayed (see Fig. 1). Like all other laboratory tests the TRH test is not invariably accurate and may occasionally be misleading. Several instances have been described of absent TSH response in patients with a hypothalamic disorder, and in others a definite TSH response in patients with hypopituitarism.

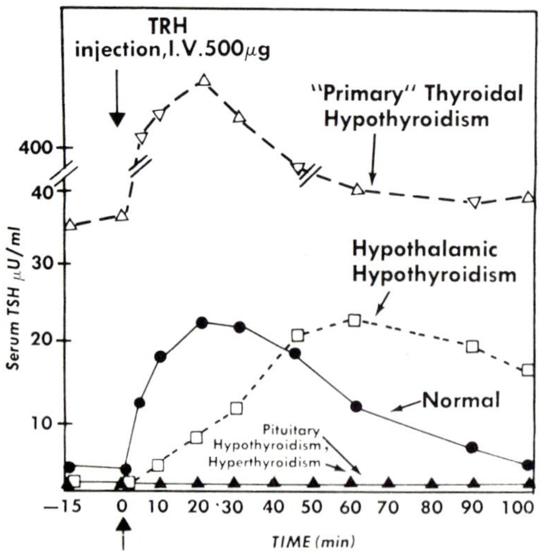

Fig. 1. From Figure 1, *Thyroid Consultation*, Vol. III, No. 2, May 1974. With permission of James A. Pittman, M. D., and Science and Medicine Publishing Co., Inc.

In hyperthyroidism TSH is low or zero and does not respond to TRH stimulation. The TRH test thus is of value in patients where the diagnosis of hyperthyroidism is vague or in doubt and may supplant the more conventional T_3 suppression test.

TRIIODOTHYRONINE (T_3)

T_3 was discovered in 1952 by Gross and Pitt-Rivers.[4] Its plasma level is 1/75 that of T_4, but its calorigenic activity is fourfold. Physiologists have argued for years concerning the relative biologic importance of T_3 and T_4, and there is considerable evidence to suggest that T_3 is the principle hormone with T_4 acting as a prehormone or precursor of T_3. Substantial support for this viewpoint derives from the observation that about 80% of circulating T_3 arises from the peripheral deiodination of T_4 (Fig. 2) and only 20% is derived from direrct thyroidal secretion. In states of altered thyroid function such as Graves' disease and iodide deficiency the thyroid contribution of T_3 is markedly increased. T_3-thyrotoxicosis is the most striking portrayal of the preferential secretion of T_3 wherein serum T_4, resin-T_3-uptake, free-thyroxine index, and thyroxine-binding-globulin all remain within normal limits in a patient with hyperthyroidism. The serum T_3 alone is elevated. Thyroidal radioiodine accumulation is increased and is not suppressed by the administration of thyroid hormone, findings typical of classical thyrotoxicosis. T_3-thyrotoxicosis has been found both in Graves' disease and in toxic nodular goiter. It is not a rare event; Hollander *et al.*[5] encountered this disorder in 4% of their hyperthyroid patients in New York City, but in Chile, an area of iodide deficiency where preferential T_3 secretion is expected, the frequency was 12.5%.

If there is a pure T_3-thyrotoxicosis, might we expect to find pure T_4-thyrotoxicosis? Such cases have been reported usually in sick thyrotoxic patients and in several otherwise well thyrotoxics. It is presumed that there is impaired T_4 to T_3 peripheral conversion, a phenomenon that is often found in sick hospitalized euthyroid patients and has come to be known as the "low-T_3 syndrome." In these individuals serum T_4 usu-

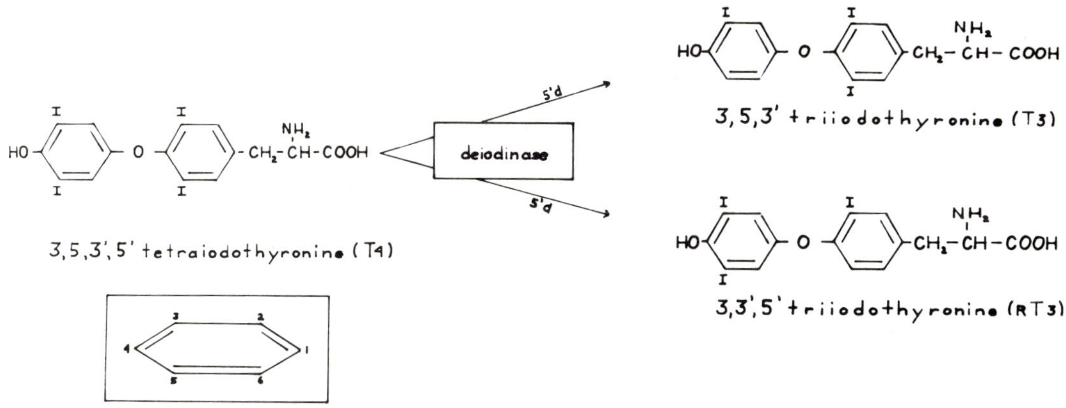

Fig. 2. The peripheral deiodination of T_4 to T_3 and reverse-T_3 (rT_3).

ally remains normal or is slightly reduced, TSH is in the normal range, and the patient does not exhibit signs of hypothyroidism. The common denominator of the low-T_3 syndrome is caloric deprivation especially for carbohydrates in the course of disseminated malignancy, infections, extensive surgery, other serious diseases, and starvation states. It is reversible if restoration of good nutrition is accomplished. In human amniotic fluid and in cord blood the T_3/rT_3 ratio is also considerably reduced. With parturition and after the physiologic rise of TSH that occurs, T_3 begins to rise reaching a peak in 48 hours. Reverse-T_3, however, also remains elevated until the fifth day when it commences its decline. Thus there is no constant ratio of T_3/rT_3 in all situations. Serum T_3 can be lowered by dexamethasone, ACTH, propylthiouracil, and propranolol.

In 1974 Chopra[6] devised a radioimmunoassay for reverse-T_3 (rT_3), a compound that differs from T_3 only in the shift of one iodine atom from the inner to the outer phenolic ring of T_3, as shown in Figure 2. In the majority of sick patients with low T_3 a proportionate increase of rT_3 occurs. Since rT_3 is biologically almost inactive, one may reasonably infer that this is a defense mechanism to protect sick tissues from excessive metabolic stimulation. The serum level of rT_3, usually about ⅓ to ¼ that of T_3 in healthy individuals, is increased in hyperthyroidism and decreased in hypothyroidism.

HYPERTHYROIDISM

There has been little progress in the past decade in elucidating the cause of Graves' disease. It has been established beyond doubt that TSH is not the responsible agent. Graves' disease presents many characteristics common to autoimmune diseases, such as thyroid-stimulating antibodies, thyroid-sensitized lymphocytes, lymphoid hyperplasia of thymus, lymph nodes, and the thyroid gland. A number of thyroid-stimulating immunoglobulins have been identified that may play a role in the induction of thyroid hypersecretion. The first thyroid stimulator thought to play a causative role in Graves' hyperthyroidism was called long-acting thyroid stimulator (LATS) since its action in stimulating guinea pig thyroids was delayed compared to the time sequence of TSH. LATS was found to be an immunoglobulin G (IgG), and, since Graves' appears to be an autoimmune disease, LATS was thought to be the, or at least, an important etiologic factor. Doubt was later cast on its importance because it could only be detected in some 60–80% of cases and its titre did not parallel the clinical course of Graves' disease. Since the discovery of LATS a number of other thyroid-stimulating IgG-fractions have been described. One intriguing fraction has been called LATS-protector (LATS-P), a substance that prevents LATS neutralization in thyroid gland homogenates, and has been found in a very large percentage of cases of Graves' disease. Another substance called human thyroid stimulator (HTS) stimulates the thyroid of humans but not those of experimental animals. It may well be that all these fractions are more or less identical, depending upon the system used to test their activity, and indeed the term "thyroid-stimulating immunoglobulins (ITSI)" has been employed to encompass all those IgG fractions.

One working hypothesis of the cause of Graves' disease is as follows:

The thyroid stimulator accomplishes its action by attaching to a TSH receptor on the thyroid cell. Graves' disease may be a defect in cell mediated immunity (CMI) that can be inherited as a genetic defect in immune surveillance. Persisting mutated T-lymphocytes that have escaped normal control because of a presumed genetic defect might give rise to forbidden clones of cells which, with the cooperation of B-lymphocytes, produce certain thyroid stimulating immunoglobulins.[7]

Jodbasedow, or iodine-precipitated thyrotoxicosis, has been known for more than a century. A considerable literature has accumulated describing hyperthyroidism following the use of iodides in the treatment of endemic goiter, from iodide-containing drugs or iodide-containing organic dyes in cholecystography and urography. One of the more recent reports[8] described hyperthyroidism appearing in four of eight patients in Boston who volunteered to be subjects of a study of the effects of iodide on thyroid hormone synthesis. Lividas *et al.*[9] found a rising serum T_4 and T_3 in patients with autonomous thyroid nodules who were given small doses of potassium iodide for three weeks. Half of the patients who were originally euthyroid showed signs of hyperthyroidism. The mechanism of Jodbasedow is unknown but, because of its rarity, one may infer that patients who become hyperthyroid must have some preexisting thyroid defect such as inactive Graves' disease. Since the synthesis of T_4 and T_3 requires available iodide, an iodide deficiency may have existed which prevented the spontaneous onset of hyperthyroidism; when iodide was supplied, thyroid hormone synthesis was abruptly accelerated to provide excessive hormone to the circulation. A related observation is that the rate of recurrence of hyperthyroidism arrested with antithyroid drugs seems to be directly proportional to the amount of available iodide. Hence patients in remission from hyperthyroidism are now warned to avoid iodides.

TREATMENT OF HYPERTHYROIDISM

When the cause of a disorder is unknown, treatment is often empiric, crude, and inexact. Until the fundamental etiology is unmasked, the treatment of hyperthyroidism must be directed primarily to reduce the excessive production and secretion of thyroid hormone rather than to the control of the primary cause. In the past three or more decades the choices of treatment have been, (1) to inhibit the formation of thyroid hormone with an antithyroid drug, (2) to remove thyroid tissue surgically, or (3) to destroy it with radioactive iodine. The selection of one of these methods in an individual case depends upon certain guidelines that have been generally accepted by thyroidologists and depend upon such factors as the age of the patient, degree of toxicity, size and nature of the goiter, and the presence of complicating medical illnesses such as heart disease. The only therapeutic refinement in the past decade has been the use of propranolol, a beta-adrenergic receptor blocker that reliably and effectively controls the sympathomimetic features of hyperthyroidism such as tachycardia, atrial arrhythymias, sweating, tremor, and hyperkinesis. Propranolol accomplishes this without altering thyroid function albeit there is some reduction in the production of T_3 from the deiodination of T_4. The patient so treated becomes clinically almost euthyroid but remains chemically hyperthyroid. It has been a life-saving drug in thyroid crisis rapidly reducing extreme tachycardia, hyperkinesis, and agitation. It has also been useful as a second line of pharmacologic attack in patients intolerant to antithyroid drugs, can be used alone or in conjunction with iodides in the preparation of hyperthyroid patients for thyroid surgery, and controls toxicity before and after radioiodine treatment. Propranolol is very useful to control thyrotoxic symptoms prior to and during thyroid laboratory studies because it does not alter the blood levels of thyroid hormones or the radioiodine uptake. The introduction of additional antithyroid drugs would be an important therapeutic advance. At present the physician only has propranolol, iodides, propylthiouracil, methylthiouracil, and methimazole for drug treatment. Carbimazole has not been approved by the FDA for use in the United States though it is widely used in Great Britain. The frequency of sensitivity reactions to antithyroid drugs appears to be on the increase. Lithium, a known goitrogen, has antithyroid properties and has been used in the treatment of hyperthyroidism[10] but has not had a widespread trial.

Antithyroid drugs were introduced in 1943 by Astwood[11] and have been used since then in selected cases for long-term therapy of hyperthyroidism and in the preparation of thyrotoxic patients for thyroidectomy. Because of their limited duration of effect the daily dose has been given in divided doses. The possibility of successful control with a single daily dose was explored by Greer *et al.*[12] and found to be effective in many cases. Greer *et al.*[13] have also challenged the rationale of the orthodox empiric selection of one year or longer for treatment of thyrotoxic patients with antithyroid drugs to insure a subsequent long term remission. Twelve of 31 patients remained in remission when the drug was stopped at or shortly after they became euthyroid, the average duration of treatment being 4½ months. They concluded that the long-term remission rate was as good with this program in many patients as when the treatment was continued for one or more years.

RADIOIODINE TREATMENT OF HYPERTHYROIDISM

The majority of patients (i.e., 80%) with hyperthyroidism are currently treated with radioiodine. Post-radiation hypothyroidism remains the only significant and apparently unavoidable adverse effect. Attempts to reduce the dose of ^{131}I to avoid this complication merely delayed its onset but added the discomfort of persistant hyperthyroid-ism for a longer post-radiation interval than occurred with larger and more orthodox doses. Trials of ^{125}I, a less penetrating isotope, produced similar results. Current thinking now advocates using full ^{131}I dosage to treat hyperthyroidism combined with careful follow-up for many years to detect post-radiation hypothyroidism. Some thyroidologists prefer to have all their patients start on thyroxine therapy once they become euthyroid reasoning that within 10 years after treatment some 40–50% will become hypothyroid anyway. This program does not obviate the need for long-term monitoring of these patients since adherance to any prolonged therapeutic program is undependable. Hedley[14] found that 15% of patients who became hypothyroid after thyroidectomy had stopped taking thyroid medication and an additional 54% were taking a suboptimal dose. Meticulous follow-up by physicians and departments of nuclear medicine must be pursued in an attempt to avoid the ravages of untreated myxedema.

OPHTHALMOPATHY

The ophthalmopathy of Graves' disease has customarily been classifed as (1) "mild" or "noninfiltrative" and (2) "severe" or "infiltrative." The mild form is manifested by stare, upper-lid retraction and lid-lag. It is benign, usually nonprogressive and ordinarily reversible with treatment of the underlying Graves' hyperthyroidism. In the severe form there is infiltration and edema of the retro-orbital space, extraocular muscles, conjunctiva, and adjacent eyelid structures. It can progress to ophthalmoplegia, corneal damage, and optic nerve involvement. Its severity may not parallel the severity of the hyperthyroid state and in fact has been observed in euthyroid patients and rarely in myxedema. It may even worsen with improvement of hyperthyroidism. In some patients the ophthalmopathy may present features of both the mild and severe forms, and there may occasionally be progression from one to the other. This suggests that the dual classification is inaccurate and that the two forms merely represent different stages of the same disease. About ten years ago a reclassification of the eye changes of Graves' disease was devised by a committee of the American Thyroid Association. Table I is an abridgement as modified in 1977.[15]

A more detailed descriptive classification is included in the same article.[15] Class 1 conforms to the older designation "mild, noninfiltrative" and Classes 2–6 to the "severe infiltrative" variety. Proptosis in excess of 22 mm, even without symptoms, belongs in Class 3. The upper limit of normal for euthyroid Japanese is 18 mm, and for blacks, 22 mm or less. With myopia, proptosis greater than 22 mm can occur in normal individuals.

The increased orbital content of Graves' disease consists of enlarged extraocular muscles and increase in fat, connective tissue, hyaluronic acid and ground substance, water, and enlarged lacrimal glands. However, it has become apparent that the major component is the swollen extraocular muscles which may increase as much as eight- to tenfold. Werner *et al.*[16] found evidence of orbital involvement, particularly of the muscles, in 44 of 47 patients with Graves' disease even though 30 were in Classes 0–1. This finding of constant involvement of the orbit suggested a common pathologic mechanism in all varieties of ophthalmopathy and also demonstrated that orbital involvement could be detected by ultrasonography in most cases of Graves' disease even when there was no clinical evidence of ophthalmopathy.

The cause of Graves' ophthalmopathy remains an enigma. Classes 0 and 1 occur in toxic nodular goiter and other forms of hyperthyroidism but 2–6 are found exclusively in Graves'. It is therefore probable that the eye change of Classes 0 and 1 are direct affects of T_4 and T_3 on the eye and the eyelids and are principally due to stimulation of the sympathetic innervation of the eyelids; Classes 2–6 add to this effect some other thyroid stimulating agent that acts upon both the thyroid gland and the eye and orbital structures. Why does the clinical course of ophthalmopathy in Classes 2–6 often fail to parallel the severity of the hyperthyroid state? Why does it sometimes worsen after treatment particularly when radioiodine has been employed? Two hypotheses have emerged in recent years to explain its pathophysiology. The one proposed by Kriss and his coworkers at Stanford[17] is in brief as follows: Thyroglobulin (Tg) continually leaks from the hyperplastic thyroid acini into lymphatics and is transferred to cervical lymph nodes. Anti-Tg antibody may be synthesized by lymphocytes within the node or within the thyroid. Retrograde lymph flow from the thyroid to the orbit has been postulated by Kriss based on evidence derived from radioisotopic thyroidolymphangiograms. ^{131}I-Tg injected into the thyroid gland was found to migrate cephalad into the superior cervical lymph nodes. Isotopes injected into extraocular muscles migrated caudad into these same nodes, indicating the potential pathway from thyroid to orbit.

Tg arriving at the orbit attaches to extraocular muscles. Tg-complexes become fixed to these muscles, and immune complexes produce muscle injury. The other theory is that of Kohn and Winand's group,[18] who visualize a reaction between an abnormal serum immunoglobulin with TSH or an exophthalmos-producing factor (EPS) derived from TSH but lacking thyroid stimulating properties. These two factors stimulate retro-orbital tissue to synthesize glycosamino-glycans, accumulate fluid, and push the globe forward. Tg-sensitized lymphocytes might react with Tg bound to extraocular muscles membrane. Thymus-derived lymphocytes (T-cells) elaborate cytotoxins and leucocyte migration inhibition factors (MIF). The cytotoxins may damage the muscle, and MIF decreasing leucocyte mobility might explain the round cell infiltration of orbital connective tissue. MIF is indicative of delayed hypersensitivity and

TABLE I.

Class[a]	Definition
0	No physical signs or symptoms
1	Only signs, no symptoms (limited to upper lid retraction, stare, lid lag)
2	Soft-tissue involvement (symptoms and signs)
3	Proptosis
4	Extraocular muscle involvement
5	Corneal involvement
6	Sight loss (optic nerve involvement)

[a] Each class usually, but not necessarily, includes the involvements in the preceding class.

is present in the serum of patients with Graves' disease. Muller *et al.*[18] showed that Tg or a related substance is present in human retro-orbital tissue. An anti-Tg reactive material was associated with extraocular muscle, and tissue homogenates obtained from the muscle were more effective antigens in the MIF assay than other orbital tissues.

It is fortunate that the severe expressions of Graves' ophthalmopathy are quite rare comprising less than 5% of patients with eye involvement since the available therapeutic measures leave much to be desired. They include local protection of the cornea, use of corticosteroids and diuretics, and surgery to correct persistent diplopia or to produce orbital decompression. In 1973 Donaldson, Bagshaw, and Kriss[19] described the use of orbital irradiation with a collimated high energy x-ray beam generated by a linear accelerator. Their aim was to selectively irradiate the swollen extraocular muscles in an attempt to ablate the sensitized lymphocytes responsible for the immune reaction. Their results in 44 patients were excellent in 13, good in 14, fair in 11 and no response in six; no patient was made worse. Confirmation of this work by others is awaited with interest.

One of the more interesting varieties of Graves' disease occurring with opthalmopathy has been called "euthyroid Graves" because hyperthyroidism is absent. It is not a rare circumstance; Hall[20] found 12 examples among 345 of his hyperthyroid cases. The usual laboratory indices of thyroid function are normal though occasional slight elevations of serum T_3 have been described. The thyroidal accumulation of radioiodine is usually normal, but in somewhat more than half the cases it is nonsuppressible and there is no TSH response to TRH stimulation, reactions typical of active Graves' hyperthyroidism. Antithyroid antibodies and thyroid stimulating immunoglobulins are also demonstrable in half of the cases. Fox and Schwartz[21] found coexisting chronic autoimmune thyroiditis (Hashimoto's) in 24 of 28 of their cases of euthyroid Graves' and reasoned that the absence of hyperthyroidism was because there was a deficiency of thyroid tissue capable of responding to a thyroid stimu-

lator. Solomon *et al.*[22] studied 17 patients with euthyroid Graves' in an attempt to identify any differences among them that could permit separation into groups. Six of their patients, classified as Group 1, showed significant titers of LATS-protector, thyroid nonsuppressibility, and antithyroid antibodies which would tend to confirm the ideas of Fox and Schwartz because these six patients combined Graves' ophthalmopathy with Hashimoto's thyroiditis and reacted as did patients with Graves' hyperthyroidism. They were not hyperthyroid because thyroid damage rendered the gland insensitive to the thyroid-stimulating IgG. Five other patients, their Group 3, showed no other evidence of Graves' disease. There was no LATS-protector, the thyroid was normally suppressible, and thyroid antibodies were absent. Solomon *et al.* speculated that perhaps these patients had a single autoimmune disease, an "isolated Graves' ophthalmopathy," with a perfectly normal thyroid gland.

SUBACUTE THYROIDITIS WITH TRANSIENT HYPERTHYROIDISM

Patients with subacute thyroiditis usually present with a tender goiter, low radioiodine uptake, and an elevated erythrocyte sedimentation rate. In about 25% of patients, circulating levels of T_4 and T_3, released into the circulation by the damaged disrupted thyroid follicles, reach a sufficient concentration to cause signs of hyperthyroidism that may last several weeks. Subacute thyroiditis is a self-limited disease, and the hyperthyroidism is transient. Recently a number of cases of hyperthyroidism associated either with a painless goiter or no thyroid enlargement at all have been reported. The disorder has been seen in a number of postpartum women. The clinical and laboratory findings otherwise conform to subacute thyroiditis and were brought to medical attention by finding low-radioiodine thyroid uptake with hyperthyroidism. In a number of similar cases chronic lymphocytic thyroiditis was found on thyroid biopsy. Jackson[23] suggested using the diagnostic term "hyper-thyroiditis" so as to include both cases of subacute and chronic thyroiditis in patients with the syndrome of "low-uptake-thyrotoxicosis-with-painless-thyroiditis." Recognition of this form of transient hyperthyroidism is essential because the usual methods of treating hyperthyroidism, i.e., antithyroid drugs, surgery, or radioiodine, are contraindicated. It adds another category in differential diagnosis when one encounters the rare combination of hyperthyroidism with low-radioiodine uptake. Other causes are exogenous iodides, thyrotoxicosis factitia, ectopic thyroid location (lingual, struma ovarii), and hyperfunctioning metastatic thyroid cancer.

HYPOTHYROIDISM

For many years clinicians have been able to choose from a variety of available thyroid hormone preparations as substitution therapy for hypothyroidism. These have included (1) Thyroid USP (desiccated thyroid), (2) Thyroglobulin from porcine thyroid glands (Proloid), (3) Sodium l-triiodothyronine (Cytomel), (4) Sodium l-thyroxine (Synthroid, Letter), (5) Liotrix, a synthetic 4:1 mixture of T_4 and T_3 (Thyrolar, Euthroid), and (6) Sodium d-thyroxine (Choloxin). In equivalent doses they all provide replacement therapy in thyroid insufficiency. However, in recent years sodium l-thyroxine has been favored by most physicians. It is a uniformly reliable synthetic product and therefore not subject to variation in potency. It lacks T_3, a deficiency once considered to be a theoretical drawback but now viewed as desirable because of its smoother more uniform effect on body metabolism and upon blood levels of T_4 and T_3. Its final acceptance as the agent of choice stems from the demonstration that fully 80% of circulating T_3 is derived not from thyroidal secretion but from peripheral deiodination of T_4. Hence the adminsitration of sodium l-thyroxine to athyroidal individuals promotes the attainment of normal blood levels of T_4 as well as T_3 and avoids the transient peaks of T_3 that often reached thyrotoxic levels when agents containing T_3 (all the above preparations except l- and d-thyroxine) were used. The average dose of sodium l-thyroxine required for replacement therapy in hypothyroid patients is from 100–200 μg daily. In rare patients, too hypersensitive to sodium l-thyroxine to tolerate therapeutic doses, sodium d-thyroxine can often be substituted. It is an effective agent in the treatment of hypothyroidism[24] and often causes less cardiovascular stimulation.

THYROID CANCER

In recent years the recognition that exposure of the thyroid gland to x-ray irradiation is associated with an increased incidence of thyroid nodularity and thyroid cancer has provoked a great deal of publicity in the lay press. Prior to 1960 x-ray treatment of infants for thymic enlargement, resistant bronchitis or pertussis, recurrent tonsillitis, cervical lymphadenitis, eczema, tinea capitis, and the treatment of adolescents for acne exposed the thyroid gland to potentially carcinogenic radiation. The subject has become an important public health problem and was the topic of a workshop in Bethesda, Maryland in September 1975,[25] and a second workshop held at the University of Chicago on September 30 to October 1976.[26] The x-ray dose bears a direct relationship to the development of thyroid nodules and cancer.[27] A dose of only 6.5 rads to the thyroid received during scalp irradiation for tinea capitis resulted in a cancer incidence of 0.1% compared to 0.02% in untreated siblings. With doses of 400–1500 rads nodular goiter was found in 27–40% and thyroid cancer in 5–9%. Larger doses caused less cancer probably because it was destructive to the thyroid nucleus. Numerous recall programs have been initiated throughout the country,[26] and physicians in practice have been alerted to aid in the search for these individuals at risk for thyroid cancer.

Needle biopsy of a thyroid nodule to refine the search for malignancy has had a revival principally since the report by Wang and his associates from the Massachusetts General Hospital.[28] Wang and others favor using a large Vim-Silverman or similar needle which extracts a core of tissue that improves the accuracy of pathologic diagnosis. Others prefer a fine needle with repetitive suction-aspiration and spreading the aspirate on slides. The pathologist must then depend on the examination of isolated cells or groups of cells, a more difficult task and in many hands a less accurate method. Needle biopsy is an office procedure that offers an additional modality in the study of the thyroid nodule.

ULTRASOUND

Ultrasound scanning of the thyroid is now a well-established procedure for the study of thyroid nodules. It very effectively can distinguish cystic from solid nodules, though it cannot differentiate malignant from benign nodules. A new technique, gray-scale ultrasonography, at first gave promise of being able to make this differentiation, but further experience has failed to substantiate the early enthusiasm.[29] Ultrasound has provided visual guidance in the aspiration of thyroid nodules. It is also helpful in estimations of the size of the thyroid gland and in serial study of nodules or goiters during suppressive therapy. Since it does not expose the patients to radiation and has no known harmful effects, it may be repeated as often as desired. Ultrasound studies of the orbit in ophthalmopathy has already been discussed.

EDITOR'S NOTE

I am continually amazed to see the difference in incidence of the syndrome of "euthyroid Graves' disease" in reports emanating from endocrinologists as compared to the patients that present to ophthalmologists. The great majority of middle-aged adults presenting with either pathologic lid retraction or acquired vertical diplopia at distance due to a tight inferior rectus muscle (simulating limitation of a superior rectus) are essentially euthyroid—clinically and chemically. Indeed, both the Werner suppression test and the TRH (thypinone) test give normal results in at least half of the patients that we see. We are thus left with a clinical diagnosis in many of these patients. It is hoped that a greater awareness of the frequency of the euthyroid state in overt thyroid ocular disease will spill over to the internists, for often the patient is caught between two opinions. The internist finding a normal thyroid function battery will state that there is no thyroid problem. The ophthalmologist encountering the classical clinical eye signs will state unequivocally—"euthyroid Graves' disease." This chapter by Dr. Schneeberg is helpful in keeping us up to date with current thyroidology. However, the diagnosis of thyroid eye disease still is a clinical one and many, many of these patients can be helped by the ophthalmologist who will take the time.

The NOSPECS classification seen in Table I has not been particularly helpful to me. Many patients have symptoms but no signs (opposite to class one). Many present with tight inferior rectus syndromes (without preceding stages). Dry eyes are not mentioned. A better classification hopefully will be forthcoming on the eye side.

JLS

REFERENCES

1. Fisher, D. A., Burrow, G. N., and Dussault, J. H., *et al.* Recommendations for screening programs for congenital hypothyroidism. Report of a committee of the American Thyroid Association. Am. J. Med. *61:*932 (1976).
2. Guillemin, R., Yamazaki, E., Jutisz, M., and Sakiz, E. Presence dans un extract des tissus hypothalamiques d'une substance stimulant la secretion de l'hormone hypophysaire thyretrope (TSH). Premier purification par filtration sur gel Sephadex. Comptes Rendus Acad. Sci. *255:*1018 (1962).
3. Bøler, J., Enzmann, F., and Folkers, K., *et al.* The identity of chemical and hormonal properties of the thyrotropin releasing hormone and pyroglutamyl-histidyl-proline amide. Biochem. Biophys. Res. Commun. *37:*705 (1969).
4. Gross, J. and Pitt-Rivers, R. The identification of 3, 5, 3'-triiodothyronine in human plasma. Lancet *1:*439 (1952).
5. Hollander, C. S., Shenkman, and L., Mitsuma, T., *et al.* T$_3$ toxicosis in an iodine deficient area. Lancet *2:*1276 (1972).
6. Chopra, I. J. A radioimmunoassay for measurement of 3,3',5'-triiodothyronine (reverse T$_3$). J. Clin. Invest. *54:*583 (1974).
7. Volpe, R. The role of autoimmunity in hypoendocrine and hyperendocrine function, with special emphasis on autoimmune thyroid disease. Ann. Intern. Med. *87:*86 (1977).
8. Vagenakis, A. G., Wang, C., and Burger, A., *et al.* Iodide-induced thyrotoxicosis in Boston. New Engl. J. Med. *287:*523 (1972).
9. Livadas, D. P., Koutras, D. A., Souvatzoglou, A., and Beckers, C. The toxic effects of small iodine supplements in patients with autonomous thyroid nodules. Clin. Endocrinol. (Oxf.) *7:*121 (1977).
10. Temple, R., Berman, M., Robbins, J., and Wolff, J. The use of lithium in the treatment of thyrotoxicosis. J. Clin. Invest. *51:*2746 (1972).

11. Astwood, E. B. Treatment of hyperthyroidism with thiourea and thiouracil, J. Am. Med. Assoc. *122:*78 (1943).
12. Greer, M. A., Meihoff, W. C., and Studer, H. Treatment of hyperthyroidism with a single daily dose of propylthiouracil. New Engl. J. Med. *272:* 888 (1965).
13. Greer, M. A., Kammer, H., and Bouma, D. J. Short-term antithyroid drug therapy for thyrotoxicosis of Graves' disease. J. Am. Med. Assoc. *297:* 173 (1977).
14. Hedley, A. J. Myxedema. Practitioner *208:*349 (1972).
15. Werner, S. C. Modification of the classification of the eye changes of Graves' disease. Recommendations of the ad hoc committee of the American Thyroid Association. J. Clin. Endocrinol. Metab. *44:*203 (1977).
16. Werner, S. C., Coleman, J. C., and Franzen, L. A. Ultrasonographic evidence of a consistent orbital involvement in Graves' disease. New Engl. J. Med. *290:*1447 (1974).
17. Kriss, J. P., Konishi, J., and Herman, M. Studies on the pathogenesis of Graves' ophthalmopathy (with some related observations regarding therapy). Recent Progr. Horm. Res. *31:*533 (1975).
18. Muller, B. R., Levinson, R. E., and Friedman, A., *et al.* Delayed hypersensitivity in Graves' disease and exophthalmos. Identification of thyroglobulin in normal human orbital muscle. Endocrinol. *100:* 351 (1977).
19. Donaldson, S. S., Bagshaw, M. A., and Kriss, J. P. Supervoltage orbital Radiotherapy for Graves' ophthalmopathy. J. Clin. Endocrinol. Metab. *37:* 276 (1973).
20. Hall, R., *et al.* Ophthalmic Graves' disease, In: *Thyrotoxicosis.* W. J. Irvine (Ed.), Williams and Wilkins, Baltimore, 1967, p 210.
21. Fox, R. A. and Schwartz, T. B. Infiltrative ophthalmopathy and primary hypothyroidism. Ann. Intern. Med. *67:*377 (1967).
22. Solomon, D. H., Chopra, I. J., Chopra, U., and Smith, F. J. Identification of subgroups of euthyroid Graves' ophthalmopathy. New Engl. J. Med. *296:*661 (1975).
23. Jackson, I. M. D. "Hyper-thyroiditis"—a diagnostic pitfall. New Engl. J. Med. *293:*661 (1975).
24. Schneeberg, N. G. The Treatment of myxedema with sodium dextro-thyroxine. Am. J. Med. Sci. *248:*399 (1964).
25. Information for Physicians on irradiation related thyroid cancer. The National Cancer Institute. Cancer *26:*150 (1976).
26. *Radiation—Associated Thyroid Carcinoma.* L. J. Degroot, L. A. Frohman, E. L. Kaplan, and S. Refetoff (Eds.). Grune and Stratton, New York, San Francisco, London, 1977.
27. Greenspan, F. S. Radiation exposure and thyroid cancer. J. Am. Med. Soc. *237:*2089 (1977).
28. Wang, C., Vickery, A. L., Jr., and Maloof, F. Needle biopsy of the thyroid. Surg. Gynecol. Obstet. *143:* 365 (1976).
29. Chilcote, W. S. Gray-Scale ultrasonography of the thyroid. Radiol. *120:*381 (1976).

37 Neuro-ophthalmic Disorders Due to Alcoholism and Malnutrition

Maurice Victor, M. D.

The abuse of alcohol gives rise to a large and diverse number of ocular disturbances. The most common of these are nystagmus and other disturbances of conjugate eye movement that occur with alcoholic intoxication and, somewhat less consistently, with abstinence from alcohol, following a period of chronic intoxication. Of greater clinical significance are the ocular muscle and gaze palsies of Wernicke's disease and the optic neuropathy of so-called tobacco-alcohol amblyopia. These latter disorders are due not to the effects of alcohol itself, but to the nutritional deficiencies engendered by alcoholism. Actually, deficiency disease occurs in only a small proportion of alcoholics, about 3% in our experience. However, the prevalence of alcoholism is of such magnitude (there are an estimated 10,000,000 alcoholics in the United States) that the nutritional disorders assume importance for this reason alone. The deficiency diseases are, of course, observed in nonalcoholics as well, as a result of dietary faddism or absorptive defects, as occur in patients with sprue, with surgical exclusion of portions of the gastrointestinal tract, and, most importantly, with pernicious anemia. Finally, attention should be drawn to an entirely different category of alcohol-induced disorder, namely to fetal damage that results from maternal alcoholism ("fetal alcohol syndrome").

ALCOHOLIC INTOXICATION

Beginning with the classical studies of

Dodge and Benedict[1] and of Miles[2] it has been repeatedly demonstrated that the acute ingestion of 1–6 oz of absolute alcohol by a nonaddicted person adversely affects all manner of motor performance—whether it be the simple maintenance of a standing posture, the control of speech, or the performance of highly organized and complex motor skills. The movements involved in these acts are not only made slower than normal but also more inaccurate and random in character and therefore less well adapted to the accomplishment of specific ends. The same pertains to eye movements. Wilkinson, Kime, and Purnell[3] recorded eye movements electrographically in healthy young people, before and after they had consumed 200 ml of 25% alcohol in 2–3 min in the fasting state. These investigators found that with relatively mild intoxication (blood alcohol levels between 80 and 110 mg %) the speed with which the eyes move from one visual target to another ("peak saccadic velocity") is reduced by alcohol and that smooth pursuit movements become interrupted and jerky due to the appearance of saccadic elements. The jerky movements of the eyes reduce the time that the target is perceived in the central part of the visual field, with presumed reduction in visual acuity. A similar slowing of saccades due to alcohol has been observed by Franck and Kuhlo.[4] Certain other sedatives, namely chlordiazepoxide and diazepam, have been shown to produce the same effects as alcohol.[5]

It has also been known for many years

that nystagmus is a characteristic symptom of alcohol intoxication and that alcohol-induced nystagmus is influenced by the position of the head. A careful analysis of this type of nystagmus has been made by Aschan and his associates,[6, 7] who recognize two forms of the disorder. One form, which they refer to as "alcohol gaze nystagmus," is brought out by eccentric fixation of gaze and becomes evident when the blood alcohol level reaches 80 mg %. The other form, designated "positional alcoholic nystagmus (PAN)," appears with much lower blood alcohol levels and consists of two phases. In the first phase (PAN I) the nystagmus appears about 30 min after a single dose of alcohol and lasts for 3–4 h; during this phase the direction of the nystagmus (named for the fast component) is to the right with the head in the right lateral position and to the left with the head in the left lateral position. There follows a silent period of 1–2 h, after which the nystagmus reappears (PAN II), but now the direction of the nystagmus is the reverse of that in the first phase. PAN II persists for several hours after the alcohol has disappeared from the blood. In a series of experiments Aschan and Bergstedt[7] have demonstrated that the latency of the nystagmus in the first phase depends upon the rate of the initial rise in blood alcohol, and that the duration and the intensity of the nystagmus in both phases are proportional to the maximal blood alcohol concentration.

Other aspects of oculomotor function are also affected adversely by alcohol. The visual suppression of vestibular nystagmus is reduced by alcohol, thus impairing the smooth oculomotor tracking of a moving target, or of a fixed target when the body is in motion.[8, 9] Mean blood alcohol levels as low as 37 mg % (produced by one or two drinks) can impair this tracking performance. These effects are of considerable practical importance for aviation. While on the ground, a pilot who drinks lightly may be unaware of any impairment of oculomotor control, but when flying, particularly in dim light, a defect in tracking performance may become evident.

In hospital practice, the oculomotor effects of alcoholic intoxication are of relatively minor importance, at least in diag-

nosis. All variety of drugs, if taken in excess, may induce nystagmus, so that the diagnosis of alcoholic intoxication depends on other criteria.

In patients with the alcohol withdrawal syndrome, nystagmus is a common but by no means consistent finding. Again, the nystagmus is overshadowed by the more dramatic manifestations of the syndrome—viz., tremulousness, seizures, hallucinations, and delirium. Frequently, the patient is so confused and uncooperative that the presence of nystagmus and other abnormalities of gaze cannot be evaluated properly. The most interesting visual abnormality of the alcohol withdrawal state, namely hallucinations, is a poorly understood phenomenon and beyond the scope of the present discussion.

THE WERNICKE-KORSAKOFF SYNDROME

Wernicke's disease or encephalopathy is a neurologic disorder of acute onset, characterized by nystagmus, abducens and conjugate gaze palsies, ataxia of stance and gait, and mental disorder. These symptoms may occur singly, but more often they occur in various combinations. For many years it was believed that Wernicke's disease was due to the toxic effects of alcohol, but now it is established that it is due to nutritional deficiency, and more specifically to a deficiency of thiamine. The pathologic changes consist essentially of symmetrically placed zones of degeneration in the paraventricular parts of the thalamus and hypothalamus, in the mammillary bodies, periaqueductal region, floor of the fourth ventricle (affecting the dorsal motor nuclei of the vagus and vestibular nuclei), and anterior lobe of the cerebellum, particularly the vermis.

Korsakoff's psychosis refers to an abnormal mental state in which learning and memory are deranged out of all proportion to other cognitive functions in an otherwise alert and responsive patient. In practically all alcoholics who present with Korsakoff's psychosis it can be demonstrated that the disease began with an acute attack of Wernicke's disease. Contrariwise, most of the patients who survive an acute attack of

Wernicke's disease are left with a permanent defect of retentive memory, i.e., Korsakoff's psychosis. Stated in another way, Korsakoff's psychosis is the chronic psychic component of Wernicke's disease. Furthermore, the neuropathologic changes in patients dying in the acute stages of Wernicke's disease and in the chronic (Korsakoff) phase are essentially the same, differing only with respect to the age of the glial and vascular reactions.

For these reasons, *Wernicke's disease and Korsakoff's psychosis in the alcoholic, nutritionally deficient patient should be regarded as the same disease, which may suitably be designated the Wernicke-Korsakoff syndrome.*

In this chapter we are concerned mainly with the ophthalmic manifestations of the Wernicke-Korsakoff syndrome, and their implications. The descriptions which follow are based on an extensive personal experience with this disease, comprising 245 carefully studied patients, the majority of whom were followed for many years and 82 of whom had complete postmortem examinations.[10] The reader is referred to this study for a more detailed account than can possibly be given here.

The ocular changes constitute the most consistent clinical manifestation of the Wernicke-Korsakoff syndrome, and the diagnosis of the illness, at least at its onset, can hardly be made in their absence. The usual ocular abnormalities are nystagmus, weakness or paralysis of the lateral recti, and palsies of conjugate gaze. The patient may present with only one of these abnormalities, but more often with two of them and in 27% of our cases, all three abnormalities were present.

Horizontal nystagmus on lateral gaze to both sides is the most common ophthalmic disorder. *Vertical nystagmus* on upward gaze is frequently associated; vertical nystagmus on downward gaze is far less common. In patients who present with complete paralysis of the lateral recti or of conjugate gaze, nystagmus may be absent, but becomes evident after treatment has been instituted and some degree of recovery of ocular movement has occurred. *Lateral rectus (abducens) palsy* of varying degree is the next most common abnormality (Fig.

1). The paralysis is always bilateral, though rarely is it perfectly symmetrical. In cases of complete or nearly complete abducens palsy, the presence of a concomitant horizontal gaze palsy is betrayed by under-adduction of the opposite eye (Fig. 1). In almost half the patients there is evidence of *paralysis or weakness of conjugate gaze*, most frequently of horizontal gaze, less often of upward gaze, and rarely of downward gaze. *Bilateral internuclear ophthalmoplegia* is a not uncommon finding (Fig. 2).

Pupillary abnormalities are uncommon as presenting signs and are rarely conspicuous, consisting usually of a sluggish reaction to light or a mild anisocoria. In patients who present with severe ophthalmoplegia and other evidence of advanced disease, the pupils may be small and nonreactive. *Funduscopic examination* occasionally discloses small retinal hemorrhages, but we have never observed papilledema in this disease. Pallor of the optic disc, a relatively rare finding, is usually attributable to an associated optic neuropathy ("tobacco-alcohol amblyopia").

Disturbances of third and fourth nerve functions are practically never observed in Wernicke's disease, except for *ptosis*, which occurred in 3% of our patients (Fig. 3).

The most notable feature of the ocular abnormalities is their sensitivity to the administration of thiamine. Recovery of ocular function often *begins* within hours after the administration of this vitamin and practically always within a day or two. Sixth nerve palsies always recover completely, within a week in most cases, occasionally longer. Ptosis and vertical gaze palsies also recover completely but somewhat more slowly. Most cases of vertical gaze paralysis recover within a week or two, but vertical nystagmus may persist for two to three months, and even longer in rare instances. Horizontal gaze palsies recover completely as a rule, but in 60% of cases, a fine horizontal nystagmus on lateral gaze remains as a permanent sequela. In this respect, horizontal nystagmus is unique among the ocular signs of Wernicke's disease, and its presence enables one to identify obscure cases of dementia in alcoholics as nutritional in nature. The response of the ocular abnormalities to the administration of thia-

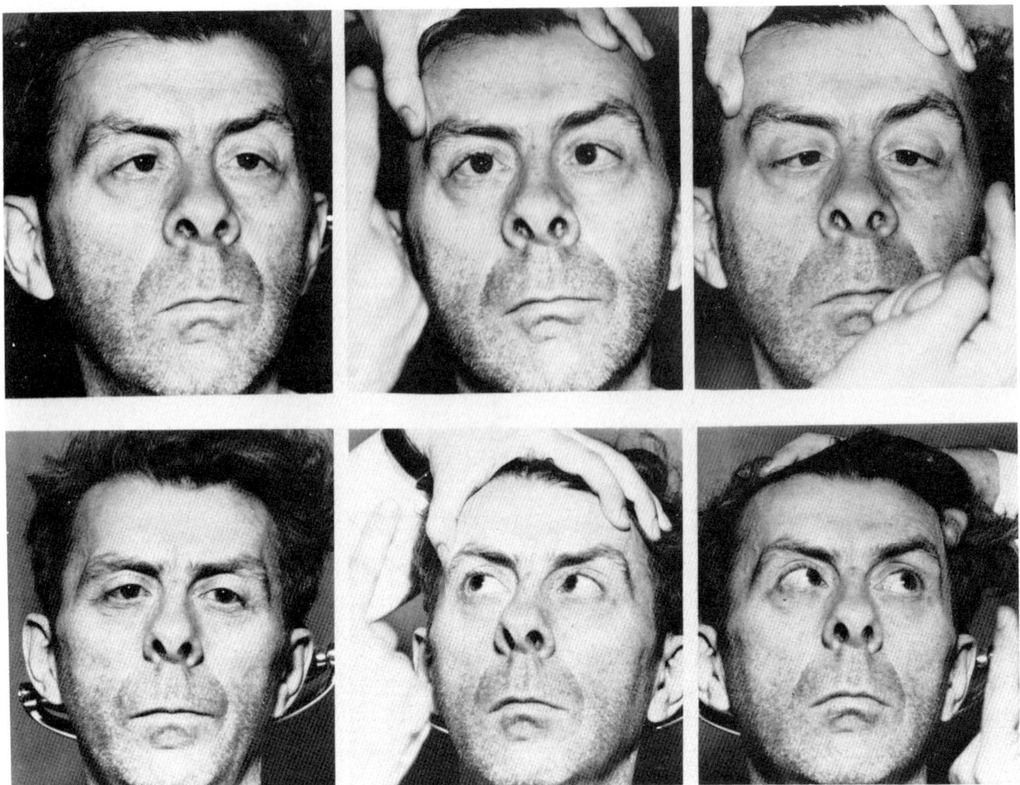

Fig. 1. Ophthalmoplegia in Wernicke's disease. *Upper Row:* At the time of admission to hospital. *Left:* Bilateral internal strabismus. *Center:* Patient is attempting to look to this right; there is a paralysis of the right lateral rectus as well as a conjugate gaze palsy manifested by an underadduction of the left eye. *Right:* Similar palsies were present on left lateral gaze, although the patient frequently converged when asked to look to his left, as in this photo. *Lower Row:* Three days later. The patient had received only glucose, water, and minerals and 50 mg thiamine intramuscularly each day. The ocular muscle and gaze palsies have receded. From Victor, *et al.*[10]

mine is so predictable that a failure of the usual response should raise doubt about the diagnosis of Wernicke's disease.

Patients with the Wernicke-Korsakoff syndrome are frequently deficient in B vitamins other than thiamine, but this does not mean that the ocular manifestations of Wernicke's disease are due to these deficiencies. We found that despite the administration of all vitamins except thiamine, the ocular muscle and gaze palsies did not improve and often worsened; only when thiamine was added did these abnormalities improve in a predictable manner.[11, 12]

Clinical-Pathologic Correlations. Our data suggest that vertical nystagmus is related to lesions in the midbrain, more specifically to lesions of the third nerve nuclei and periaqueductal region. Horizon-

tal nystagmus correlates closely with lesions of the vestibular complex, particularly of the medial vestibular nuclei.

The anatomic basis of the gaze palsies is difficult to determine because these ocular abnormalities are so readily reversible; most likely they are related to the pretectal and periaqueductal lesions. Undoubtedly, the lateral rectus palsies are due to lesions of the sixth nerve nuclei, and ptosis and pupillary abnormalities to lesions of the third nerve nuclei, although discrete examples of these relationships are difficult to document. A problem in clinical-pathologic correlation arises in relation to patients who showed no ocular abnormalities at the time of death but in whom autopsy discloses lesions of the third and sixth nerve nuclei. Either the lesions in such cases were

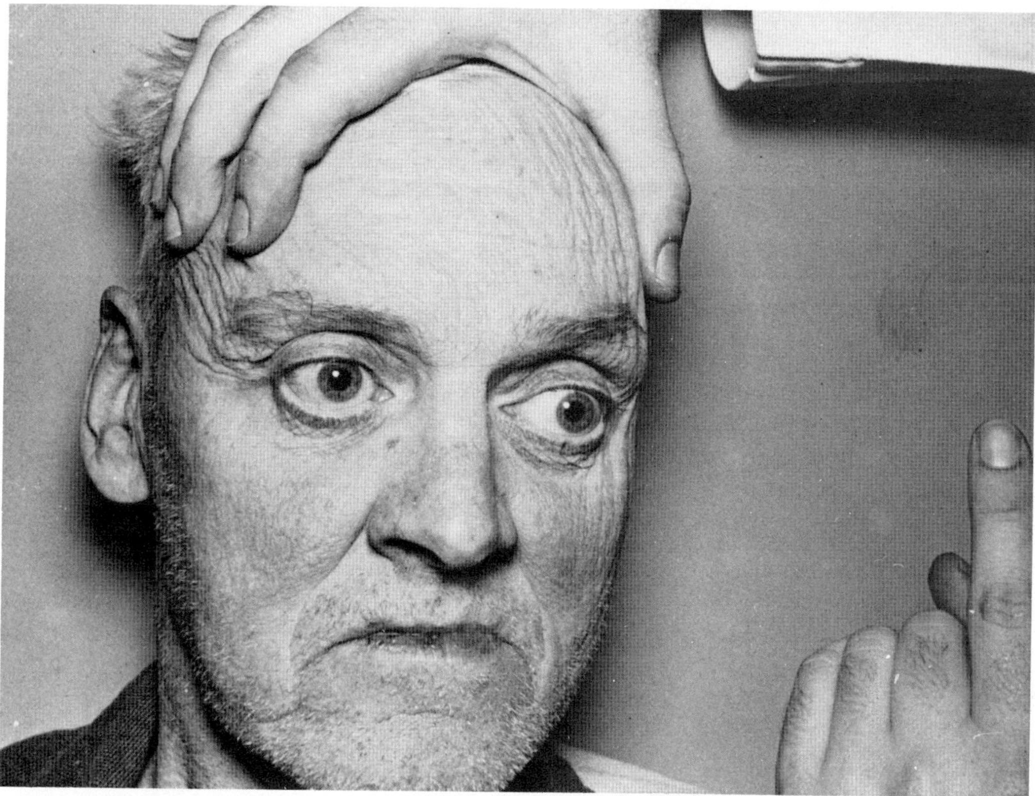

Fig. 2. Ophthalmoplegia in the acute phase of Wernicke's disease. The patient is attempting to look to his left. There is a moderate degree of weakness of the left lateral rectus. The presence of a gaze palsy, probably internuclear ophthalmoplegia, is indicated by a failure of the adducting eye to move more than a few degrees medial to the midline. Identical abnormalities were present on attempted right lateral gaze. From Victor, *et al.*[10]

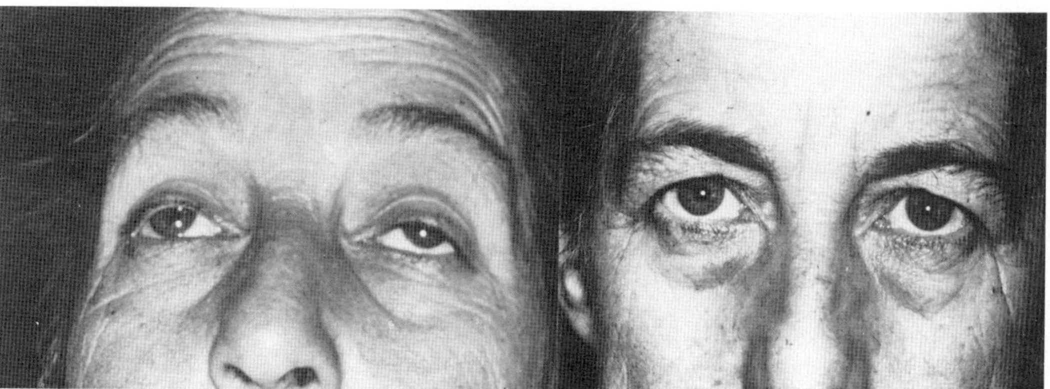

Fig. 3. Ophthalmoplegia in Wernicke's disease. *Above:* Bilateral ptosis, left greater than right. The patient is attempting to look upward, as indicated by the wrinkled forehead, and manifests a paralysis of conjugate movement in that direction. *Below:* Three days after the administration of glucose, minerals and thiamine (50 mg intramuscularly each day). The ptosis has disappeared. Also, the gaze palsy had improved. From Victor, *et al.*[10]

not large enough to cause clinically evident weakness or the number of surviving cells ("margin of safety") was sufficient to allow restoration of oculomotor function.

Treatment of the Wernicke-Korsakoff Syndrome. Wernicke's disease represents a medical emergency and its recognition demands the immediate administration of thiamine. Although 2–3 mg of this vitamin are sufficient to modify the ocular signs, much larger doses are usually employed—50 mg intravenously and 50 mg intramuscularly—the latter dose being repeated each day until the patient resumes a normal diet. The prompt use of thiamine prevents progression of the disease and reverses those lesions, or portions thereof, in which permanent damage has not yet occurred, i.e., the biochemical lesions. As indicated above, the remarkable sensitivity of the ocular palsies to the administration of thiamine constitutes an important diagnostic as well as therapeutic measure. In patients who show only ocular and ataxic signs, the prompt administration of thiamine is crucial in preventing the development of an amnesic psychosis.

A particular danger attends the treatment of depleted alcoholics with glucose solutions. Characteristically, such patients subsist on a diet low in thiamine and disproportionately high in carbohydrate, to which they add the carbohydrate calories derived from alcohol itself (alcohol is burned almost entirely as carbohydrate). The intravenous administration of glucose in these circumstances may exhaust the patient's thiamine stores and precipitate Wernicke's disease or cause an early form of the disease to worsen rapidly. The occurrence of Wernicke's disease that has been observed to follow intravenous hyperalimentation[13] and refeeding of prisoners of war[14] and in patients who had been on a starvation diet[15] is probably due to a similar mechanism, i.e., an increment of calories with a decrease in the thiamine to calorie ratio. For this reason it is good practice to add large amounts of B vitamins in all cases requiring parenteral glucose or hyperalimentation, even though the alcoholic disorder under treatment, e.g., delirium tremens, is not primarily due to vitamin deficiency.

"TOBACCO-ALCOHOL" AMBLYOPIA

This is an unfortunate but entrenched term which is widely used to designate a characteristic disorder of vision among alcoholics and smokers and which is not due to a lesion of the cornea or other parts of the eye concerned with refraction. *Deficiency amblyopia* would be a preferable term insofar as the disorder is almost certainly due to nutritional deficiency and not to the toxic effects of alcohol or tobacco. Alternately, one might use the term *nutritional optic neuropathy* which indicates both the cause and the probable site of the primary lesion.

Typically, the patient complains of a blurring of vision for near and distant objects, developing gradually over a period of several days or weeks. Examination discloses a reduction in visual acuity and the presence of bilateral and roughly symmetrical central *or* centrocecal scotomas, which have sloping diffuse edges and are greater for colored than for white test objects. Within the scotoma are one or more nuclei of intense defect, situated on the horizontal meridian of the retina. Most often the scotoma begins on the nasal side of the blind spot and gradually extends toward the point of fixation, which it finally overlaps (Fig. 4). Or it may begin and remain most prominent at the point of fixation (Fig. 5). The proposition that tobacco amblyopia can be distinguished from alcoholic (or nutritional) amblyopia on the basis of small differences in the location of the most intense defect (paracentral vs. central) is simply not in keeping with the observed facts.[20]

Funduscopic abnormalities are observed occasionally in this form of amblyopia. These vary from mild papillitis with slight hyperemia and blurring of the disc margins to pallor of the optic disc in the most advanced cases. Retinal hemorrhages occur rarely. Untreated, the disorder may progress to irreversible optic atrophy. Under the influence of a nutritious diet and B vitamin supplements, improvement occurs in all but the most chronic cases, the degree of recovery depending upon the severity of the disease and its duration before therapy was instituted.

The pathologic changes have been stud-

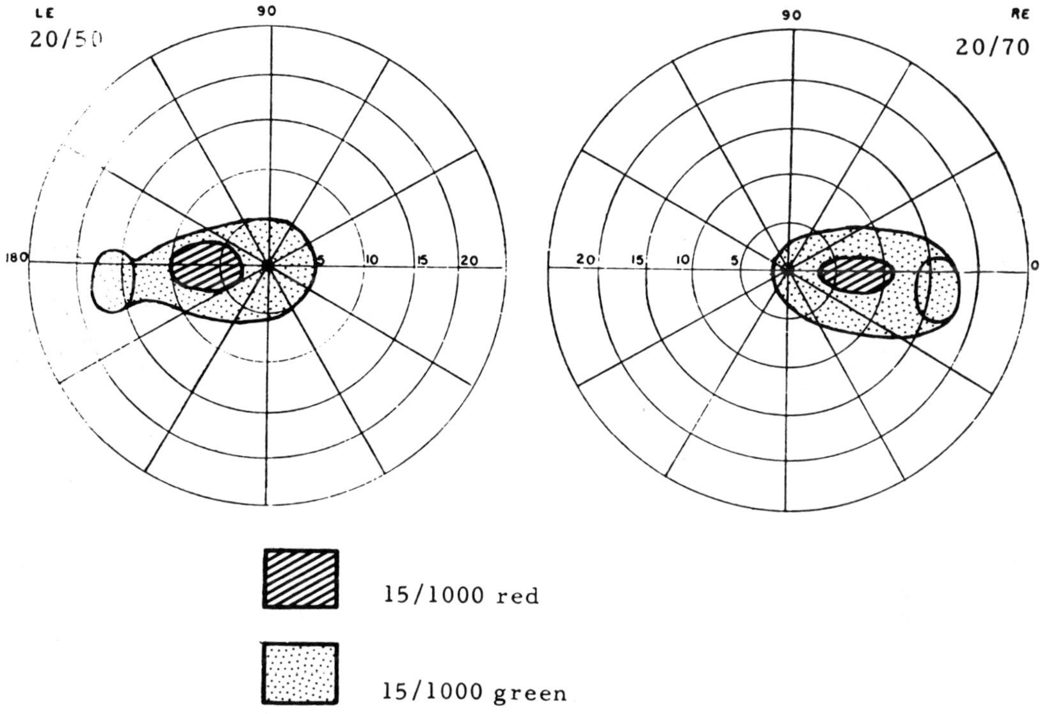

15/1000 red

15/1000 green

Fig. 4. Centrocecal scotomas in a 54-year-old malnourished alcoholic. Vision had deteriorated progressively during the two months preceding the visual field examination. The most intense defects are paracentral. For clinical and pathologic details of this case see Victor *et al.*[16]

ied in only a few cases.[16, 17] Essentially the changes consist of a degeneration of the optic nerves, chiasm, and tracts, more or less confined to the papillomacular bundles, associated with a loss of retinal ganglion cells, particularly in the region of the macula (Figs. 6–8). The primary lesion is probably in the optic nerve rather than in the retinal ganglion cells, although this point has not been settled completely.[17]

The evidence is overwhelming that so-called tobacco-alcohol amblyopia is due to nutritional deficiency and not, as some ophthalmologists still believe, to the toxic effects of alcohol or tobacco. The data supporting this view have been documented in detail by Potts[18] as well as by ourselves.[19, 20] The importance of nutritional factors in the genesis of retrobulbar neuropathy became apparent soon after the Second World War, when numerous reports appeared, describing a uniform type of amblyopia that had occurred among prisoners-of-war in the Far East.[21–26] This amblyopia did not differ clinically or pathologically (Fig. 9) from so-

called tobacco-alcohol amblyopia, although the prisoners had had access neither to tobacco nor alcohol. Actually, convincing experimental evidence for a nutritional etiology of tobacco-alcohol amblyopia had been supplied earlier by Carroll.[27] He studied 25 patients with the latter disorder under controlled dietary conditions. These patients were allowed to drink and smoke in their usual manner, providing that they ate a nutritious diet supplemented with B vitamins. All of these patients recovered vision completely or almost completely, to the same extent as any previous group of 25 patients who had simply stopped smoking and drinking.

In 1958, Heaton, McCormick, and Freeman[28] introduced a new concept of the pathogenesis of tobacco amblyopia, namely that in persons with even mild vitamin B_{12} deficiency the retina or the optic nerve is unduly sensitive to tobacco. Wokes[29] theorized further that cyanide generated in tobacco smoke combined with body stores of hydroxycobalamins to form cyanocobala-

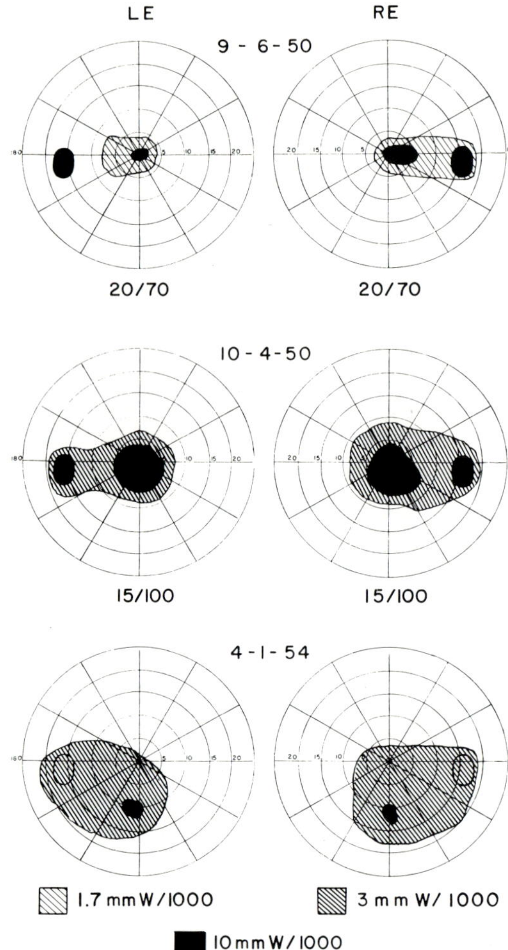

Fig. 5. Progressive visual impairment in a 60-year-old alcoholic. The most intense defect during the first two examinations was at the fixation point. For clinical and pathologic description of this case see Victor and Dreyfus.[17]

min which then "acted as a brake on respiratory enzymes such as cytochrome oxidase." These reports, in Potts' words, "sent a pack of ophthalmologists baying down a tobacco trail, which they still pursue."[18] Indeed, the ophthalmologic literature is replete with articles that seem to have accepted without question the notion that low concentrations of vitamin B_{12} reduce the capacity to bind cyanide which then is free to damage the optic nerves (see the review of Potts[18] for a complete list of references).

That vitamin B_{12} deficiency may cause optic neuropathy cannot be doubted (see below), but the idea that cyanide in tobacco smoke has a damaging effect on the optic nerves is supported neither by logic nor by experimental data. A rather complete critique of this subject appeared in a previous monograph in this series[20] so that a detailed argument need not be presented here. However, several points bear repetition. For one thing, vitamin B_{12} binding of cyanide is neither the only mechanism by which cyanide is metabolized, nor the most important one. Alternate pathways include excretion by the lungs, combination with cystine, and oxidation to carbon dioxide and water. By far the largest portion of absorbed cyanide is converted by rhodanese (an enzyme that is *not* dependent upon vitamin B_{12}) to the relatively innocuous thiocyanate ion, and is excreted in this form. Also one should be clear about the significance of the nervous system lesions that have been produced experimentally by the chronic administration of cyanide. These lesions involved the cerebral white matter preferentially; the optic nerves were affected relatively infrequently and to a mild degree.[30–36] More importantly, the concentrations of cyanide that were required to damage myelinated structures are infinitely greater than the concentrations which could possibly be achieved through smoking.

Potts[18] has written a highly informative and critical essay on tobacco amblyopia, which should be read by everyone interested in this subject. He identifies the many discrepancies and internal inconsistencies that characterize the writings on tobacco-alcohol amblyopia and make it impossible to adduce that either alcohol or tobacco is the primary toxic agent in so-called tobacco-alcohol amblyopia. On the basis of the best experimental evidence, Potts concludes also that tobacco-alcohol amblyopia cannot be attributed to the toxic effects of cyanide but that it is a disease of nutritional deficiency.

The specific nutritional factor that is responsible for tobacco-alcohol amblyopia may be difficult to determine. Some observations in prisoners of war implicated a deficiency of riboflavin.[25] Other studies[27, 37] indicate that thiamine may be the essential factor. The most readily defined cause is vitamin B_{12} deficiency (see below), but this factor is operative in only a small propor-

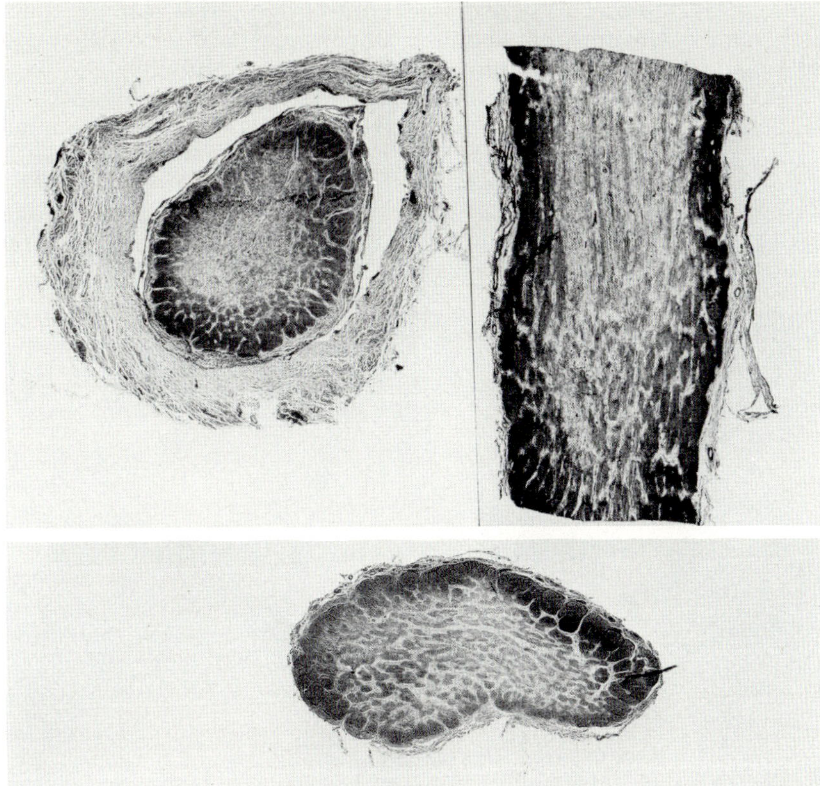

Fig. 6. Optic nerve lesions of the patient whose fields are illustrated in Figure 5. *Upper left:* Cross section through the optic nerve just behind orbit. *Upper right:* longitudinal section at same level. *Below:* cross section through the optic nerve anterior to the chiasm. Each section shows extensive destruction of medullated fibers in the area of the papillomacular bundle. Spielmeyer stain for myelin.

tion of patients with amblyopia. One may speculate that under certain conditions of dietary deprivation a deficiency of any one of several B vitamins, or perhaps a combination of deficiencies, may produce retrobulbar neuropathy. In this respect the effect of nutritional deficiency on the optic nerves is like the effect on the peripheral nerves.

OPTIC ATROPHY DUE TO VITAMIN B₁₂ DEFICIENCY

Pernicious anemia and its neurologic manifestations are unique among nutritional diseases, insofar as they result not from a lack of vitamin B_{12} in the diet but from a failure to transfer minute amounts of this nutrient across the intestinal mucosa—"starvation in the midst of plenty," as Castle has aptly put it. This type of nutritional disease is referred to as a "conditioned deficiency"; in the case of pernicious anemia the disease is conditioned by a lack of intrinsic factor in the gastric secretions.

Involvement of the nervous system is common in pernicious anemia. Usually this takes the form of a degeneration of the posterior and lateral funiculi of the spinal cord (subacute combined degeneration). In a small proportion of patients the spinal cord disease is associated with lesions of similar histologic type in the cerebral white matter.[38] A symmetrical, predominantly distal polyneuropathy of metabolic ("dying-back") type occurs in somewhat less than 5% of patients with pernicious anemia.[39]

Visual impairment, clinically indistinguishable from so-called tobacco amblyopia, is an uncommon manifestation of Addisonian pernicious anemia but a well-documented one, nevertheless.[40–46] Furthermore, an amblyopia of this type may be the initial or sole manifestation of vitamin B_{12} deficiency.[47–51] Clinically, the amblyopia of vitamin B_{12} deficiency is characterized by varying degrees of pallor of the temporal portions of the optic discs and the presence of bilateral central or centrocecal scotomas. On the basis of these findings, one is probably correct in assuming that the visual impairment is due to degeneration of the optic nerves and that the papillomacular bundles are predominantly affected. A pathologic study of the optic nerve lesions in pernicious anemia has not been made, however.

Our studies of experimentally induced vitamin B_{12} deficiency in monkeys have

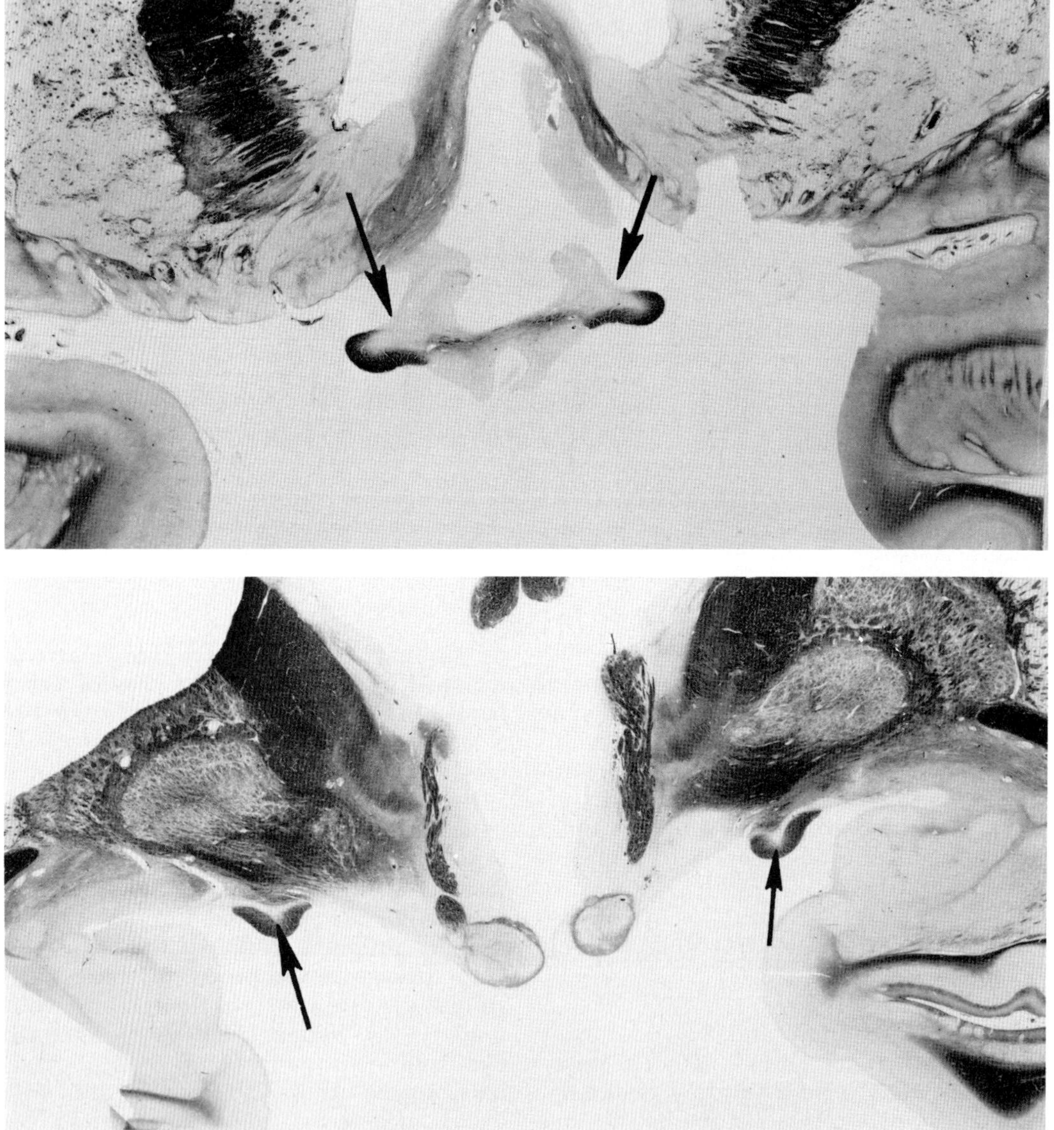

Fig. 7. Lesions of the chiasm and optic tracts from the case illustrated in Figures 5 and 6. Coronal sections of the brain at the level of the posterior part of the chiasm (*above*) and the proximal portions of the optic tracts (*below*). Arrows point to the zones of demyelination, corresponding to the distribution of the papillomacular bundles. Spielmeyer stain for myelin.

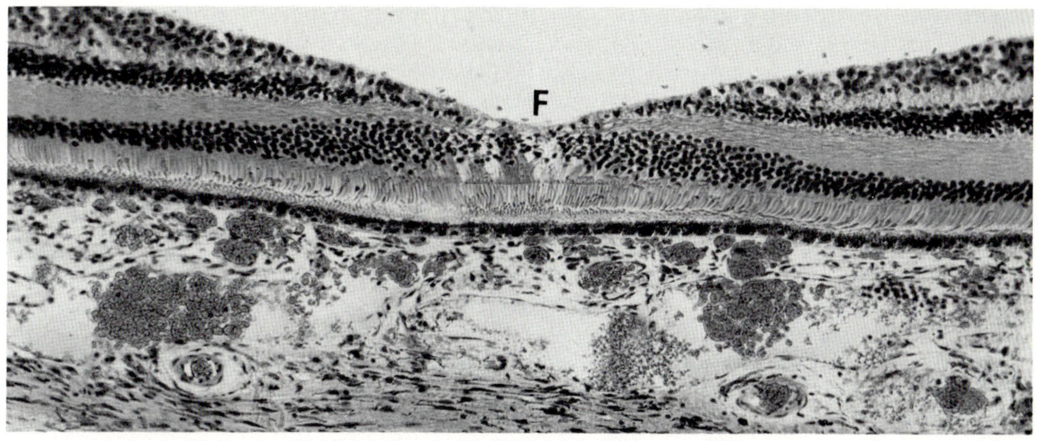

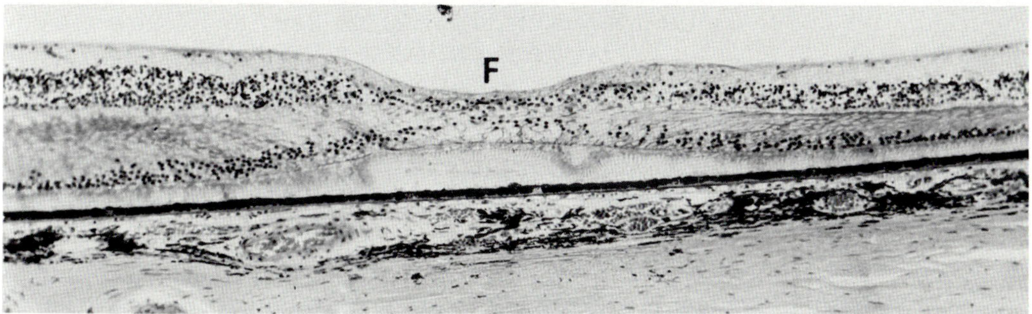

Fig. 8. Retinal lesion from case illustrated in Figures 5–7. Sections through the macula, stained with hematoxylin and eosin. *Above:* Normal control; the most superficial (ganglion cell) layer of the retina is several cells thick. *Below:* Section from retina of patient with "tobacco-alcohol" amblyopia; there is almost complete loss of ganglion cells in parafoveal portions of the macula. (F) fovea.

cast some light on the nature of the optic nerve lesions.[52–55] A severe degree of vitamin B_{12} deficiency was produced in nine rhesus monkeys by maintaining them on a carefully controlled experimental diet that supplied less than 500 pg of B_{12} daily but adequate amounts of all other nutrients and vitamins. Over a period of 13–21 months, the B_{12} levels fell gradually in the serum (to 10 pg/ml), the red cells (to 72 pg/ml) and the liver (to 5% of control levels). Interestingly, none of the animals developed an anemia or a megaloblastic bone marrow, even though some of them were maintained on the deficient diet for longer than five years.

The initial clinical manifestation of deficiency was an impairment of vision, which appeared between 33 and 45 months after the institution of the vitamin B_{12} deficient diet. In three monkeys, the visual loss progressed to a state of complete blindness with loss of pupillary reflexes. Funduscopic examination, at the onset of the visual disturbance, disclosed pallor of the temporal part of the disc; later the entire disc appeared pale (Fig. 10). Pallor of the optic discs was accompanied by a reduction in the number of small blood vessels crossing the disc margin and a loss of retinal nerve fibers radiating from the disc margin (Fig. 10). Three to four months after the onset of visual symptoms, the animals developed a progressive spastic paralysis of their hind limbs. The relatively early onset of the visual symptoms, which clearly preceded the symptoms of spinal cord disease, is noteworthy, since in humans these manifestations of vitamin B_{12} deficiency usually occur in the reverse order. Also, the universal occurrence of visual loss in vitamin B_{12} deficient monkeys is unlike the human condition, in which amblyopia is a relatively rare complication.

At the time of writing, eight of the deficient monkeys have been sacrificed and studied pathologically (one is still living). Degenerative changes in the peripheral visual pathways were found in each of the autopsied animals. Similar changes were also observed in the spinal cord white matter, but these will not be discussed here, except to state that they are indistinguishable from the spinal cord lesions of pernicious anemia (Fig. 11).

Sections at different levels of the optic nerves showed a loss of myelinated fibers in a discrete patch occupying about 30–50% of the cross sectional area (Fig. 12). Both myelin and axis cylinders were involved, the former earlier and to a greater extent than the latter. Near the globe, the lesion occupied the temporal portion of the nerve (Fig. 13) whereas posteriorly it occupied a central position; thus, its location corresponded to the distribution of the papillomacular bundle. In two monkeys with relatively mild involvement of the peripheral visual pathways the lesions were confined to the territory of the papillomacular bundle, and in one of them to the retrobulbar portion of the optic nerve. In the remaining cases, the degeneration in the optic nerves could be followed back into the chiasm and optic tracts. In some cases the lesions in the chiasm and tracts were confined to the distribution of the papillomacular bundle, but in others the lesions were much more extensive (Fig. 14).

The degenerative changes in the visual pathways ranged from vacuolization of tissue and spongy change to frank cavitation. Myelin was completely absent in the central part of the lesion and fragmented into ovoids in the margins of the lesions. Axons were lost to a much lesser degree (Fig. 15). The lesions in the papillomacular bundle of the optic nerves were old and inactive as judged by their histopathology, and features of active degeneration, such as spongy

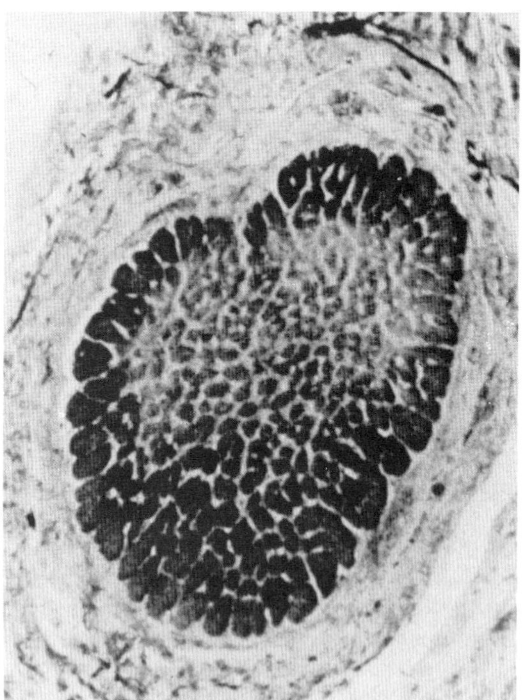
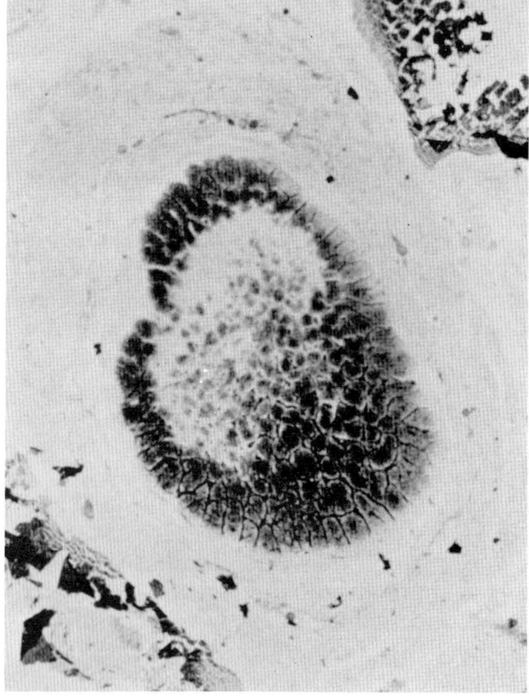

Fig. 9. Sections of the retro-orbital portion of the optic nerve from a Canadian soldier held prisoner of war by the Japanese. In October 1942 he rapidly lost vision, to the point of almost total blindness. He was treated sporadically with thiamine and yeast tablets and vision recovered partially, but remained less than 6/60 bilaterally. He died of myocardial infarction in 1953. *Left:* Myelin-stained cross section, showing marked degeneration of the papillomacular bundle. *Right:* Silver stain for axons; the loss of fibers corresponds to the demyelinated zone seen on the left. From Fisher, C. M.[23]

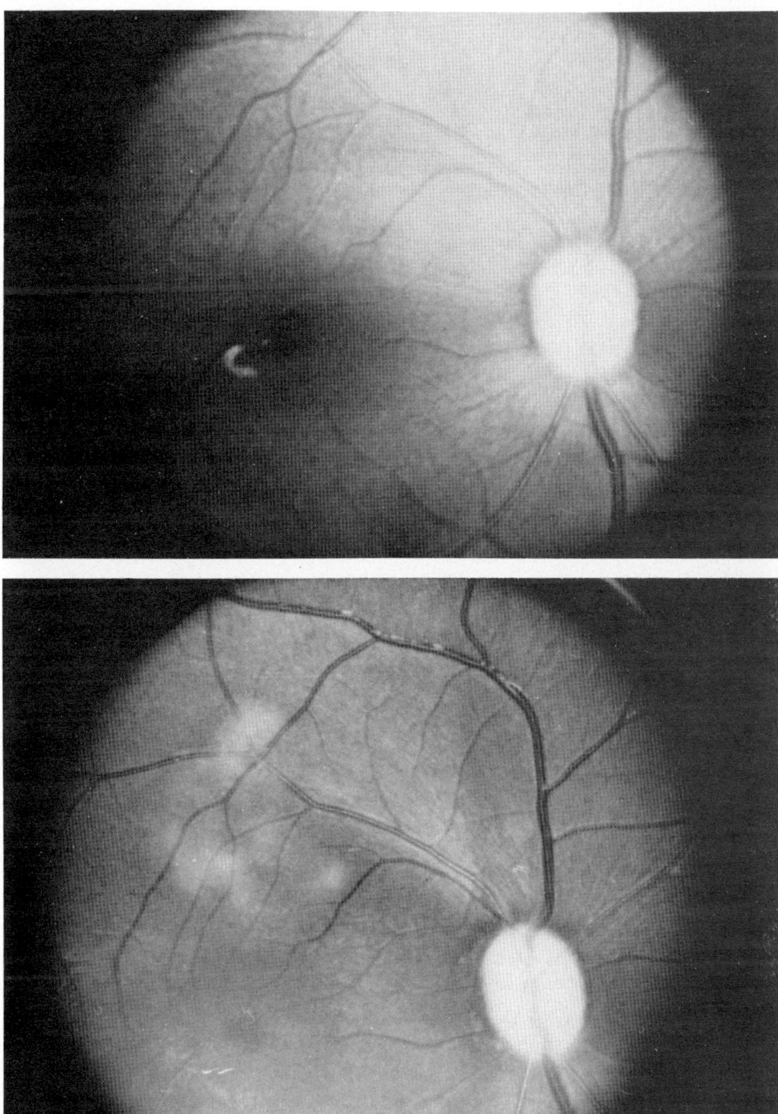

Fig. 10. *Above:* Retinal photographs of right eye of normal monkey. Note the arching myelinated fibers converging onto the disc from the temporal portion of the retina. *Below:* Retina of the right eye of a vitamin B$_{12}$ deficient monkey. The disc is sharply outlined and atrophic. The myelinated fibers are absent except for a small number superiorly. The light areas in the temporal parts of each fundus are artefactual. From Chester, *et al.*[55]

change and the presence of sudanophilic macrophages (phagocytosis), became progressively more prominent as the lesion was traced caudally. There was no inflammatory reaction. The vessels were normal and connective tissue was not increased. *In summary,* the appearance of the lesions in the optic nerves, chiasm, and tracts suggests that the degeneration begins in the papillomacular bundle in the retrobulbar portion of the optic nerves, and that it subsequently spreads caudally and beyond the confines of this bundle.

In the lateral geniculate bodies there was evidence of trans-synaptic degeneration, characterized by loss of some neurons and

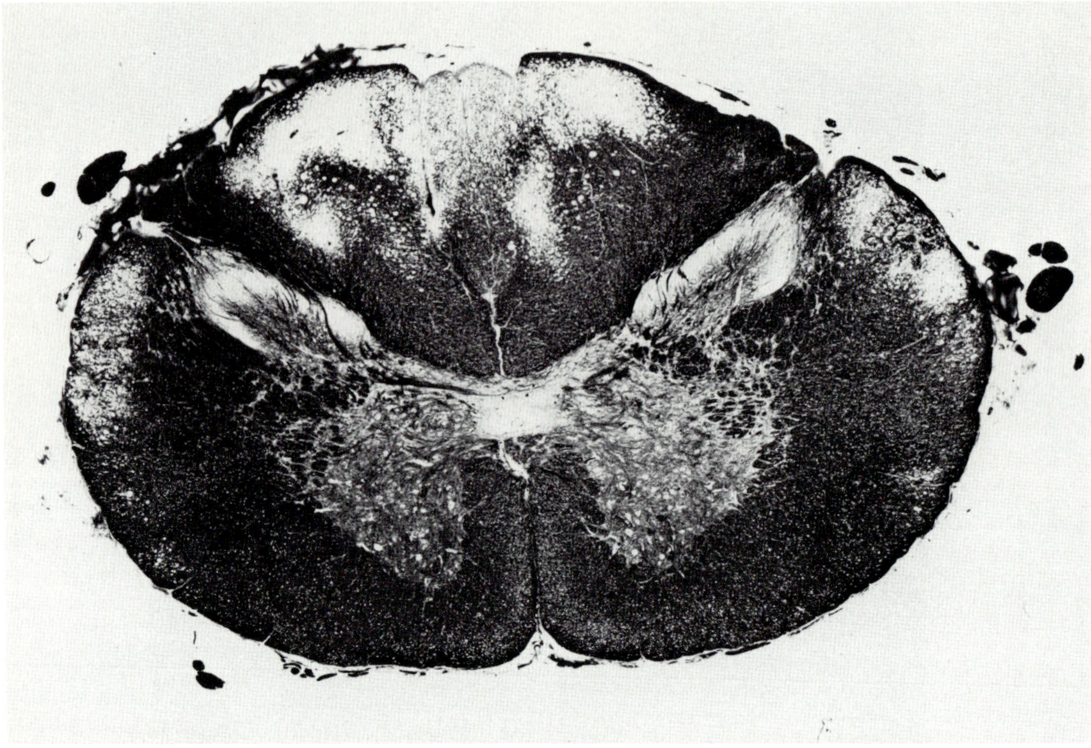

Fig. 11. Degeneration of the posterior and lateral columns of the cervical portion of the spinal cord, from a vitamin B_{12} deficient monkey. Myelin Stain. From Agamanolis, Victor, *et al.*[53]

shrinkage and dense staining of the remaining ones. No pathologic changes were observed in the optic radiations and visual cortices of any of the deficient animals.

To date, the retina has been studied in only two of our deficient monkeys.[55] In both there was a marked depletion of ganglion cells in the perifoveal macula, where normally the ganglion cell layer is several cells thick (Fig. 16). Other parts of the retina showed no abnormalities. The degeneration of the macular ganglion cells is probably secondary (retrograde) to the lesion in the optic nerve and not a primary effect of B_{12} deficiency. One cannot be certain about this point, but the study of early lesions in the spinal cord suggests that the primary effect of vitamin B_{12} deficiency is on the myelinated fiber. In these lesions the initial ultrastructural alterations consisted of a separation of myelin lamellae and the formation of intramyelinic vacuoles, leading to complete destruction of the myelin sheath and eventually to the destruction of the axon. Further studies of the retina are underway and may help to resolve this question.

The *pathogenesis* of the central nervous system lesions in vitamin B_{12} deficiency is not known. Vitamin B_{12} plays an important role in DNA synthesis, and it appears likely that impairment of DNA synthesis in B_{12} deficiency is responsible for the hematologic abnormalities, particularly for the production of megaloblasts. Since neurons do not divide, this factor does not appear to be operative in regard to central nervous system degeneration. The notion that the central nervous system of vitamin B_{12} deficient individuals is poisoned by the chronic action of cyanide is untenable, for reasons indicated above. One of the better understood functions of vitamin B_{12} is its role as a coenzyme in the methylmalonyl CoA mutase reaction. In this reaction, which is a key step in propionate metabolism, methylmalonyl CoA is transformed to succinyl CoA, which subsequently enters the Krebs cycle. It has been shown that impairment of this metabolic step may lead to production of abnormal fatty acids.[56] Since fatty acids are important building blocks of cell membranes and, therefore, of myelin, it is possible that this abnormality may in some way be responsible for the central nervous system degeneration.

FETAL ALCOHOL SYNDROME

That parental alcoholism may damage the offspring has been a recurrent theme in medical lore. The documented occurrence of such a relationship was lacking, however, until the turn of the century, when Sullivan[57, 58] showed that the mortality among the children of drunken mothers was almost two and one-half times greater than among children of nondrinking women of "similar stock." The increased mortality was attributed by Sullivan and later by Haggard and Jellinek[59] to postnatal influences such as poor nutrition and chaotic home environ-

ment rather than to intrauterine effects of alcohol. Following Sullivan's studies there appeared isolated clinical reports of damage to the fetus as a result of alcoholism in the mother (see Jones and Smith[60] and Warner and Rosett[61] for historical surveys), but in general this notion was rejected and relegated to the category of superstitions about alcohol and alcoholism. Thus, as late as 1959, Keller wrote: "the old notions about children of drunken parents being born defective can be cast aside, together with the idea that alcohol can directly irritate and injure the sex glands."[62]

In the past decade, the effects of alcohol abuse on the fetus have been rediscovered, so to speak. Lemoine *et al.*[63] in France, and Ulleland[64] and Jones, Smith, and their colleagues[65, 66] in this country, have described a distinctive pattern of abnormalities in infants born of severely alcoholic mothers. This congenital disorder, which Jones *et*

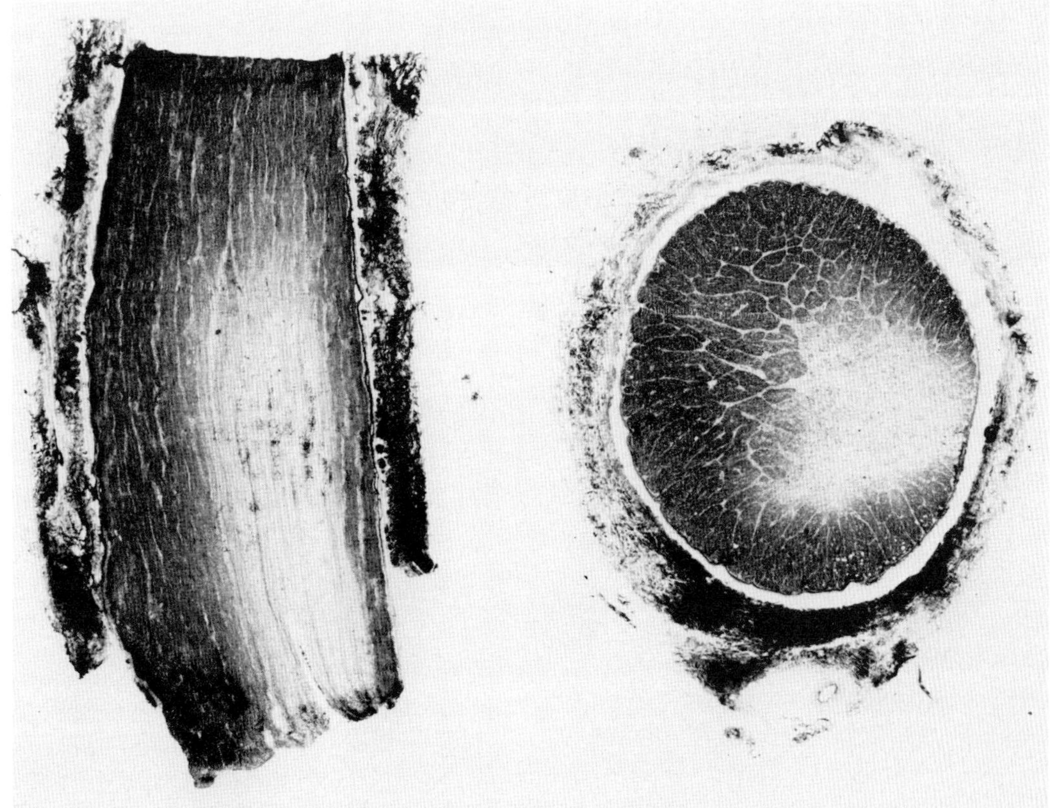

Fig. 12. Longitudinal and cross sections of the optic nerve in a vitamin B_{12} deficient monkey, showing loss of medullated fibers in distribution of papillomacular bundle. Myelin stain. Compare with Figures 6 and 9. From Agamanolis, Victor, *et al.*[53]

al.[65] have termed the "fetal alcohol syndrome" is characterized by a failure of intrauterine growth and of postnatal development, often combined with craniofacial malformations and less regularly with defects of the limbs, heart, and other organs. The early descriptions of the fetal alcohol syndrome have been corroborated by several subsequent studies, based on observations of substantial numbers of patients.[67, 68]

The affected infants are small in length in comparison to weight and most of them fall below the third percentile for head circumference. The ocular abnormalities are particularly distinctive and comprise short palpebral fissures, which are probably a reflection of microphthalmia, and epicanthal folds (Fig. 17). Less consistent abnormalities are maxillary hypoplasia, micrognathia, and cleft palate; dislocation of the hips, flexion deformities of the fingers, and a limited range of motion of other joints; cardiac anomalies (usually spontaneously closing septal defects); anomalous external genitalia; and capillary hemangiomata. The newborn infants suck and sleep poorly, and many of them are irritable, hyperactive, and tremulous; the latter symptoms resem-

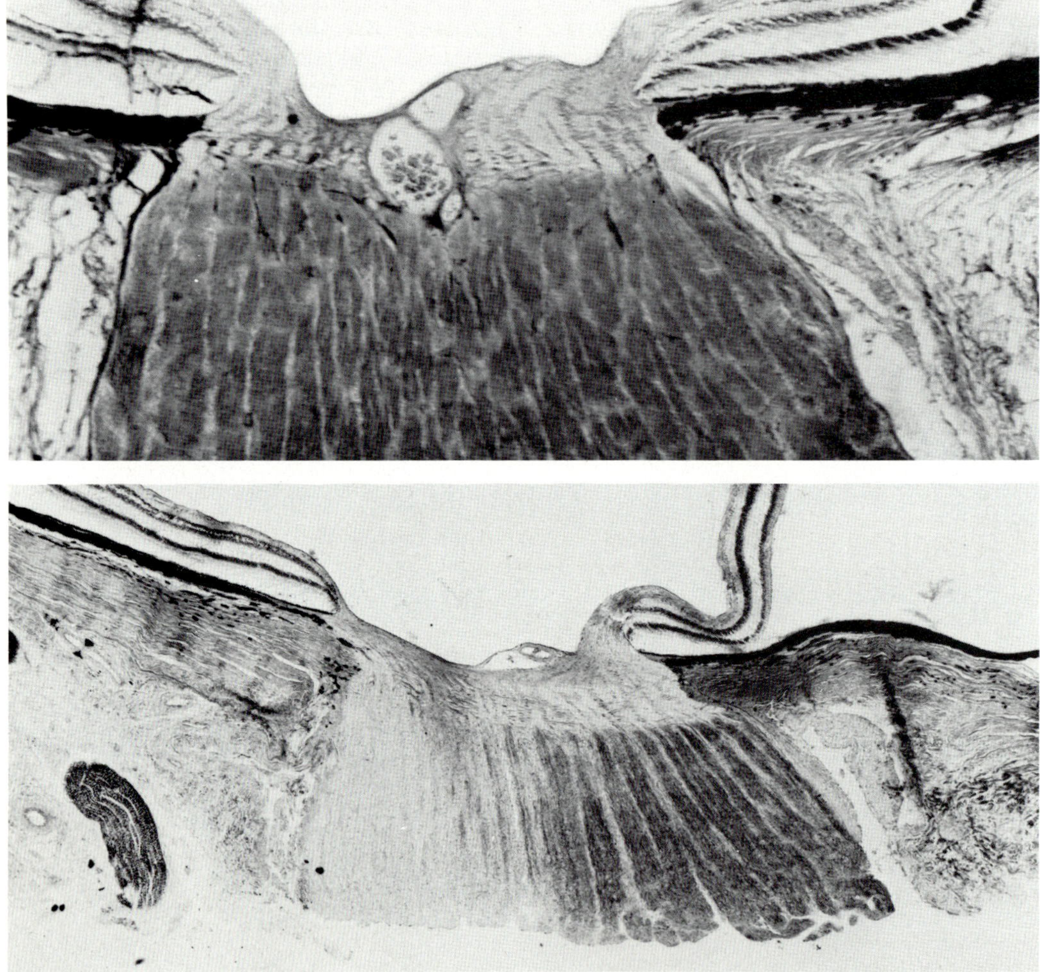

Fig. 13. Optic nerve lesion in vitamin B_{12} deficiency. Sections through the disc and retrobulbar portion of the optic nerve. *Above:* Normal monkey. *Below:* B_{12} deficient monkey. Note that the optic nerve is reduced in size (sections photographed at same magnification) and that medullated fibers have degenerated in the temporal half of the nerve. Myelin stain. From Agamanolis, Victor, *et al.*[53]

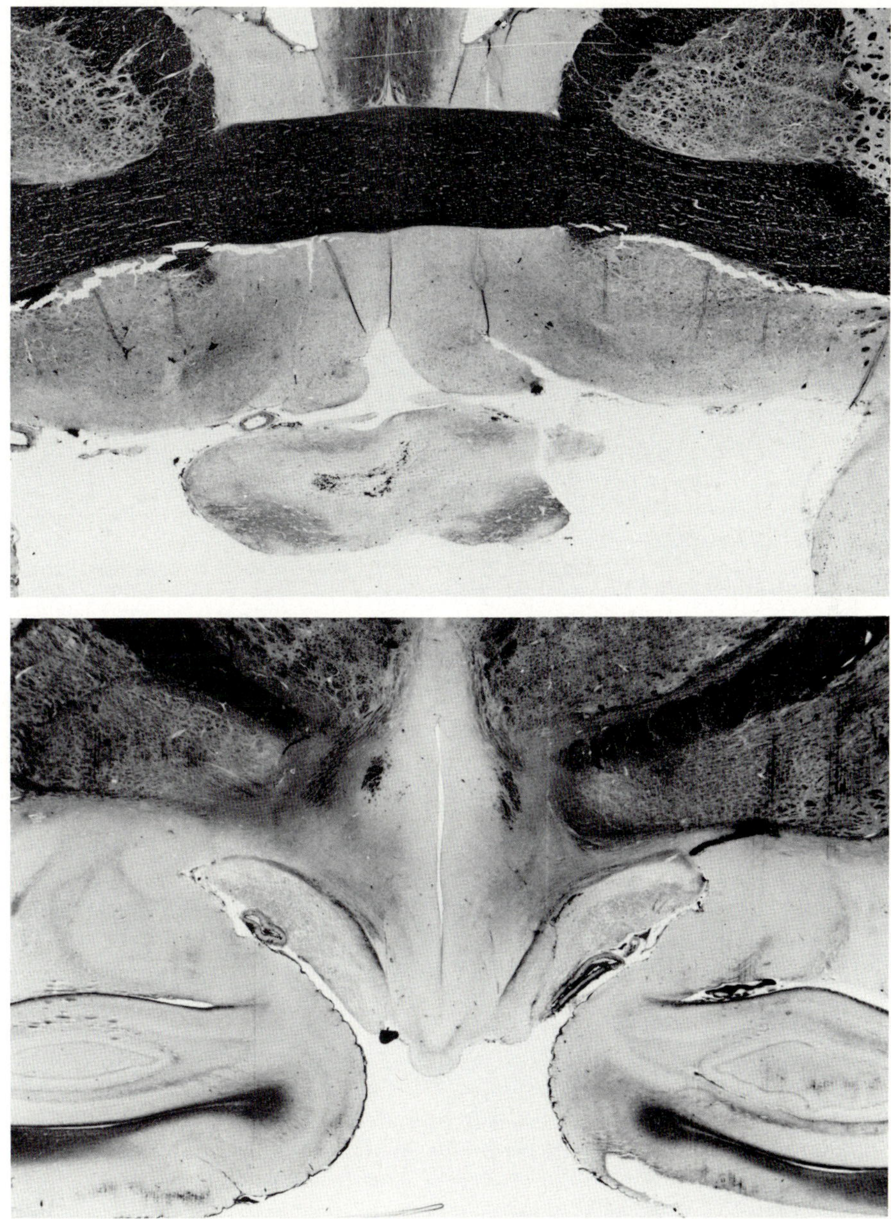

Fig. 14. Lesions of the optic chiasm and tracts in vitamin B$_{12}$ deficient monkey. Note extensive degeneration of the chiasm (*above*) and optic tracts (*below*). Myelin stain. From Agamanolis, Victor, *et al.*[53]

ble those of alcohol withdrawal, except that they persist. In one series of such infants there was a neonatal mortality of 17%.[66] Furthermore, seriously affected infants who survive the neonatal period fail to achieve normal weight, length, and head circumference and remain backward mentally to a varying degree, even under optimal environmental conditions.

To date, the neuropathologic findings have been described in only one newborn infant.[60] The brain in this case weighed only 140 g, and histologic examination disclosed numerous abnormalities of neuronal migration, lack of cortical sulcation (lissencephaly), and agenesis of the corpus callosum—findings which indicate that the developmental abnormality occurred in the

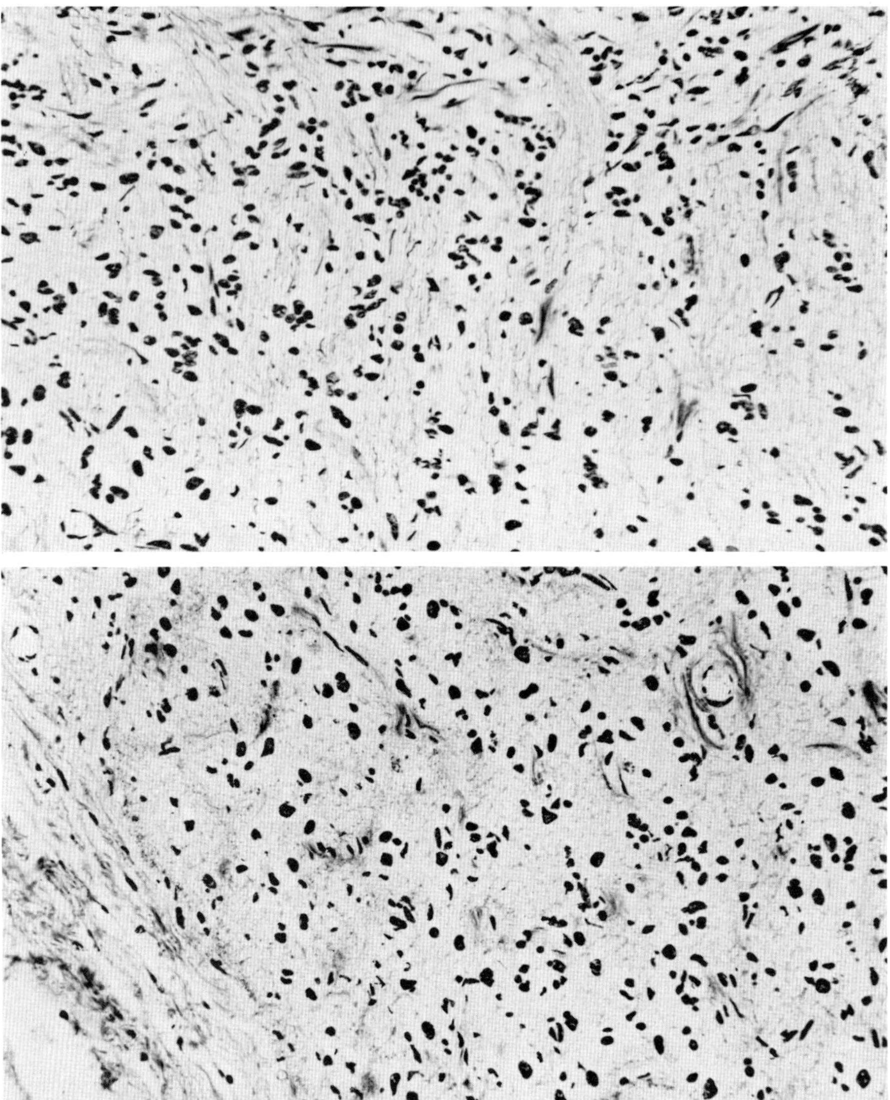

Fig. 15. Sections through the papillomacular bundle of the optic nerve of vitamin B$_{12}$ deficient monkeys, stained by the Bodian (silver) method for axons. *Above:* Relatively mild deficiency; despite a severe degree of demyelination, some bundles of axis cylinders remain throughout section. *Below:* Severe deficiency; axis cylinders are absent.

first few months of fetal life. Whether these changes are representative will only be determined by the examination of more cases.

Although the relationship of this syndrome to severe maternal alcoholism seems undoubted, the precise mechanism by which alcohol produces its effects is not understood. The limited evidence to date favors a toxic effect of alcohol or perhaps one of its metabolites or contaminants rather than a nutritional or genetic factor.

The critical degree of maternal alcoholism that is necessary to produce the fetal alcohol syndrome and the critical stage in gestation during which it occurs are not known. Instances of the syndrome observed to date have occurred only in children born to severely alcoholic mothers who continued to drink heavily throughout their pregnancy—an average of 6 oz of absolute alcohol (or 12 oz of 86 proof whiskey) daily, according to Rosett *et al.*[69] Preliminary data, derived from the collaborative study being sponsored by the National Institutes of Health, indicate that about one-third of the offspring of such women have the syndrome. Prospective studies of these problems, and of the effects on the fetus of lesser degrees of maternal alcoholism, are in progress in several centers.

EDITOR'S NOTE

Dr. Victor is the world authority on the neurologic complications of alcohol. I quite agree with him that the theory relating cyanide from tobacco exposure to nutritional amblyopia should go out with high button shoes! One interesting new point for me has been relating heavy alcohol intake with hypertensive vascular disease. A reference in this regard is: Klatsky, A. L., Friedman, G. D., and Siegelaub, A. B., "Alcohol and Hypertension," which appeared in *Compr. Ther.* 4(12):60–68, Dec. 1978.

I like to keep the following table in mind when seeing a patient in consultation with a history of alcoholism:

Neuro-ophthalmologic Aspects of Alcohol
1. trauma
2. syphilis
3. subdural hematoma
4. alcoholic cerebellar ataxia
5. Wernicke-Korsakoff syndrome
6. nutritional amblyopia
7. bleeding varices and ischemic retinopathy and optic atrophy
8. delirium tremens
9. "rum fits"
10. alcoholic peripheral neuropathy
11. alcoholic myopathy
12. fetal alcohol syndrome
13. Marchiafava-Bignami disease
14. central pontine myelinolysis
15. optic atrophy due to methanol contamination
16. toxic optic atrophy from contaminants

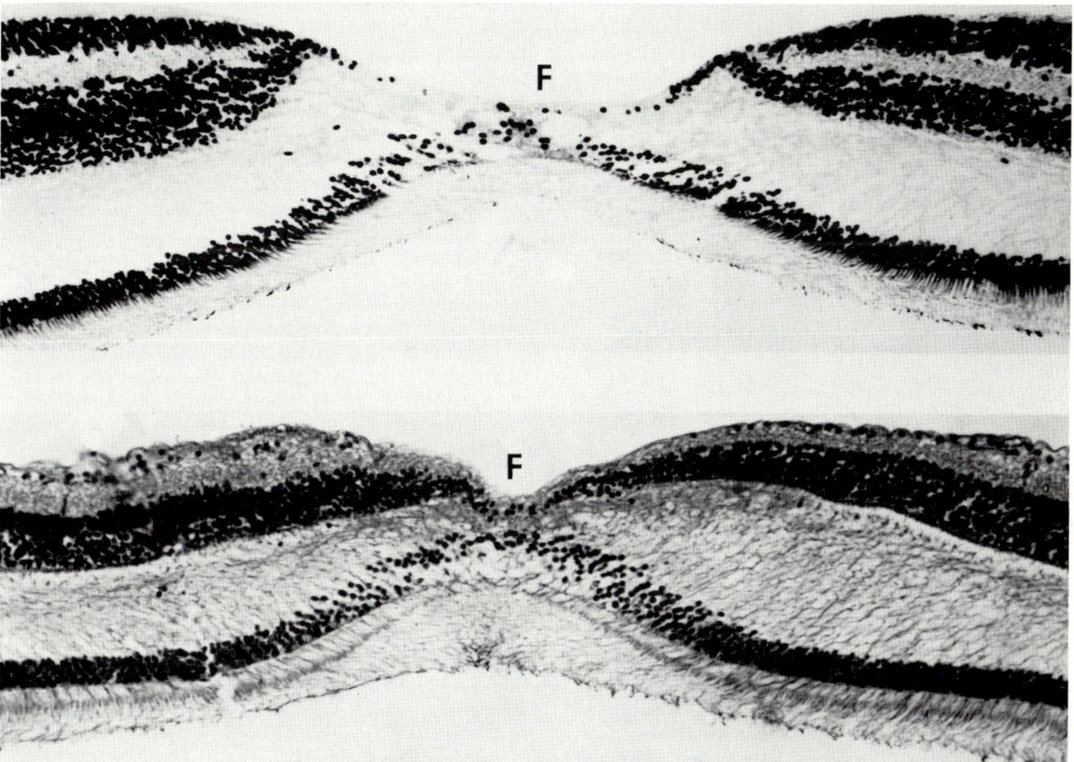

Fig. 16. Retinal lesion in vitamin B$_{12}$ deficiency. The sections are through the macula and stained with hematoxylin and eosin. *Above:* Normal control monkey; the parafoveal ganglion cell layer is several cells thick. *Below:* B$_{12}$ deficient monkey; severe loss of ganglion cells in parafoveal parts of the macula. Compare with Figure 8. (F) fovea. From Chester, *et al.*[55]

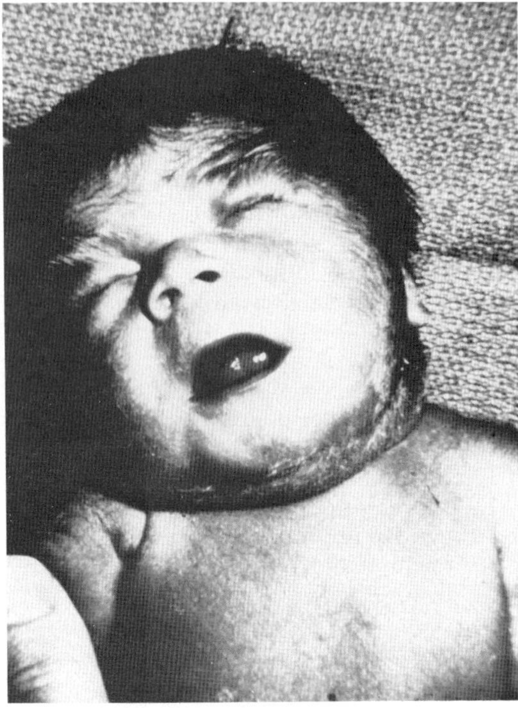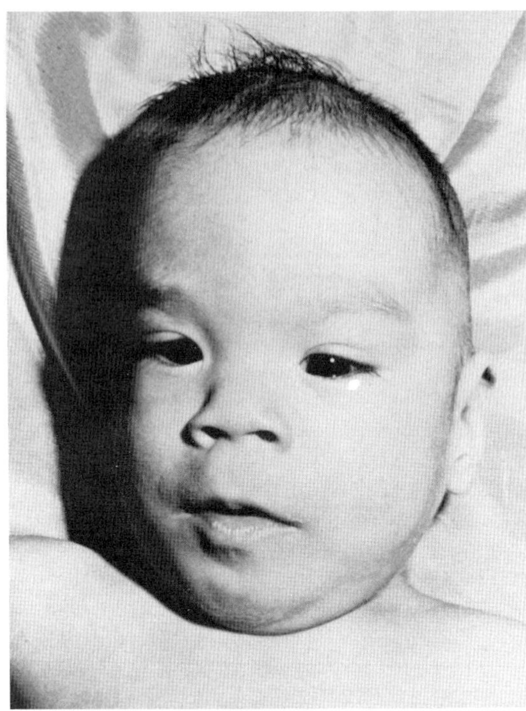

Fig. 17. The fetal alcohol syndrome. Note the hirsutism in the newborn (left) and the epicanthal folds and short palpebral fissures at 10 months of age (right). Courtesy of Dr. D. W. Smith, University of Washington, Seattle.

17. drugs associated with alcohol abuse
18. hypertension

I am sure there are others, but it does help to recall that the alcoholic is more often exposed to trauma, other drugs, venereal infections, seizures, and the like, so the above has helped me. Dr. Victor caused me to add the fetal alcohol syndrome to this list!

JLS

REFERENCES

1. Dodge, R. and Benedict, F. G. *Psychological Effects of Alcohol.* Carnegie Institution of Washington, Washington, D.C., 1915, Pub. No. 232.
2. Miles, W. R. *Effects of Alcohol on Psycho-physiological Functions.* Carnegie Institution of Washington, Washington, D.C., 1918, Pub. No. 266.
3. Wilkinson, I. M. S., Kime, R., and Purnell, M. Alcohol and human eye movement. Brain 97:785–792 (1974).
4. Franck, M. C. and Kuhlo, W. Die Wirkung des Alkohols auf die raschen Blickzielbewegungen beim Menschen. Arch. Psychiatr. Nervenkr. *213:*238–245 (1970).
5. Gentles, W. and Llewellyn, T. E. Effect of benzodiazepines upon saccadic eye movements in man. Clin. Pharmacol. Ther. *12:*563–574 (1971).
6. Aschan, G. Different types of alcohol nystagmus. Acta Otolaryngal. Suppl. *140:*69–78 (1958).
7. Aschan, G. and Bergstedt, M. Positional alcoholic nystagmus (PAN) in man following repeated alcohol doses. Acta Otolaryngol. Suppl. *330:*15–29 (1975).
8. Gilson, R. D., Schroeder, D. J., Collins, W. E., and Guedry, F. E., Jr. Effects of different alcohol dosages on tracking performance during vestibular stimulation. Aerospace Med. *43:*656–660 (1972).
9. Guedry, F. E., Jr., Gilson, R. D., Schroeder, D. J., and Collins, W. E. Some effects of alcohol on various aspects of oculomotor control. Aviation Space Environ. Med. *46:*1008–1013 (1975).
10. Victor, M., Adams, R. D., and Collins, G. F. *The Wernicke-Korsakoff Syndrome. A Clinical and Pathological Study of 245 cases, 82 with Postmortem Examinations.* F. A. Davis, Philadelphia, 1971.
11. Phillips, G. B., Victor, M., Adams, R. D., and Davidson, C. S. A study of the nutritional defect in Wernicke's syndrome: The effect of a purified diet, thiamine, and other vitamins on the clinical manifestations. J. Clin. Invest. *31:*859–871 (1952).
12. Victor, M. and Adams, R. D. On the etiology of the alcoholic neurologic diseases: With special references to the role of nutrition. Am. J. Clin. Nutr. *9:*379–397 (1961).
13. Baughman, F. A., Jr. and Papp, J. P. Wernicke's encephalopathy with intravenous hyperalimentation: Remarks on similarities between Wernicke's

encephalopathy and the phosphate depletion syndrome. Mt. Sinai J. Med. N.Y. *43*:48–52 (1976).

14. Cruickshank, E. K. Wernicke's encephalopathy. Q. J. Med. *19*:327–338 (1950).

15. Drenick, E. J., Joven, C. B., and Swenseid, M. E. Occurrence of acute Wernicke's encephalopathy during prolonged starvation for the treatment of obesity. New Engl. J. Med. *274*:937–939 (1966).

16. Victor, M., Mancall, E. L., and Dreyfus, P. M. Deficiency amblyopia in the alcoholic patient: A clinicopathologic study. Arch. Ophthalmol. *64*:1–33 (1960).

17. Victor, M. and Dreyfus, P. M. Tobacco-alcohol amblyopia. Further comments on its pathology. Arch. Ophthalmol. *74*:649–657 (1965).

18. Potts, A. M. Tobacco amblyopia. Surv. Ophthalmol. *17*:313–339 (1973).

19. Victor, M. Tobacco-alcohol amblyopia: A critique of current concepts of this disorder, with special reference to the role of nutritional deficiency in its causation. Arch. Ophthalmol. *70*:313–318 (1963).

20. Victor, M. Tobacco amblyopia, cyanide poisoning and vitamin B_{12} deficiency: A critique of current concepts. In: *Miami Neuroophthalmology Symposium*. J. L. Smith (Ed.), Huffman, Hallandale, Fla., 1970, Vol. 5, Chap. 3, pp. 33–48.

21. Crawford, J. N. and Reid, J. A. G. Nutritional disease affecting Canadian troops held prisoner of war by the Japanese. Can. J. Res. *25*:53–85 (1947).

22. Denny-Brown, D. E. Neurological conditions resulting from prolonged and severe dietary restriction. Medicine *26*:41–113 (1947).

23. Fisher, C. M. Residual neuropathological changes in Canadians held prisoners of war by the Japanese. Can. Serv. Med. J. *11*:157–199 (1955).

24. King, J. H., Jr. and Passmore, J. W. Nutritional amblyopia: A study of American prisoners of war in Korea. Am. J. Ophthalmol. *39*:173–186 (1955).

25. Smith, D. A. and Woodruff, M. F. A. *Deficiency Diseases in Japanese Prison Camps*, Med. Res. Counc. Spec. Rep. No. 274. Her Majesty's Stationery Office, London, 1951.

26. Spillane, J. D. *Nutritional Disorders of the Nervous System*. Williams & Wilkins, Baltimore, 1947.

27. Carroll, F. D. The etiology and treatment of tobacco-alcohol amblyopia. Am. J. Ophthalmol. *27*:713–725 (1944a); 847–863 (1944b).

28. Heaton, J. M., McCormick, A. J. A., and Freeman, A. G. Tobacco-amblyopia: A clinical manifestation of vitamin B_{12} deficiency. Lancet *2*:286–290 (1958).

29. Wokes, F. Tobacco amblyopia. Lancet *2*:526–527 (1958).

30. Ferraro, A. Experimental toxic encephalomyelopathy (diffuse sclerosis following subcutaneous injections of potassium cyanide). Psychiatr. Q. *7*:267–283 (1933).

31. Hurst, E. W. Experimental demyelination of the central nervous system. 1. The encephalopathy produced by potassium cyanide. Aust. J. Exp. Biol. Med. Sci. *18*:201–223 (1940).

32. Hicks, S. P. Brain metabolism in vivo. 1. The distribution of lesions caused by cyanide poisoning insulin hypoglycemia, asphyxia in nitrogen, and fluoroacetate poisoning in rats. Arch. Pathol. *49*:111–137 (1950).

33. Lumsden, C. E. Cyanide leucoencephalopathy in rats and observations of the vascular and ferment hypotheses of demyelinating diseases. J. Neurol. Neurosurg. Psychiatr. *13*:1–15 (1950).

34. Hirano, A., Levine, S., and Zimmerman, H. M. Experimental cyanide encephalopathy: electron microscopic observations of early lesions in white matter. J. Neuropathol. Exp. Neurol. *26*:200–213 (1967).

35. Levine, S. Experimental cyanide encephalopathy: gradients of susceptibility in the corpus callosum. J. Neuropathol. Exp. Neurol. *26*:214–222 (1967).

36. Bass, N. H. Pathogenesis of myelin lesions in experimental cyanide encephalopathy. Neurol. *18*:167–177 (1968).

37. Rodger, F. C. Experimental thiamine deficiency as a cause of degeneration in the visual pathway of the rat. Br. J. Ophthalmol. *37*:11–29 (1953).

38. Adams, R. D., and Kubik, C. S. Subacute combined degeneration of the brain in pernicious anemia. New Engl. J. Med. *231*:1–9 (1944).

39. Woltmann, H. W. The nervous system in pernicious anemia; an analysis of one hundred and fifty cases. Am. J. Med. Sci. *157*:400–409 (1919).

40. Hamilton, H. E., Ellis, P. P., and Sheets, R. F. Visual impairment due to optic neuropathy in pernicious anemia: report of a case and review of the literature. Blood *14*:378–385 (1959).

41. Courville, C. B. and Nielsen, J. M. Optic atrophy associated with subacute combined degeneration of the spinal cord: report of 2 cases. Bull. Los Angeles Neurol. Soc. *3*:83–87 (1938).

42. Kampmeier, R. H. and Jones, E. Optic atrophy in pernicious anemia. Am. J. Med. Sci. *195*:633–638 (1936).

43. Turner, J. W. A. Optic atrophy associated with pernicious anemia. Brain *63*:225–236 (1940).

44. Benham, G. H. H. Visual field defects in subacute combined degeneration of the spinal cord. J. Neurol. Neurosurg. Psychiatr. *14*:40–46 (1951).

45. Hyland, H. H., and Sharpe, V. J. H. Optic nerve degeneration in pernicious anemia. Can. Med. Assoc. J. *67*:660–665 (1952).

46. Enoksson, P. and Norden, A. Vitamin B_{12} deficiency affecting the optic nerve. Acta Med. Scand. *167*:199–208 (1960).

47. Cohen, H. Optic atrophy as presenting sign in pernicious anemia. Lancet *2*:1202–1203 (1936).

48. Box, C. R. Amaurosis in pernicious anemia. Lancet *2*:1269 (1936).

49. McAlpine, D. and Goldsmith, A. J. B. Optic atrophy and pernicious anemia. Arch. Middlesex Hosp. *1*:109–118 (1951).

50. Lerman, S. and Feldmahn, A. L. Centrocecal scotomata as the presenting sign in pernicious anemia. Arch. Ophthalmol. *65*:381–385 (1961).

51. Olivarius, B. deF. and Jensen, L. Retrobulbar neuritis and optic atrophy in pernicious anemia. Acta Ophthalmol. (Kbh.) *30*:190–197 (1961).

52. Kark, J., Victor, M., Hines, J., and Harris, J. Nutritional vitamin B_{12} deficiency in rhesus monkeys. Am. J. Clin. Nutrition *27*:470–478 (1974).

53. Agamanolis, D. P., Victor, M., *et al.* Neuropathology of experimental vitamin B_{12} deficiency in monkeys. Neurol. *26*:905–914 (1976).

54. Agamanolis, D. P., Victor, M. *et al.* An ultrastructural study of subacute combined degeneration of

the spinal cord in vitamin B_{12} deficient rhesus monkeys. J. Neuropathol. Exp. Neurol. *37:*273–299 (1978).

55. Chester, E. M., Agamanolis, D., *et al.* Optic atrophy in experimental vitamin B_{12} deficiency in monkeys. Neurol. (in press).

56. Frenkel, E. P., Kitchens, R. L., and Johnston, J. M. The effect of vitamin B_{12} deprivation on the enzymes of fatty acid synthesis. J. Biol. Chem. *248:*7540–7546 (1973).

57. Sullivan, W. C. A note on the influence of maternal inebriety on the offspring. J. Ment. Sci. *45:*489–503 (1899).

58. Sullivan, W. C. The children of the female drunkard. Med. Temperance Rev. *3:*72 (1900).

59. Haggard, H. W. and Jellinek, E. M. Alcohol Explored. Doubleday, Doran and Co., Garden City, N.Y., 1942.

60. Jones, K. L. and Smith, D. W. Recognition of the fetal alcohol syndrome in early infancy. Lancet *2:*999–1001 (1973).

61. Warner, R. H. and Rosett, H. L. The effects of drinking in offspring: An historical survey of the American and British literature. J. Stud. Alcohol *36*(11):1395–1420 (1975).

62. Keller, M. Other effects of alcohol. In: *Drinking and Intoxication, Part I: Physiological and Psychological Effects of Alcohol.* R. G. McCarthy (Ed.), The Free Press, Glencoe, Ill., 1959, pp. 13–17.

63. Lemoine P., Harrousseau, H., Borteyru, J. P., and Menuet, J. C. Les enfants de parents alcooliques: Anomalies observees: A propos de 127 cas. Ouest Med. *25:*477 (1968).

64. Ulleland, C. The offspring of alcoholic mothers. Ann. N.Y. Acad. Sci. *197:*167–169 (1972).

65. Jones, K. L., Smith, D. W., Ulleland, C. N., and Streissguth, A. P. Pattern of malformation in offspring of chronic alcoholic mothers. Lancet *1:*1267–1271 (1973).

66. Jones, K. L., Smith, D. W., Streissguth, A. P., and Myrianthopoulos, N. C. Outcome in offspring of chronic alcoholic women. Lancet *1:*1076–1078 (1974).

67. Hanson, J. W., Jones, K. L., and Smith, D. W. Fetal alcohol syndrome. Experience with 41 patients. J. Am. Med. Assoc. *235:*1458–1460 (1976).

68. Mulvihill, J. J. and Yeager, A. M. Fetal alcohol syndrome. Teratol. *13*(3):345–348 (1976).

69. Rosett, H. L., Ouellette, E. M., and Weiner, L. A pilot prospective study of the fetal alcohol syndrome at the Boston City Hospital. Part I: Maternal drinking. In: *Work in Progress on Alcoholism.* F. A. Seixas and S. Eggleston (Eds.). Ann. N.Y. Acad. Sci. *273:*118–122 (1976).

Cockayne's Syndrome. Neuro-ophthalmic, CAT Scan, and Endocrine Observations

Steven Coker, M. D.,
John Susac, M. D.,
James Sharpe, M. D.,
and Robert Smallridge, M. D.

In 1936, Cockayne[1] described two dwarfed siblings (a six-year-old male and a seven-year-old female), with small heads, sunken eyes, and prominent maxillae. Both children were mentally deficient, had decreased hearing, scaly dermatitis, pigmentary retinal degeneration, large hands, thickening of the cranial vault on x-ray, and long extremities. These children were active and described as good tempered, laughing with slight provocation. Subsequent examination[2] of these children at ages 16 and 17 revealed a decrease in visual acuity, cataracts, and multiple joint contractures. The girl reached a height of three feet, four and one-half inches, the boy, three feet, eight and one-half inches, and both had some pubertal changes.

Since the report by Cockayne of these two cachectic dwarfs, more than thirty similar children have been described and additional features reported. Intracranial calcification, osteoporosis, posterior tapering of the vertebral bodies, and slender ribs may be seen on x-ray.[3] Truncal and extremity incoordination, spasticity, nystagmus, and peripheral neuropathy also occur. The onset of clinical symptoms is usually in the second year of life, although developmental milestones are often somewhat delayed earlier. Deterioration progresses with blindness, deafness, mental deficiency, paralysis, and incoordination. The children with Cockayne's syndrome usually die in adolescence or early adult life from inanition and infection.[5-7]

The neuro-ophthalmic findings and results of computerized axial tomography (CAT) in four children with Cockayne's syndrome are described. One child had retinal vascular complications, not previously documented in this disease. This child also underwent extensive endocrine evaluation.

CASE REPORTS

Case 1. K. A. is a 9½-year-old female product of a 35-week gestation with birth weight of 4 lb, 15 oz. Developmental milestones were abnormal: she crawled at five months, walked at 18 months, put words together at three years, and toilet trained at three and one-half to four years. Frequent stumbling and falling was noted at two years, and this gradually worsened so that she stopped walking at four years of age. Dysarthria has been present since the onset of speech development. At present she knows most of the alphabet, can name colors, and count to 10. She cannot read. The family history reveals three children of a maternal great uncle with nanism who all died in their twenties. Two normal brothers of these dwarfs had a total of three dwarfed children. This child is a second cousin to these three children herein described with Cockayne's syndrome.

Physical examination revealed a thin 22-

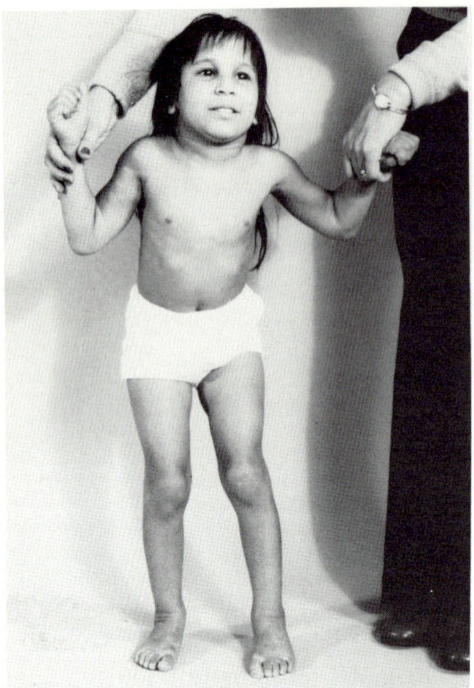

Fig. 1.

pound, dwarfed female, 36 in. tall, with a prominent maxilla (Fig. 1). Head circumference is 18 in. She has large hands in relation to her body size and flexion contractures of the knees, ankles, and hips bilaterally. Neurologic examination revealed horizontal pendular and gaze evoked nystagmus, truncal ataxia, intention tremor of all four extremities, hyperreflexia of the lower extremities, and bilateral Babinski reflexes. Funduscopic examination under anesthesia revealed a gross vitreous hemorrhage in the right eye, precluding examination of the retina. In the left eye, dilated, tortuous veins with intraretinal and subhyaloid hemorrhages were found. The disc was pale and sheathed. Narrowed arterioles were noted.

Routine laboratory data, including CBC, electrolytes, urinalysis, T_4, cholesterol, triglycerides, CPK, and serum protein electrophoresis, were normal. Chromosomal analysis with banding revealed a normal karyotype. EKG, chest x-rays, and bone age were normal. There was decreased vertebral body height, long diaphyseal with prominent metaphyseal segments of the long bones as well as increased density of the skull with intracranial calcifications by

x-rays. Nerve conduction velocity studies were normal. An EEG showed slowing of the background rhythm. A CAT scan revealed bilateral basal ganglia calcifications (Fig. 2). The cerebrospinal fluid was completely normal.

Endocrine and metabolic studies revealed the following results*: T_4, T_3RU, TSH, cholesterol, triglycerides, urinary 17 OHCS, and 17 ketosteroids were normal. Alpha amino nitrogen and amino acid profile were normal. An oral glucose tolerance test (1.75 gm/kg) produced a rise in plasma glucose from 61 mgm% to a peak of 112 mgm% at 30 min. The basal insulin level was 15 U/ml and rose to 55 U/ml at 60 min. Her basal growth hormone was 4 ng/ml and rose to 32 ng/ml following intravenous insulin (0.1 u/kg). Serum somatomedin activity was 1.4 u/ml as determined in a rat costal cartilage bioassay. The patient's serum was capable of stimulating (^{3}H) thymidine incorporation into the DNA of chick embryo fibroblast.

Case 2. A. C. is a 10-year-old cachectic dwarf. She is the product of a normal pregnancy, labor, and delivery. Initial growth and development were normal. Postural unsteadiness was noted with the onset of walking and her intellectual development has been delayed.

Examination. The maxilla is prominent. There is low amplitude, horizontal pendular nystagmus on forward fixation, and jerk nystagmus on lateral gaze. There is truncal instability and inability to perform tandem walking. Cranial nerves, motor strength, muscle tone, reflexes, and upper extremity cerebellar testing are normal. Funduscopic examination was normal, but the electroretinogram (ERG) was reduced to 10% of normal. Bilateral calcifications of the basal ganglia were present on CAT scans (Fig. 3).

Case 3. A. C. is a 14-year-old dwarfed, mentally deficient female with a prominent maxilla, disproportionately large feet and hands, and large ears. She was considered normal until one to two years of age when delayed gross motor development and

* Insulin and growth hormone levels were kindly measured by Dr. C. Ronald Kahn, National Institutes of Health. Somatomedin was measured by Dr. William Daughaday, St. Louis, MO, and chick embryo fibroblast studies performed by Dr. S. Peter Nissley, NIH.

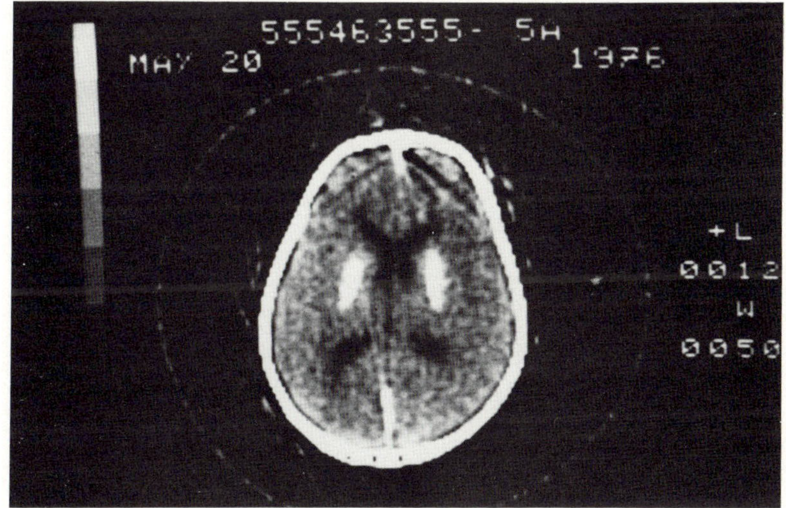

Fig. 2.

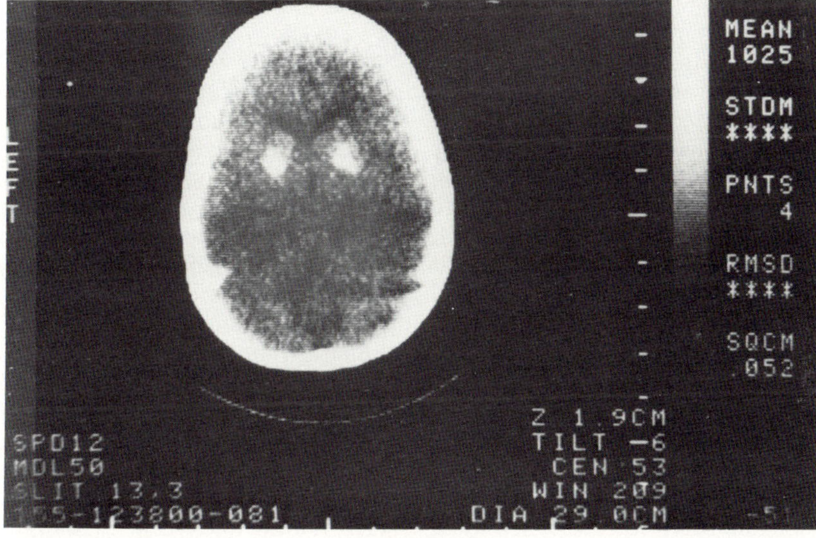

Fig. 3.

growth were noted. Her gait has become progressively unsteady.

Examination. Cranial nerves were normal, including hearing to whispered voice. There is a mild spastic quadriparesis, moderate truncal and extremity ataxia, hyperactive deep tendon reflexes, and bilateral extensor plantar responses. The fundus was normal on ophthalmoscopic examination, but the electroretinogram was only 10% of normal amplitude. A CAT scan revealed bilateral calcification of the basal ganglia, occipital lobes, and right frontal calcification (Fig. 4).

Case 4. N. C. was a 23-year-old male with cachectic nanism and prominent maxillae. His early development was normal up until the age of 30 months when nystagmus and incoordination were detected.

Examination. He was 45 in. tall, appeared old, and had marked intellectual deterioration with speech limited to dysarthric "yes" or "no" responses to questions. The eyes were deeply set. Visual acuity was limited to finger counting at 4 ft. Funduscopic examination revealed optic atrophy. Although the retina appeared normal, the electroretinogram was reduced to 10% of

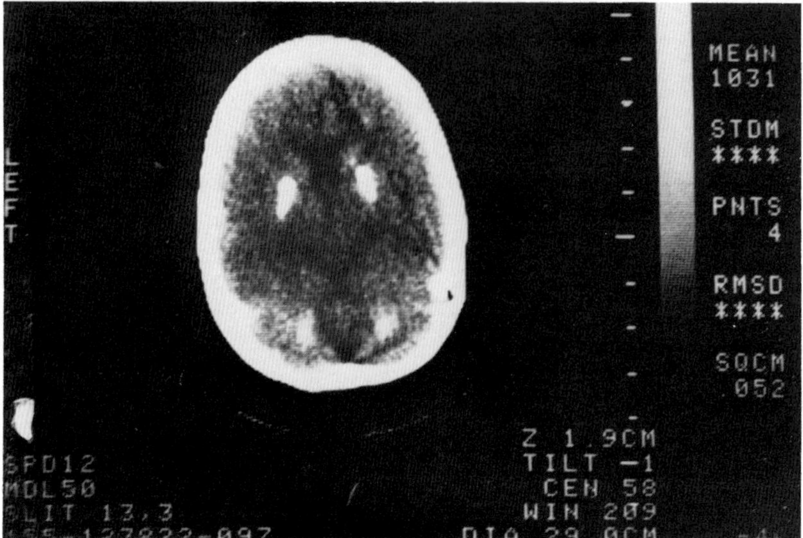

Fig. 4.

the normal amplitude. The pupils were 4 mm and reacted well to light. He had bilateral paralytic exotropia. Adduction of each eye to the midposition was achieved only to oculocephalic maneuvers. Abducting jerk nystagmus of each eye occurred during lateral gaze. Upward gaze was paralyzed and downward gaze was limited to about 20°. Levator palpebrae function was intact. He had mild bilateral central facial paresis. Hearing was intact to loud speech. Spastic quadriparesis prevented his standing without assistance. Deep tendon reflexes were increased and both plantar responses were extensor. Ataxia was marked in the upper limbs. He had moderate kyphosis. The right testicle was small and left undescended. CAT scanning revealed bilateral calcification in the basal ganglia, frontal and occipital hemispheres as well as enlargement of the ventricular system (Fig. 5).

The patient died six months later from progressive inanition. Postmortem examination performed at another medical center confirmed typical pathologic features of Cockayne's syndrome with widespread cerebral, brain stem, and cerebellar involvement.

DISCUSSION

Cockayne's syndrome may be described as an autosomal recessively inherited dis-order manifested by cachectic dwarfism, progeroid appearance with prominent maxillae, and a progressive neurologic disorder that includes mental deficiency, incoordination, spasticity, hearing loss, and degeneration of the retina. The neuropathologic changes consist of widespread patchy demyelination with relative preservation of axis cylinders and variable neuronal loss in the cerebral cortex and cerebellum. Siderocalcific deposits in the brain and its vessels are characteristic.[5, 7, 8] The pathogenesis of Cockayne's syndrome is unknown.

Attempts to find an endocrine abnormality to explain nanism in this entity have been unsuccessful. Fujimoto *et al.*[9] described one patient who had an elevated fasting insulin level, hypercholesterolemia, and renal disease. Cotton *et al.*[10] studied a child who had a large rise in growth hormone levels after only a mild reduction in blood glucose and a large rise in insulin during glucose and tolbutamide tolerance tests. With these two exceptions, there have been no metabolic abnormalities described that might explain the dwarfism in these children. In Case 1, all the usual laboratory studies were normal, including the patient's insulin response during a glucose tolerance test and her growth hormone response to hypoglycemia. The presence of normal serum somatomedin-like activity excludes a mechanism such as seen in Laron's dwarf-

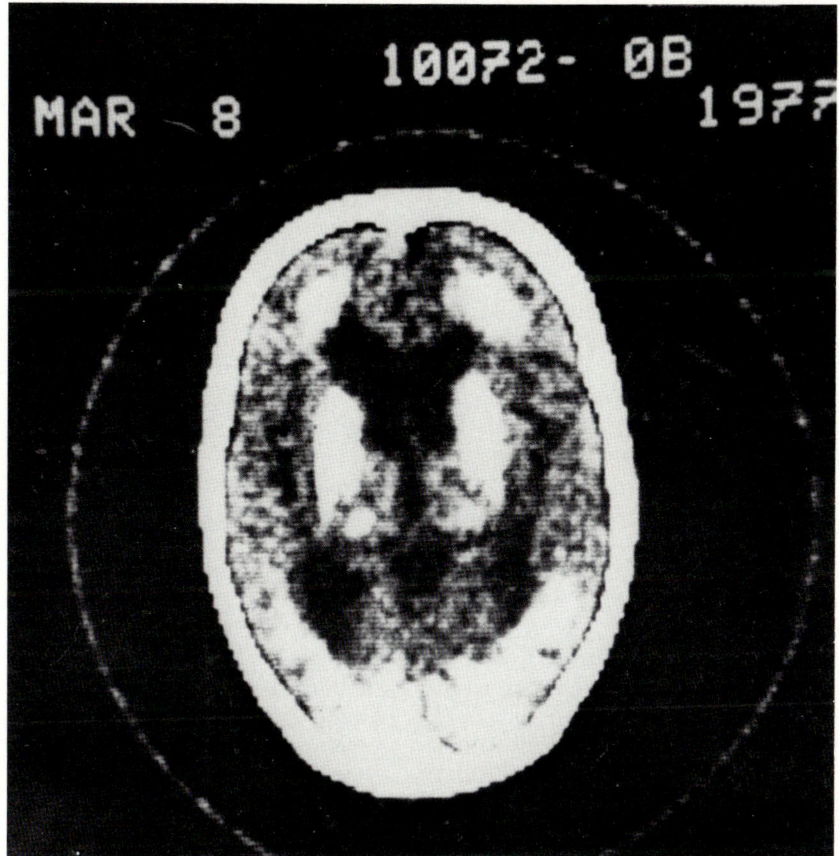

Fig. 5.

ism, where somatomedin levels are low.[11] Additional evidence of biologically active somatomedin is provided by finding that the patient's serum is capable of stimulating (^{3}H) thymidine incorporation into DNA of chick embryo fibroblasts.[12] These studies do not rule out the possibility that the patient's dwarfism is due to end-organ resistance to somatomedin.

There are specific x-ray findings in Cockayne's syndrome, and the radiologist may be the first to suggest the diagnosis.[3] The earliest x-ray findings become noticeable in the second and third years of life, and include thick skull, thin, flared ribs, shortened vertebral bodies, and long diaphysis and widened metaphysis of long bones. Calcifications on skull x-ray have been described periventricularly and in the basal ganglia in roughly one-half of the reported cases. Since the CAT scan is much more sensitive in detecting intracranial calcification, prob-ably more cases could be detected at an earlier age by its use. In each of our patients, the CAT scan revealed extensive calcifications which were more widespread than previously detected by skull x-ray. Two patients had calcifications of the frontal and occipital lobes, as well as the basal ganglia.

Neuro-ophthalmic manifestations were prominent in our cases. Pigmentary retinal degeneration and optic atrophy are a recognized cause of visual loss in Cockayne's syndrome.[1, 6, 8] Although none of our patients had the fundus appearance of retinitis pigmentosa, typical or atypical, three (Cases 2, 3, and 4) had subnormal ERG's and one had optic atrophy (Case 4). Our first patient, who had a normal ERG, had a most unusual venous stasis retinopathy which has not been previously reported. This process led to vitreous hemorrhage in one eye. We postulate the deposition of calcium in the walls of central retinal veins, similar to that occurring in cerebral vessels, may cause this venous stasis retinopathy. Visual loss may result from damage to occipital cortex as identified pathologically by Moosey.[5] The prominent subcortical occipital lobe calcifications in two of our patients (Cases 3 and 4) indicate that involvement of the visual radiations can also be responsible. None of our patients had impaired pupillary responses to mydriatics or the defective tearing described in a few such cases.[16, 17]

Pendular nystagmus in all four of our cases can be explained by the cerebellar and brain stem demyelination typical of Cockayne's syndrome.[8, 18] Acquired pendular nystagmus in multiple sclerosis correlates with the occurrence of limb and truncal ataxia[19]; ataxia was present in all of our cases. In Case 4, ocular motor dysfunction progressed to bilateral paralytic exotropia with abducting nystagmus of each eye. This wall-eyed bilateral internuclear ophthalmoplegia (WEBINO Syndrome) has been attributed to combined involvement of medial rectus neurons and the medial longitudinal fasciculae.[20] Vertical ophthalmoplegia with sparing of upper lid and pupillary constrictor function in Case 4 signified prenuclear involvement of the rostral midbrain or bilateral damage to the paramedian pontine reticular formation.[21]

In its advanced stages, Cockayne's syndrome can be diagnosed readily by the constellation of dwarfism, skeletal changes, psychomotor deterioration, and intracranial calcification. Although no treatment to prevent growth failure and progressive nervous system damage is available, early diagnosis is important for genetic counselling. Detection of intracranial calcification by CAT scanning and awareness of the distinctive neuro-ophthalmic manifestations illustrated by our cases will facilitate prompt recognition of this unique heredofamilial disease.

EDITOR'S NOTE

I have never personally seen a case of Cockayne's syndrome, or at least I have never recognized it as such if I did! Therefore, after reading this paper I called Dr. John Susac on the telephone and asked him this question—"John, if I were on a desert island and a child with Cockayne's syndrome swam up on shore, how could I really make that diagnosis?" He said—"Well, they are little old people… they look like progeria!" I looked at the bibliography of this paper and saw that the first two papers by Cockayne mentioned dwarfism with retinal atrophy and deafness. I asked Dr. Susac if his cases had retinal atrophy and deafness, and he replied "No." I said—"Well, how am I going to tell the ophthalmologist out there in practice, how to really diagnose this thing?" Dr. Susac then replied—"Well, when these cases first came in, we didn't know what they had either! However, when we got the CT scans, they showed basal ganglia calcification and that is how we made the diagnosis!" Now, we are warming up—if you have a funny-looking child who obviously has some syndrome that you are not familiar with, you can get a CT scan—and if they have basal ganglia calcification, you may have a Cockayne's syndrome on your hands! I think that is the point of this chapter.

Dr. Fredie Gargano tells me on the phone that the differential diagnosis of basal ganglia calcification in a young patient on computed tomographic scan is: hypoparathyroidism, pseudohypoparathyroidism, idiopathic, and familial. He told me that in cytomegalic inclusion disease all the calcification is periventricular, but that, in toxoplasmosis, they have calcification not only in basal ganglia but in other areas (as noted in frontal and occipital lobes in the cases here reported).

I must admit I'm still not an expert on Cockayne's syndrome after having read the chapter. I spoke with Dr. Norman Schatz on the phone after beginning this note. He told me he had never seen a case of Cockayne's syndrome himself, but that he had been a visiting lecturer some place and they showed him one. He told me that after he had seen the case, he still wasn't sure what he had seen! Walsh and Hoyt mention on page 907— "In 1936, Cockayne described in two siblings dwarfism, partial deafness, retinal degeneration, mental deficiency, photosensitivity of the skin, deformities of the joints, and cataracts." Apparently dwarfism, photosensitivity, progeria, large ears, and large hands and feet are major points. However, I believe the real contribution of this chapter is that the computed tomographic scan may lead you to this unusual diagnosis if you find basal ganglia calcification in a young patient who reminds you of progeria!

JLS

REFERENCES

1. Cockayne, E. A. Dwarfism with retinal atrophy and deafness. Arch. Dis. Child. *11:*1–8 (1936).
2. Cockayne, E. A. Case reports: dwarfism with retinal atrophy and deafness. Arch. Dis. Child. *21:*52–54 (1946).
3. Alton, D. J., McDonald, P., and Rielly, B. J. Cockayne's syndrome: report of three gases. Radiology *102:*403–406 (1972).
4. Moosa, A. and Dubowitz, V. Peripheral neuropathy in Cockayne's syndrome. Arch. Dis. Child. *45:*674–677 (1970).
5. Moosey, J. The neuropathology of Cockayne's syndrome. J. Neuropath. Exp. Neurol. *26:*654–660, (1967).
6. Neill, C. A. and Dingwall, M. M. A syndrome resembling progeria: a review of two cases. Arch. Dis. Child. *25:*213–223 (1950).
7. Paddison, R. M., Moosey, J. *et al.* Cockayne's syndrome: a report of five new cases with biochemical, chromosomal, dermatologic, genetic and neuropathology observations. Derm. Trop. *2:*195–203 (1963).
8. Sugarman, G. I., Landing, B. H., and Reed, W. B. Cockayne syndrome: clinical study of two patients and neuropathologic findings in one. Clin. Pediatr. (Phila.) *16:*225–232 (1977).
9. Fujimoto, W. Y., Greene, M. L., and Seegmiller, J. E. Cockayne's Syndrome: report of a case with hyperlipoproteinemia, hyperinsulinemia, renal disease and hormonal growth hormone. J. Pediatr. *75:*881–884 (1969).
10. Cotton, R. B., Keats, T. E., and McCoy, E. E. Abnormal blood glucose regulation in Cockayne's syndrome. Pediatrics *45:*54–60 (1970).
11. Daughaday, W. N., Laron, Z., Pertzelan, A., and Heins, J. N. Defective sulfatron factor generation: a possible etiological link in dwarfism. Trans. Assoc. Am. Physicians *82:*129–140 (1969).
12. Moses, A. C. *et al.* Contribution of human somatomedin activity to the serum growth requirement of human skin fibroblasts and chick embryo fibroblasts in culture. J. Clin. Endocrinol. Metab. *46:* 937 (1978).
13. Norman, R. M. and Tingey, A. H. Syndrome of micrencephaly, stio-cerebellar calcifications and leukodystrophy. J. Neurol. Neurosurg. Psychiatr. *29:*157–163 (1966).
14. Pearce, W. G. Ocular and genetic features of Cockayne's syndrome. Can. J. Ophthalmol. *7:*435–444 (1972).
15. Coles, W. H. Ocular manifestations of Cockayne's syndrome. Am. J. Ophthalmol *67:*762–764 (1969).
16. Lieberman, W. J., Schimek, R. A., and Snyder, C. H. Cockayne's disease: a report of a case. Am. J. Ophthalmol. *52:*116–118 (1961).
17. Spark, H. Cachectic dwarfism resembling the Cockayne-Neil type. J. Pediatr. *66:*41–47 (1965).
18. Rowlatt, U. Cockayne's syndrome: report of case with necropsy findings. Acta Neuropathol (Berl.) *14:*52–61 (1969).
19. Aschoff, J. G., Conrad, B., Kornhuber, H. H. Acquired pendular nystagmus with oscillopsia in multiple sclerosis: a sign of cerebellar nuclei disease. J. Neurol. Neurosurg. Psychiatr. *37:*570–577 (1974).
20. Daroff, R. B. and Hoyt, W. F. In: *Supranuclear Disorders of Ocular Control Systems in Man: Clinical, Anatomical and Physiological Correlations in the Control of Eye Movements.* P. Bach-Y-Rita, C. C. Collins, and J. E. Hyde (Eds.), Academic, New York, 1971, p. 223.
21. Christoff, N. A clinicopathologic study of vertical eye movements. Arch. Neurol. *31:*1–8 (1974).
22. Riggs, W., Jr. and Seibert, J. Cockayne's syndrome: roentgen findings. Am. J. Roentgenol. *116:* 623–33 (Nov. 1972).
23. Land, V. J., and Nogrady, M. B. Cockayne's syndrome. J. Can. Assoc. Radiol. *20:*193 (1969).

39 Ocular Findings in Kenny Syndrome

James R. Boynton, M.D.,
Thomas R. Pheasant, M.D.,
Bruce L. Johnson, M.D.,
Daniel B. Levin, M.D.,
and Barbara W. Streeten, M.D.

In 1966 Kenny and Linarelli described an unusual congenital syndrome.[1] A mother and son exhibited the following characteristics: low birth weight, dwarfism, delayed closure of the anterior fontanel, uniquely thickened long bone cortex with stenotic medullary cavities,[2] transient hypocalcemia with hyperphosphatemia leading to tetany, and normal mentation. Since this original description only two additional case reports of this syndrome have appeared.[3,4] The ophthalmic examination in all cases has been inaccurate or incomplete, and actually refers to hypermetropia. This chapter describes the ocular findings in four patients with Kenny syndrome, including histologic examination of one case.

CASE REPORTS

Case 1. The patient was first admitted to the hospital at age nine months with fever, tetany, dwarfism, and retarded bone age. A diagnosis of hypoparathyroidism was made and vitamin D therapy instituted. Multiple admissions for fever and convulsions followed, usually accompanied by upper respiratory disease. Hypocalcemia and hyperphosphatemia were documented repeatedly. Intelligence and tests of pituitary function were normal. At age 10, height and bone age were both retarded. Skull roentgenograms showed bilateral temporal lobe calcifications. X-rays of the long bones revealed internal cortical thickening and stenotic medullary cavities.

The patient appeared miniature with prominent forehead, microphthalmos, and micrognathia (Fig. 1). Height was 40 in.

At age three she was seen with a large right esotropia. The right disc was noted to be blurred, and the macular area of each eye was described as gray. At age five, vision was recorded as counting fingers at four feet in the right eye, and 20/200 in the left eye. The retina of the right eye was elevated and gray inferotemporally.

The patient was not seen again until she was age nine. Vision in the right eye was hand motion due to a dense cataract. An early band keratopathy was noted. Shortly thereafter the patient developed an acute glaucoma in the right eye with a flat anterior chamber. A posterior sclerotomy and lens aspiration were performed.

We first examined the patient at age twelve. Her best corrected vision was 20/800 in the right eye and 20/200 in the left eye. The refractive error in the left eye was +24.00 diopters. The fundus of the right eye was obscured by a secondary membrane after lens extraction. Corneas measured 8 mm in diameter and exhibited band keratopathy, greater on the right. The left fundus was filled with multiple, dilated, tortuous vessels. The entire retina appeared swollen and abnormal, especially in the region about the optic nerve. The vascular pattern combined with these highlights presented the deceptive picture of an accessory optic nerve head (Fig. 2).

Photographs, however, revealed a single elevated optic nerve head with tortuous, redundant retinal circulation simulating an accessory optic disc above. The retinal pigment epithelium was prominent in the posterior pole with pigment clumping in the parafoveal region. Fluorescein angiography

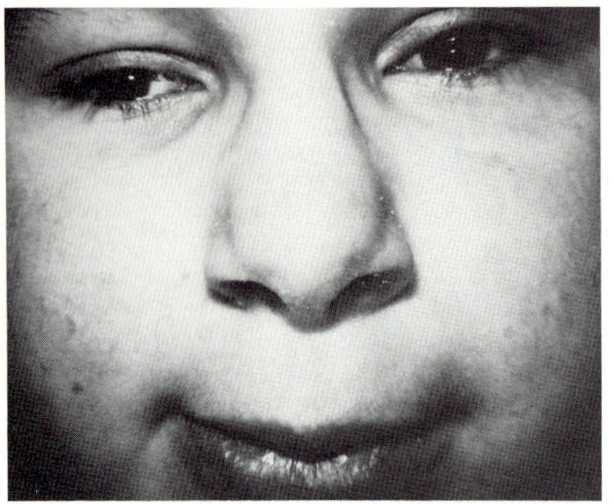

Fig. 1. Case 1. Facial appearance characteristic of Kenny syndrome in a 13-year-old girl.

confirmed a single retinal circulation (Fig. 3). Dye transit demonstrated dilated tortuous arterial and venous systems. There was no leakage or loss of competence of the retinal vasculature. The retina appeared crowded, as if confined to a smaller than normal space.

B-scan ultrasonography showed a single nerve pattern and a globe 13 mm in length. The nerve pattern appeared slightly enlarged relative to the size of the globe. Roentgenograms of the optic foramina were unremarkable.

Case 2. The mother and son originally described by Kenny in 1966[1] were recently examined. Their systemic findings are detailed in that report. The thirteen-year-old boy had a facial appearance similar to the first patient (Fig. 4). He was 53 in. in height. Best corrected vision was 20/30 in each eye with a +9.25 sphere in the right eye and a

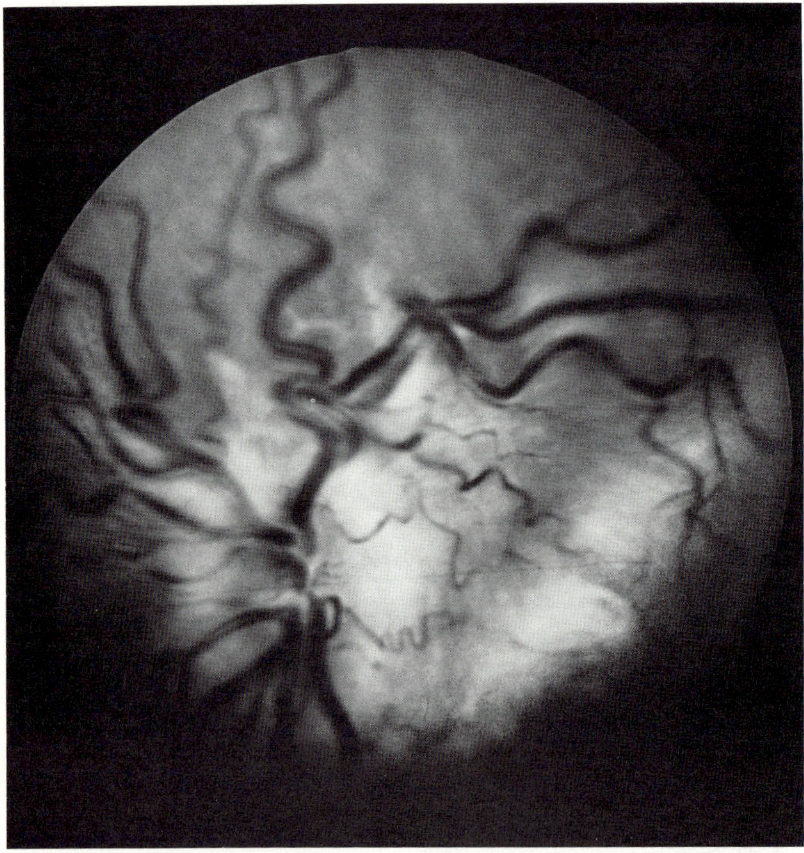

Fig. 2. Case 1. OS. The retinal vessels are tortuous and dilated. The disc is blurred and elevated. A confluence of vessels combined with unusual retinal highlights simulates an "accessory disc" superotemporal to the nerve head. The macular area is deeply pigmented and poorly defined.

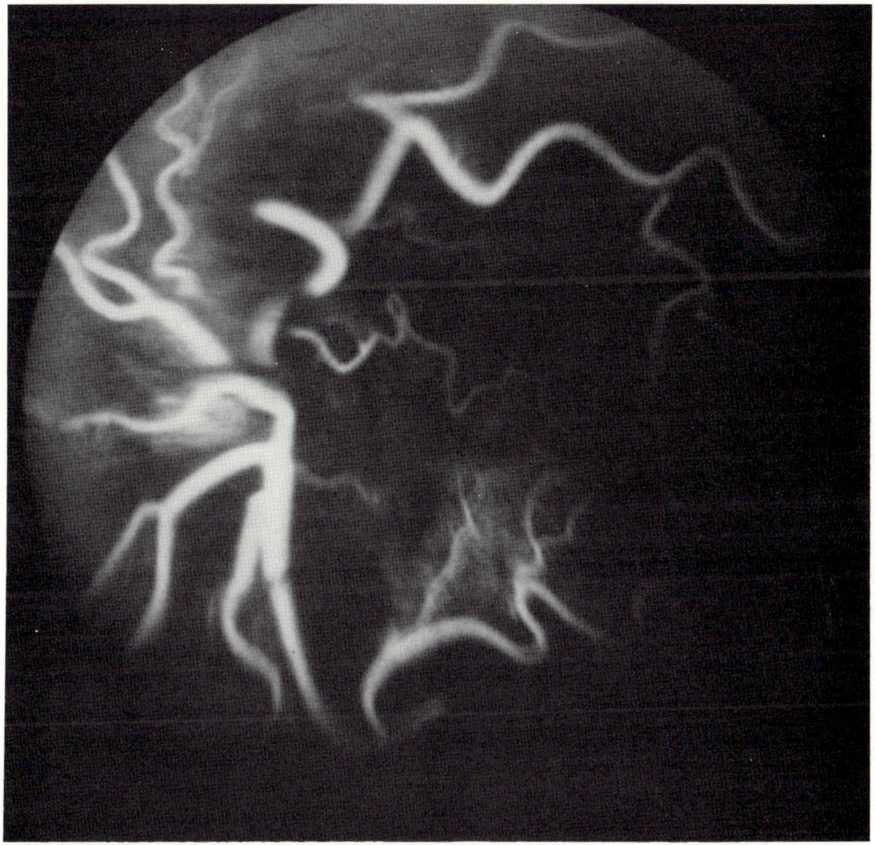

Fig. 3. Case 1. OS. Fluorescein angiogram, arterial phase. A single tortuous vascular system is present. There was no leakage of fluorescein in later photographs.

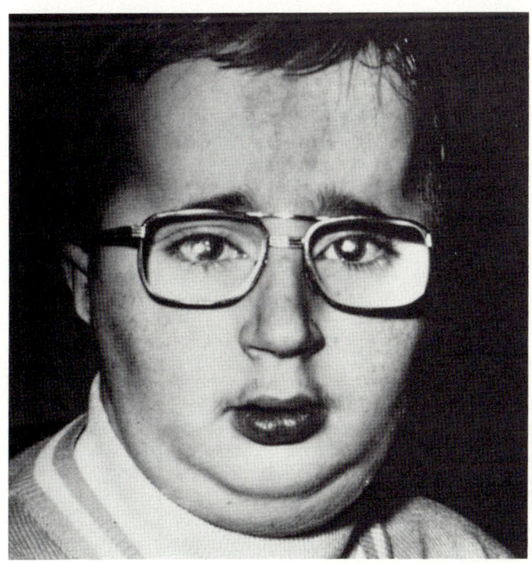

Fig. 4. Case 2. Characteristic facial appearance of Kenny syndrome in a 13-year-old boy.

+9.75 sphere in the left eye. Corneas measured 9 mm in diameter. Optic discs appeared slightly elevated with blurred margins and tortuous retinal vessels. The remainder of the ocular examination was normal.

Case 3. The fifty-year-old mother of the above patient was also examined. She had a history of mild diabetes and was under 46 in. in height. Vision was 20/25 with a +5.75, +1.75 × 130° in the right eye and 20/40 with a +6.50, +1.25 × 60° in the left eye. Corneas measured 10 mm in diameter. The fundi were unremarkable.

Case 4. The patient enjoyed good health until age five at which time he experienced an episode of tetany which was treated successfully with oral calcium. He was subsequently begun on vitamin D therapy. At age eight, growth retardation was apparent. Extensive clinical testing revealed undetectable levels of parathyroid hormone in the presence of serum hypocalcemia and hyperphosphatemia. X-rays showed internal cortical thickening of the long bones with medullary stenosis.

The only ophthalmic record available indicated a vision of 20/40 in each eye, achieved with a +9.00, +2.00 × 90° in the right eye and a +11.00, +1.50 × 90° in the left eye. The fundi were noted to show "pseudoneuritis" with tortuous vessels.

At age 19 he suffered a respiratory and cardiac arrest during an upper respiratory illness. At the time of his death blood chemistries were: sodium 123 mEq/L, potassium 2.6 mEq/L, chloride 85 mEq/L, CO_2 22 mM/L, and calcium 6.9 mEq/L.

At autopsy all organs were small, consistent with dwarfism. Extraocular abnormalities were limited to the bones, brain, and a total absence of any parathyroid tissue. The bones showed internal cortical thickening with medullary stenosis. The calvarium was thin and the anterior fontanel was open. Brain abnormalities included brachycephaly, and a partial Arnold-Chiari malformation with congenital tonsillar herniation. There was considerable calcification of the basal ganglia. Calcospherites and psammoma-like bodies were found in this region, and many capillaries contained calcific deposits (Fig. 5). Multiple hemispheric gyral abnormalities were present. The cerebellum showed bilateral calcification of the dentate nuclei, gliosis, and shrinkage of the folia.

The enucleated eyes were nanophthalmic, the right measuring 17.5 × 17.5 × 16.5 mm and the left 17 × 17 × 16.5 mm. The clear corneas measured 9.5 × 8.5 mm. No intraocular abnormalities were noted on gross examination. Microscopically, hematoxylin-eosin stained sections showed elevated optic discs associated with slightly narrow scleral apertures. The discs appeared swollen with lateral displacement of the peripapillary retina due to a bulging of the edge of the disc tissue usually seen in papilledema. Capillaries were slightly increased in this lateral bulge. The left disc contained several small calcified drusen-like bodies within the nerve fiber bundles

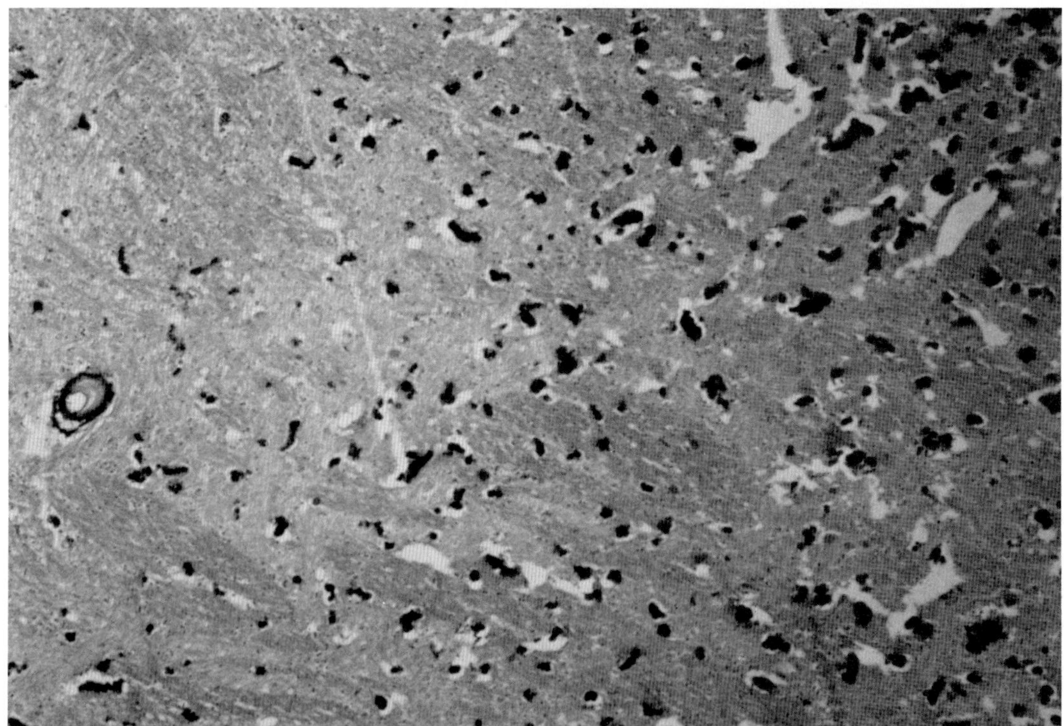

Fig. 5. The basal ganglia contains numerous irregular calcium deposits and a mineralized thick-walled vessel (hematoxylin-eosin, original magnification ×60).

anterior to the fibrous portion of the lamina cribrosa.

Histochemical stains (Von Kossa and Dahl's modification of the alizarin red) for the demonstration of the calcium indicated prominent amounts within the cornea. The corneal epithelium contained abundant calcium within both the nuclei and cytoplasm. Bowman's layer was spared. The central stroma showed no detectable deposits within its superficial one-quarter. The deeper stromal layers, however, revealed prominent calcification which was most pronounced throughout the central mid-stroma. Descemet's membrane was spared throughout its length. Heavy deposits of calcium were present in the corneal endothelium. Less numerous granules were seen within the endothelium cells lining the trabecular meshwork beams. Calcium was demonstrated in the iris and ciliary epithelium. Rather heavy deposition of calcium was present within the inner one-half of the pre-equatorial retina. No calcium was detected within the outer retina. Small amounts were present in occasional astrocytes on the disc surface, and, except for the calcified drusen-like bodies noted in the hematoxylin-eosin sections, none was seen in the disc substance or attached optic nerves.

COMMENT

There is a related spectrum of ocular findings in the above cases. Case 3 had moderate nanophthalmos and hyperopia, but otherwise normal eyes. Cases 2 and 4 exhibited high hyperopia, nanophthalmos with pseudopapilledema, and retinal vascular tortuosity. Case 1 demonstrated severe microphthalmos of 13 mm with extreme pseudopapilledema and macular crowding. Although nanophthalmic eyes may be predisposed to angle closure glaucoma,[5] the only such case was seen in an eye which developed a mature cataract. The anterior chamber angles examined histologically in Case 4 appeared small, but normally open. These eyes were 17 mm in diameter.

A congenitally full disc, elevated, with blurred margins and tortuous vessels, was seen in three patients and histologically confirmed in one case. This type of nerve head is common in hyperopic eyes, although extreme hyperopia and microphthalmos may exist with relatively normal appearing discs.[6] Optic nerve head sections in Case 4 showed pseudopapilledema resulting from a crowding or compression of the glial and nervous tissue in the region of the disc. Presumably a small scleral canal must accommodate a normal number of axons and supporting elements.

It is also possible that a small scleral aperture could compromise the flow of axoplasm. Altered axoplasmic flow may be a factor in the production of optic disc drusen.[7] The small focal drusen present in Case 4 are certainly consistent with this hypothesis. If indeed a small scleral canal causes a hold-up of axoplasmic flow which in turn results in swelling of the nerve fibers anterior to the lamina cribrosa, there may be an element of true disc swelling present. Perhaps some cases regarded in the past as pseudopapilledema are in fact a very low grade papilledema secondary to local anatomic factors. Similar cases in children have been termed "buried drusen." It may be that early in life there is mild disc swelling which later results in drusen deposition.

The fundus picture in Case 1 is an example of extreme pseudopapilledema. Convergence of tortuous vessels combined with light reflexes from the unusual retinal topography produce the deceptive picture of a doubling of the optic nerve head (Fig. 1). Fluorescein angiography shows a single extremely hypervascular retinal circulation with reduplications simulating a "double papilla." There is pigment epithelial clumping in the macula and a crowded appearance of the posterior retinal circulation. Many macular abnormalities have been described in microphthalmic and nanophthalmic eyes.[6, 8–12] It is possible that some of these macular conditions are due to crowding of the retinal elements into a small scleral shell. Folds in the retina have been seen in small eyes, presumably on this basis.[6]

Case 1 represents an example of pseudo-doubling of the optic nerve. A number of articles report duplicated or doubled optic discs and nerves.[13–18] Analysis of these papers reveals not one convincingly documented case. Duke-Elder's volume on congenital abnormalities[19] simply quotes the literature on the subject, devoting a section to double optic nerves without questioning the entity. We believe that true duplication of the optic nerve head does not exist.

Abnormal calcium metabolism is a prominent feature of Kenny syndrome. The exact nature of these abnormalities has not been determined, but several features have emerged. Bouts of hypocalcemia are easily triggered by minor systemic insults and respond to calcium and vitamin D therapy. At the present time the relationship of this therapy to tissue calcium deposition is unknown.

Case 4 is the only known patient with Kenny syndrome to be studied at autopsy. There was a total absence of parathyroid tissue despite an extensive search of the soft tissues of the neck including histological step sectioning. All long bones sampled revealed marked cortical thickening and severe medullary stenosis. Numerous central nervous system calcifications were present within the basal ganglia and dentate nuclei and focal mineralization was seen in the white matter of the cerebral hemispheres and cerebellar folia.

The ocular manifestations of these calcium abnormalities are of interest. Case 4 showed an unusual pattern of corneal calcification which was not visualized on clinical examination or in the routine hematoxylin-eosin sections, but was detectable only with the aid of special histochemical stains for calcium.

The tiny focal drusen deposits in the optic nerve head may relate to the disc swelling, although it is possible they are an incidental finding.[20] Their relationship to the other central nervous system calcifications is uncertain.

It is important for ophthalmologists and neurologists to be aware of this syndrome since they may be called upon to examine such a patient because of seizures, poor vision, small eyes, "papilledema," or other ocular abnormalities. If the diagnosis of Kenny syndrome is not known or suspected, dangerous electrolyte abnormalities may go undetected or their effects treated incorrectly.

Kenny syndrome bears a superficial resemblance to pseudohypoparathyroidism. Classically, the latter patients tend to be mentally retarded, are stocky, disproportionate dwarfs, and lack the characteristic x-ray picture of the long bones seen in Kenny syndrome. However, as this condition becomes better defined, it may well be classified as a hypoparathyroid variant, possibly even coming to represent the prototype of congenital hypoparathyroidism.

SUMMARY

In 1966 Kenny reported two cases with an unusual congenital syndrome including dwarfism, thickened long bone cortex, transient hypocalcemia, and normal intelligence. Ocular findings ranged from uncomplicated nanophthalmos with hyperopia to extreme pseudopapilledema, vascular tortuosity, and macular crowding.

In the case autopsied, calcium deposits demonstrable only by special histochemical stains were uniquely distributed in the cornea. Retinal calcification was also an unusual feature.

Because one patient exhibited a pseudo-doubling of the optic papilla, the literature reporting cases of double optic nerves was reviewed. We conclude that no convincing case of true doubling of the optic nerve has been described.

Neurologists and ophthalmologists should be aware of Kenny syndrome and be alert for undiagnosed electrolyte abnormalities, especially hypocalcemia, in such patients.

EDITOR'S NOTE

I have never seen a case of Kenny's syndrome and indeed had never heard of it until Dr. Boynton gave this paper at the Bascom Palmer Residents Day last year. Nanophthalmos means a "dwarf eye," and I presume is even much, much smaller than a microphthalmic eye. The interesting point to me about this paper is that this syndrome somewhat resembles pseudohypoparathyroidism. We saw in the chapter on Cockayne's syndrome that this was also in the differential of children with basal ganglia calcification. One would be interested in the computed tomographic scan of a child with Kenny's syndrome, too. This is an interesting paper, however, and will help us when we encounter a young patient with small eyes, high hypermetropia, pseudopapilledema, tortuous vessels in the fundus—and will remind us to check the serum calcium and phosphorus and look for intracranial calcification—both by plain skull films and by computed tomographic scan.

JLS

ACKNOWLEDGMENT

Some of the material in this chapter was taken from Boynton, J. R. *et al.* Ocular findings in Kenny's syndrome. Arch. Ophthalmol. *97:*896–900 (1979). Copyright 1979, American Medical Association.

REFERENCES

1. Kenny, F. M. and Linarelli, L. Dwarfism and cortical thickening of tubular bones. Am. J. Dis. Child. *111:*201–207 (1966).
2. Caffey, J. Congenital stenosis of medullary spaces in tubular bones and calvaria in two proportionate dwarfs—coupled with transitory hypocalcemia tetany. Am. J. Roentgenol. *100:*1–11 (1967).
3. Frech, R. S. and McAlister, W. H. Medullary stenosis of the tubular bones associated with hypocalcemic convulsions and short stature. Radiology *91:*457–461 (1968).
4. Wilson, M. G., Maronda, R. F., Mikity, V. G., and Shinno, N. W. Dwarfism and congenital medullary stenosis (Kenny syndrome). Birth defects. *10*(12), 128–132 (1974).
5. O'Grady, R. B. Nanophthalmos. Am. J. Ophthalmol. *71:*1251–1253 (1971).
6. Boynton, J. R. and Purnell, E. W. Bilateral microphthalmos without microcornea associated with unusual papillomacular retinal folds and high hyperopia. Am. J. Ophthalmol. *79:*820–826 (1975).
7. Spencer, W. H. Drusen of the optic disk and aberrant axoplasmic transport. Am. J. Ophthalmol. *85:*1–12 (1978).
8. Mohamed, M. A. Tapeto-retinal degenerations. Report of a new syndrome. Bull. Ophthalmol. Soc. Egypt *63:*223–227 (1970).
9. Duke-Elder, S. and Abrams, D. Ophthalmic optics and refraction. In: *System of Ophthalmology.* S. Duke-Elder (Ed.), C. V. Mosby, St. Louis, 1970, p. 298.
10. Reber, M. Microphthalmic complique d'hypermetropie excessive et d'anomalies de la macula observée chez trois soeurs. Ann. Oculistique *119:* 445–446 (1898).
11. Malbran, E., Priani, P., and Lombardi, A. Macroquistes de retina, retinosquises e hipermetropia elevada. Arch. Oftalmologia Buenos Aires. *45:*180–185 (1970).
12. Von Zuccoli, A. Neuer beitrag zum bild der makrozysten bei der hohen hypermetropie. Ophthalmologica *145:*419–424 (1963).
13. Lamba, P. A., Prakash, P., and Dayal, Y. Duplication of the optic papilla. Orient Arch. Ophthalmol. *6:*87–90 (1968).
14. Aouchiche, M., Boyer, R., and Fetchi, A. A propos du diagnostic, des doubles papille. Bull. Soc. Ophthalmol. Fr. *84:*625–635 (1971).
15. Straburzynski, J. Double optic disc in patient with Marfan's syndrome. Klin. Oczna *42:*913–915 (1972).
16. Bajan, Von M. and Holmay, O. Doppelte sehnervenscheibe bei einem jugendlichen. Klin. Monatsbl. Augenheilkd. *151:*207–210 (1967).
17. Bonamour, M. G. A propos des "Double Papille." Bull. Soc. Ophthalmol. Fr. *64:*802–805 (1964).
18. Lamba, P. A. Doubling of the papilla. Acta Ophthalmol. *47:*4–9 (1969).
19. Duke-Elder, W. S. *Duke-Elder System of Ophthalmology.* C. V. Mosby, St. Louis, 1963, Vol. 3, Pt. 2.
20. Friedman, A. H., Beckerman, B., Gold, D. H., *et al.* Drusen of the optic disc. Surv. Ophthalmol. *21:* 375–390 (1977).

40 Voluntary and Reflex Vertical Gaze

Lawrence R. Jenkyn, M. D.
Alexander G. Reeves, M. D.

INTRODUCTION

The clinical utility of examination of horizontal eye movements, both voluntary (saccadic or pursuit) and reflex (oculovestibular or optokinetic), is well known. Less emphasis has been stressed on dysfunction of gaze in the vertical plane[5, 9] except for descriptions of lesions typified by Parinaud's syndrome. This chapter will attempt to summarize what is known about the neuroanatomical substrates of voluntary and reflex vertical gaze and the implications of abnormalities in this subsystem of conjugate eye movements.

NEUROANATOMY

It is presumed that the neocortex is the site of origin of impulses to the oculomotor and trochlear nuclei during voluntary up- or downgaze.[42] While saccadic horizontal eye movements appear to begin principally in the frontal eye field (Area 8 of Brodman), saccadic vertical eye movements can be elicited by double simultaneous stimulation of homologous points of the neocortex bilaterally from almost any region. It is typical that these evoked versions are not perpendicular to the horizontal, but rather take diagonal vectors, up or down.[42] Regional cerebral blood flow (rCBF) analysis of one patient making vertical saccades demonstrated focal increases in mean rCBF in the frontal eye fields simultaneously.[30] Nashold and Gills[31] elicited downward vertical eye movements from unilateral stimulation of the posterior sensory nucleus of the thalamus. Spiegel *et al.*[38] obtained ver-

tical eye movements from stimulation in the fields of Forel. Additionally, evidence is available to suggest that the basal ganglia are interposed between neocortical and primary motor cortex neurons (Area 4 of Brodman).[8] Outflow from the motor cortex then proceeds through the internal capsule to the pretectal region. Whether synapses occur directly with the oculomotor and trochlear nuclei or not is unclear. Selective loss of voluntary downgaze has been reported with lesions just dorsal to the red nuclei.[4, 10, 12, 17, 22] Selective loss of voluntary upgaze occurs with posterior commissure and dorsal pretectal lesions.[4, 10, 33, 34] Thus there is a separation of functional pathways in the pretectum for voluntary up- and downgaze.

Christoff[9] provided evidence that integrity of the rostral paramedian pontine reticular formation (PPRF) is also necessary for voluntary vertical eye movements. Bilateral neoplastic invasion of the rostral PPRF was associated with impaired voluntary horizontal gaze and upgaze. Thus, polysynaptic connections from neocortex to oculomotor and trochlear nuclei include the basal ganglia, pretectum, and rostral pons. These findings are summarized in Figure 1.

As little is known about the neuroanatomical connections of reflex vertical gaze as for voluntary vertical gaze.[4, 5, 35–37] Best defined are the extraocular responses following semicircular canal stimulation.[2, 8, 13, 40] Bilateral ampullofugal flow in the posterior canals and ampullopetal flow in the anterior canals results in tonic, conjugate downgaze whether elicited by double simultaneous ice water caloric irrigation of the external ear canal in the supine subject, by hyperextension of the neck (oculocephalic maneuver in the vertical plane), or appropriate Barany chair rotation. Conversely, ampullofugal flow in the anterior canals and ampullopetal flow in the posterior canals produces tonic conjugate upward deviation of the eyes. This follows double-simultaneous hot water irrigation of the external ear canals in the supine subject, hyperflexion of the neck, or Barany chair rotation.[3] As hot water tends either to be too noxious a stimulus or insufficiently warmer than body temperature to elicit thermal currents in the endolymph of the semicircular canals, cold or ice water is the optimal stimulus to use. The connections between the vestibular nuclear complex and the oculomotor and trochlear nuclei are through the medial longitudinal fasciculus (MLF). This has been demonstrated both experimentally in monkeys[15, 26] and in one human example.[24] These connections are crossed with the major contribution to the left MLF coming from the right vestibular nuclei and vice-versa. Innervation then of the right superior rectus and the left

inferior oblique muscles (both with neuronal cell bodies in the left third nerve nucleus) arrives through the left MLF without further internuclear decussations. Similarly, the left inferior rectus and the right superior oblique would be innervated by axons traveling from the right vestibular nucleus via the left MLF. The level of the decussation of vestibular efferents is unknown but may be in the region of the sixth nerve nucleus.[2] Because of the simultaneous stimulation of both vestibular nuclei during vertical oculocephalic or double simultaneous ice water caloric irrigation, integration of both sides occurs.[29, 33, 40] These concepts are summarized in Figure 2. Whether ancillary connections in the pontine tegmentum exist other than in the MLF is not known. Evidence at present favors the MLF as necessary for transmission of reflex messages to the midbrain nuclei while loss of tegmental integrity sparing only the MLF has been reported to spare at least reflex downgaze.[18]

DISORDERS OF VOLUNTARY VERTICAL GAZE

This discussion will confine itself to pathologic involvement of the central nervous system. It should be recognized that a host of neuromuscular problems will impair voluntary and reflex vertical gaze, usually equally, and often will give rise to similar disorders of horizontal gaze. Extraocular defects are monocular or binocular. These diseases include myasthenia gravis, ocular myopathies, thyroid disease, Guillain-Barré syndrome, Miller-Fisher syndrome, ophthalmoplegic migraine, meningitis, and meningeal carcinomatosis. Monocular paralysis of gaze follows intraorbital or superior orbital fissure invasion by tumor or granulomatous disease, or mono- or polyneuropathies of cranial nerves.

Diffuse cerebral dysfunction is probably the most common cause of impaired voluntary vertical gaze. This observation has been made in patients with dementia (from any cause including degenerative disease, multi-infarct dementia, or hydrocephalus) or metabolic encephalopathy, and has also been attributed to normal aging.[1, 14, 21, 25] As the cortex diffusely seems to play a role in

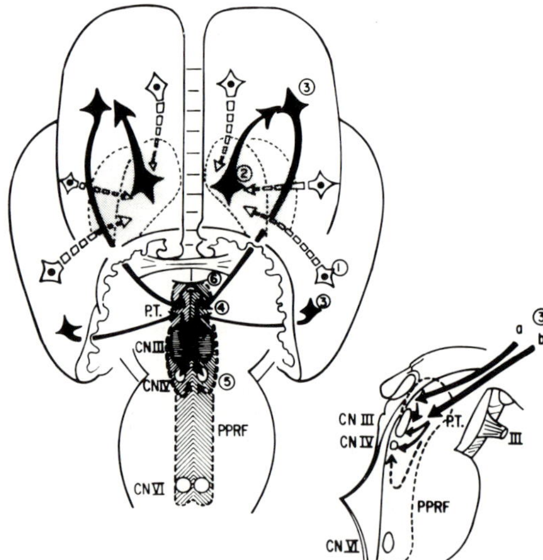

Fig. 1. Proposed pathways for voluntary vertical gaze. 1 and 2. Diffuse cortical and basal ganglia initiation of motor activity. 3. Frontal and occipito-parietal pathways to pretectal region. 4. Pretectum (PT). 5. Rostral paramedian pontine reticular formation (PPRF). 6. Posterior commissure. III = oculomotor complex. IV = trochlear nucleus. VI = abducens nucleus. a. dorsal input to pretectum for upgaze. b. ventral input to pretectum for downgaze.

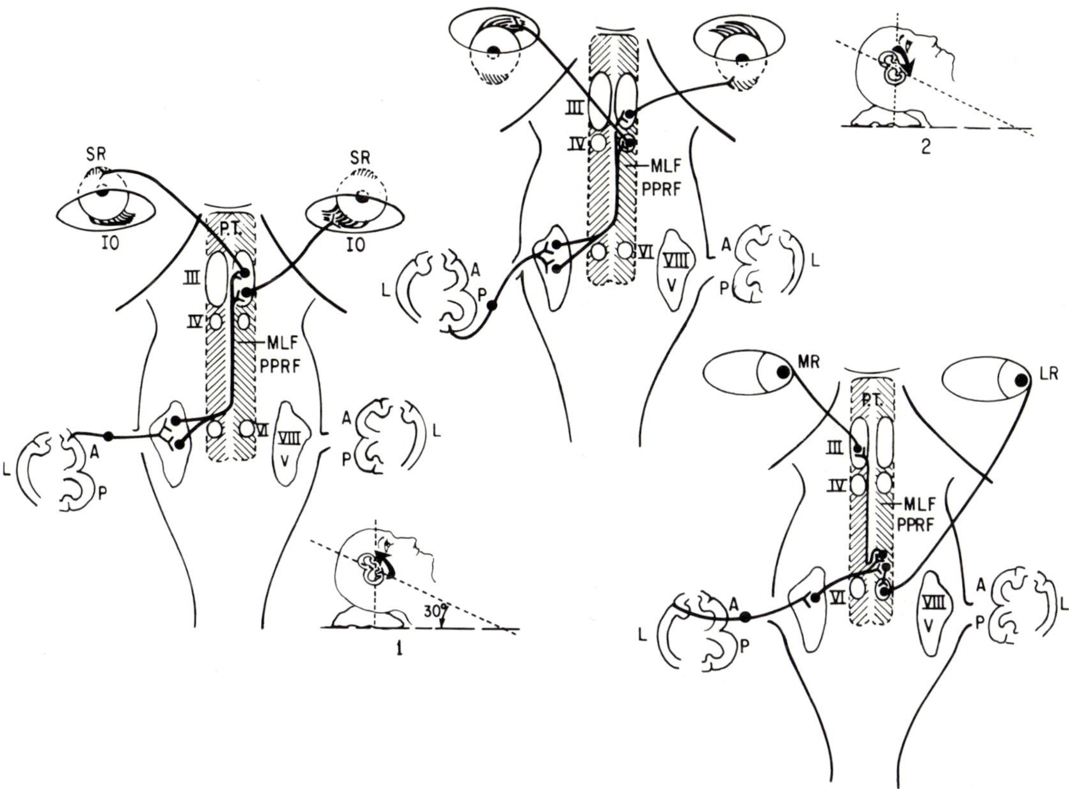

Fig. 2. Excitatory pathways between the individual semicircular canals and extraocular muscles (reflex vertical gaze). A = anterior semicircular canal. P = posterior semicircular canal. L = lateral semicircular canal. SR = superior rectus. IR = inferior rectus. SO = superior oblique. IO = inferior oblique. III = oculomotor complex. IV = trochlear nucleus. VI = abducens nucleus. MLF = medial longitudinal fasciculus. PT: pretectum. PPRF = paramedian pontine reticular formation. VIII v. = vestibular nuclear complex. *Inset* = orientation of the anterior and posterior semicircular canals with patient supine for caloric testing. 1. Vectors of endolymphatic flow in anterior and posterior semicircular canals with double simultaneous hot caloric irrigation of the external auditory canals (reflex upgaze). 2. Vectors of flow with double simultaneous cold caloric irrigation (reflex downgaze).

eliciting vertical eye movements, diffuse impairment of cortical neurons would logically impair vertical gaze. Upgaze seems more sensitive to this phenomenon than downgaze. This is possibly due to the fact that upgaze is an uncommon voluntary movement as opposed to down- or horizontal gaze. Hence, this function would be less well learned and more sensitive to early diffuse cortical dysfunction.

Diseases of the basal ganglia are associated with impaired vertical gaze as well. This is especially true for downgaze in Parkinsonian patients,[11, 12] although we have observed limited upgaze in these patients frequently. Similar defects are seen in Wilson's disease,[27] kernicterus,[19, 20] and Huntington's chorea.[39] These illnesses are also often associated with cortical lesions diffusely (Parkinson's disease), pretectal lesions (kernicterus), and brainstem nuclear lesions (Wilson's disease). Thus, the exact role of the basal ganglia lesions in impairing eye movements is unclear.

Infarction in the pretectum is associated with defective vertical gaze. As mentioned above, lesions dorsomedial to the red nuclei selectively impair downgaze, while more dorsal lesions involving the posterior commissure and dorsal pretectal region selectively impair upgaze. The latter is the presumed site of dysfunction of expanding neoplasms of the pineal region, originally described by Parinaud. Other pathologic states that particularly may involve the pretectal substrate of voluntary gaze include progressive supranuclear palsy,[41] Whipple's disease,[16] a sphingomyelin storage disease associated with sea-blue histiocytes in the bone marrow,[32] cephalic tetanus,[7] metastatic or primary tumor, and stereotactic lesions made for relief of pain or extrapyramidal dysfunction.[31, 38] Excluding progressive supranuclear palsy and Whipple's disease, these have been poorly documented pathologically and much speculation has followed the very little solid data which has been obtained. Of interest are two reports of supranuclear paralysis of upgaze in one eye only.[23, 28] Unilateral rostral midbrain lesions were observed in each, suggesting that prenuclear, precommissural integration of upgaze occurs ipsilaterally for each eye.

It appears that lesions in the rostral paramedian pontine reticular formation also impair voluntary vertical gaze. Experimental ablation evidence in monkeys and observations in patients with bilateral tumors of the region support this.[6, 9] It is rare to observe this defect, however, as most patients with lesions here are comatose due to rostral reticular formation damage and are thus untestable.

DISORDERS OF REFLEX VERTICAL GAZE

While labyrinthine, vestibulo-cochlear nerve or vestibular nuclear lesions impair reflex vertical gaze, other clinical features accompanying such lesions provide adequate accurate diagnostic data, and, hence, vestibulo-ocular dysfunction is rarely tested or observed. Pontine infarction or hemorrhage would be expected to spare voluntary vertical eye movements (if the patient is alert) while eliminating reflex gaze if vestibular nuclear or MLF lesions occur. The MLF may also be involved in isolation by multiple sclerosis, tumor, infarction, or metabolic suppression.

Of interest in this regard is the observation that MLF lesions in the monkey impair maintenance of voluntary upgaze once the saccade has taken place.[15, 26] This phenomenon is observed in man with bilateral MLF lesions as upward-beating nystagmus. This implies a role for the vestibular nuclei in sustaining vertical saccades once they are initiated. As vertical nystagmus is also seen with cerebellar lesions, it is tempting to postulate that connections from the cerebellum via the fastigial nuclei and inferior cerebellar peduncle to the vestibular nuclei are important in sustaining conjugate vertical eye movements.

CONCLUSIONS

Disorders of vertical gaze can be separated anatomically into specific reflex and voluntary components. Detailed evaluation of each component of vertical eye movements will provide accurate localization of pathologic processes. Further observations of these components will increase our understanding of the neuroanatomic correlates of these eye movements specifically as well as cortical and brainstem function in general.

EDITOR'S NOTE

The authors have given a concise neuroanatomical background to understand the various disordered forms of eye movements seen in neurological patients. I find that a simple clinical presentation of some of the forms of eye movement disorder is at times more helpful for the young physician with a bit less emphasis on the neuroanatomy. For example, if you walk into a patient's room, and the patient is sitting there with both eyes deviated to his right and rather consistently maintains that position, there really are only four possible things that one needs to think of: (1) there is an irritative lesion of Area 8 on the left; (2) or there is a paralytic lesion of Area 8 on the right; (3) or there is an irritative lesion of the paramedian pontine reticular formation on the right; or (4) there is a paralytic lesion of the paramedian pontine reticular formation on the left. More simply stated, horizontal eye movements are contralaterally represented when one stimulates the hemisphere—but ipsilaterally represented when one stimulates the pons. Thus, *stimulate left prefrontal* optomotor eye field and *eyes* go to the *right*. Stimulate *right pons*, and *eyes* go to the *right*. Now, you may wonder—how can you differentiate the irritative from the paretic lesions? "On the hoof" they really are rather easy to differentiate by simply looking at the patient for a moment or two. If there is an irritative left cortical lesion at work, one will note that the patient's eyes are usually to the right, but there is a bit of drift back towards the midline and then they are driven on out there to the right again. In other words, there is a bit of gaze paretic nystagmus going on. On the other hand, if there is simply a tonic imbalance, the patient's eyes will just sit over there to the right—"like a dead hog in the sunshine," so to speak. So, if the problem is irritative, they will "irritate"—and if the problem is paralytic, they will just look "paralyzed" over to that side—for practical purposes.

Now, let's consider a patient on that neurologic ward whose eyes are looking straight ahead in the primary position when you look at him, and who can look fully to the left, up, and down when you ask him to do so—but who simply cannot look at all to his right. Now, we have a problem with a marked weakness of right conjugate gaze, even though there is no apparent deviation of the eyes in the primary position. The first thing we do is to ask the patient to look to his right (or test right conjugate gaze to *command*). The next thing we do is to ask the patient to follow a light or a finger as we slowly move this towards his right (or test right conjugate gaze on *following*). If we still get no movement, we have the patient look at our flashlight and then turn the patient's head to his left (to test the oculovestibular responses and/or tonic neck reflex). This is called the *"doll's head maneuver."* If the eyes come over promptly with the doll's head maneuver, obviously the problem with right gaze is supranuclear. If the eyes do NOT come over promptly with the doll's head maneuver, then we should irrigate the patient's *RIGHT ear* with *COLD* water, while he is lying back on his hospital bed with one or two pillows. This will elicit a *slow* phase to the *right* (which is what we are trying to bring out in the first place). Obviously, it will also induce a rapid phase to his left, which is called a left nystagmus since all nystagmus is named by the rapid phase. We are not looking for that in this patient. We are trying to get his eyes over to his right—by

hook or crook! If the eyes go over to the right after cold water in the right ear, then we have a supranuclear right gaze paresis. There are many, many pearls that can come out of instilling ice water into the neurologic patient's ear, and we cannot go over all of them in this little note. The point I'm trying to make is that we also need more simple office motility pearls to tell the young physician *how* to do it, and many times they get so confused trying to remember that the tract of Darkschewitsch passes from the optic tract to the habenular ganglion, then through the posterior commissure to the oculomotor nucleus (and I just copied that out of *Wolff* to be sure)—that they really don't know the simple maneuvers of evaluating ocular motility in the neurologic patient. Finally, it would be a wonderful thing if neurologists and neurosurgeons could be taught how to do the screen and cover test. A basic knowledge of eye motility patterns is *essential* in knowing whether a deviation of the eyes is simply a strabismus pattern or is an acquired neuro-ophthalmologic motility disorder. One hates to see patients admitted to hospital for 10 days of neurologic investigation when they have only an A or V pattern esotropia in childhood, and really needed only an "OV" (office visit) by an ophthalmologist knowledgeable of that problem. On the other hand, if the ophthalmologist misses the pattern and refers it to the neurologist or neurosurgeon, one really cannot blame the latter for the workup. We do need better communication between eye men seeing these problems, however, and young men in neurology and neurosurgery—for otherwise the patient is the one who gets the excessive and often unnecessary workup.

JLS

REFERENCES

1. Adams, G. F. and Hurwitz, L. J. *Cerebrovascular Disability and the Aging Brain.* Churchill Livingstone, Edinburgh and London, 1974, pp. 28–50.
2. Baloh, R. W. and Honrubia, V. *Clinical Neurophysiology of the Vestibular System.* F. A. Davis, Philadelphia, 1979.
3. Bender, M. B. (Ed.). *The Oculomotor System.* Harper and Row, New York, 1964.
4. Bender, M. B. Pathways mediating vertical eye movements. *Trans. Am. Neurol. Assoc.* 84:159–161 (1959).

5. Bender, M. B. Comments on the physiology and pathology of eye movements in the vertical plane. *J. Nerv. Ment. Dis. 130:*456–466 (1960).

6. Bender, M. B. and Shanzer, S. Oculomotor pathways defined by electric stimulation and lesions in the brainstem of monkey. In: *The Oculomotor System.* M. B. Bender (Ed.), Harper and Row, New York, 1964, pp. 81–140.

7. Biglan, A. W., Ellis, F. D., and Wade, T. A. Supranuclear oculomotor palsy and exotropia after tetanus. *Am. J. Ophthalmol. 86:*666–668 (1978).

8. Carpenter, R. H. S. *Movements of the Eyes.* Pion Ltd., London, 1977.

9. Christoff, N. A clinico-pathologic study of vertical eye movements. Arch. Neurol. *31:*1–8 (1974).

10. Christoff, N., Anderson, P. J., and Bender, M. B. A clinicopathologic study of associated vertical eye movements. Trans. Am. Neurol. Assoc. *87:* 184–186 (1962).

11. Cogan, D. G. Brain lesions and eye movements in man. In: *The Oculomotor System.* M. B. Bender (Ed.), Harper and Row, New York, 1964, pp. 417–427.

12. Cogan, D. G. Paralysis of downgaze. Arch. Ophthalmol. *91:*192–199 (1974).

13. Cohen, B. Vestibulo-ocular relations. In: *The Control of Eye Movements.* P. Bach-y-Rita and C. Collins (Eds.), Academic, New York, 1971, pp. 105–148.

14. Critchley, M. Neurologic changes in the aged. J. Chronic Dis. *3:*459–477 (1956).

15. Evinger, L. C., Fuchs, A. F., and Baker, R. Bilateral lesions of the medial longitudinal fasciculus in monkeys: effects on the horizontal and vertical components of voluntary and vestibular induced eye movements. Exp. Brain Res. *28:*1–20 (1977).

16. Finelli, P. F., McEntee, W. J., Lessell, S., Morgan, T. F., and Copetto, J. Whipple's disease with predominantly neuroophthalmic manifestations. Ann. Neurol. *1:*247–252 (1977).

17. Halmagyi, G. M., Evans, W. A., and Hallinan, J. M. Failure of downward gaze. Arch. Neurol. *35:* 22–26 (1978).

18. Hawkes, C. H. "Locked-in" syndrome: report of seven cases. Br. Med. J. *4:*379–382 (1974).

19. Haymaker, W. Pathology of kernicterus and posticteric encephalopathy. In: *Kernicterus and Its Importance in Cerebral Palsy.* C. A. Swinyard (Ed.), Charles C. Thomas, Springfield, Ill., 1961.

20. Hoyt, C. S., Billson, F. A., and Alpins, N. The supranuclear disturbances of gaze in kernicterus. Ann. Ophthalmol. *10:*1487–1492 (1978).

21. Hurwitz, L. J. Neurological aspects of old age and capacity. Gerontol. Clin. *10:*146–156 (1968).

22. Jacobs, L., Anderson, P. J., and Bender, M. B. The lesions producing paralysis of downward but not upward gaze. Arch. Neurol. *28:*319–323 (1973).

23. Jampel, R. S., and Fells, P. Monocular elevation paresis caused by a central nervous system lesion. Arch. Ophthalmol. *80:*45–57 (1968).

24. Jenkyn, L. R., Margolis, G., and Reeves, A. G. Reflex vertical gaze and the medial longitudinal fasciculus. J. Neurol. Neurosurg. Psychiatr. *41:* 1084–1091 (1978).

25. Jenkyn, L. R., Walsh, D. B., Culver, C. M., and Reeves, A. G. Clinical signs in diffuse cerebral dysfunction. J. Neurol. Neurosurg. Psychiatr. *40:* 956–966 (1977).

26. King, W. M., Lisberger, S. G., and Fuchs, A. F. Responses of fibers in medial longitudinal fasciculus (MLF) of alert monkeys during horizontal and vertical conjugate eye movements evoked by vestibular or visual stimuli. J. Neurophysiol. *39:* 1135–1149 (1976).

27. Kirkam, T. H. and Kamin, D. F. Slow saccadic eye movements in Wilson's disease. J. Neurol. Neurosurg. Psychiatr. *37:*191–194 (1974).

28. Lessell, S. Supranuclear paralysis of monocular elevation. Neurolog. (Minneap.) *25:*1134–1136 (1975).

29. McMasters, R. E., Weiss, A. H., and Carpenter, M. B. Vestibular projections to the nuclei of the extraocular muscles. Am. J. Anat. *118:*163–194 (1966).

30. Melamed, E. and Larsen, B. Cortical activation patterns during saccadic eye movements in humans: localization by focal cerebral blood flow increases. Ann. Neurol. *5:*79–88 (1979).

31. Nashold, B. S. and Gills, J. P. Ocular signs from brain stimulation and lesions. Arch. Ophthalmol. *77:*609–618 (1967).

32. Neville, B. G. R., Lake, B. D., Stephens, R., and Sanders, M. D. A neurovisceral storage disease with vertical supranuclear ophthalmoplegia, and its relationship to Niemann-Pick disease. Brain *96:*97–120 (1973).

33. Pasik, P., Pasik, T., and Bender, M. B. The pretectal syndrome in monkeys. I. Disturbances of gaze and body posture. Brain *92:*521–534 (1969).

34. Pasik, T., Pasik, P., and Bender, M. B. The pretectal syndrome in monkeys. II. Spontaneous and induced nystagmus and "lightning" eye movements. Brain *92:*871–884 (1969).

35. Shanzer, S. Effects of semicircular canal stimulation in monkeys with lesions of the medial longitudinal fasciculus (MLF). Fed. Proc. *23:*414 (1964).

36. Shanzer, S. and Bender, M. B. Oculomotor responses on vestibular stimulation of monkeys with lesions of the brainstem. Brain *82:*669–682 (1959).

37. Shanzer, S., Goto, K., Cohen, B., and Bender, M. B. Medial longitudinal fasciculus and vertical eye movements. Trans. Am. Neurol. Assoc. *89:*255–256 (1964).

38. Spiegel, E. A., Wyeis, H. T., Szekely, E. G., Soloff, L., Adams, J., Gildenberg, P., and Zanes, C. Stimulation of Forel's field during stereotaxic operations in the human brain. Electroencephalogr. Clin. Neurophysiol. *16:*537–548 (1964).

39. Starr, A. A disorder of rapid eye movement in Huntington's chorea. Brain *90:*545–555 (1967).

40. Szentagothai, J. The elementary vestibulo-ocular reflex arc. J. Neurophysiol. *13:*395–407 (1950).

41. Troost, B. T. and Daroff, R. B. The ocular motor defects in progressive supranuclear palsy. Ann. Neurol. *2:*397–403 (1977).

42. Walsh, F. B., and Hoyt, W. F. *Clinical Neuro-Ophthalmology.* 3rd ed. Williams and Wilkins, Baltimore, 1969.

41 The Sylvian Aqueduct Syndrome as a Sign of Thalamic Vascular Malformation

Frank J. Bajandas, M.D.
Michael Aptman, M.D.
and Steve Stevens, M.D.

INTRODUCTION

There are few clinical entities that can compete with the Koerber-Salus-Elschnig sylvian aqueduct syndrome in helping the physician to localize a neurological disease process. It directs the clinician's attention to the dorsal, rostral midbrain and suggests various possible etiologies, all of which affect the pretectum of the upper mesencephalon. We report two patients with vascular malformations of the thalamus and with clinical presentations that included the sylvian aqueduct syndrome.

CASE REPORTS

Case 1. A 30-year-old right-handed white male was in good health until June 10, 1976, when he noted numbness of the right tongue, gums, face, head, neck, and hand. Ten days later, he noted the additional symptom of difficulty walking, with a tendency to fall to the right side. He had no visual complaints.

One month after onset, he noted mild, intermittent numbness of the right hand and the right face. On August 14, 1976, he experienced sudden, severe, left-sided headaches, awkward gait, tendency to fall to the right side, and numbness of the right half of the body. The following morning he noted double vision and sought medical attention.

Neurological evaluation revealed right-sided hypalgesia and right upper extremity hyperreflexia with a pronator drift. The gait was ataxic with a tendency to fall to the right.

Neuro-ophthalmological examination revealed visual acuity of 20/15 in both eyes. The pupils measured 4 mm in both eyes and exhibited 1+ reaction to light and 3+ reaction to near. He demonstrated retraction of both upper lids and preferred to keep his head extended because of double vision in the primary position and on up gaze. He was found to have 5 prism diopters of right hypertropia in the primary position and no vertical deviation on gaze down.

The remainder of the eye motility measurements showed enough incomitance to suggest that the right hypertropia was due to relative weakness of the left superior rectus muscle. He exhibited marked limitation of upward gaze and bilateral retraction nystagmus on attempted upward gaze and while observing downgoing optokinetic targets. The upward excursions of the eyes could be increased by vertical doll's head maneuvers (Fig. 1). Visual fields and ophthalmoscopy were normal.

Lumbar puncture revealed normal opening pressure with normal glucose, protein, and no cells. Computerized tomography (CT) scan demonstrated an abnormal density, exhibiting slight enhancement with contrast material and appearing to be located in the left thalamus (Fig. 2).

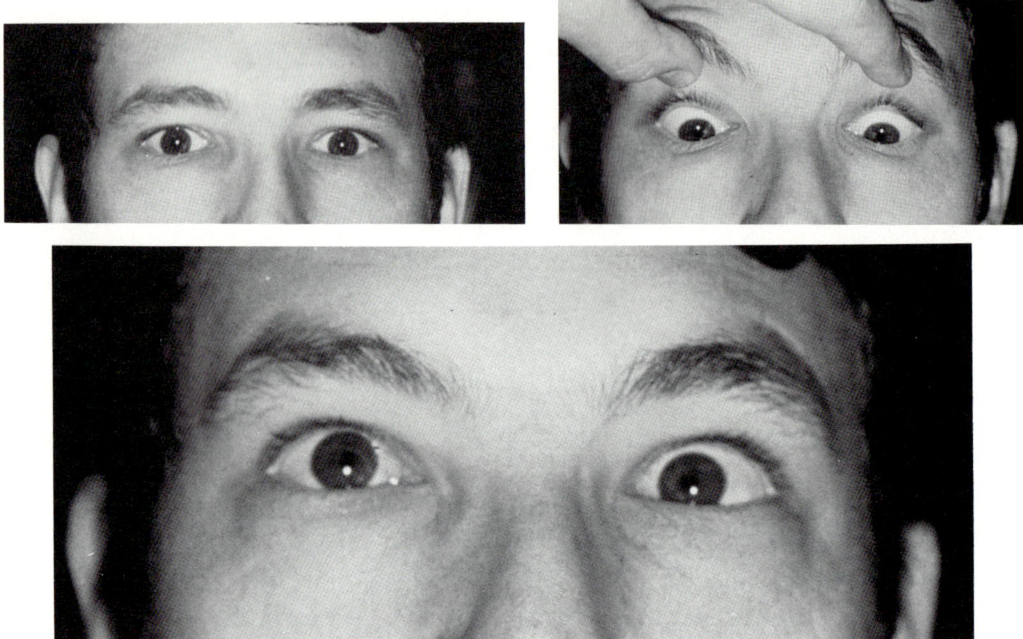

Fig. 1. (Bajandas, Aptman, and Stevens). Case 1. Top left, upper eyelid retraction (Collier's sign). Top right, normal gaze down. Center left, markedly reduced gaze up, with right hypertropia.

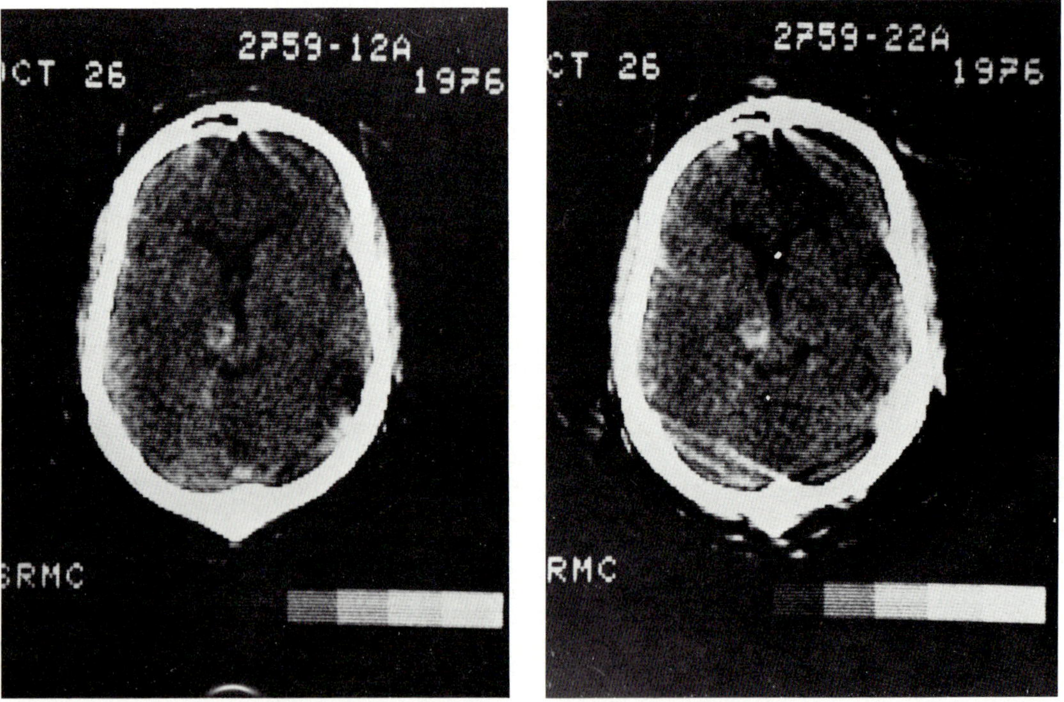

Fig. 2. (Bajandas, Aptman, and Stevens). Case 1. Computerized tomography (CT scan). Left, before intravenous injection of contrast material, abnormal density in the area of the left thalamus. Right, after intravenous injection of contrast material, slight enhancement of the left thalamic density.

Arteriography demonstrated stretching of the left anterior thalamo-perforating artery and a stellate venous malformation in the area of the left thalamus (Fig. 3).

The patient experienced gradual and nearly complete clearing of his symptoms during the subsequent two months. He was seen one year later and complained only of slight numbness of the right hand and minimal difficulty with his right hand when playing the organ in concert (Fig. 4). The findings were completely normal except for decreased right arm-swing during heel-to-toe walking. Repeat CT scan demonstrated possibly a slight decrease in the size of the left thalamic density.

Case 2. A 34-year-old right-handed Mexican-American male was in good health until September 23, 1976, when he experienced sudden loss of consciousness. On examination the same day, he was found to be comatose, demonstrating a dilated, unreactive left pupil, and decerebrate posturing, with Cheyne-Stokes respiration. His neck was stiff. Ophthalmoscopy was normal. He had bilateral Babinski responses.

Arteriography demonstrated an arteriovenous malformation of the left thalamus (Fig. 5). Right lateral ventricular tap yielded bloody cerebrospinal fluid. A right lateral ventricular drainage procedure was performed. The patient had a hospital course complicated by infection, possible rebleed, and a blocked shunt.

He subsequently showed gradual improvement and was discharged on October 27, 1976. He reported continued improvement and became able to ambulate by himself. By February 1977, he complained only of mild residual weakness and numbness of the left lower extremity, some difficulty with coordination, double vision, and difficulty looking up.

Examination of February 15, 1977 revealed a corrected visual acuity of 20/20−2 in the right eye and 20/15−2 in the left eye. The right pupil measured 4 mm and demonstrated 1–2+ reaction to light. No Marcus Gunn pupillary phenomenon was noted. Both pupils showed 3+ reaction to near.

The upper lids rested just below the upper limbus and demonstrated retraction, exposing 1–2 mm of sclera when the patient concentrated on a small near target.

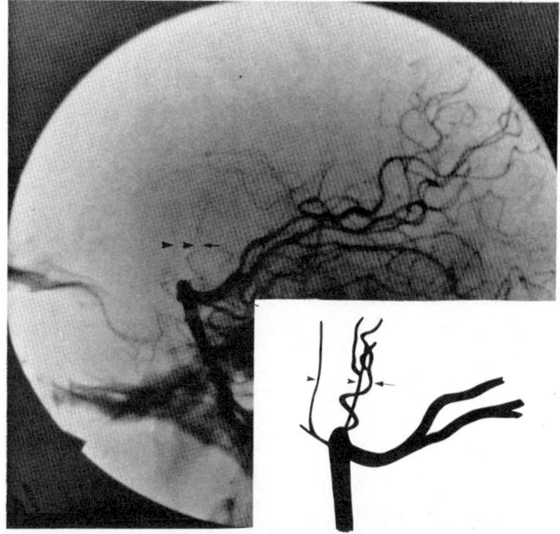
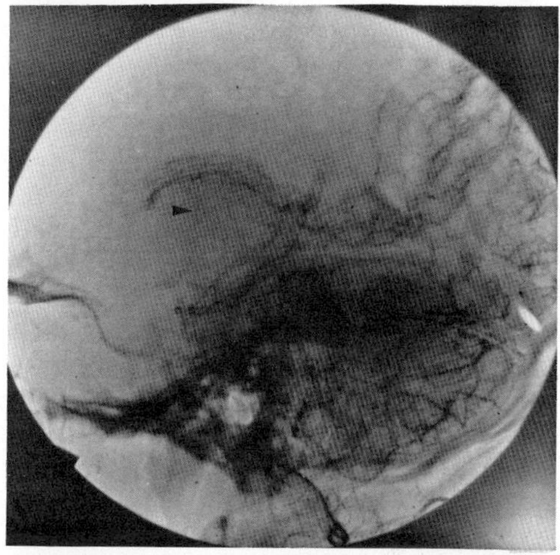
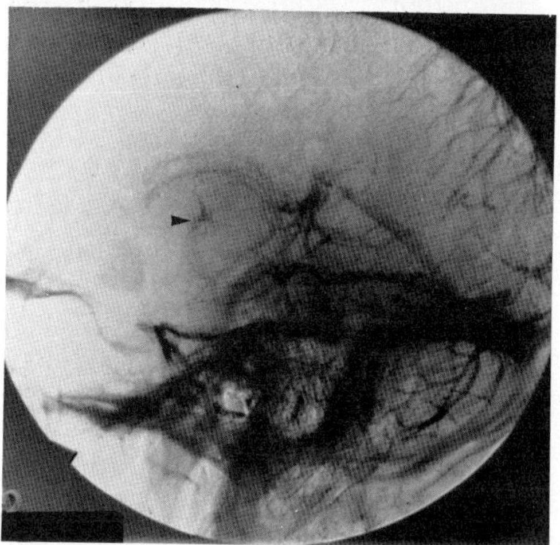

Fig. 3. (Bajandas, Aptman, and Stevens). Case 1. Vertebral angiogram. Top, arterial phase. Bottom, late venous phase, residual staining of the stellate venous malformation of the left thalamus (arrow).

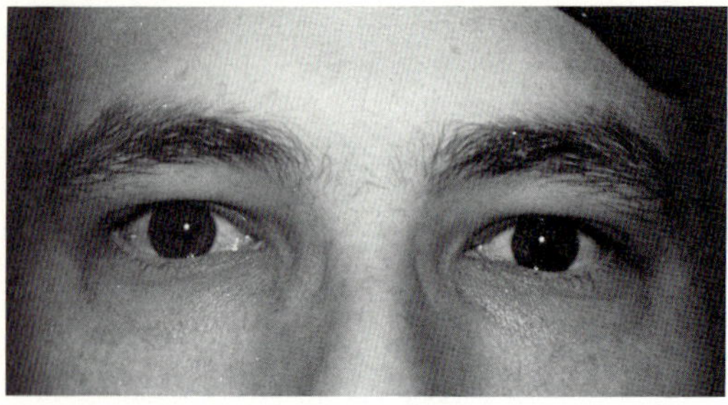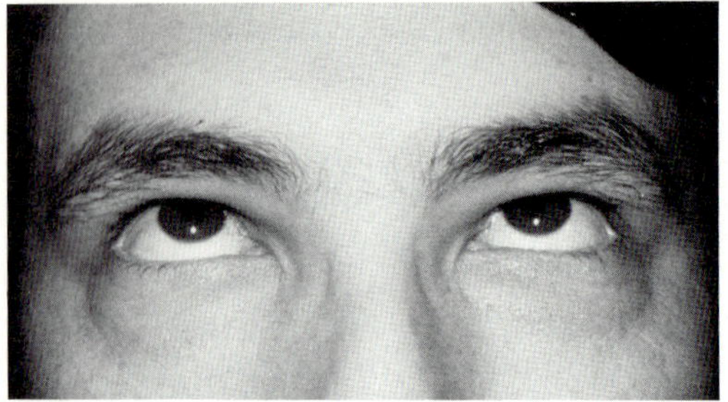

Fig. 4. (Bajandas, Aptman, and Stevens). Case 1. One year after onset of symptoms. Left, no longer demonstrates lid retraction. Right, now able to voluntarily execute full gaze up.

He was unable to look above the primary position, but the upward excursions of the eyes could be improved with vertical doll's head maneuvers. Convergence retraction nystagmus was present on attempted upward gaze and while observing down-going targets.

He was found to have 5 prism diopters of left hypertropia with incomitance that suggested relative weakness of the right inferior oblique muscle. The hypertropia disappeared on gaze down. He also demonstrated 22 prism diopters of exotropia that remained comitant in the cardinal position of gaze. He was unable to converge his eyes.

Visual field and ophthalmoscopic examinations were normal. The neurological examination was normal except for mild weakness and hypalgesia of the left lower extremity and slight gait ataxia.

The initial CT scan, performed in February 1977, failed to show any abnormality despite repeated testing, with and without enhancement.

In March 1978, the patient reported continued improvement. The neurological and neuro-ophthalmological examinations revealed no change.

DISCUSSION

The sylvian aqueduct syndrome is frequently referred to as the pretectal or dorsal-rostral-midbrain syndrome. Eponymically it is known as the Koerber-Salus-Elschnig syndrome, although the first component was described by M. H. Parinaud[1] in 1883. Table I provides a historical outline of the sequential recognition of the varied components of the syndrome and lists some of the case reports and experimental studies

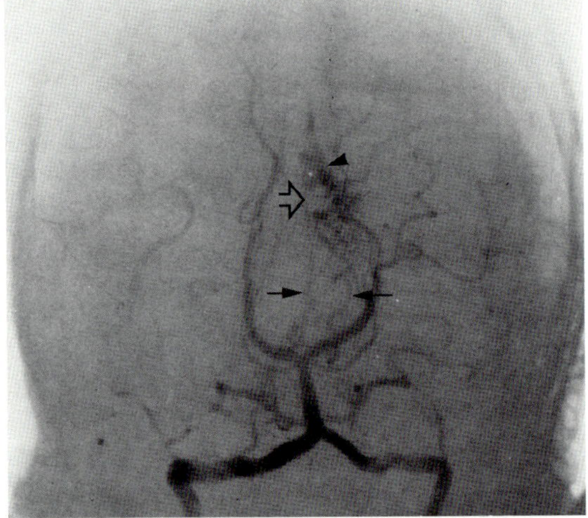

Fig. 5. (Bajandas, Aptman, and Stevens). Case 2. Vertebral angiogram, subtraction technique. Left, lateral projection, arteriovenous malformation in the area of the left thalamus (arrow). Right, anteroposterior projection, arteriovenous malformation near the midline on the left side (arrow).

that have confirmed the diagnostically localizing value of these clinical findings.

The syndrome is generally thought to include the following clinical findings:

1. paresis of vertical gaze (especially upward)
2. paresis of convergence
3. convergence and/or retraction nystagmus (either spontaneous, on attempted upward gaze, or while observing down-going optokinetic targets)
4. light-near dissociation of the pupils
5. upper eyelid retraction (Collier's sign)
6. skew deviation

More than 60 cases of the sylvian aqueduct syndrome have been reported and attributed to a variety of disease processes.

Smith has noted that each of the major etiologies tends to have an age predilection.[12] The clinician may find it helpful to remember this age related classification of the more common causes of this syndrome (Table II).

The pathology is usually reported as being localized to the dorsal rostral midbrain in the pretectum or periaqueductal gray matter. However, the effect in this area may also be produced by an abnormality in the posterior portion of the third ventricle (immediately superior to the pretectum) and may be due to a pineal tumor, a thalamic lesion, or simply dilatation of

TABLE I. *Historical review of clinical and experimental reports of the sylvian aqueduct syndrome*

Date	Author	Clinical and experimental observations
1883	Parinaud[1]	Paresis of upward gaze and of convergence
1903	Koerber[2]	"Nystagmus retractorius"
1910	Salus[3]	Echinococcal cyst, fourth ventricle
1913	Elschnig[4]	Glioma, pineal and midbrain
1923	De Monchy[5]	Convergence nystagmus and light-near dissociation of the pupils; pinealoma
1927	Collier[6]	Lid retraction
1959	Fisher[7]	Paresis of upward gaze and of convergence, with tonic downward deviation of the eyes and skew deviation, in patients with thalamic hemorrhage
1959	Smith[8]	Retraction nystagmus elicited by down-going optokinetic targets
1961	Smith[9]	Paresis of upward and downward gaze and nystagmus retractorius in a patient with stereotactic lesion of the thalamus
1967	Nashold[10]	Sylvian aqueduct syndrome in patients with stereotactic periaqueductal lesions
1969	Pasik[11]	Paresis of upward and downward gaze and of convergence in monkeys with pretectal lesions.

TABLE II. *Age-predilection of etiologies of sylvian aqueduct syndrome*[12]

Age (years)	Etiology
1	Congenital aqueductal stenosis
10	Pinealoma
20	Head trauma
30	Arteriovenous malformation
40	Multiple sclerosis
50	Midbrain ischemia

the third ventricle in patients with hydrocephalus.[13, 14]

Our patients demonstrated the sylvian aqueduct syndrome and were found to have vascular malformations of the thalamus. Ralston and Papatheodorou[15] reported a patient who demonstrated paresis of upward gaze and vertical nystagmus and was found to have a thalamic arterovenous malformation. The patient underwent successful treatment of the vascular malformation by direct, transventricular visualization and coagulation with bipolar forceps.

Askenasy, Wijsenbeck, and Herzberger[16] described a patient with retraction nystagmus and lid retraction secondary to an arterovenous aneurysm of the midbrain.

Gil Peralta, Alberca, Escudero, and Touzon[17] reported the case of a patient with Rendu-Osler-Weber (familial telangiectasia) disease with developed retraction nystagmus, paresis of upward and downward gaze, and paresis of convergence. The patient was found to have an arterovenous malformation of one of the posterior cerebral arteries.

Sochoky[18] described a patient with paresis of vertical gaze due to a vascular malformation of one of the superior cerebellar arteries.

The reports of Fisher[8] and Smith[9] have emphasized the tendency for lesions of the thalamus to present with components of the sylvian aqueduct syndrome (Table I).

SUMMARY

We report the cases of two patients with vascular malformations of the thalamus and with clinical findings that included the (Koerber-Salus-Elschnig) sylvian aqueduct syndrome. These cases confirm the diagnostic value of this syndrome in directing the clinician to a study of the dorsal rostral midbrain.

REFERENCES

1. Parinaud, M. H. Paralysie des mouvements associés des yeuz. Arch. Neurologie *5*(14):145–172 (1883).
2. Koerber, H. Uber drei Falle von Retraktionsbewegung des Bulbus (Nystagmus retractorius). Ophthalmolog. Klin. *7*:65–67 (1903).
3. Salus, R. On acquired retraction movements of the eyes. Arch. Ophthalmol. *42*:34–44 (1913).
4. Elschnig, A. Nystagmus retractorius, ein cerebrales Herdsymptom. Med. Klin. *9*:8–11 (1913).
5. De Monchy, S. J. R. Rhythmical convergence spasm of the eyes in a case of tumour of the pineal gland. Brain *46*:179–188 (1923).
6. Collier, J. Nuclear ophthalmoplegia, with especial reference to retraction of the lids and ptosis and to lesions of the posterior commissure. Brain *50:*488–498 (1927).
7. Fisher, C. M. Pathologic and clinical aspects of thalamic hemorrhage. Trans. Am. Neurol. Assoc. *84:*56 (1959).
8. Smith, J. L., Zieper, I. Gay, A. J., and Cogan, D. G. Nystagmus retractorius. Arch. Ophthalmol. *62:*864–867 (1959).
9. Smith, J. L., Nashold, B. S., and Kreshon, M. J. Ocular signs after stereotactic lesions in the pallidum and thalamus. Arch. Ophthalmol. *65:*532–535 (1961).
10. Nashold, B. S. and Gills, J. P. Ocular signs from brain stimulation and lesions. Arch. Ophthalmol. *77:*609–618 (1967).
11. Pasik, P., Pasik, T., and Bender, M. B. The pretectal syndrome in monkeys. I. Disturbances of gaze and body posture. Brain *92:*521–534 (1969).
12. Smith, J. L. Nystagmus. Neuro-Ophthalmology Tapes, No. 4.
13. Chattha, A. S. and Delong, G. R. Sylvian aqueduct syndrome as a sign of acute obstructive hydrocephalus in children. J. Neurol. Neurosurg. Psychiatr. *38:*288–296 (1975).
14. Swash, M. Periaqueductal dysfunction (the Sylvian Aqueduct Syndrome): a sign of hydrocephalus? J. Neurol. Neurosurg. Psychiatr. *37:*21–26 (1974).
15. Ralston, B. L. and Papatheodorou, C. A. Vascular malformation of the left thalamus. Report of a case of successful treatment, with a note on occlusion of the left internal cerebral vein. Neurosurg. *17:*505–510 (1960).
16. Askenasy, H., Wijsenbeck, H., and Herzberger, E. Retraction nystagmus and retraction of the eye lids due to arteriovenous aneurysm of the midbrain. Arch. Neurol. Psychiatr. *69:*236–241 (1953).
17. Gil Peralta, A., Alberca, R., Escudero, L., and Touzon, M. J. Nystagmus retractorious: Malformacion arteriovenosa cerebral y enfermedad de Rendu-Osler. Rev. Clin. Esp. *129:*195–200 (1973).
18. Sochoky, S. Arteriovenous fistula of the lung. Lancet *82:*12 (1962).

42 Syringobulbia and Its Neuro-Ophthalmological Manifestations

John A. Costin, M. D.
J. Lawton Smith, M.D.

INTRODUCTION

Syringobulbia is an insidious neurologic disorder with many ophthalmologic signs and symptoms. Briefly defined, syringobulbia is a progressive degenerative disorder characterized pathologically by central cavitation of the medulla oblongata. It is uniformly associated with syringomyelia,* an identical condition involving usually the cervical and high thoracic segments of the spinal cord.

In the brainstem, the cavitation is variable in size and shape, leading to symptoms that are predominantly unilateral. Involvement of the oculomotor system, the sympathetics, and the trigeminal nucleus, as well as other structures of neuro-ophthalmologic significance, are highlighted by the following case reports and subsequent discussion.

Case 1

A 21-year-old, right-handed, black man presented with horizontal diplopia and transient blurring of vision of one year's duration. He also had a three-year history of voice change and the inability to stand straight. For two years he had progressive numbness of his left upper extremity to the point that he cut his hand accidentally on several occasions and was totally unaware of this until he saw blood.

Neuro-ophthalmologic examination was remarkable for bilateral abducens weakness, left weaker than right. Furthermore, gaze evoked jerk nystagmus was present with the fast component beating toward the side of horizontal gaze. In down gaze, dissociated downbeating vertical nystagmus was noted with the left eye beating more rapidly than the right. A rotary component was seen as well.

Corneal sensation was absent on the left (Fig. 1) and greatly diminished on the right. Light touch and pain sensation were similarly markedly diminished on the left side of the face in all three trigeminal divisions, but were intact on the right. There was weakness of the left orbicularis oculi. The uvula moved up and to the right, and the gag reflex was absent bilaterally. There was marked hemiatrophy of the left side of the tongue associated with coarse fasciculations (Fig. 2).

Other findings included obvious wasting of both upper extremities and neck muscles, as well as fasciculations in the forearm and platysma. Scoliosis was also present (Fig. 3).

The patient was admitted to the hospital with a diagnosis of syringobulbia. A pantopaque myelogram demonstrated an enlarged cervical spinal canal and enlargement of the spinal cord (Fig. 4). Subsequently, an air myelogram was performed and showed collapse of the cervical spinal cord with gross spaces between the dura and arachnoid (Fig. 5).

The patient was surgically treated with a terminal ventriculostomy and regained

---

* The word "syrinx" is derived from the Greek word for "pipe," and thus syringomyelia is a "pipe" or cavity in the marrow (myelia) of the spinal cord.

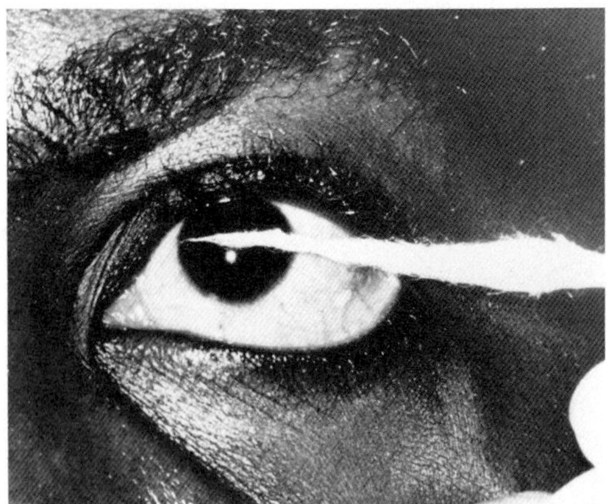

Fig. 1. Corneal anesthesia (Case 1).

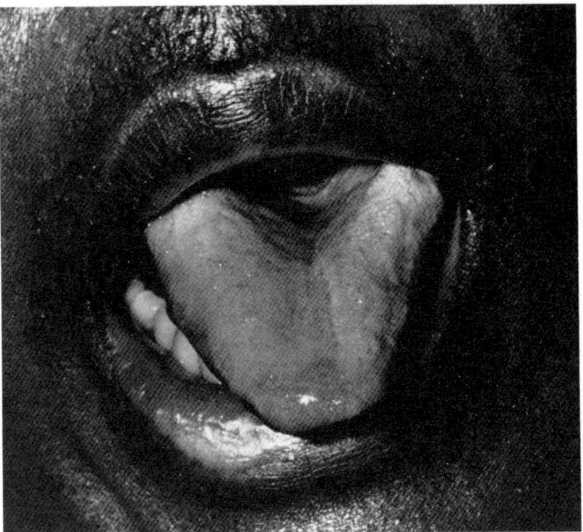

Fig. 2. Hemiatrophy of the tongue with deviation toward the left (Case 1).

some corneal and facial sensitivity in the immediate postoperative period.

Case 2

A 35-year-old, right-handed, white female presented with a 13-year history of numbness in the thumb and first two digits of her right hand. This slowly progressed, leading to anesthesia of the right upper extremity. Vertical diplopia was noticed two years prior to the initial examination, and difficulty with speech, a mild right ptosis, and numbness of the left hand were present for one year.

Neuro-ophthalmological examination revealed a right ptosis and miosis (Fig. 6). A diagnosis of a right Horner's syndrome was confirmed by cocaine testing (Fig. 7). Hor-

izontal gaze evoked jerk nystagmus was present with a rotary component. On downgaze, the nystagmus converted to dissociated downbeating with the right eye beating faster than the left. Motility examination revealed a right hypertropia with a skew deviation.

Sensory examination of the face was normal except for hypesthesia to pin prick in the second division of the trigeminal nerve on the right. Visual fields showed lower bitemporal defects breaking out from the blind spot. The discs were normal.

Minimal dysphonia was present, and gag reflexes were absent bilaterally. Fasciculations of the tongue were noticed, as well as a slight right-sided hemiatrophy of the tongue.

Inspection of the upper extremities revealed marked wasting of the intrinsic muscles of the hands and a "claw" hand on the right (Fig. 8).

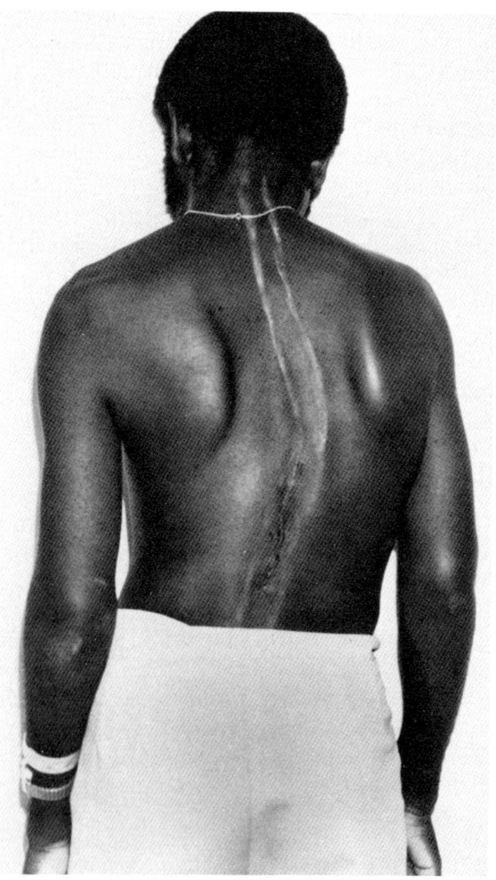

Fig. 3. Scoliosis (Case 1).

Suboccipital craniotomy and cervical laminectomy with decompression of the syrinx cavity were subsequently performed. This resulted in a resolution of her skew deviation and a decrease in her nystagmus.

The patient's findings were essentially unchanged at a 15-year following-up examination.

Case 3

A 39-year-old black man was seen in consultation and gave a history of pain and paresthesias in his left hand for ten years. A similar process began in his right hand two years prior to examination. Progressive weakness of the upper extremities caused him to seek a medical opinion.

Simple inspection revealed rather marked kyphoscoliosis of the spine with the left shoulder higher than the right. On neuro-ophthalmologic examination he was found to have a left Horner's syndrome, proven by a cocaine test. He had 20/15 vision in each eye. Gaze evoked rotary nystagmus, most prominent in right gaze, was also seen. No vertical nystagmus was present. Versions were full without any tropias.

Ophthalmoscopy was of interest. The right disc was flat and showed a slight scleral conus (Fig. 9). The left disc showed atrophy and a notch temporally (Fig. 10).

Further examination showed bilateral "claw" hands and a trophic ulcer on the left hand. Obvious wasting of the intrinsic muscles of the hands was present. He was areflexic in the upper extremities and hyperreflexic in the lower extremities. Dissociated sensory loss was present from C3 to T4 bilaterally.

Myelography revealed a markedly enlarged spinal canal and cord. Diffuse communicating hydrocephalus was found on pneumoencephalography. A diagnosis of syrinx was made, and surgery was performed. The syrinx was decompressed via a posterior fossa approach. The base of the fourth ventricle or obex was packed with muscle fragments.

On the sixth postoperative day, the patient died suddenly of a myocardial infarction. Autopsy revealed: (1) Symmetrical dilatation of the lateral and third ventricles to three times normal size. (2) The enlarged

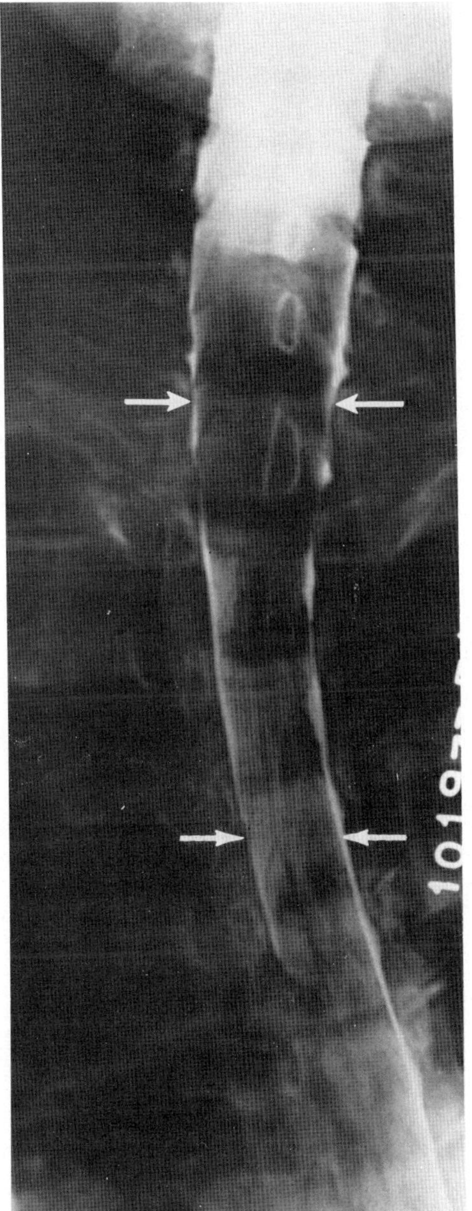

Fig. 4. Pantopaque myelogram showing a widened spinal canal (upper white arrows) with dye outlining an enlarged cervical and upper thoracic spinal cord. Lower thoracic spinal canal (lower white arrows) is one-third less in size than cervical canal (upper white arrows).

third ventricle was protruding forward abutting the optic chiasm. When viewed from above (Fig. 11), the optic nerves and third ventricle can be seen. Upon opening

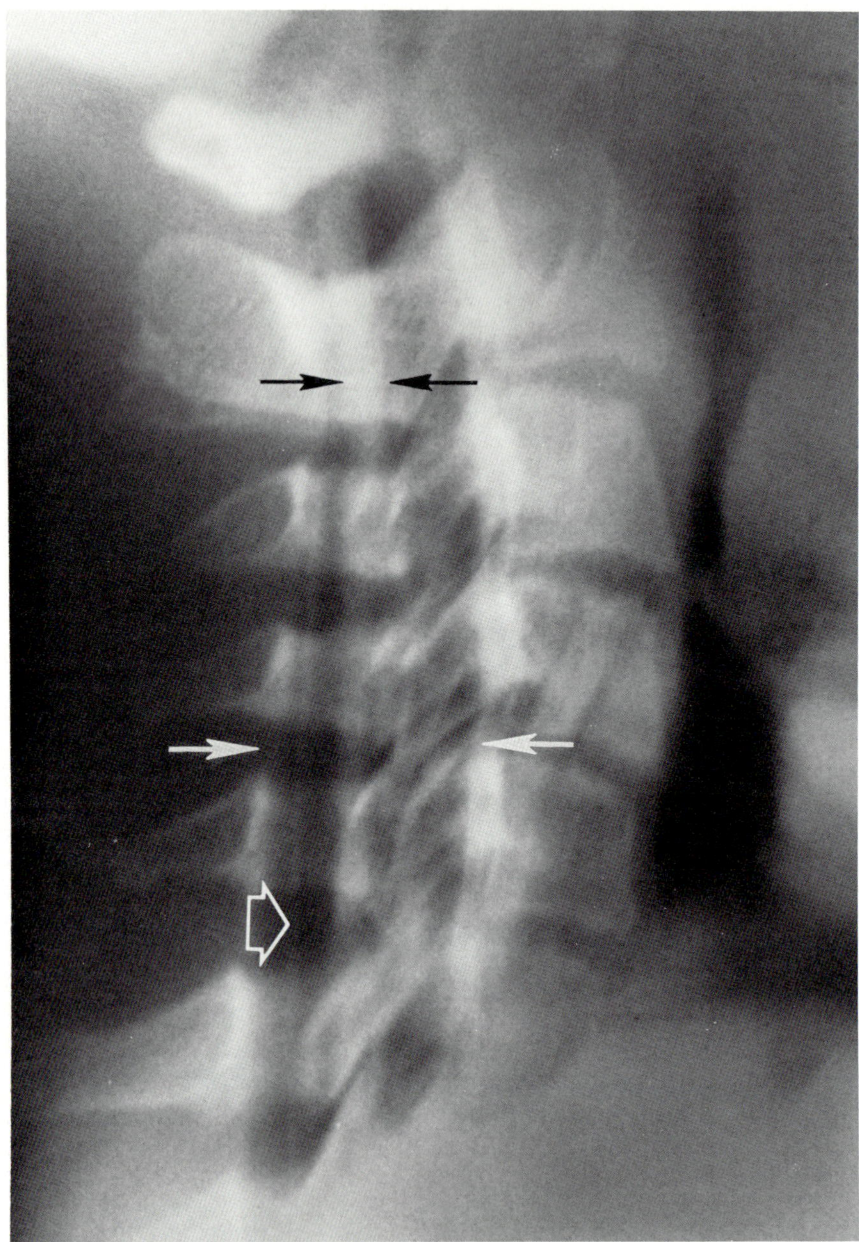

Fig. 5. Air myelogram showing collapse of the spinal cord (black arrows) with a widened spinal canal (white arrows). Dura appears as a faint white line (large open arrow) (Case 1).

the third ventricle (Fig. 12) and viewing the chiasm from above, a notch can be seen in the middle of the chiasm. (3) A syrinx was found beginning with a slit-like prolongation of the fourth ventricle at the obex. This cavity extended caudally to the sixth thoracic segment.

NEURO-OPHTHALMOLOGIC MANIFESTATIONS

1. Sensory Loss

Upper Extremities. Although a syrinx can involve any tract in the spinal cord, the one characteristic finding is dissociated sen-

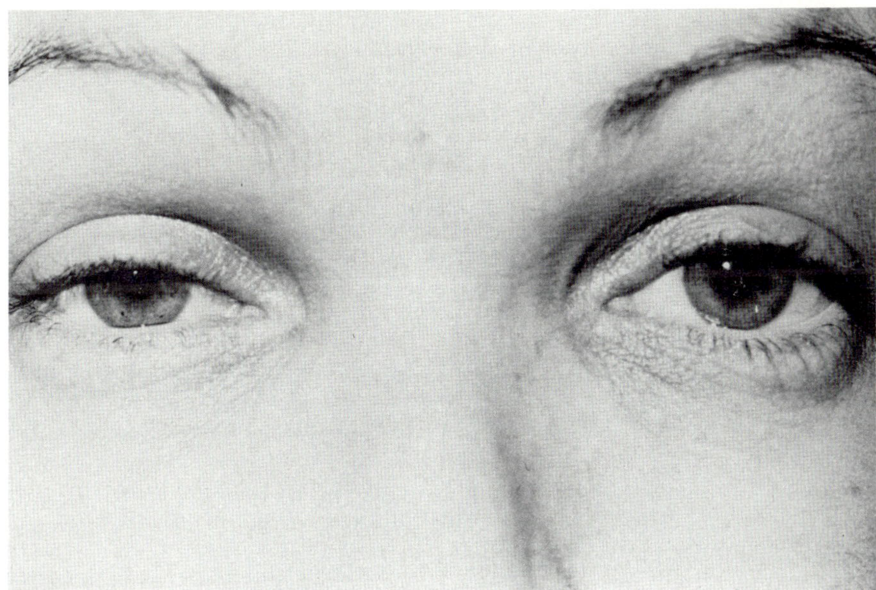

Fig. 6. A right Horner's syndrome with miosis and ptosis (Case 2).

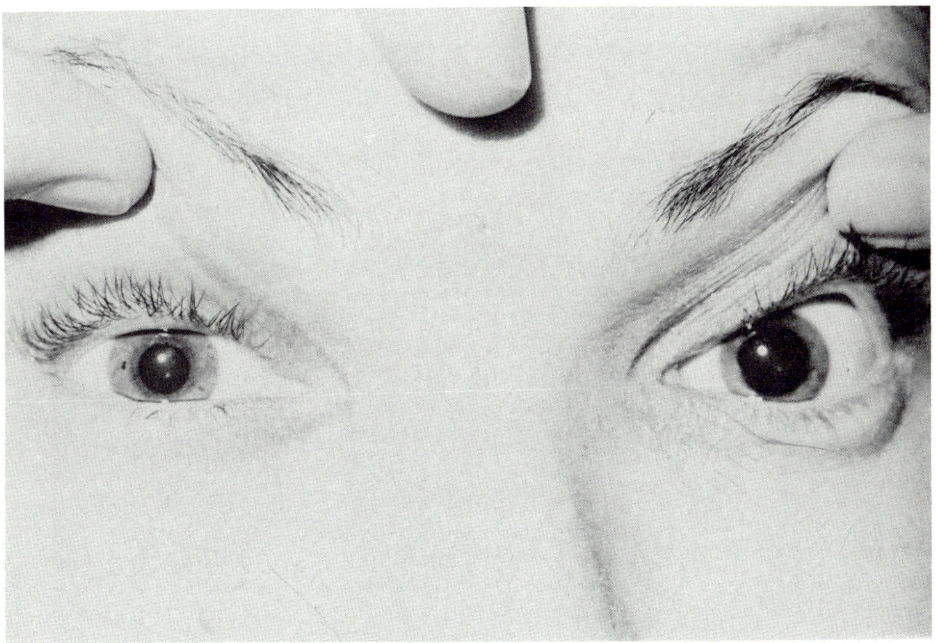

Fig. 7. A right Horner's syndrome after cocaine testing (Case 2).

sory loss. This refers to the loss of pain and temperature but with intact light touch, vibration, and position sense. With syringomyelia, this process most commonly involves the upper extremities. It begins in the hands and marches insidiously upwards, eventually involving the classical cloak or veil distribution. The patient may be unaware of the sensory loss, and a history of painless cuts and burns about the hands can often be obtained.

Trigeminal Divisions. In syringobulbia, sensory dissociation similarly occurs. Involvement of the descending root of the trigeminal nucleus causes diminished pain and temperature about the face, but leaving light touch intact. As the process continues, all sensory modalities are affected in the trigeminal distribution.

Thus, in syringobulbia, ipsilateral corneal hypesthesia is not uncommon, but total anesthesia is less common.

2. Motor Involvement

Upper Extremities. Damage to the anterior horn cells is responsible for the motor abnormalities. The hands frequently show the sequelae first. There are varying amounts of atrophy of the intraosseous muscles, as well as the thenar and hypothenar muscles. The end result of this may be a "claw" hand as seen in Figure 8 from Case 2. Later, the muscles of the arm and shoulder girdle may become affected.

XII Cranial Nerve. Involvement of the hypoglossal nucleus leads to fasciculations of the tongue and eventual ipsilateral hemiatrophy of the tongue (Fig. 2). On protru-

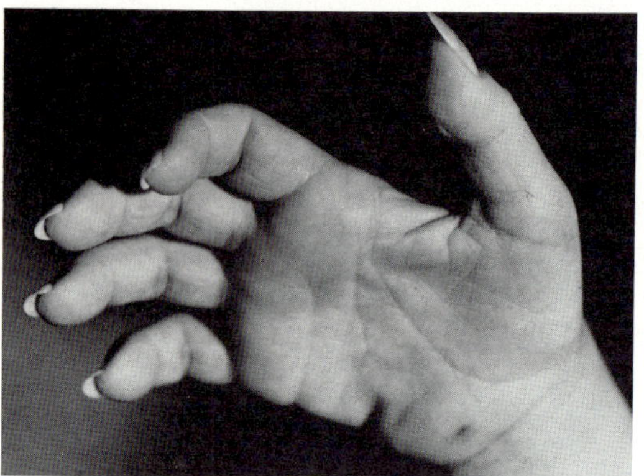

Fig. 8. "Claw" hand with wasting of the thenar and hypothenar muscles (Case 2).

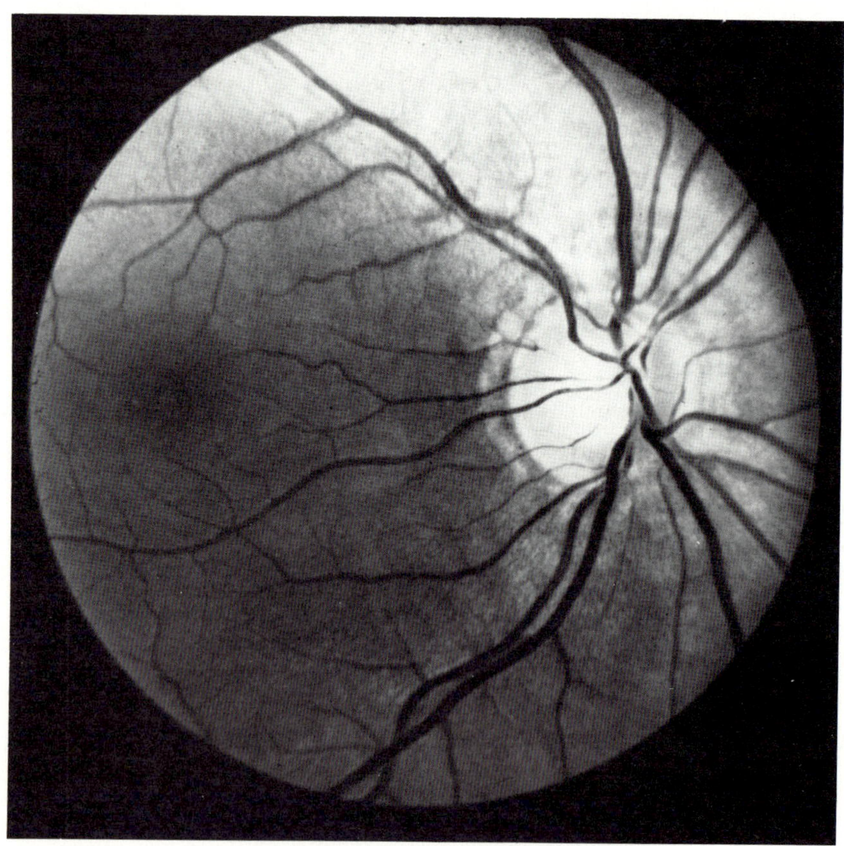

Fig. 9. Normal right disc (Case 3).

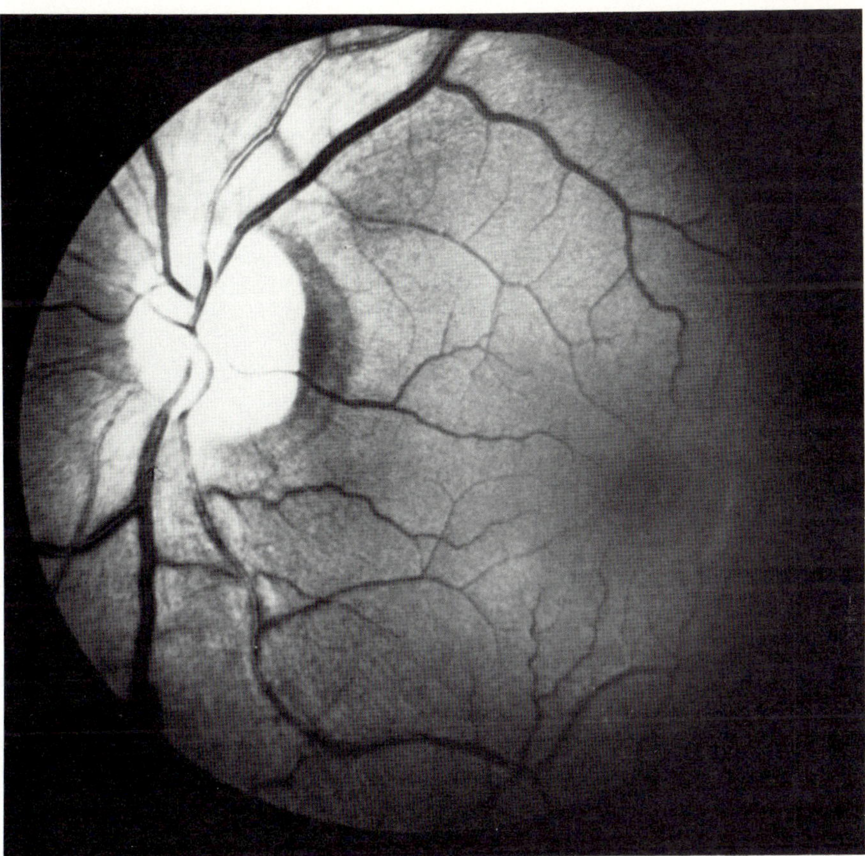

Fig. 10. Atrophic left disc (Case 3).

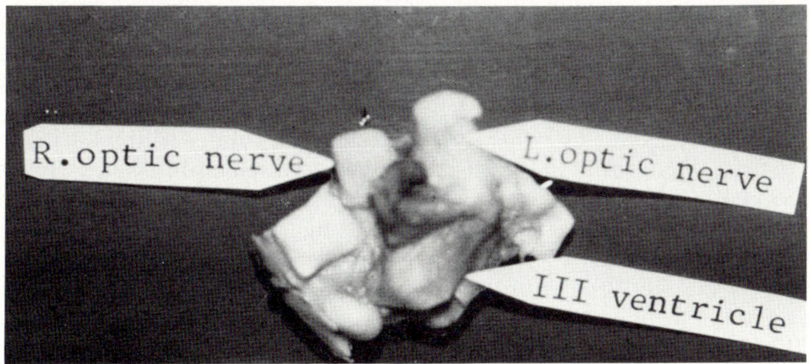

Fig. 11. Optic nerves and third ventricle viewed from above (Case 3).

sion, the tongue will deviate toward the side of the syrinx.

XI Cranial Nerve. Weakness of the sternocleidomastoid and trapezius muscles results from involvement of the accessory nucleus.

X and IX Cranial Nerves. Moving cephalad, dysphagia, dysphonia, and deviation of the uvula are seen when the syrinx compromises the glossopharyngeal and vagus nuclei. Interestingly, dysphonia is one of the most disconcerting symptoms, and patients seem to identify easily its time of onset historically.

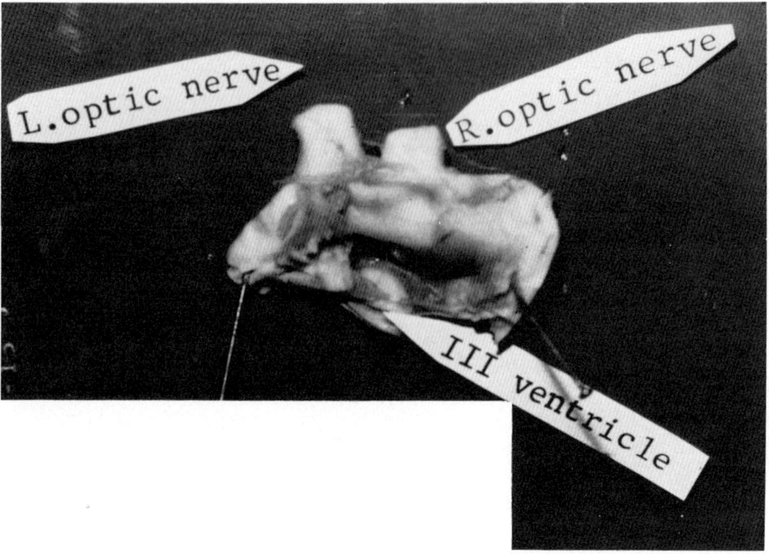

Fig. 12. Chiasm and optic nerves viewed from above after opening the third ventricle (Case 3).

VIII Cranial Nerve. There have been reports of decreased tearing due to involvement of the superior salivatory nucleus as well as decreased saliva production.[1] The facial nucleus is only rarely involved clinically. The explanation for this is not clear.

VI, IV, and III Cranial Nerves. Paralysis of the extraocular muscles is not uncommon and has been reported to occur in 11% of 300 cases of syringobulbia as reported by Schlesinger. The abducens nucleus is involved most commonly. This produces uncrossed diplopia and may lead to a head turn. Often this is the most distressing symptom to the patient. The ophthalmologist may first encounter the patient because of the symptomatic diplopia. The trochlea and oculomotor nucleus are less commonly involved.

II Cranial Nerve. Optic atrophy and papilledema have been reported by several authors.[1, 2, 4] The mechanisms for this have heretofore been unknown (see Pathophysiology below). Involvement of the optic nerves is difficult to understand unless one considers Gardner's hypothesis on the etiology of syringomyelia.[5]

Horner's Syndrome. Interruption of the cervical sympathetic fibers in the ciliospinal center of Budge leads to a Horner's syndrome.[6, 7] This is a rather characteristic finding in syringobulbia. The Horner's syndrome may be "full-blown" with obvious ptosis, miosis, and anhidrosis (Fig. 6). Usually, however, the diagnosis is more subtle, with mild to minimal ptosis and slight anisocoria, thus necessitating the performance of a cocaine test in all suspected cases of syringobulbia with anisocoria.

Nystagmus. Nystagmus is a frequent finding in syringobulbia.[8] Just as a dissociated sensory loss is rather pathognomonic, so is dissociated nystagmus. This refers to oscillations of different amplitudes or frequencies or even different directions when comparing one eye to the other. Cogan[9, 10] first popularized the association of dissociated nystagmus with posterior fossa lesions. He stated that the eye on the same side as the lesion showed the greater oscillations, and this proved to be the case in two of our three patients.

Although rotary nystagmus as well as horizontal jerk nystagmus are seen in syringobulbia, downbeating nystagmus seems characteristic. In our cases, the downbeating was accentuated by downgaze. Surgical relief of the syrinx may lessen or even abolish the nystagmus.

PATHOGENESIS

Although this condition has been recognized for over 210 years, the pathogenesis remains obscure.

The term "hydromyelia" was introduced

by Virchow[11] in 1863, since he believed the origin of the cavity was due to abnormal expansion of the central canal secondary to fluid produced by the central canal. Others have since differentiated between dilation of a central canal, or hydromyelia, and a spinal cord cavity independent of the central canal, or syringomyelia. For practical purposes, this differentiation is not made, since most of the time separating the two entities is difficult and because of the probability that they share the same underlying etiology.

Since Virchow's time, numerous hypotheses have come and gone.[12-16] The one which has received the most support has been proposed by Gardner.[5, 17] He suggests that all of these cavitations have a common denominator—the inadequate escape of cerebrospinal fluid during critical developmental periods. To better understand this theory, one must review a bit of the dynamics of cerebrospinal fluid production and flow (Fig. 13).

Fluid is produced in the choroid plexus of the lateral ventricle, choroid plexus of the third ventricle, and the choroid plexus of the fourth ventricle. This fluid then exists at the foramen of Luschka and the foramen of Magendie. The choroid plexuses begin secreting cerebrospinal fluid at the fourth or fifth week of gestation; however, foramina are not yet patent at this time.[5, 18] The fluid then permeates through the roof of the fourth ventricle and into the central canal, causing a syrinx of hydromyelia. At the eighth to ninth week of gestation, the foramina of Lushka and Magendie become patent, thus allowing cerebrospinal fluid egress into the subarachnoid space and similarly decompresses the hydromelia, or dilated central canal. As a result, the central canal becomes a small vestigial structure.

It is Gardner's contention that a number of things can go wrong in this critical developmental period. The foramina may fail to open at the critically appropriate time, or the roof of the fourth ventricle may not be as permeable as necessary to relieve the cerebrospinal fluid pressure. The result is the same, i.e., the cerebrospinal fluid is then transmitted from the floor of the fourth ventricle through the obex or opening into the central canal of the spinal cord. This

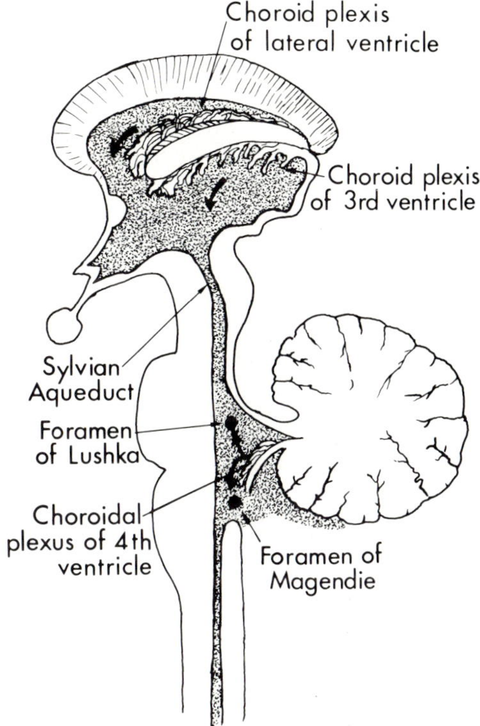

Fig. 13. Pathway of cerebrospinal fluid flow.

resultant dilation leads to a widened spinal cord and subsequent widened spinal canal. The ependyma is then damaged by the pressure, and a false diverticulum forms, or syrinx cavity. The elevated cerebrospinal fluid pressure similarly dilates the ventricular system (as seen in Case 3), but since the ventricles are lined by firmer white matter, they yield less, thus leading to a less consistent finding of hydrocephalus on autopsy or radiographic examination.

In those cases where hydrocephalus is present (Case 3), the dilated third ventricle may compress the chiasm and optic nerves. This process could lead to disc edema and eventual optic atrophy. This mechanism could account for the findings in Case 3. This patient had unilateral optic atrophy, and on necropsy a dilated third ventricle was found with compression and notching of the chiasm.

Gardner's theory with its underlying hydrocephalus could be the common denominator to explain involvement of the optic nerves in syringobulbia.

NEURO-RADIOGRAPHIC STUDIES

Plain x-rays of the spine will frequently show kyphoscoliosis. This often will precede any other signs and symptoms, suggesting possibly that the axial muscles may be affected before others. Plain x-rays will also reveal widening of the spinal canal in the area of the syrinx. This then brings up the differential diagnosis of a wide canal which for practical purposes is between a syrinx and a neoplasm.[19, 20]

Computerized tomography is helpful in the syrinx patient to define ventricular dilatation. Indeed, the syrinx itself has been reportedly demonstrated by computed tomography,[21] but this is technically very difficult and often impossible with the usually available equipment. The definitive test, however, is myelography.[22-25] In a syrinx this will show again widening of the spinal cord and a fusiform dilatation of the spinal cord in the involved area (Fig. 4). An Arnold-Chiari malformation may also be found in association with syringomyelia. Still, the myelogram does not accurately differentiate an intramedullary spinal cord tumor from a syrinx. *Air myelography is necessary.* In this test, air injected into the spinal canal will collapse the syrinx and thus the spinal cord (Fig. 5).

SURGERY

A number of surgical approaches have been advocated for the treatment of a syrinx.[26-28] Basically two techniques prevail:

1. Obex Tamponade. Posterior fossa exploration with a high cervical maninectomy is performed, and obex tamponade is done by using muscle fragment or other suitable material.

2. Terminal Ventriculostomy (Syringoperitoneal Shunt). A shunt decompresses the syrinx and retards progression by allowing egress of fluid from the cavity.

From a neuro-ophthalmologic point of view, several considerations regarding surgical treatment are important.

1. The motility may improve after surgery. An example is seen in Case 2 where the preoperative skew deviation resolved and remained absent for 15 years postoperatively

2. The nystagmus may improve. That is, the amplitude and frequency may diminish as was true in Case 1
3. The cranial nerve deficits may remain stable. The outlook in this condition may then be more optimistic than previously pictured

SUMMARY

Syringobulbia is a chronic cavitating process which is treated by surgery. The signs and symptoms involve virtually every cranial nerve, including the optic nerves. As a result, a plethora of neuro-ophthalmologic findings may be present in these patients. Early diagnosis and treatment are important, since many of these patients are helped by surgery.

REFERENCES

1. Posey, W. C. and Spiller, W. G. *The Eye and Nervous System.* J. B. Lippincott, Philadelphia, 1906, pp. 572–578.
2. Hermann, G. Anatomischer Befund bei Syringomyelie mit Opticus-Atrophie. Z. Gesamte Neurol. Psychiatr. *111:*713–721 (1927).
3. Coste, F., *et al.* Syringomyelie et syringobulbie atrophie optique unilaterale. Rev. Neurol. (Paris) *65:*360–374 (1936).
4. Alpers, B. J. and Bernard, C. I. Syringomyelia with choked disc. J. Nerv. Ment. Dis. *73:*577–587 (June 1931).
5. Gardner, W. J. Hydrodynamic mechanism of syringomyelia: Its relationship to myelocele. J. Neurol. Neurosurg. Psychiatr. *28:*247–259 (1965).
6. Furukawa, T. and Toyokura, Y. Alternating Horner syndrome. Arch. Neurol. *30:*311–313 (April 1974).
7. Amyot, R. Atypical clinical aspects of syringomyelia: The importance of sympathetic troubles. Can. Med. Assoc. J. *29:*60–63 (July 1933).
8. Thrush, A. C. and Foster, J. B. An analysis of nystagmus in 100 consecutive patients with communicating syringomyelia. J. Neurol. Sci. *20:*381–386 (1973).
9. Cogan, D. G. Dissociated nystagmus with lesions in the posterior fossa. Arch. Ophthalmol. *70:*361–368 (1963).
10. Cogan, D. G. and Barrows, L. J. Platybasia and Arnold Chiari malformation. Arch. Ophthalmol. *52:*13–22 (1954).
11. Virchow, R. Die Betheiligung des Ruckenmarhes an der Spina Bifida und die Hydromyelia. Virchows Arch. [Pathol. Anat.] *27:*575 (1863).
12. Conway, L. W. Hydrodynamic studies in syringomyelia. J. Neurosurg. *27:*501–514, (1967).
13. Batnitzhy, S., *et al.* Meningomyelocele and syringohydromyelia. Neuroradiology *120:*315–357 (August 1976).

14. Williams, B. The distending force in the production of "communicating syringomyelia." Lancet *2:* 189–193 (July 26, 1969).
15. Williams, B. Pathogenesis of syringomyelia. Lancet *2:*969–970 (Nov. 4, 1972).
16. Ball, M. J. and Dayan, A. D. Pathogenesis of syringomyelia. Lancet *2:*799–801 (October 14, 1972).
17. Gardner, W. J. and McMurry, F. G. "Non-Communicating" syringomyelia: A non-existent entity. Surg. Neurol. *6:*251–256 (October 1976).
18. Weed, L. H. *Development of Cerebro-spinal Spaces in Pig and Man.* Carnegie Institute, Washington, D.C., 1917, pub. #225.
19. Dolan, K. D. Expanding lesions of the cervical spinal canal. Radiol. Clin. North. Am. *15*(2):203–214 (Aug. 1977).
20. Hertel, G. The width of the cervical spinal canal and the size of the vertebral bodies in syringomyelia. Eur. Neurol. *9:*168 (1973).
21. DeChiro, G. *et al.* Axial tomography in syringomyelia. New Engl. J. Med. *292*(1):13–16 (1975).
22. Tjaden, R. J. *et al.* Iodoventriculography in hydromyelia. J. Can. Assoc. Radiol. *20:*265–267 (December 1969).
23. Narwood-Nash, D. C. and Fitz, C. R. Myelography and syringohydromyelia in infancy and childhood. Radiol. *113:*661–669 (December 1974).
24. Heinz, E. R. *et al.* Radiologic signs of hydromyelia. Radiol. *86:*311–318 (February 1966).
25. Conway, L. W. Radiographic studies of syringomyelia. Trans. Am. Neurol. Assoc. *86:*205 (1961).
26. Krayenbuhl, H. Evaluation of different surgical approaches in the treatment of syringomyelia. Clin. Neurol. Neurosurg. *77*(2):111–128 (Dec. 1975).
27. Krayenbuhl, H. and Benini, A. A new surgical approach in the treatment of hydromyelia and syringomyelia. J. R. Coll. Surg. Edinb. *16:*147–161 (1971).
28. Wetzel, N. and Davis, L. Surgical treatment of syringomyelia. Arch. Surg. *68:*570 (1954).

43 Immunity, Cytomegalovirus, and the Eye

Bernard H. Doft, M.D.

The increasing use of immunosuppressives in neoplastic diseases, organ transplantation, and rheumatology has led to the occurrence of previously unknown ocular infections. These opportunistic infections are ones which occur with organisms which ordinarily are nonvirulent. They may be fungi such as Candida, Aspergillus, or Cryptococcus, parasites such as Toxoplasma gondii, or viral organisms such as the herpesvirus group, which includes herpes simplex, varicella-zoster, and cytomegalovirus. Of the viruses, cytomegalovirus is a relatively common cause of opportunistic ocular infection. Advances in knowledge about immune defense mechanisms have led to a greater understanding of the setting in which these ordinarily nonvirulent viruses cause disease and provide the basis for understanding current therapeutic approaches to infections with these organisms.

THE IMMUNE SYSTEM

The immune defense system is complex. Two important components are B-cells and T-cells. *B*-cells are lymphocytes derived from *bone* marrow or gut associated lymphoid tissue. These lymphocytes (with help) produce circulating antibodies, which are molecules which have the ability to selectively bind specific antigens. Collectively they are responsible for circulating or *humoral* immunity. *T*-cells are lymphocytes which are derived from or "educated" by the *thymus*. They are responsible in large part for *cellular immune responses*, which are mediated by living cells rather than circulating antibodies. As an example, the common PPD skin test for tuberculosis represents a type of cell mediated immune response called delayed hypersensitivity.

Both B-cell and T-cell functions are important in protecting the human host from invading organisms, but the two systems have different roles.[1] *Humoral immunity is not effective against many viral infections.* Infections with the viruses of the herpes group, including cytomegalovirus, may occur even when extremely high serum antibody levels against the virus are present. High antibody levels prove the humoral immune system is intact.[2-4] Conversely, patients whose humoral immune responses are impaired are fully able to defend against many viral infections.[5]

Cellular immunity, on the other hand, is *essential* to provide protection from these *viruses*.[3] Individuals who have diminished cellular immunity are extremely susceptible to these viral infections, in spite of the presence of a normal humoral immune system.[5] Depressed cellular immunity may result in reactivation of latent viral infections.

What then are the factors which lead to suppression of the immune response and susceptibility to the viral diseases in question? (Table I.) The human fetus is immunologically immature, and therefore is at risk for opportunistic infection. There are rare congenital defects of the immune response. Neoplastic diseases are associated with immunosuppression and an increased incidence of cytomegalovirus infections.[6-8] In large part, though, an increased incidence of opportunistic infections follows iatrogenic suppression of normal immune responses. A host of different immunosuppressive cytotoxic agents or corticosteroids are being used with neoplastic disease, autoimmune, and rheumatologic conditions, as well as with organ transplants. An increased incidence of cytomegalovirus infections occurs when these agents are used, even when the underlying disease is one which does not in itself predispose to cytomegalovirus infection.[9, 10]

CLINICAL MANIFESTATIONS OF CYTOMEGALOVIRUS INFECTIONS

Approximately 2–3% of infants are culture positive for cytomegalovirus at the time of birth, the virus having been acquired transplacentally.[2] However, most culture positive infants have no signs or symptoms of disease. A few may have mental retardation or deafness attributable to cytomegalovirus infection. Only rarely does the syndrome of acute cytomegalovirus disease of infancy present. This is an acute fulminating illness resulting in devastating central nervous system, hepatic, pulmonary, and hematologic involvement. Neonatal cytomegalovirus retinitis occurs as part of this syndrome in one-quarter of cases, and rarely it is the only clinical manifestation of neonatal infection.[11]

Cytomegalovirus is an ubiquitous organism. By the age of 35, over 80% of adults have been exposed to it.[12] It is important to understand that in the normal adult, primary infection most commonly occurs without symptoms and causes no apparent illness. The virus may cause a benign short-lived viral syndrome or respiratory illness, and it may cause a heterophil negative infectious mononucleosis-like syndrome. Isolated specific organ involvement with cytomegalovirus in a healthy adult can occur, but is uncommon. There is only a single reported case of cytomegalovirus retinitis in a healthy adult.[13]

The manifestations of cytomegalovirus infections in the immunocompromised adult are different, however. Severe disseminated infections may occur, or the virus may seem to focus on one or a limited number of target organs. Infection may be primary or may represent reactivation of dormant or latent virus which the patient may have acquired years before. Without preexisting serological studies it can be impossible to tell. Illness may manifest itself with fever, arthralgias, and atypical lymphocytosis,[14] hepatitis, central nervous system involvement, pneumonitis, gastrointestinal bleeding from vasculitis induced ulcers, skin lesions secondary to vasculitis,[15] or with a characteristic ocular picture.

OCULAR INVOLVEMENT WITH CYTOMEGALOVIRUS

Obviously, ocular involvement with cytomegalovirus does not occur in all immunosuppressed patients, and it occurs in only a limited percent of patients with other systemic evidence of cytomegalovirus infection. For example, 60% of renal transplant patients on immunosuppressives manifest some morbidity from cytomegalovirus infections, but only 4%–5% of the same group develop cytomegalovirus retinitis.[16] In a prospective study of 61 renal transplant patients, just less than one-half developed cytomegalovirus viremia. The viremia was self-limited in 22 cases, but chronic (lasting greater than six months) in five. Two of these five developed cytomegalovirus retinitis. It is interesting that both cases which developed retinitis had intense viremia which lasted greater than 11 months, but none of the patients who manifested self-limited viremia developed retinitis. Cytomegalovirus retinitis should be looked for as a late manifestation of intense cytomegalovirus infection. High antibody titers may be present, and aid in diagnosis, but they are not protective.[17]

The ocular manifestations of cytomegalovirus infection are characteristic. The clinical course may be short, or it may last months or years. Initial lesions are characterized by granular white dots or patches surrounded by otherwise normal retina (Fig. 1). These patches represent areas of viral involvement.[18] Adjacent retinal vessels may appear sheathed, or as white cords. As the process evolves over weeks to months, the localized granular dots and patches appear to coalesce (Fig. 2), and the involved retina appears necrotic and thick-

TABLE I. *Factors associated with opportunistic infections*

1. Prematurity
2. Rate congenital defects of the immune system
3. Neoplasia
4. Iatrogenic suppression of the immune system
   a. Cytotoxic agents
   b. Steroids
   c. Organ transplant recipients

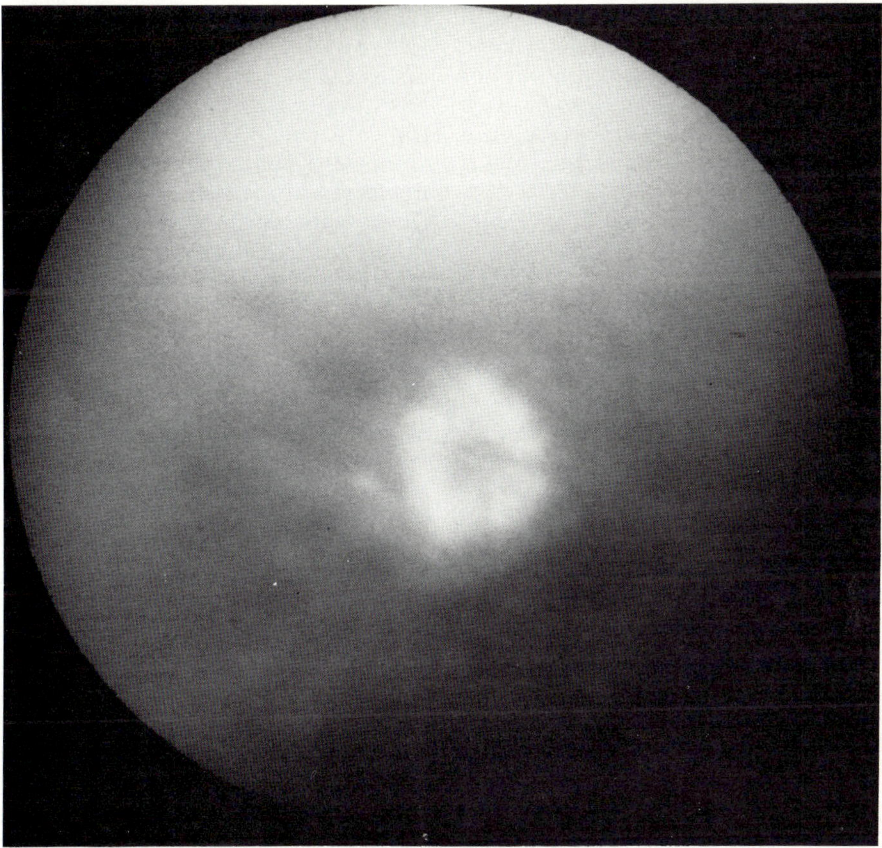

Fig. 1. Granular white retinal lesions of cytomegalic retinitis.

ened. Superimposed areas of hemorrhage within the necrotic area may occur and can falsely give the impression of a branch vein occlusion. As the process develops, necrotic areas of retina become gray-brown, thinned, and atrophic (Fig. 3). An only minimally pigmented scar develops, perhaps due to such extensive necrosis of the retinal pigment epithelium that no further proliferation is possible. While the center of the lesion atrophies and scars, the surrounding advancing edge may demonstrate the characteristic early changes with small white granular satellite lesions.[18] This inflammation-scarring process may march through different areas of the retina. Along with the retinitis, a mild to moderate uveitis and vitritis may occur. Visual function is significantly affected if the macula becomes involved with the necrotizing retinitis, if enough of the peripheral retina is involved to severely limit visual field, or if retinal detachment occurs.[4]

The pathologic picture may suggest the mechanism of viral spread. Endothelial cells of the retinal blood vessels are markedly involved, and this suggests hematogenous spread of the virus to the retina. Endothelial cell sloughing may lead to hemorrhage or to narrowing or occlusion of the local retinal vessels, giving the white cord-like picture seen on ophthalmoscopy. The white satellite lesions adjacent to coalesced areas of retinal involvement suggest that intraretinal progression occurs by direct cell to cell spread, the type of spread for which humoral immunity has little protective benefit, and for which functioning cellular immunity may be protective. Sharply demarcated areas of necrotic tissue are seen adjacent to normal areas of retina. In involved areas of retina, all retinal layers and the retinal pigment epithelium are involved with virus. Light microscopy shows characteristic enlargement (cytomegaly) of the cells, intranuclear and intracytoplasmic inclusions. There is often a clear zone around the nuclear inclusions, giving an owl eye appearance, and there is margination of nuclear chromatin.[19] On electron microscopy, viral particles are seen within the intranuclear and intracytoplasmic inclusions.

DIAGNOSIS

The diagnosis of cytomegalovirus retinitis in large part depends upon recognizing the clinical appearance in the appropriate patient setting. Though clinical appearance is characteristic, it is not diagnostic, for on the basis of ophthalmoscopic appearance it is impossible to differentiate the retinitis of cytomegalovirus from that of herpes simplex, varicella zoster, or toxoplasma gondii.

When clinical examination suggests one of these opportunistic infections, one should obtain serum antibody titers to cy-tomegaloviruses. A fourfold change in titer, either increasing or decreasing, or the presence of any titer when it can be documented that none was present before, may help indicate the presence of recent infection. Generally, the complement fixation test is most readily available, although indirect fluorescent antibody and other techniques may also be employed. (These tests may be available from your local hospital laboratory. If not, for $19.90 you can obtain the Complement Fixation titer from Bio Science Laboratories, 7600 Tyrone Avenue, Van Nuys, California 91405, if you send them 1 cc of serum in a red top tube. The Indirect Fluorescent Antibody test can be obtained for $9.00 by sending 1 cc of serum in a red top tube to National Health Science Laboratories, 1 N.E. 19 Street, Miami, Florida 33130.) Titers from patients on steroids may not be reliable.

Additional tests may be available at cer-

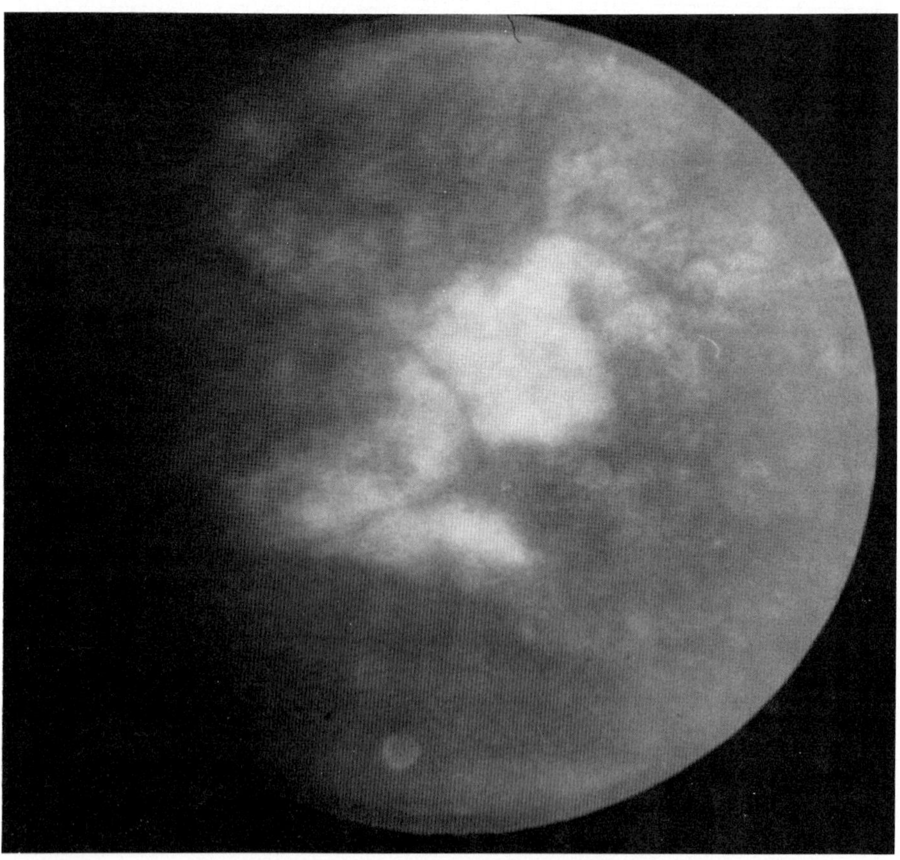

Fig. 2. Coalescence of cytomegalic retinal lesions.

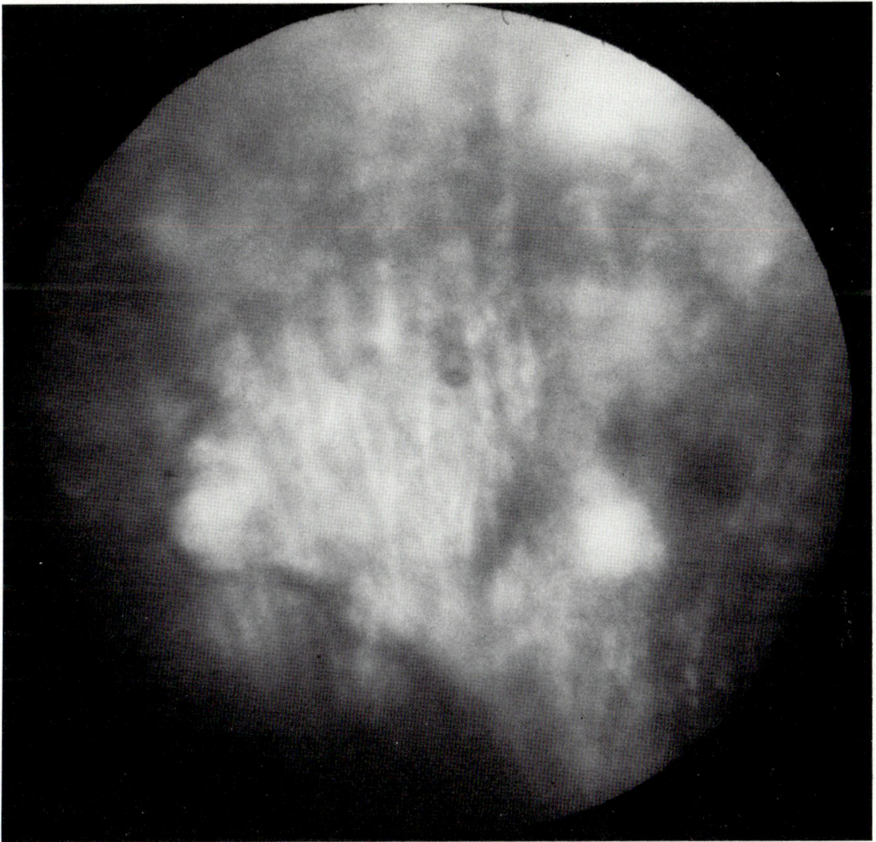

Fig. 3. Central atrophic retinal scar with areas of active cytomegalovirus retinitis at borders.

tain academic centers. These include viral cultures of blood leukocytes, urine, and throat to confirm the presence of cytomegalovirus. Cultures in isolated cases have been positive from aqueous,[10] subretinal fluid in a case with retinal detachment,[4] and from tears.[20] Exfoliative cytology to look for cytomegalic cells, as for example in urine sediment, is not reliable.

TREATMENT

A large number of ocular infections with cytomegalovirus are iatrogenically induced with immunosuppressive agents. The rationale for the use of these agents is that cure or palliation of the underlying disease may make tolerable the infectious complications, and that hopefully improved management of these infections will be developed.[21] This is not possible, as the cytomegalovirus is ubiquitous. A second approach would be the use of antiviral chemotherapy. Interferon is an agent which may limit viral infections. However, thus far it has not shown definite beneficial effect with cytomegalovirus infections.[22-27] Adenine arabinoside (Vidarabine) may transiently suppress cytomegalovirus, but its effect is minimal in immunosuppressed patients.[28, 29] A third possible therapeutic approach would be to augment the hosts immune response to invading virus, as with vaccination. At present, an approved live virus for human vaccination is not available. Passive administration of hyperimmune globulin would not likely be helpful as the role of antibodies in preventing cytomegalovirus disease is limited.

What about boosting cellular immune responses? We have previously seen that cellular immunity provides the bulwark of defense against cytomegalovirus.[30, 31] Augmentation of the cellular immune system could therefore be expected to be of benefit in cytomegalovirus infections. Transfer factor is a low molecular weight nonimmunogenic substance derived from leukocytes of donors who are sensitive to certain antigens. The substance confers on recipient lymphocytes the ability to perform T-cell functions against antigens to which the recipient was not previously sensitive. Transfer factor has been used in cytomegalovirus retinitis with apparent success.[32] This form of treatment holds immense potential on theoretical grounds, but a great deal more favorable data is needed before it can be accepted as clinically useful.

What we have seen is that there is no proven or accepted form of active intervention with cytomegalovirus, though several areas merit further exploration. However, there is something the physician can do. If the host is immunosuppressed because of pharmacological agents, the immune response can be boosted—*simply decrease or withdraw the offending immunosuppressive agents*. Thus, improvement or remission in cytomegalovirus retinitis has been observed when doses of steroids or immunosuppressives have been decreased.[4, 32] Any patient with cytomegalovirus retinitis should be carefully evaluated if he is being treated with immunosuppressive agents or steroids. If consistent with the underlying systemic disease for which the patient is being treated, attempts to reduce or eliminate these drugs should be initiated.

REFERENCES

1. Allison, A. C. Immunity and immunopathology in virus infections. Ann. Inst. Pasteur Lille *123*:585 (1972).
2. Stagno, S., Reynolds, D. W., Eng-Shang, H., *et al.* Congenital cytomegalovirus infection. New Engl. J. Med. *296*:154 (1977).
3. Rand, K. H., Rasmussen, L., Pollard, R. B., *et al.* Cellular immunity and Herpes virus infections in cardiac transplant patients. New Engl. J. Med. *296*:1372 (1977).
4. Aaberg, T. M., Cesarz, T. J. and Rytel, M. W. Correlation of virology and clinical course of cytomegalovirus retinitis. Am. J. Ophthalmol. *74*:407 (1972).
5. Glasgow, L. A. Cellular immunity in host resistance to viral infections. Arch. Intern. Med. *126*:125 (1970).
6. Duvall, C. P., Casazza, A. R., Grimley, P. M., *et al.* Recovery of cytomegalovirus from adults with neoplastic disease. Ann. Intern. Med. *64*:531 (1966).
7. Henson, D., Siegel, S. E., Fuccillo, D. A., *et al.* Cytomegalovirus infections during acute childhood leukemia. J. Infect. Dis. *126*:469 (1972).
8. Rosen, P. and Hajdu, S. Cytomegalovirus inclusion disease at autopsy of patients with cancer. Am. J. Clin. Pathol. *55*:749 (1971).
9. Dowling, J. N., Saslow, A. R., Armstrong, J. A., *et al.* Cytomegalovirus infection in patients receiving immunosuppressive therapy for rheumatologic disorders. J. Infect. Dis. *133*:399 (1976).
10. Chumbley, L. C., Robbertson, D. M., Smith, T. F., *et al.* Adult cytomegalovirus inclusion retino-uveitis. Am. J. Ophthalmol. *80*:807 (1975).
11. Lonn, L. I. Neonatal cytomegalic inclusion disease chorioretinitis. Arch. Ophthalmol. *88*:434 (1972).
12. Rowe, W. P., Hartley, J. W., Waterman, S., *et al.* Cytopathogenic agent resembling human salivary gland virus recovered from tissue cultures of human adenoids. Proc. Soc. Exp. Biol. Med. *92*:418 (1956).
13. Chawla, H. B., Ford, M. J., Munro, J. F., *et al.* Ocular involvement in cytomegalovirus infection in a previously healthy adult. Br. Med. J. *858*:281 (1976).
14. Suwansirkul, S., Rao, N., Dowling, J. N., *et al.* Primary and secondary cytomegalovirus infection. Arch. Intern. Med. *137*:1026 (1977).
15. Minars, N., Silverman, J. F., Escobar, M. R., *et al.* Fatal cytomegalic inclusion disease. Arch. Dermatol. *113*:1569 (1977).
16. Fiala, M., Payne, J. E., Berne, T. V., *et al.* Epidemiology of cytomegalovirus infection after transplantation and immunosuppression. J. Infect. Dis. *132*:421 (1975).
17. Fiala, M., Chatterjee, S. N., Carson, S., *et al.* Cytomegalovirus retinitis secondary to chronic viremia in phagocytic leukocytes. Am. J. Ophthalmol. *84*:567 (1977).
18. de Venecia, G., ZuRhein, G. M., Pratt, M. V., *et al.* Cytomegalic inclusion retinitis: a clinical, histopathologic and ultrastructural study. Arch. Ophthalmol. *86*:44 (1971).
19. Boniuk, I. The cytomegaloviruses and the eye. Int. Ophthalmol. Clin. *12*:169 (1972).
20. Cox, F., Meyer, D., and Hughes, W. T. Cytomegalovirus in tears from patients with normal eyes and with acute cytomegalovirus chorioretinitis. Am. J. Ophthalmol. *80*:817 (1975).
21. Levin, M. J. and Zaia, J. A. Immunosuppression and infection, Progress? New Engl. J. Med. *296*:1406 (1977).
22. Strander, H., Cantell, K., Carlstroem, G., *et al.* Acute infections in Interferon-treated patients with osteosarcoma: preliminary report of a comparative study. J. Infect. Dis. *133*:245 (1976).
23. Merigan, T. C., Rand, K. H., Pollard, R. B., *et al.* Human leukocyte interferon for the treatment of Herpes zoster in patients with cancer. New Engl. J. Med. *298*:981 (1978).
24. O'Reilly, R. J., Everson, L. K., Emoedi, G., *et al.* Effects of exogenous interferon in cytomegalovirus infections complicating bone marrow transplantation. Clin. Immunol. Immunopathol. *6*:51 (1976).
25. Arvin, A. M., Yeager, A. S. and Merigan, T. C. Effect of leukocyte interferon on urinary excretion of cytomegalovirus by infants. J. Infect. Dis. *133*:205 (1976).

26. Hirsch, M. S. Interferon—its hour come at last? New Engl. J. Med. *298*:1022 (1978).

27. Wadell, J. Hazards of human leukocyte interferon therapy. New Engl. J. Med. *296*:1295 (1977).

28. Rytel, M. W. and Kauffman, H. M. Clinical efficacy of adenine arabinoside in therapy of cytomegalovirus infections in renal allograft recipients. J. Infect. Dis. *133*:202 (1976).

29. Ch'ien, L. T., Cannon, N. J., Whitley, R. J., *et al.* Effect of adenine arabinoside on cytomegalovirus infections. J. Infect. Dis. *130*:32 (1974).

30. Rola-Plesczynski, M., Frenkel, L. D., Fucillo, D. A., *et al.* Specific impairment of cell-mediated immunity in mothers of infants with congenital infection due to cytomegalovirus. J. Infect. Dis. *135*:386 (1977).

31. Starr, S. E. and Allison, A. C. Role of T lymphocytes in recovery from Murine cytomegalovirus infection. Infect. Immun. *17*:458 (1977).

32. Rytel, M. W., Aaberg, T. M., Dee, T. H., *et al.* Therapy of cytomegalovirus retinitis with transfer factor. Cell. Immunol. *19*:8 (1975).

44 Acute Cerebellar Infarction—A Potential Surgical Emergency

Henry H. Schmidek, M. D.
Murali Guthikonda, M. D.

Acute cerebellar infarction is an infrequently diagnosed clinical syndrome which only sporadically has been recognized as having important surgical implications. The realization that an infarcted and swollen cerebellum can produce life threatening brainstem compression was first reported in 1956.[2] To date 16 cases reportedly have been treated by surgical decompression because of progressive neurologic deterioration. We are reporting the present case because this entity deserves earlier recognition and treatment than has been the experience to date.

CASE REPORT

A 51-year-old right-handed white male experienced the sudden onset of severe bifrontal headache, severe dizziness, and difficulty with vision. He was brought to the emergency room, where he was nauseous and vomiting. Admission blood pressure was 164/102. The pulse was 60 and the respirations were 16 per minute. The patient was somnolent and disoriented but easily arousable. There was a horizontal nystagmus, especially on the right lateral gaze. The clinical impression was of acute cerebellar hemorrhage or acute cerebellar infarction. A CT scan performed immediately after admission showed no evidence of ventricular dilation, hemorrhage, infarction, or tumor. Over the next 36 hours, the patient became progressively less responsive and lapsed into coma. Angiography performed on the second day after admission showed an old occlusion of the right internal carotid artery at the bifurcation of the internal and external carotid arteries.

The right posterior inferior cerebellar artery was occluded distally at the junction of the retromedullary and pretonsillar segments (Fig. 1). There was a mass effect on the right side of the posterior fossa. The venous phase of the carotid angiogram revealed a prominent degree of hydrocephalus. The patient immediately was taken to the operating room, and a posterior fossa craniotomy and Cl laminectomy were performed. The initial ventricular tap revealed clear cerebro-spinal fluid under greatly increased pressure. The right cerebellar hemisphere was extremely swollen and bone-white in color. On incision the pia, the cerebellum, and the right tonsil were found to have liquified, and were removed by aspiration. Following resection of the inferomedial right cerebellar hemisphere, the posterior inferior cerebellar artery was examined and found thrombosed. Postoperatively, the patient regained consciousness within 24 hours of surgery. At that time he had a persistent horizontal nystagmus and dysmetria of the right upper extremity. His postoperative course required a ventriculoatrial shunt because of a large pseudomeningocele that developed at the operative site. An isotope cisternogram showed evidence of ventricular reflux and a markedly delayed cerebro-spinal fluid circulation. Following the shunt, the patient continued to improve and was discharged home without evidence of cerebellar or brainstem dysfunction.

DISCUSSION

This case is typical in most of its characteristics of a definable syndrome, that of

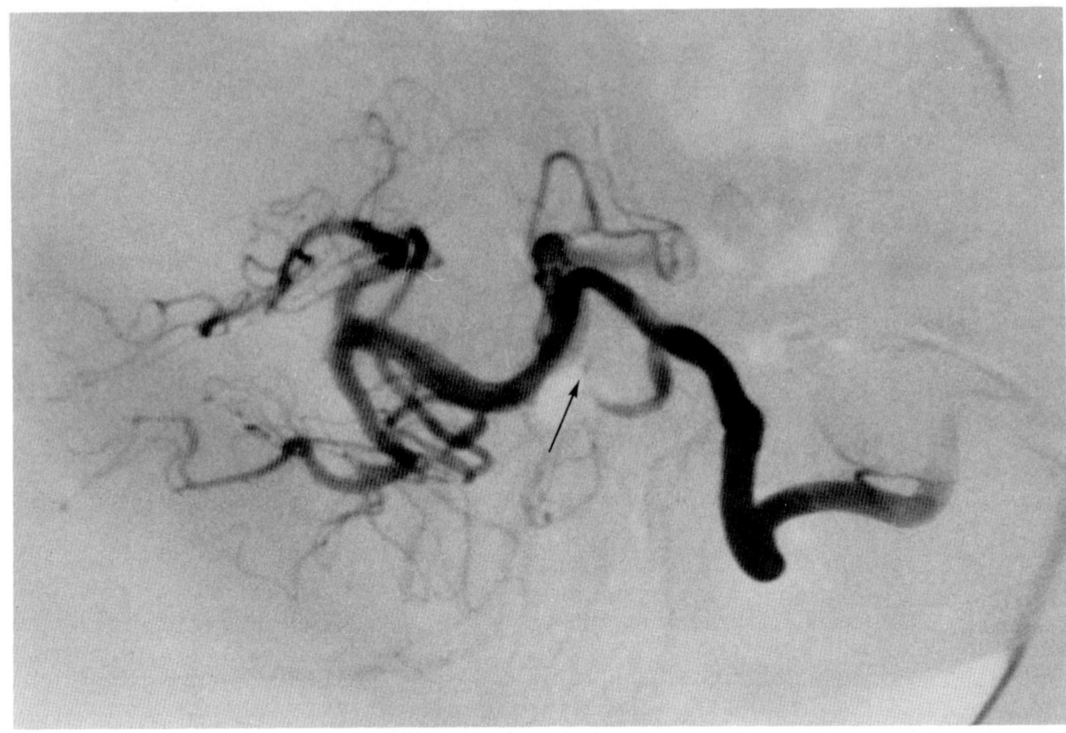

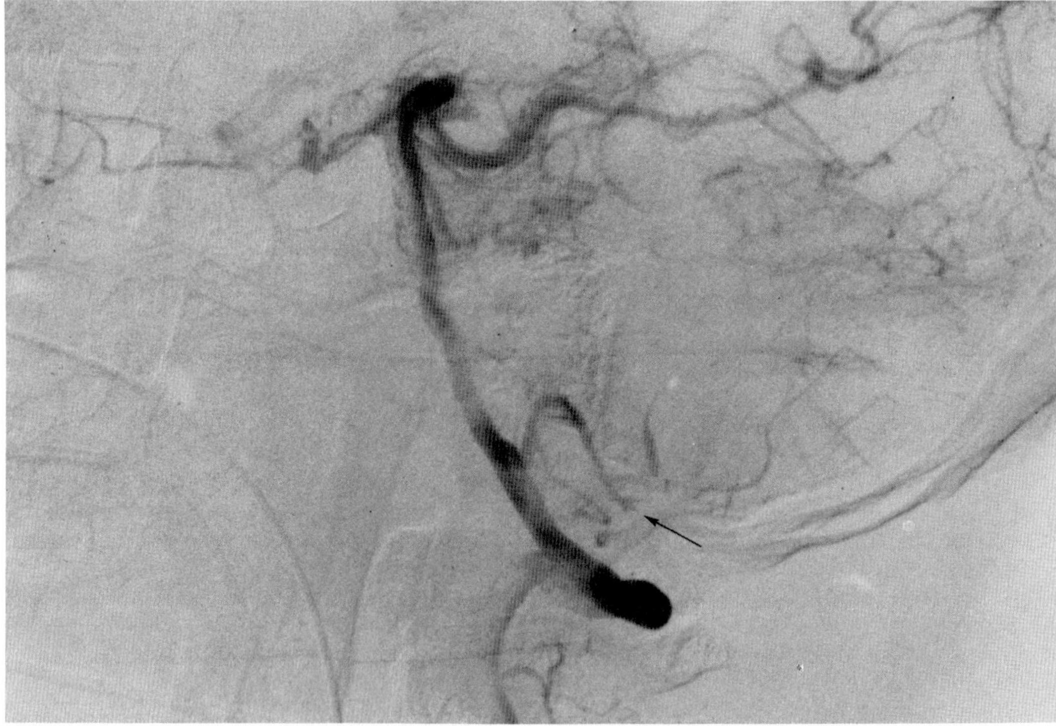

Figs. 1A and 1B. Angiographic demonstration of occlusion of the posterior inferior cerebellar artery in case of acute cerebellar infarction.

acute cerebellar infarction with brainstem compression (Table I). The vast majority of cases reported to date have occurred in males ages 40–60, presenting with the abrupt onset of headache, nausea, vomiting, dizziness, horizontal nystagmus, and inability to stand. The patients do not usually have a history of hypertension antedating the stroke. When hypertension is present, this finding suggests direct brainstem compression of the floor of the fourth ventricle with resultant neurogenic hypertension. Within 24–96 hours of the ictus, the neurologic deficit either plateaus at this level or there is steady neurologic deterioration associated with progressive obtundation (Table II). If this neurologic progression occurs, examination at this stage usually will reveal an obtunded patient, with horizontal nystagmus often in association with either paralysis of gaze to the side of infarct, deviation of the eyes to the opposite side, or skew deviation of the eyes. Papilledema may now be present, and the plantar reflexes are extensor. Cerebellar ataxia and dysarthria also may be present, in the absence of motor paralysis or sensory deficit. Although the rare case exists of a patient who has recovered from comatose state without surgery but treated with steroids, the expected event is that of steady deterioration until the death of the patient unless posterior fossa decompression is performed.

The CT scan appearance of cerebellar infarction is of a hypodense area of about 20 Houndsfield units involving a significant portion of the cerebellar hemisphere (Fig. 2). The inability to identify this abnormality of this patient's first CT scan is not unusual, with the infarct not becoming apparent for 36–48 hours after the stroke. In these cases, posterior fossa angiography may help in establishing the diagnosis if time and progression of illness does not allow the CT scan to be repeated. The second CT scan will often show the low-density lesion, with a mass effect in the posterior fossa, and a degree of associated hydrocephalus. There is little experience with the diagnosis of the condition angiographically, and the studies of this case showing occlusion of the distal posterior inferior cerebellar artery is unusual, al-

TABLE I. *Clinical characteristics—isolated cerebellar infarction (Fisher)*

   A. Initial phase
       Nystagmus
       Rotatory dizziness
       Nausea, vomiting
       Inability to stand
   B. Later phase
      I. Cerebellar
          Dysmetria
          Intention tremor
          Rebound phenomenon
     II. Brain stem signs
          Obtundation
          Contralateral eye deviation
          Small pupils
          Ataxic respirations

TABLE II. *Clinical course of cerebellar infarction*

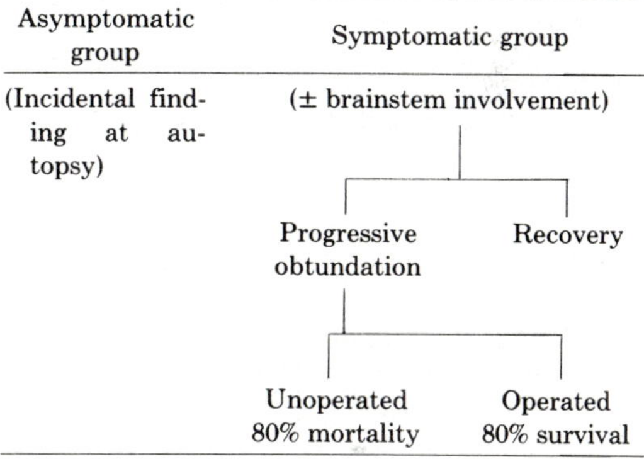

though from pathological studies one may expect to find occlusion of either the posterior inferior cerebellar, vertebral, superior cerebellar, or posterior cerebral arteries.[7] Ventriculography was used in making the diagnosis of posterior fossa mass in the pre-CT-scan era and would not need to be resorted to at present. In this case, as in most other cases that have been reported, there was no evidence of associated lateral medullary infarction manifested by lower cranial nerve pareses, long tract signs, or a Horner's syndrome. Since the prognosis for survival after isolated lateral medullary infarction is good, associated cerebellar infarction and swelling with brainstem compression may explain some of the deaths in this condition within 48–96 hours of the ictus.

Pathological studies[7] have shown that acute cerebellar infarction results most

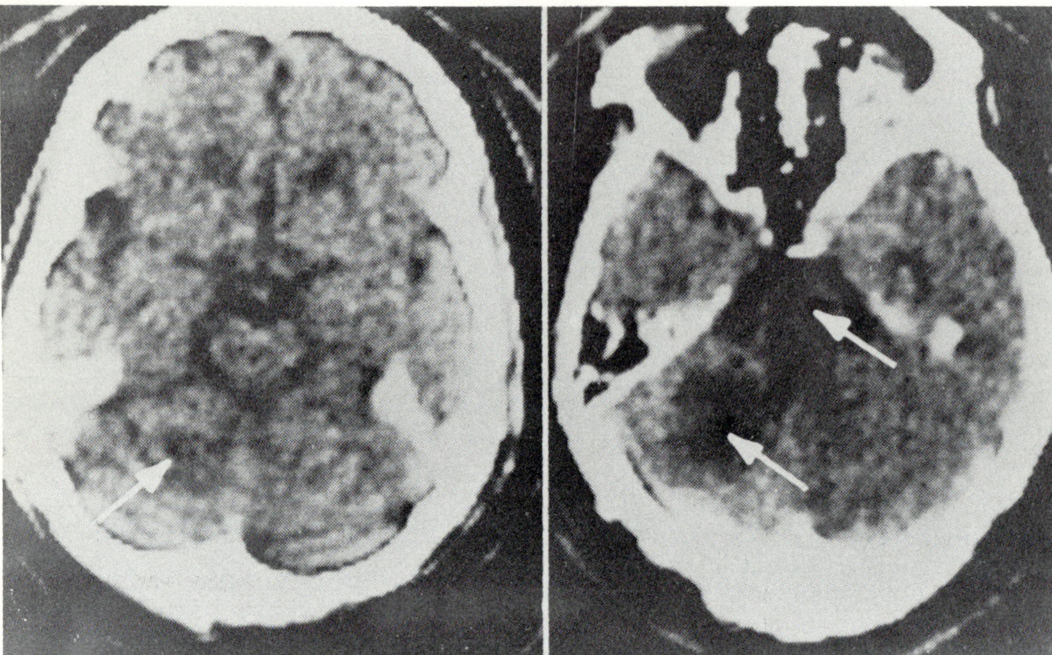

Fig. 2. Appearance on CT scan of acute cerebellar infarction.

commonly from thrombotic vascular occlusion of the posterior inferior cerebellar artery, and this occlusion may produce cerebellar infarction without brainstem involvement. To be symptomatic, the infarction usually involves more than one-third the mass of the cerebellar hemisphere, and the swelling evolves over two to five days, and probably explains the onset of the delayed clinical deterioration. In a review of 5,494 autopsies,[7] acute cerebellar infarction was found to have an incidence approximating that of acute cerebellar hemorrhage. In 28 cases of pure acute cerebellar infarction from this series, 10 patients were awake and alert on admission and eventually lapsed into coma and died. A single case was operated upon after the patient already was comatose and this patient died following surgery. In no case was the correct diagnosis made premortem. Only five of these 28 cases had associated brainstem infarction. In this same series there were 24 previously uncategorized cases of "old cerebellar infarction" found among the autopsy material (Table III). In reviewing the clinical data, 13 of these cases had a substantial, unexplained dementia with hydrocephalus

TABLE III. *Cerebellar infarction. Autopsy series (Alvord, 1975)*

Total cases autopsied	5,494
Cerebellar hemorrhage	39
Cerebellar infarction	82
Pure massive cerebellar infarction	28
Large old cystic infarctions	24
Combined cerebellar and brainstem infarcts	30

whose substrate may well have been an unrecognized cerebellar infarction with a degree of obstructive hydrocephalus, and nine cases had important clinical findings attributable to the acute cerebellar infarction. The mortality rate in this group of cases attributable to acute cerebellar infarction was greater than 50%, and, once the patient exhibited progressive deficits, the mortality exceeded 80%. Acute cerebellar infarction is an identifiable clinical entity, almost identical in its features with those of acute cerebellar hemorrhage, and like acute cerebellar hemorrhage often requires surgical decompression as a life saving measure (Table IV). The reported surgical experience to date with acute cerebellar infarction has been of 17 cases, including the one presented in this report (Table V).

TABLE IV. *Cerebellar strokes*

	Cerebellar hemorrhage	Cerebellar infarction
Age	Elderly	Elderly
Associated Medical problems	HBP, ASCVD	HBP, ASCVD
Acuteness	Acute	Acute
Symptoms	Headache, nausea, vomiting, dizziness	Headache, nausea, vomiting, dizziness
Progression of clinical picture	Minutes to hours	Hours to days
LP	Bloody	Clear
CT	Blood (high-density lesion)	Normal or low-density lesion

TABLE V. *Cerebellar infarction. Clinical case reports—Surgical experience*

Year	Authors	No. of cases
1956	Fairburn et al.[2]	2
1956	Lindgren[4]	2
1959	Pomme[5]	2
1960	Wood and Murphy[8]	5
1970	Lehrich et al.[3]	3
1975	Duncan et al.[1]	1
1977	Savitz et al.[6]	1
1978	Schmidek	1
	Total	17

The diagnosis prior to operation in all but two of these cases has been of a posterior fossa tumor. The realization that cerebellar infarction can produce a surgical emergency was first reported in 1956 by Fairburn.[2] Two of these cases were operated on with recovery. The third case in this report died suddenly before surgery. The other cases reported between 1956 and 1975 all exhibited the typical features of the syndrome as discussed, an exception being the 1977 report by Savitz[6] of a case in which the cerebellar infarction was associated with brainstem findings. This patient was operated on after lapsing into coma. This patient recovered but with persistent brainstem signs (Table VI).

The differential diagnosis of this condition includes acute labyrinthitis, with dizziness often being the most troublesome complaint early in the illness evolution; acute cerebellar hemorrhage is identical to acute cerebellar infarction in its anatomic involvement and in most of its clinical features. Two important distinctions, however, are that the patient with an acute cerebellar infarction is often not known to be hypertensive prior to the illness and that the neurologic deterioration in acute cerebellar hemorrhage classically is more rapid, occurring over a period of hours rather than days as is the case in acute cerebellar infarction. The CT scan should allow these conditions to be distinguished immediately, although occasionally a hemorrhagic infarction may occur in the cerebellum and confuses the issue. Posterior fossa subdural or epidural hematoma may occur without a demonstrable occipital fracture and present a diagnostic problem, particularly if it is not possible to get a history of trauma.

CONCLUSION

Acute cerebellar infarction is a distinct and recognizable clinical entity with an incidence comparable to that of acute cerebellar hemorrhage. To date, however, only 16 surgically treated cases have been reported, and in only two of these cases was the diagnosis made preoperatively. Untreated, the condition is almost invariably fatal. If the patient is comatose at the time of surgery, the operative mortality exceeds 50%, whereas none of the patients operated on before they lapsed into coma died. This entity deserves earlier recognition and treatment than has been the experience to date, and to accomplish this requires a high index of suspicion of the condition. The initial CT scan may not be helpful in establishing the diagnosis, and repeat CT scan and angiography may be necessary; however, if the tempo of deterioration is rapid, immediate surgical intervention should be undertaken based on the history and physical examination alone.

EDITOR'S NOTE

The "pearl" to me in this paper is that if

TABLE VI. *Cerebellar infarction—Surgical experience*

Authors	No. of cases	Symptoms	Mode of Dx	Days of OR	Recovery
Fairburn *et al.*[2]	2	F.V.	Ventriculography	26	+
		HA, V	Ventriculography	5	+
Lindgren[4]	2	HA, D, V	Ventriculography	4	−
		HA, D, V	Ventriculography	5	+
Pommes[5]	2	HA	Ventriculography		+
		HA, V, A			−
Wood and Murphy[8]	5	HA, N, V, D	Ventriculography	3	+
		HA, D	Ventriculography	3	+
			Ventriculography	2	−
			Ventriculography	3	−
		HA, D, N	Ventriculography	3	+
Lehrich *et al.*[3]	3	HA, D		4	+
		HA, D, V	Angio + Ventriculography	2	+
		Blurred vision	Angio + PEG + ventriculography	10	−
Duncan[1]	1	D, N, V, HA		2	+
Savitz[6]	1	HA, D, A	Angio	1	+

HA: Headache; D: Dizziness; A: Ataxia; N, V: Nausea, Vomiting

you suspect a patient of having either an acute cerebellar hemorrhage or an acute cerebellar infarction, the first thing to get is a good computed tomographic scan. Now, it is apparent that if there is a hematoma present, it would or should be seen on the first study. However, Dr. Schmidek points out in this chapter that the first study may not show the lesion in an acute cerebellar infarction—so that the computed tomographic scan may need to be repeated 24 or 48 hours later, depending upon the patient's clinical course—to establish the diagnosis of an acute cerebellar infarction. That single point and his surgical experience warrants further consideration by clinicians. In his letter with this chapter, Dr. Schmidek states that he has seen four cases of acute cerebellar infarction in the last month before sending the manuscript. That reminds me of a story that many years ago a famous British neurologist was visiting Johns Hopkins Hospital and Dr. David Clark showed him a patient with Kinnier Wilson's sign of an ectopic pupil with a pinealoma. When Dr. Clark asked the distinguished physician if he had ever seen this before—he replied: "Yes, David, I have *seen* this several times before, but this is the first time that I have *observed* it." This is so true in medicine. Prophet Isaiah tells us in chapter 6, verse 9—"And he said, Go, and tell this people, Hear ye indeed, but understand not; and *see* ye indeed, but *perceive* not." And again

in chapter 42, verse 20—"*Seeing* many things, but thous *observest* not; opening the ears, but he heareth not." We often *see* things in medicine for a long time before we *perceive* them or before we *observe* them. It is hoped that this study by Dr. Schmidek will allow us to have more perception in the management of patients with acute posterior fossa emergent syndromes!

JLS

REFERENCES

1. Duncan, G., Parker, S., Fisher, C. M. L. Acute Cerebellar infarction in the PICA territory. Arch. Neurol. *32:*364–368 (1975).
2. Fairburn, B. and Oliver, L. Cerebellar softening—a surgical emergency. Br. Med. J. *1:*1335–1336 (1956).
3. Lehrich, J. R., Winkler, G., and Ojemann, R. G. Cerebellar infarction with brain stem compression—diagnosis and surgical treatment. Arch. Neurol. *32:*490–498 (1970).
4. Lindgren, S. Infarctions simulating brain tumors in the posterior fossa. J. Neurosurg. *13:*575–581 (1956).
5. Norris, J., Eisen, A. A., and Branch, C. L. Problems in cerebellar hemorrhage and infarction. Neurol. *19:*1043–1050 (1969).
6. Savitz, M., Katz, S., and Nakasawa, H. Acute cerebellar infarction producing brain stem compression. Mt. Sinai J. Med. N.Y. *44*(2):299–303 (1977).
7. Sypert, G. and Alvord, E. Cerebellar infarction—a clinicopathological study. Arch. Neurol. *32:*357–363 (1975).
8. Wood, M., and Murphy, F. Obstructive Hydrocephalus due to infarction of a cerebellar hemisphere. J. Neurosurg. *30:*260–263 (1969).

45 Downbeat Nystagmus—A Clinical Update

Harold E. Shaw, Jr., M.D.
J. Lawton Smith, M.D.

INTRODUCTION

Since Cogan's classic paper in 1968, little has been written about downbeat nystagmus, a vertical jerk nystagmus with the fast phase downward, which has been associated with lesions at the craniocervical junction.[1] In this chapter we discuss the clinical features of downbeat nystagmus and suggest guidelines for the management of patients with this disorder.

SUBJECTS AND METHODS

Thirty-nine cases of downbeat nystagmus collected from the files of one of us (J. L. S.) and seen during the period 1966–1978 at the Bascom Palmer Eye Institute were reviewed. Patient selection was based upon the presence of vertical nystagmus with the fast component downward. All of the patients were personally examined by one or both of us. Follow-up information was available in 37 of the 39 cases and ranged from one month to 11 years with an average of 17.4 months.

RESULTS

Patient Characteristics

Twenty-four females and 15 males comprise this series. Thirty-seven were white and two were black. Their ages ranged from 11 to 75 years, and the average was 48 years.

Characteristics of Downbeat Nystagmus

The nystagmus was symptomatic in 21 of the 39 patients; however, only 11 patients described oscillopsia. The others in whom the nystagmus was symptomatic complained of blurring of vision or difficulty reading. In 16 cases, the chief complaint was related to the nystagmus. In 25 cases, downbeat nystagmus was present either historically or by previous documentation elsewhere from four to 72 months, with an average of 22 months, prior to our initial examination.

Downbeat nystagmus was clinically evident in the primary position of gaze in only 17 patients. In two of those patients the nystagmus was detectable in the primary position alone. The nystagmus was greatest in downgaze in 30 cases and eccentrically in 28. In three cases the nystagmus was most prominent in upgaze, and in two cases was equal in upgaze and downgaze. The amplitude and frequency of the nystagmus were highly variable.

Associated Neuro-ophthalmologic Findings

The visual acuity in most patients was normal or nearly normal. Thirty-two had 20/40 acuity or better in the worse eye. Four had less than 20/40 in the better eye. The visual acuity was not specified in three cases. The visual fields were normal in 33 patients. One patient had a left homonymous hemianopia, and another had a central scotoma. In four cases the fields were not recorded.

Other ocular motor disturbances were commonly associated with downbeat nystagmus. Seven patients had upbeat nystagmus in up gaze, five had rotary nystagmus, four had horizontal nystagmus, one had periodic alternating nystagmus, and one had inverse latent macro square wave jerks.[2] Fourteen patients had ocular dysmetria. A skew deviation was present in 10 patients. Abnormal optokinetic responses, particularly to vertical targets, occurred in 22 patients.

Other Clinical Signs and Symptoms

A prominent finding in 22 of our 39 patients was ataxia. Some were grossly ataxic, whereas in others the ataxia was subtle. Romberg testing in 12 patients was positive in four, negative in four, and equivocal in four. Finger-to-nose testing in nine patients was abnormal in four, normal in three, and equivocal in two. Tandem walking was abnormal in all 12 patients tested with this maneuver. Frequently, the patients complained of dizziness, and some had true vertigo. Diplopia was common.

Diagnostic Evaluation

In addition to the clinical examination, 34 patients had skull x-rays, 17 had computerized axial tomograms, seven had arteriograms, eight had myelograms, and nine had pneumoencephalograms. Five patients had posterior fossa operations.

Causes of Downbeat Nystagmus

Spinocerebellar degeneration was diagnosed in 15 patients and was the most common disorder associated with downbeat nystagmus. Included in this group were seven familial cases from two families. Three patients had Arnold-Chiari malformations. Brain stem vascular lesions accounted for three cases, two of which were due to brain stem ischemia and one due to a vascular abnormality related to hereditary hemorrhagic telangiectasia. Three patients had syringobulbia. Two patients had posterior fossa neoplasms—one was a pontine tumor and the other a posterior fossa tumor of unspecified type removed surgically many years before we first saw her. Two patients had basilar meningitis, and one had severe demyelinating disease. In 10 cases the cause for the downbeat nystagmus was undetermined, but in none of the 10 could a structural lesion be identified. Table I depicts the causes of downbeat nystagmus according to age groups.

DISCUSSION

Downbeat nystagmus is a vertical jerk nystagmus with a fast phase beating downward, which is considered indicative of an abnormality at the craniocervical junction. The Arnold-Chiari malformation or basilar impression are the specific lesions which have been most often associated with downbeat nystagmus, but miscellaneous other causes have also been reported.[1, 3-9] It is now obvious that the differential diagnosis in a patient with downbeat nystagmus encompasses many possibilities. The most common cause of downbeat nystagmus in our series was spinocerebellar degeneration. Approximately half of our cases of downbeat nystagmus due to spinocerebellar degeneration were familial. These patients had a wide spectrum of neurologic signs and symptoms, and in some the downbeat nystagmus was the predominant or only detectable abnormality. Arnold-Chiari malformations, neoplasms, vascular lesions, meningitis, syringobulbia, and demyelinating disease were also causes of downbeat nystagmus in our series. It is important that in a significant number of cases a specific cause for the downbeat nystagmus could not be found despite extensive investigation and careful follow-up.

TABLE I. *Etiology of downbeat nystagmus*

Age group	No.	Spinocerebellar degeneration[a]	Arnold-Chiari	Neoplasm	Vascular	Infection	Syrinx	Demyelinating	?
Under 30	8	2	1	—	—	1	1	1	2
30–60	17	4	2	2	2	1	2	—	4
Over 60	14	9	—	—	1	—	—	—	4
Total	39	15	3	2	3	2	3	1	10

[a] Includes seven familial cases from two families.

Surgically amenable lesions must always be considered as a cause of downbeat nystagmus. However, our experience indicates that, in most cases, downbeat nystagmus results from nonsurgical intrinsic brain stem disease at the level of the craniocervical junction. The clinical course is typically one of insidious onset and slow or minimal progression. A number of patients in our series have been followed for years with little evidence of neurologic deterioration. Others have made similar observations in patients with downbeat nystagmus.[1, 10]

We believe that all patients with downbeat nystagmus should have a thorough ophthalmologic and neurologic evaluation, including careful examination of family members. The following case history illustrates the importance of this point.

A 39-year-old woman had oscillopsia and episodic diplopia of six years duration. She reported that her mother, age 79, had a ten-year history of progressive intellectual deterioration and difficulty walking. A sister, age 59, had a gait disturbance also. A maternal aunt became demented in her later years and died in a mental institution. Neuro-ophthalmologic examination revealed that the patient had downbeat nystagmus, skew deviation, and mild difficulty with tandem walking. Her 18-year-old daughter was present during the examination, and she too was found to have subtle downbeat nystagmus. She had no other neurologic abnormalities and was clinically asymptomatic. Subsequent examination of the patient's mother and sister revealed both had downbeat nystagmus. The diagnosis of hereditary spinocerebellar degeneration was established.

A true lateral skull x-ray should be obtained in all patients with downbeat nystagmus, asking the radiologists to look specifically for abnormalities at the craniocervical junction. Further workup is dictated by the clinical situation. In many cases, periodic follow-up may be all that is indicated. In some cases, more intensive neuroradiologic investigation may be necessary. In our experience, CT scanning is inade-

quate for evaluating the craniocervical junction. Posterior fossa angiography may occasionally be helpful. High cervical myelograms can provide useful information in some cases. However, the most definitive neuroradiological procedure for assessing the structures at the craniocervical junction is posterior fossa pneumoencephalography with frontal and lateral tomograms.[11, 12] Although rarely necessary, this procedure should be considered in those patients with progressive neurologic signs and symptoms referable to the craniocervical junction which cannot otherwise be explained.

SUMMARY

We reviewed 39 cases of downbeat nystagmus and found a variety of causes for this condition. The most common cause of downbeat nystagmus in our series was spinocerebellar degeneration, which often was familial. Downbeat nystagmus is frequently associated with ataxia and generally reflects nonsurgical brain stem disease at the level of the craniocervical junction. Many patients with downbeat nystagmus have a relatively benign clinical course. In those with progressive neurologic symptomatology, true lateral skull x-rays, and, if necessary, posterior fossa pneumoencephalography with frontal and lateral tomography should be performed to rule out surgically amenable lesions.

EDITOR'S NOTE

For years, all we taught about vertical nystagmus was three things: (1) the commonest cause of vertical nystagmus is drugs; (2) with the exception of drugs, vertical nystagmus always posterior fossa dysfunction; and (3) vertical nystagmus with the rapid phase down (i.e. downbeat nystagmus) points to a low level brain stem lesion at about the cervicomedullary junction. We then went into an era of appreciating the fact that downbeat nystagmus was pointing to Arnold Chiari malformation, basilar impression, high cervical cord meningiomas, and other *surgical* lesions at foramen magnum level and we would even at times advise suboccipital craniectomy explorations on such cases, if the neuroradiologic studies were equivocal. The point of this paper, however, is to emphasize that the commonest cause of downbeat nystagmus now seen in our office practice of neuro-ophthalmology is *familial.* The first thing one should do when encountering a case of downbeat nystagmus is to check the relatives by having them look down and right and down and left (in extremes of gaze) and looking very carefully. Many of them also have subclinical downbeat nystagmus, and usually they do *NOT* know they have it. Since it is usually *NOT* present in primary position, or even in straight down gaze, you will have to look for it yourself to make sure whether it is there or not. If they have trouble walking tandem, you probably have a familial spinocerebellar degeneration presenting as downbeat nystagmus. If the family studies are negative, you should get a true lateral plain skull film, and you may then have to proceed to either a pneumoencephalogram with PA and lateral tomography or a metrizamide computed tomographic study or both. The air study is the definitive study for these cases, however, and it must be done by a good neuroradiologist using tomography to be adequate. However, although some of these cases are due to surgical lesions and one certainly does not want to miss them, the differential diagnosis is very, very large and the majority of cases (about ⅔'s) are due to medical (non-surgical) causes. They do better with two pair of glasses, avoiding

bifocals, and having a separate pair of reading glasses. Dr. Costin wonders if this can be seen with alcoholic cerebellar ataxia and this warrants further study.

JLS

REFERENCES

1. Cogan, D. G. Down-beat nystagmus. Arch. Ophthalmol. *80:*757 (1968).
2. Doft, B. H., Smith, J. L., and Ugarte, T. R. Inverse latent macro square wave jerks and downbeat nystagmus. In: *Neuro-ophthalmology Update.* J. L. Smith (Ed.), Masson, New York, 1977, pp. 339–343.
3. Cogan, D. G. and Barrows, L. J. Platybasia and the Arnold-Chiari malformation. Arch. Ophthalmol. *52:*13 (1954).
4. Mahaley, M. S. Ocular motility with foramen magnum syndromes. In: *Neuro-ophthalmology.* J. L. Smith (Ed.), C. V. Mosby, St. Louis, 1968, Vol. 4, pp. 110–116.
5. Hart, J. D. and Sanders, M. D. Down beat nystagmus. Trans. Ophthalmol. Soc. U. K. *90:*483 (1970).
6. Zee, D. S., Friendlich, A. R., and Robinson, D. A. The mechanism of downbeat nystagmus. Arch. Neurol. *30:*227 (1974).
7. Keane, J. R. Periodic alternating nystagmus with downward beating nystagmus. Arch. Neurol. *30:* 399 (1974).
8. Zee, D. S., Yee, R. D., Cogan, D. G., Robinson, D. A., and Engel, W. K. Ocular motor abnormalities in hereditary cerebellar ataxia. Brain *99:*207 (1976).
9. Daroff, R. B., Troost, B. T., and Dell'Osso, L. F. Nystagmus and related ocular oscillations, In: *Neuro-ophthalmology.* J. S. Glaser (Ed.), Harper and Row, Hagerstown, 1978, p. 232.
10. Daroff, R. B. Personal communication.
11. Newton, T. H. Personal communication.
12. Gargano, F. P. Personal communication.

46 Hypertension

Barry J. Materson, M. D.

Ophthalmologists encounter hypertension in four ways. First, owing to the *prevalence* of hypertension in the population, there is about a 20% chance of any given patient having hypertension. Second, patients with a chief complaint of *headache* may be hypertensive. Treatment of the hypertension will not relieve a headache due to some other cause but, if the headache is specifically due to hypertension, control of the blood pressure may cure the headache. Third, some patients complain of *visual disturbances* which turn out to be due to hypertensive retinopathy. Treatment of the hypertension will usually reverse these symptoms. Finally, hypertension and its treatment may pose problems for ophthalmologic *surgery*.

Essential hypertension has no principal defined cause and is completely asymptomatic. It can be detected only by routine sphygmomanometry. It is known that about half of all hypertensive patients were never aware that they had elevated blood pressure. The intensive educational campaign of both the public and physicians since 1972 has greatly reduced such ignorance, but the majority of hypertensive individuals in the United States still do not have their pressure under control. All health care professionals should measure the blood pressure of every patient on every visit or delegate this to a nurse or even properly trained office clerical personnel. It is easy to buy or make up a stethoscope with one head and two sets of ear pieces so that the teacher and trainee can hear the Korotkoff sounds simultaneously.

Untreated hypertension has an unacceptable morbidity and mortality in the form of strokes, cardiovascular, and end-stage kidney disease. The cost in human misery as well as dollars is staggering. Adequate treatment can prevent much of this morbidity and mortality. Hypertension is the *only* major cardiovascular disease for which treatment has been proven not only to be effective, but also cost effective. This is in contrast to diabetes mellitus for which insulin has resulted in considerable prolongation of life but has not prevented the numerous complications including blindness.

One of the major problems in treating hypertension is that side effects of medications may convert a totally asymptomatic patient into an unhappy one. The skillful physician will accomplish successful lowering of the blood pressure with minimal interference with the patient's normal life.

TECHNIQUES

Diagnosis of hypertension may cause patients to develop a morbid preoccupation with their blood pressure, lose excessive time from work without justification, be denied life insurance, or even lose a job. It is, therefore, crucial that the label of "hypertension" not be erroneously applied.

Three or more readings should be taken at least one week apart in order to establish the diagnosis. Keep in mind that pain of any kind, including headache, can elevate the blood pressure. Patients should be relaxed and comfortable in a room neither too warm or too cold. They should avoid eating, drinking, and smoking at least 30 min prior to the measurement. Bowel, bladder, and stomach should be empty. Neither the patient nor the examiner should engage in conversation during the measurement since this elevates blood pressure. Except for severely elevated pressures, no single determination should make the diagnosis of hypertension.

Place the blood pressure cuff snugly on the bare arm with the lower edge one inch above the antecubital fossa. Use a special large or thigh cuff for very large muscular or obese arms. Holding the arm at heart level, inflate the cuff 30 mm Hg above the point where the radial pulse disappears and allow it to deflate at about 2–3 mm Hg per second. Listen with the stethoscope bell over the brachial artery for the first Korotkoff sound (systolic), muffling of the sounds (phase IV diastolic), and disappearance (phase V diastolic). If phase IV and V differ by more than 5 mm Hg, record both. Take the pressure in both arms on the first occasion to ascertain that it is similar. If not, use the higher pressure and make a note always to use that arm. Take the readings with the patient supine and after standing 2 min. If the patient is normotensive and not on any medication, the seated position is more convenient for subsequent visits.

SEQUELAE OF HYPERTENSION

Hypertension is clearly a disease of quantity: the higher the pressure, the worse the consequences. We consider a diastolic pressure of 115 mm Hg or greater to represent *severe* hypertension. Identification demands immediate treatment. *Moderate* hypertension spans diastolic pressure of 105–114 mm Hg and also demands treatment although the urgency is not nearly so great. *Mild* hypertension is defined by diastolic pressures between 90 and 104 mm Hg. Hypertension is mild in perhaps 70% of cases. Here the risks of no treatment have been clearly defined, but the benefits of drug therapy are much less certain. This lack of certainty prompted the series of guidelines displayed in Table II. Dr. Edward D. Freis has proposed a simple point system (Table III) to assist in decision making. In any case, treatment vs. nontreatment in the mild range is an individual decision. These patients will most likely benefit from the "hygienic" treatments discussed below. In any case, it is clear that any kind of hypertension, regardless of cause, age, race, sex, labile, or fixed is a risk. The best operational

Table I. *Classification of hypertension*

Type	Definition	Five-year survival untreated (%)	Benefit of treatment demonstrated
Malignant	Severe hypertension with papilledema (K-W-B IV)	0–1	Yes
Accelerated	Severe hypertension with retinal hemorrhages and/or exudates (K-W-B III)	20	Yes
Severe	Diastolic pressure over 114 mm Hg	40	Yes
Moderate	Diastolic pressure between 105 and 114 mm Hg	55	Yes
Mild	Diastolic pressure between 90 and 104 mm Hg	79	Controversial

Table II. *Treatment guidelines for hypertension*

Must treat:
- Malignant hypertension
- Accelerated hypertension
- Hypertensive crisis
- Patients with definite target organ damage

Should treat:
- Men and women of any age with diastolic pressure over 104 mm Hg

Probably should treat:
- Women with BP over 160/95
- Men over 45 with BP over 140/95
- Men under 45 with BP over 130/90
- Black men and women with BP over 140/90
- Patients with positive family history of hypertension and BP over 140/90

Table III. *Risk score for treatment of patients with diastolic pressures 90–104 mm Hg*

Risk	Score
Male	1
Black	1
Less than 45 years old	1
Diastolic always above 95 mm Hg	1
Systolic always above 165 mm Hg	1
Family history of complicated hypertension	1
Hyperlipidemia	1
Diabetes mellitus	1
Target organ damage	2

If diastolic pressure is	Treat if total risk factor score is
90–94 mm Hg	4 or more
95–99 mm Hg	3 or more
100–104 mm Hg	2 or more

definition of hypertension is that level of arterial pressure elevation above which diagnosis and treatment do more good than harm.

Hypertension is a life-long disease which does not become "cured" at any single point and blood pressure control does not signal permission to stop treatment or cease observation. One physician who can provide long-term care should be responsible for the patient. Ordinarily, the ophthalmologist cannot render primary care. Most patients should be referred onward to a physician willing and able to provide long-term treatment. When severe or malignant hypertension demands immediate hospitalization and/or more than routine baseline diagnostic studies, refer to a physician or group that is capable of assuming full responsibility for directing workup and treatment. However, the ophthalmologist should not be a flaccid appendage to the health care team and should be prepared to assume some of the treatment responsibilities when the patient is under his aegis and, importantly, to be aware of the implications of various drug regimens upon his management of the patient.

WORKUP

Ninety-four per cent of all adult patients with hypertension have no defineable secondary cause; i.e., they have *essential hypertension*. Another 5% have some type of *chronic renal disease*. The remaining 1% is the sum of all other causes including primary aldosterone secreting tumors, pheochromocytoma, coarctation of the aorta, Cushing's syndrome, and others. One important cause of hypertension is *oral contraceptive* and postmenopausal *estrogens*. Only a small number of women taking these hormones develop significant hypertension, but it may be severe and it is usually totally reversible. All hypertensive women should be queried about hormonal use. If the drug is stopped, it may be many months before the blood pressure returns to normal and drug treatment may be necessary in the meantime. It is essential to provide an alternative means of contraception to these patients.

A good history seeking the onset of known hypertension (ask about military and employment physicals, insurance exams, blood pressure taken prior to donating blood), drug and alcohol use, family history, and history of renal disease may provide important diagnostic clues. Physical examination should reveal the classic habitus of Cushing's syndrome. Patients with pheochromocytoma are rarely obese, and they may have orthostatic hypotension. Nearly 60% of patients with renal vascular hypertension have abdominal bruits, but so do 7% of the normal population. Palpate the abdomen for large polycystic kidneys. If the use of beta blockers is anticipated, there should be no evidence of asthma or obstructive airway disease. Listen to the heart for an atrial diastolic gallop (S_4). Check the peripheral pulses for delay due to aortic coarctation.

The basic laboratory tests are listed in Table IV. An intravenous pyelogram should be done only in patients in whom renal vascular hypertension is strongly suspected. It is an exceedingly poor screening test with about 15% each of false positives and false negatives. Indications for a more extensive workup are in Table V.

HYGIENIC MEASURES

"Hygienic" instructions should be given to all patients to increase the effectiveness of drug treatment and occasionally eliminate the need for it in some patients with mild hypertension. These include the rational restriction of dietary salt, reduction of overweight, alcohol avoidance, proper exercise, and stress avoidance.

Reduction of dietary salt is important because salt restriction may lower the blood pressure sufficiently to avoid drug therapy, will increase the efficacy of diuretic drugs, and reduces the risk of hypokalemia. By salt restriction we mean consumption of a

TABLE IV. *Recommended basic hypertension laboratory workup*

- Complete blood count (CBC)
- Routine urinalysis
- Serum creatinine and/or urea nitrogen
- Serum potassium
- Serum glucose, uric acid, and cholesterol
- Baseline electrocardiogram

TABLE V. *Workup for selected secondary causes of hypertension*

Indication	Special test
1. Abnormal urinalysis or family history of polycystic kidneys or palpable kidneys or symptoms referable to geritourinary system	Intravenous pyelogram (IVP)
2. Bacteriuria or history suggesting infection	Quantitative midstream, clean-catch urine culture and sensitivity
3. Onset of hypertension before age 25 or diastolic pressures 110 mm Hg or more or sudden onset of hypertension or accelerated/malignant hypertension or true drug resistance *and* patient is a surgical candidate	Renal arteriogram. If positive for renal artery stenosis, confirm with bilateral renal vein renins
4. Unprovoked hypokalemia	24-hour urine potassium. If over 30 mEq/L, then plasma renin activity. If low, then 24-hour urine aldosterone. If high, treatment for primary aldosterone secreting tumor
5. Paroxysmal hypertension or family history of pheochromocytoma or evidence of multiple endocrine neoplasia	Urinary metanephrine or VMA

4–6 g salt (67–103 mEq sodium) diet. Basically, this means no cooking with salt, no use of salt at the table, no canned or processed foods, limiting dairy products, and avoiding condiments and snacks that are obviously salty. Potassium-containing salt substitutes may be of value.

Consumption of excessive alcohol is associated with an increased risk for hypertension independent of race or sex. Alcohol abuse may not only increase the blood pressure, but potentiate central nervous system depression caused by many antihypertensive drugs.

Weight reduction will reduce blood pressure but is difficult to achieve. Very obese patients will usually require initial drug therapy.

Good physical conditioning will lower the blood pressure. However, people who are poorly conditioned must take great caution in entering an exercise program.

DRUG THERAPY

The National Commission on Hypertension Education protocol is a stepwise addition of drugs to each other. Step 1 is the administration of a *diuretic*. If that fails to control the blood pressure, then Step 2 is the *addition* of a drug which acts primarily on the *adrenergic* nervous system. If the blood pressure is still not controlled, then Step 3 is the *addition* of a *vasodilator* drug to the other two.

Diuretics have been the cornerstone of antihypertensive therapy for the past two decades. They should be the first step in virtually all patients because they are convenient to take once a day, are relatively inexpensive, have very few side effects, and about 70% of hypertensive patients can be expected to respond to them alone.

Ophthalmologists often employ carbonic anhydrase inhibitor diuretics for the treatment of glaucoma. They are not useful as antihypertensives.

Table VI lists a few selected diuretics. The so-called loop diuretics have great natriuretic potency, but relatively short duration of action. They must be given at least twice daily. Loop diuretics should be limited to patients with renal failure or edema which does not respond to less potent drugs.

The "thiazide" group is most commonly used to treat hypertension. This group contains the benzothiadiazines of which hydrochlorothiazide (HydroDiuril[R], Esidrix[R], Oretic[R] and others) is the prototype. It is a medium duration of action drug and usually requires twice daily dosing, but is the least expensive. Chlorthalidone (Hygroton[R]) and metolazone (Zaroxolyn[R], Diulo[R]) have an action similar to the thiazides. Chlorthalidone has the longest duration of action (about 48 hr). Metolazone acts for about 24 hr and seems to be effective even in the face of decreased renal function.

There are two potassium sparing diuret-

TABLE VI. *Selected antihypertension diuretic drugs*

Drug	Dose (mg/day)	Advantages
Hydrochlorothiazide (Hydro-Diuril[R], Esidrix[R], Oretic[R], and others)	25–150 mg (usually BID)	Least expensive
Chlorthalidone (Hygroton[R])	25–100 mg (once daily)	Very long acting (48 hrs)
Metolazone (Zaroxolyn[R], Diulo[R])	2.5–20 mg (once daily)	Long acting (24 hrs) Effective even with decreased renal function
Ticrynafen (Selacryn[R])	250–1000 mg (usually BID)	Uricosuric
Furosemide (Lasix[R])	20 mg and up (at least BID)	Potent "loop blocker." Use for severe edema, renal failure
Spironolactone (Aldactone[R])	100–200 mg (usually BID or QID)	Potassium-sparing
Triamterene (Dyrenium[R])	100–300 mg (usually BID or TID)	Potassium-sparing non-steroidal. Not antihypertensive

ics currently available in the United States. Spironolactone (Aldactone[R]) is a steroid inhibitor of aldosterone which has a three to five day onset of action and an equal duration of offset. Be careful when giving potassium to patients who have recently been on this drug to avoid hyperkalemia. Triamterene (Dyrenium[R]) is independent of aldosterone, and, while it is not a good antihypertensive agent alone, it is useful combined with a thiazide to protect against hypokalemia. These drugs should be avoided or used with great caution in the elderly and in patients with diabetes or decreased renal function.

Start with the lowest effective dose of diuretic and increase about once a month as necessary. Use the once daily longer acting ones to enlist the greatest degree of cooperation from your patients. The full therapeutic effect may take six to 12 weeks. If the pressures at the end of one month at the higher dose levels are close to goal and there are no side effects, it may be worth waiting another month or two to see if that one drug alone will do the job. The most predominant of the side and adverse effects are hypokalemia and hyperuricemia. In general, we are not too concerned about serum potassium levels down to 3.0 mEq/l in asymptomatic patients not taking digitalis. Patients on digitalis must have their potassium replenished. Do not give potassium routinely, especially to older patients, those with diabetes or patients with renal failure. They may become seriously hyperkalemic. Treat only those patients who require treatment If a patient presents for

surgery and has hypokalemia, the potassium may be replaced in the intravenous solutions prior to and during surgery. Hyperuricemia is rarely a problem in that it generally does not result in gout or other discernible disease. If the uric acid levels are high preoperatively, the patient should be kept well hydrated to avoid monosodium urate precipitation.

The Step 2 (antiadrenergic) group of drugs is the most difficult to use and causes the most problems for both the physician and the patient. Table VII is a simplified list of these drugs grouped for convenience of discussion and intelligent use. In general, no more than one of these drugs should be used at the same time from the same subgroup.

Reserpine when combined in low doses (0.1–0.25 mg) with a diuretic drug has the advantage of once a day administration, long duration of action, and low cost. If a patient taking reserpine is to undergo general anesthesia, it is essential that the anesthesiologist be aware of the drug. It is possible to compensate for the effects of reserpine during anesthesia, and surgery need not be delayed because a patient has been taking the drug.

Methyldopa is effective drug which most people can take twice daily. Its major side effects include drowsiness, disturbances of sexual function, positive Coomb's test, fever, and idiosyncratic hepatitis. Methyldopa is also available in an intravenous preparation which may simplify postoperative management. However, there is no other specific advantage of the intravenous

TABLE VII. *Antiadrenergic antihypertensive drugs*

Major site of action	Dose (mg/day)	Special features
Central nervous system		
Reserpine (Serpasil[R] and others)	0.1–0.25 mg (QD)	Once daily dosage, very effective
Methyldopa (Aldomet[R])	500–3000 mg (BID)	Very effective
Clonidine (Catapres[R])	0.2–0.8 mg (BID)	Effective, good for anxious patients
Peripheral nervous system		
Guanethidine (Ismelin[R])	10–600 mg (QD)	Once daily dosage
Alpha adrenergic blockers		
Prazosin (Minipres[R])	3–20 mg (BID)	Cardiac unloader; use in renal failure
Beta adrenergic blockers		
Propranolol (Inderal[R])	80–480 mg (BID)	Well tolerated
Metoprolol (Lopressor[R])	100–200 mg (BID)	Cardioselective

route. The dose range is variable from 500 to 3000 mg per day.

Clonidine is similar to methyldopa but has less orthostatic hypotension and disturbances of sexual function. It may cause dry mouth, parotid swelling, and postural dizziness as well as drowsiness. Give clonidine twice daily (0.2–0.8 mg with a maximum of 2.4 mg), but do not discontinue it abruptly because of the possibility of rebound hypertension.

Prazosin dilates both the resistance arterioles and the capacitance veins thereby causing orthostatic hypotension. If therapy is initiated with 1 mg and gradually increased, the chance of hypotension is minimized. Prazosin does not seem to increase the heart rate or cardiac output, can be used in patients with renal failure, and is, in our opinion, the drug of choice for patients with both hypertension and congestive heart failure. The usual dose is 6–20 mg divided twice daily.

Beta adrenergic blocking drugs are used for treatment of migraine headaches and glaucoma in addition to hypertension. For hypertension propranolol is given twice daily in doses starting at 80 mg/day up to 320 or 480 mg. Doses up to 3000 mg have been used with safety, but the tablet sizes are 10, 40, or 80 mg, and while convenience decreases at these doses, the cost escalates. The dose may be increased every one to two weeks for outpatients or more frequently in the hospital. Side effects are lethargy, sleep disturbances, cold extremities, a tendency toward bronchoconstriction, some changes in carbohydrate metabolism, and decreased cardiac output and A-V conduction. Propranolol is contraindicated in patients with asthma, congestive heart failure, insulin-dependent diabetes mellitus, more than first degree heart block, and symptomatic occlusive peripheral vascular disease. Metoprolol is beta$_1$ selective and has less propensity for bronchoconstriction. However, in the higher doses (100–200 mg/day or more) required for the treatment of hypertension, this beta selectivity may be decreased or lost. When treating patients who are at risk for bronchoconstriction with metoprolol, it is essential to follow the manufacturer's directions with great care. Timolol is used for the treatment of glaucoma by direct installation into the conjunctival sac. Practolol is a beta blocker which was used for years in Europe before it was discovered to have a significant incidence of both ophthalmic and cutaneous complications. Practolol has been taken off the world market, but the FDA remains concerned about the possibility of similar lesions with the currently marketed drugs as well as those undergoing trial. Ophthalmologists are likely to be the first to note any association of corneal ulcerations or other ocular lesions in patients under treatment with beta blockers.

There has been a great deal of concern about the effects of sudden discontinuation of the beta blockers. This stems from the fact that they were originally used for the treatment of angina pectoris and, therefore, preselected a population of patients with symptomatic coronary artery disease. When the drug was discontinued, heart rate increased and some patients experienced a worsening of angina or even myocardial infarction. However, in the hospital setting, especially in patients who are postoperative, there is much less likelihood that the patients will be able to exert themselves enough to generate dangerous heart rates. The current recommendations are to decrease the amount of beta blocker preoperatively if the surgery is elective or, alternatively, to continue it up to the time of surgery and begin it as soon as possible afterwards. Again, the anesthesiologist must be aware of the fact that the patient is taking beta blockers so that potential problems with hypotension or bradycardia can be dealt with easily.

Guanethidine has a long duration of action, but causes sexual dysfunction, orthostatic hypotension, and diarrhea. The dose ranges from 10–600 mg/day. The anesthesiologist must be notified that the patient is taking guanethidine, but surgery need not be delayed.

The direct vasodilators are listed in Table VIII. They increase the heart rate and cardiac output which may cause palpitations, angina pectoris, and headache. Combination with a beta blocker decreases this side effect.

A new experimental group of drugs which interfere with the renin-angiotensin system is of tremendous interest and have received so much publicity in both the lay and scientific press that they should be mentioned. One new type of drug, saralasin, is a competitive antagonist of angiotensin II at the arteriolar receptor site. Saralasin was thought to be an ideal drug for the diagnosis

and perhaps treatment of renin dependent hypertension, but it has limitations and only a parenteral preparation is available at this time. Drugs which inhibit the conversion of inactive angiotensin I to active angiotensin II in the lung have excited considerable interest. Teprotide (SQ20881) is a preparation for parenteral use. It markedly increases renin although it lowers the blood pressure and has been used to increase the specificity of differential renal vein renins in patients with renal artery stenosis. It might prove to be useful in hypertensive crisis. Captopril (SQ14225) is an oral converting enzyme inhibitor which could prove to be very useful for the treatment of all kinds of hypertension irrespective of the initial renin levels. Very early data suggest that it is much more effective when used in combination with a diuretic drug.

There are a number of drugs which can be used for the treatment of hypertensive emergencies, but hydralazine and diazoxide (Hyperstat[R]) are most useful until the patient can be moved to a monitored area. Hydralazine is an excellent drug for treatment of severe hypertension in situations where intensive monitoring is not available or only a temporary effect is required. Generally, it is given in doses of 10–20 mg intravenously (it can also be given intramuscularly) and has an effect within a few minutes which may last for minutes to hours. Diazoxide may be given intravenously either as a 300-mg rapid bolus or as a series of 30-mg doses about 5 min apart. The latter method will take more time and more total drug, but is safer. The blood pressure may stay down for many hours and this is again useful in situations where intensive monitoring is not at hand. It also causes reflex tachycardia in addition to marked volume retention and the possibility of hyperglycemia. Patients should be pretreated with intravenous furosemide (20–40 mg should be sufficient for most patients). Glucose levels in the serum should be monitored closely in diabetics and insulin given as needed. Like hydralazine, it must be used with caution in patients with stroke or dissecting aneurysms.

The reviews of drugs and their use in this chapter are necessarily brief and incom-

TABLE VIII. *Vasodilator antihypertensive drugs*

Drug	Dose (mg/day)	Special features
Hydralazine (Apresoline[R])	50–200 mg (BID)	Excellent with beta blocker and diuretic May be used as a Step 2 drug
Minoxidil (Loniten[R])	5–40 mg (QD or BID)	Extremely potent Must be used with a diuretic and antiadrenergic
Diazoxide (Hyperstat[R])	300 mg IV	Emergency use only

plete. The full manufacturer's instructions must be consulted before use of any of these potent medications. When the experience of the ophthalmologist is not commensurate with the demands of the situation or the particular drug under consideration, expert consultation must be sought.

In summary, the ophthalmologist has both the opportunity to detect and initiate the treatment of hypertension. It is a crucial role in the over-all well-being of patients who are seen for diagnosis and treatment of symptoms of eye disease.

CASE HISTORIES

Case 1. A 75-year-old man is almost literally dragged into your office by his wife because of his obvious progressive decrease in visual acuity. You determine that he has dense lenticular cataracts and advise surgery. However, his blood pressure is 160/106. He denies a history of hypertension. What do you do?

Answer. First, attempt to determine his prior blood pressure reading. Usually a quick call to his primary care physician will generate this information. If he has been normotensive, chances are that this is "office hypertension" generated by anxiety related to fear of blindness, surgery, surgical failure, and even death. If possible, repeat the measurement later (a well-trained office clerk can do this). Pressures at this level should be confirmed at least two additional occasions before deciding to treat. There is no emergency, and he can have surgery. He will probably require substantial reassurance and antianxiety medication.

Case 2. A 22-year-old woman is self-referred because of recent onset of severe headaches and vague, visual complaints. She denies a history or family history of hypertension. Her blood pressure is 200/130. She denies using oral contraceptives and further relates that when her IUD was inserted only three months prior, her blood pressure was normal. A call to her gynecologist confirms this. Ophthalmologic examination shows marked retinal arteriolar spasm but is otherwise normal. What do you do?

Answer. Sudden onset of severe hypertension in a young, previously normotensive patient is strongly suggestive of secondary hypertension. She requires immediate treatment and diagnostic procedures. She should be hospitalized that day by a physician prepared to assume full responsibility for her management. There is a strong likelihood of her having renal artery stenosis due to fibromuscular dysplasia. However, we know of a similar acute presentation by a 17-year-old boy who, it turned out, had consumed the leftover brine from a jar of pickled pigs feet. He was cured in one day with a diuretic.

Case 3. You are called to see a 45-year-old construction worker who came to the Emergency Room because of a foreign body in his eye. The nurse tells you that his blood pressure is 170/100. He is in severe pain and badly frightened. He was once told his blood pressure was "a little bit elevated," but that he did not need treatment. You remove the foreign body, treat his eye, and arrange for him to see you in the office in three days. What do you do about the blood pressure?

Answer. Nothing yet. Remember that pain—any kind of pain—may elevate blood pressure. Low back pain, a toothache, or headache are common causes of temporary increase of blood pressure above baseline. Perhaps elevated blood pressure is more often due to headache than the converse. However, he should be rechecked at the return office visit. If his blood pressure is more than 140/90, he should be checked again at a third visit. Persistent elevation demands follow-up by a physician willing to assume primary care responsibilities.

Case 4. A patient is referred to you for ophthalmic surgery. He is a known hypertensive but is well controlled on medication. You schedule him for surgery in ten days but, on admission to the hospital the evening before, his blood pressure is 210/140. He is asymptomatic. The patient explains that he "assumed" he should stop taking his medication prior to surgery and has been untreated for nine days. What do you do?

Answer. Reschedule the surgery. There is a definite risk to operating on a severely hypertensive patient. Usually, the previous medications can be restarted at lower dose and increased fairly quickly as needed. The anesthesiologist must be informed. Usually the medication can be restarted after surgery. Be very careful with potassium administration to patients taking spironolactone (Aldactone[R]) because the drug effect may last three to five days making hyperkalemia a risk.

Case 5. A 72-year-old man with adult onset, non-insulin-dependent diabetes mellitus is hospitalized for glaucoma surgery. He has been taking hydrochlorothiazide 50 mg and propranolol 160 mg twice daily for hypertension. His blood pressure on admission is 180/105 mm Hg. Because of marked anxiety the patient insists on general anesthesia. However, during anesthesia with halothane there is excessive bleeding. Can you use 2% lidocaine (Xylocaine[R]) with 1: 100,000 epinephrine locally?

Answer. Try to avoid it if at all possible. The epinephrine can be absorbed and cause marked hypertension in the presence of propranolol. If you must use it, use as little as possible after alerting the anesthesiologist. Parenteral dosing must be avoided.

EDITOR'S NOTE

It is surprising how often a patient is referred for a neuro-ophthalmologic consultation because of headaches or blurred vision and on routinely checking their blood pressures in our office the reading is found to be 210/125. I then ask the patient how long the blood pressure has been up, and they usually reply that they didn't know this at all or that they had not had their pressure measured in a long time. This is a very, very common experience. Dr. Materson is at the Miami Veterans Hospital on the medical service and is an expert in hypertension. We had him come over to the Saturday Neuro-ophthalmology Conference and he gave a superb lecture on hypertension—and even an ophthalmologist could understand his approach! Therefore, I invited him to summarize this data for you, and you have this in this chapter.

The moral of the story is this: (1) have someone in your office check the blood pressure on every new patient; (2) they should have the patient's arm at the level of their heart when this is done (if the arm is up, the reading will be too low; if the arm is down, the reading will be too high); (3) if there are any neurologic complaints, both arms should be measured (this is an excellent test for vertebrobasilar disease when you may often find a significant difference in the two arms); and (4) again with symptoms, one should check the blood pressure with patient supine and standing, or sitting and standing. Now, I don't want to scare the ophthalmologist off—so *please*—have someone in your office check the blood pressure on at least one arm and in one posture on every new patient! We get excited when we consider that 2% of the population over 40 has glaucoma and check applanation tensions like mad looking for that! Well, we need to remember that 6% of the population has had syphilis—10% of the population has migraine—and that 20% of the adult population has hypertension! So, common things are common, and rare things are rare—and that sphygmomanometry is going to pay off 10 times as often as that applanation tonometer! Furthermore, it is not even enough to refer them to an internist or general physician and ask that they be treated for hypertension. You should check up on that patient when he or she returns and make sure they have done this. This is one of the most significant treatable things in neurology. I have seen many patients present with an acute subarachnoid hemorrhage—have a big workup and subsequently have surgery for their aneurysm—pull through and go home and everybody is happy. However, they may often come back 18 months later, or two to three years later, with a big intracerebral hematoma due to the hypertension which was not adequately treated nor followed up, and that is important! Where there is smoke, there is fire—and where there are aneurysms, there are cases of hypertension. It really doesn't do the patient much good for you to find that "white without pressure" in the periphery with indirect, and miss the fact that he went out of your office with an undetected 220/125 blood pressure. Thank you, Dr. Materson, for helping us being reminded about the problem of hypertension!

JLS

Index